A CONCISE REPERTORY

OF

HOMOEOPATHIC MEDICINES

(*Arranged Alphabetically*)

by

Dr. S. R. Phatak, M.B.B.S.

Author of Repertory of Biochemic Remedies (English)
Homoeopathic Materia Medica and Repertory of Homoeopathic
Medicines (in Marathi); Materia Medica of Homoeopathic
Medicines (English)

THIRD EDITION
(Revised and Enlarged)
by
Dr. D. S. Phatak, M.B.B.S.

B.Jain Publishers Pvt. Ltd.
New Delhi (India)

Distributed by
Aggarwal Book Centre
A-147, Shankar Garden, Vikas Puri,
New Delhi-18 (India)Ph.: 091-11-25612013
E-mail aggarwal@vsnl.com
Website : www.homoeopathic.com

Reprint edition 2001

B. JAIN'S PRICE RS. 160.00

Printed & Published by

KULDEEP JAIN

for

B. Jain Publishers (P) Ltd.

1921, St. No.10, Chuna Mandi,
Paharganj, New Delhi-110 055.
Phones : 3683200, 3683300, 3670430, 3670572
FAX : 011-3683400 & 3610471
Email : bjain@vsnl.com
Website : www.bjainindia.com

PRINTED IN INDIA
by
J. J. Offset Printers
7, Wazirpur, Printing Press Area
Delhi-110 035.

ISBN-81-7021-757-1
BOOK CODE: B - 5457

To my friend
Late Mr. S. L. KAPADI

PREFACE

Prescribing in Homoeopathy is both Sciene and Art. But it is a difficult Art. Good case-taking, sound knowledge of Materia Medica and skilful use of the reference books are the three prerequisites.

This repertory is intended to serve as a handy and useful reference book. It is an attempt to lessen the difficulties of the prescriber. No originality can be claimed in a book of this type, except that of presentation. There are advantages and in the traditional type of repertory. The author feels that the present arrangement will minimise the disadvantages. Remedies for a particular rubric are reduced to minimum possible by a careful selection. No drug is given unless the author has used it in his own practice or unless there is strong justification provided for it, by authorities like Dr. Boger, Dr. Kent, Dr. Clarke's Dictionary etc.

A concise repertory cannot take the place of exhaustive repertories of Kent, Boeninghausen and others. It is aimed at reducing the burden of the prescriber, in every sense of the word.

In this repertory, the headings mentals, generals, modalities, organs, and their sub-parts are all arranged according to their alphabetical order. All the physiological and **Plan of the Book & How to Use it** pathological conditions such as appetite, aversions, desires, nausea, vomiting, thirst, fever, pulse etc. are also included in alphabetical order. Cross references are given where-ever necessary. In such arrangement there will be no difficulty in finding the appropriate rubrics. In each such rubric all important symptoms, their concomitants and their modalities are given. But the prescriber should not entirely depend on the particulars, for

finding out the correct remedy. If he can find the correct remedy, according to the totality of symptoms, under the particular organ or sub-part of it, so much the better, otherwise he has to find the remedy considering the general conditions and general modalities. For all the general modalities, the words Agg. and Amel. are printed AGG. and AMEL. For the modalities under particular rubric only, these should be no difficulty in finding out as to which modality is general and which is particular. For example "Eyes closing Agg". Though this modality is given under eyes, it modifies the general symptoms as well as those of the eyes.

Dr. Boger has a remarkable knack of coining a general rubric from some particular symptom. (Those who have used his Synoptic Key must have noticed it). For example, take the rubric 'Awkwardness'. This symptom is given by Dr. Kent in his repertory under, 'Extremities'. There it shows that the patient either drops things from his hands or walks stumbling. But when Dr. Boger made it a general rubric, it means that the patient's mental and/or physical behaviour may be awkward. All such headings coined by Dr. Boger are included in this repertory. Not only that but the author himself has coined a few new headings from his own experience. For example the rubric "unsteady sensation". Once a patient consulted the author for this sensation. This patient, whenever he used to stand for more than a few minutes, used to feel unsteady, not giddy, but as if he was not standing firmly on the ground. The author found for him the remedy from those given under unsteady gait.

Every homoeopathic practitioner is aware that modalities and concomitants are the most important factors for finding a correct remedy. The author has garnered all useful modalities from different standard repertories and has included those in this book. The modality "Holding the breath Amel", is given only by Dr. Boenninghausen in this Therapeutic Pocket Book. This modality gave the author, once an opportunity to cure remarkably an ulcer on the dorsum of the foot due to Thrombo-angiitis obliterans.

The repertories are compiled for finding out as far as possible a correct remedy by referring to the various symptoms given under various organs; along with the circumstances, conditions and timing which modify them. In order to arrive at the suitable remedy, the remedies given under a particular symptoms are graded according to their importance. The prescriber, however, should bear in mind that every remedy–high grade or low grade– becomes equally important when it is connected with peculiar concomitant or with an unusual condition or circumstance. **Repertorization does not mean Mechanical Repertorization. Totality of Symptoms does not mean Numerical Totality, but Qualitative Totality.** One peculiar concomitant or an unusua condition may determine the totality of the case.

Patients do not always tell their symptoms according to the rubric used in the repertory. Nor do they give all the information required by the prescriber. The prescriber has to find much of the information regarding modalities and concomitants by appropriate questioning and confirm it by cross-questioning. After this, the prescriber with his logical mind has to sift, evaluate and interpret the meaning of the symptom or symptoms correctly, to enable him to refer to the appropriate rubric in the repertory. All the modalities in a case are not equally important. The modality regarding the position or posture of a patient may sometimes be more valuable. If a patient says that he feels better only when he assumes some strange position, this condition should be considered first. This modality is not given in any standard repertory, though some positions in sleep are given. But Dr. Boger with his remarkable knowledge of behaviour of drugs has coined a heading, "Attitudes bizarre" given under generalities. The meaning is obvious. The patient's disposition whether mental or physical is bizarre, i.e. strange or unusual. Again some modality may be common, but when associated with the diseased condition, with which it has absolutely no connection, becomes uncommon or unusual. Once the author was consulted by a patient who was suffering from what is known as peripheral neuritis. He was not suffering from diabetes, nor were there any untoward incidents preceding that condition. The patient felt pain in both the legs, below the knees. The pain was better by moving the legs, while walking and by hard pressure. But the patient told the author that when he belched or passed flatus, he felt much relief. If the prescriber will try to find a remedy for this group of symptoms from any other repertory, he is probably liable to miss the mark. But Dr. Boger has given the modality "Passing flatus up and down, Amel" under the rubric "Flatulence". The author has elevated the rank of this particular to the general rubric.

The aversions, desires, mental attitudes, causation, have their own place in the selection of the remedy, when they are very marked. Causations will be found under Agg's either general or particular. Mental attitudes will be found under mental conditions. Sometimes the appearance of symptoms on one side, or going upwards or downwards etc., give a right clue to the selection of remedy, when they are very marked. All these conditions are given under 'Directions' of symptoms. The prescriber should be alert; he should look everywhere to arrive at the correct remedy.

Everything cannot be explained in the preface. But the author hopes, that the few instances given above will enable the prescriber to understand what to look, where to look, and how to look. As said in the beginning, prescribing in homoeopathy is an Art. And one can only achieve sort of proficiency in this Art by constant and diligent study of the remedies given in various standard materia medica, with reference to their place value given in the repertory.

The author conceived the idea of preparing and arranging the repertory in one alphabetical order when he used to discuss the uses of various repertories, with the doctors who **Story of** came to him for guidance in the study of **This Book** Homoeopathy. The repertory had also to be a concise and handy one. Though this idea took root, the author on account of his indifferent health was reluctant to undertake this task. But his friend Mr. S. L. Kapadi, who knew about the idea, unexpectedly came to his help. One day he came to the author with a skeletal copy of this work and asked the author to fill up the gaps, check and recheck it. This skeleton work was prepared by Mr. Kapadi from author's rough draft, notes etc. of Marathi repertory. The author was surprised. This was more than what was expected from a layman.

The author had to consent. He arranged the work properly, re-wrote it and made many additions. Dr. (Miss) Homai A. Merchant who used to come to the author for guidance in the study of Homoeopathy saw this hand-written copy. She herself very kindly offered to type it. The typed copy was lying with the author for nearly ten years. During this interval, many useful additions were made. But on account of various reasons, the author did not consider getting it printed. Mr. Kapadi induced my son to get it printed. When it was decided to publish it, my son approached Mr. D. P. Datay, who promised all help and undertook the composing work. Then the author had no choice left.

Dr. (Miss) Merchant again came to the rescue. When requested, very willingly she typed the whole work again for the press and made some valuable suggestions.

No work is ever complete. But it can be rightly claimed that considering the object of writing a compact, handy repertory useful for prompt reference, no effort was spared to make this work as complete as is possible.

Thanks are due to Dr. (Miss) Merchant for her neat typing. My son Dr. D. S. Phatak did the preliminary spadework. He went **Thanks** through all the cross references, looked the final **giving** proofs carefully and deserves all praise. Mr. Datay gave useful suggestions about everything connected with the printing. His lino-operators, Mr. Sane, Mr. Ranade, Mr. Mhaiskar and Mr. Damle showed immense patience with the author's never-ending correction and additions. Thanks are also due to the proprietors of the Mouj Printing Press for agreeing to print the book.

The author does not know how to thank Mr. Kapadi, without whose preliminary help and persistence later, the book may not have seen the light of the day. Prescribers who find this book useful owe a great deal to his interest in it.

Finally the author is gratefully indebted to all those masters of Homoeopathy from whose works he has drawn freely to make this book as useful as possible.

The author is well aware of the mistakes which have crept in, inspite of careful proof reading. Lines under some rubrics are misplaced while printing. The prescriber is requested to correct the book as per errata and refer to the list of abbreviations when necessary.

Sept. 1963   **S.R. Phatak**

PREFACE TO THE SECOND EDITION

While compiling a Materia Medica as a companion volume to my repertory, I have had to go through different materia medicas written by various authors like Drs. Hering. Clarks, Boger, Boericke, Kent and many others.

While doing this I found many new clinical and pathological symptoms. So I have taken this opportunity to add these symptoms in this edition of my repertory. Very few changes were found necessary while revising the book.

My repertory was well received not only in India, but even abroad in America and England. The demand for it was persistent and increasing, but if my colleague Dr. P. Sankaran had not undertaken the responsibility of publishing it, the book in this second edition would not have seen the light so soon. Not only I thank him but users of this book must thank him also for this.

My friend Dr. (Miss) Homai Merchant has been kind enough to offer her services and type out the whole manuscript without a single murmur. For this I am grateful to her.

No repertory, whether exhaustive or concise, is ever complete. Yet, I hope this book will be more useful to prescribers to find the correct remedy in most of their daily routine cases. And if they know the techniques of Dr. Boger, they will have occasion to refer to the exhaustive repertories very rarely.

I am thankful to M/s Jokap Printers for doing the printing so patiently and painstakingly.

Lastly I must thank God for preserving me in spite of my old age and poor health to see this edition published.

Bombay, 21 Oct. 1977 **S. R. Phatak**

PREFACE TO THE THIRD EDITION

I am happy that after about 23 years this third edition is being published. The total period for the revision was about seven years.

The number of pages has increased partly because of bigger type, still the book remains handy. New aditions one marked with '+' mark.

B. Jain Publishers deserve my thanks for the publication.

Please see the note prepared for the third edition.

June 2000   **Dr. D. S. Phatak**

ABBREVIATIONS

The abbreviations which are well known or self-explanatory such as Sul. for Sulphur; Sil. for Silica etc. are not listed below. The list given below represents those drugs where misunderstanding and mistakes are liable to occur.

Remedies with their abbreviations

Abies Canadensis	Ab-c
Abies Nigra	Ab-n.
Acalypha Indica	Acaly.
Aceta Racemosa	See Cimicifuga.
Adonis Vernalis	Adon.
Agnus Cactus	Agn.
Allium Cepa	See Cepa.
Allium Sativum	All-s.
Alumen	Alum.
Alumina	Alu.
Alumina Silicata	Alu-sil.
Ambrosia	Ambro.
Ammonium Bromatum	Am-br.
Angustura Vera	Ang.
Apium Graveolens	Ap-g.
Apocynum Cannabinum	Apoc.
Aralia Racemosa	Aral.
Arum Triphyllum	Aru-t.
Asclepias Tuberosa	Ascl.
Astacus Fluviatilis	See Cancer fluviatilis.

Avena Sativa	Avena.
Berberis Aquifolium	Berb-aq.
Berberis Vulgaris	Berb.
Bothrops	Both.
Bursa Pastoris	Bur-p.
Cadmium Sulph	Cadm.
Calendula	Calen.
Cancer Fluviatilis	Canc-fl.
Cannabis Indica and Sativa	Cann.
Castor Equi	Castr-eq.
Castoreum	Castr.
Ceanothus	Cean.
China	Chin.
Chininum Arsenicosum	Chin-ars.
Chloral Hydrate	Chlo-hyd.
Chlorum	Chlor.
Cinconha	See China.
Cimex Acanthia	Cimex.
Cocculus	Cocl.
Coccus Cacti	Coc-c.
Codeinum	Codei.
Comocladia	Como.
Curare	Cur.
Dioscorea Villosa	Dios.
Dulcamara	Dul.
Epiphegus	Epip.
Euonymus Atropurpurea	Euon.
Eupatorium Perfoliatum	Eup-p.
Eupatorium Purpureum	Eup-pur.
Euphorbrium Off	Euphor.
Euphrasia	Euphr.
Eupion	Eupi.

Fagopyrum	Fago.
Ferrum Picricum	Fer-pic.
Guaiacum	Guai.
Gymnocladus	Gym.
Helianthus	Helin.
Hepar Sulphuris Calcareum	Hep.
Hyoscyamine Hydrobrom	Hyo-hydro.
Iberis	Iber.
Indigo	Ind.
Iodoformum	Iodf.
Jaborandi	Jab.
Kali Permanganatum	Kali-per.
Kalmia Latifolia	Kalm.
Lachnantes	Lachn.
Lactic acid	Lact-ac.
Lactuca Virosa	Lact-v.
Lapis Albus	Lap-alb.
Lappa Arcticum	Lapp.
Lithium Carb	Lith.
Lobelia Inflata	Lob.
Lolium Temulentum	Lol-t.
Lycopersicum	Lycoper.
Lycopus Virginicus	Lycops.
Lyssin	Lyss.
Mancinella	Manc.
Manganum	Mang.
Melilotus	Meli.
Millefolium	Mill.
Myrica	Myr.
Niccolum	Nicc.
Nitro-muriatic acid	Nit-m-ac.
Ocinum Canum	Oci-c.

Passiflora Incarnata	Passif.
Petroleum	Petr.
Pilocarpus Microphyllus	See Jaborandi.
Plantago	Plant.
Prunus Spinosa	Pru-sp.
Ranunculus Bulbosus	Ran-b.
Ranunculus Scleratus	Ran-s.
Radium Bromide	Radm.
Sabadilla	Saba.
Sabal Serrulate	Sabal.
Salix Nigra	Salix.
Sanguinaria	Sang.
Sarracenia Purpurea	Sarr.
Scilla	Scil.
Secale Cornutum	Sec.
Senecio Aureus	Senec.
Senega	Seneg.
Sinapis	Sinap.
Solanum Nigrum	Sol-n.
Spigelia	Spig.
Squilla	See Scilla.
Succinum	Succi.
Sulfonal	Sulfo.
Symphytum	Symph.
Tarentula Cubensis	Tarn-c.
Tarentula Hispania	Tarn.
Thlapsi Bursa Pastoris	See Bursa Pastoris.
Thyroidinum	Thyr.
Trombidium	Tromb.
Zingiberis	Zing.

ABDOMEN Affections In
GENERAL : Aeth; Arg-n; ARS;
Bry; *Calc;* Carb-v; *Chin;* Colo;
Lach; LYC; NUX-V; PHO; PUL;
Sep; Sil; SUL; Ver-a.
UPPER : Caus; *Cham;* Chin;
Cocl; Nux-v; Pul.

Drawn, in : Thu.

LOWER : See Hypogastrium.

SIDES : Asaf; Carb-v; Chin;
Ign

Right : Ars; Lach; *Lyc; Rhus-t*

heavy : Tab.

left, to : Sep.

Left : Alu; Arg-m; Asaf;
Bro;Dul; Flu-ac; Hep;
Plb; Rhe; *Sil; Sul;* Tarx.

right, to : Nux-v.

heavy object,as if,in : Lyc.

rigidity : Nat-m.

Alternating : Arn; *Pul;* Sul.

Distension : Caus; *Nat-m.*

Flowing towards :

genitals, from : Colo.

Sticking, in: Ign.

running, when : Tub.

BACKWARD : Arn; ARS; BELL;
Bor; Carb-v; Chel; Con;
Cup; Fer; Kali-p; Lyc; Nux-v;
PHO; Plb; Pul; Sep; Sul; *Tab.*

CHEST, To: Aeth; *Cham;* Lach.

FORWARD, Into : Thu.

GROINS, To : Pul.

ILEOCOECAL REGION : See
Appendicitis.

LIMBS, with : Aeth.

SCROTUM, To : Ver-v.

THIGHS, To : Lil-t; Mag-p;

Sabal; Sabi; *Stap;* Thyr.

TRANSVERSELY, Across : *Chel.*

UPWARD : Aco; ARS; Calc;
Carb-v; Kali-bi; Kali-c;
Lac-ac; Saba.

Right : Aco; Kali-c; Mag-m;
MURX; Seneg; Sep.

Left : Alu; Ign; *Naj; Nat-s;*
Spo; Zin.

Diagonally : Lach.

AFTERNOON Agg : Am-m.

Amel : Nat-s.

ALTERNATING, Head, with :
Alo; Bry; Calc; Cina; Pod;
Thu.

Chest, with : Radm; Ran-b.

Ear, with : Radm.

Eye, with : Euphr.

Other organs, with : Bry;
Colo; Nux-v; Radm; Ran-b.

ANXIETY, emotions, felt, in :
Ars; Aur; Carb-v; Cham;
Cup; *Kali-c;* Mez, Nux-v;
Pho; Ver-a.

BALL : See Lump.

BAND, ABOUT : Caus; *Chel;*
Chio; Lyc; Nux-v; Plb; *Pul;*
Sul.

BANDAGING Amel : Cup; Flu-ac;
Nat-m; Nit-ac.

BREATH, Holding Agg: Dros;
Spig.

BREATHING Deep Agg: *Arg-n;*
Caus; Kre; Pul.

Amel : Card-m; Flu-ac; Thu.

BUBBLING : *Lyc;* Pul; Sul-ac;
Tarx.

BURNING, In (See Stomach) :

Caps; *Caus; Iris;* Manc; Terb; Ver-a.

Digestive tract, whole : *Iris.*

Hot coals, as from : Ver-a.

Water, running down : Chin.

Steam passing through, as if : Ascl.

CHANGING About, in : Dios; Mur-ac; Nux-v.

CLAWING : Bell; Lyc.

COITION, After, Agg : Caus; Pho-ac; Ther.

COLDNESS, In : Amb; *Ars;* Cadm; Calc; Colch; Grat; Kali-br; Kali-c; *Meny;* Pho; Sec; Sep; Sul-ac; *Ver-a;* Zin.

Burning, with : Pho.

Colic, with : Calc; Kali-s.

Eating, after : Pul.

Icy : Colch; Crot-h.

Pressure Agg : Meny.

Throat, rising to : Carb-an.

CONCUSSION Agg : Bry.

CONTRACTED : Mag-p.

Hour-glass : Rhus-t.

CONVULSIVE Motions, Spasms, after : Buf.

COUGHING Agg : Anac; Ant-t; Bry; Dros; Lyc; *Nux-v;* Pall; Pho.

COVERING, Lifting up, Amel : Bell; Lac-c; *Lach;* Lil-t; Pho; Sec; Stap; Tab.

DIARRHOEA, Sense of : Bry; Dul; Hyds; NUX-V; Pul; Ran-sc.

DISTENDED, Tympanitic, inflated, etc. : *Abro; Aco;* Agar; Alo; ARG-N; Ars; CALC; CARB-V;

Cham; CHIN; Cic; Cocl; *Colch;* Colo; *Grap;* Hep; Hyo; KALI-C; Lach; Lil-t; LYC; Mag-c; *Merc; Nat-c; Nat-m;* Nat-p; Nux-m; NUX-V; *Pho;* Pho-ac; Raph; Rhus-t; Stram; Sul; *Terb;* Vario; *Ver-a*

Children, in : Bar-c; Calc; Caus; Sul.

Clothes feel tight : Mos.

+ loosened, amel : Onos.

Contracts, when touched : Colch.

Epilepsy, before : Cup;

Fontanelles, open with : Sil.

Hard : *Kali-c.*

Hot : Merc-d.

Hysterical : Tarx.

Legs, stretch, cannot : Colch.

Lying Agg : Carb-v.

Menses, during : Chin; *Cocl;* Kali-c; Nat-c; *Sul.*

Milk, after : *Con.*

Operation, after : Carb-an; Hypr.

Painful : Aco; Ars; Bry; Caus; Lach; Merc; Rhus-t.

amenorrhoea, with : Castr.

Parturition, after : Lyc; *Sep.*

+ Pregnancy, as if : Vario.

+ Sides : Caus; *Nat-m.*

Stools, after : Carb-v; Grap; *Lyc.*

Amel : Hypr.

Sudden : Nat-m.

Whooping cough, with :

2

Kali-s.

DRAWING, As if : Caps; Pul; Sep.

DRAWN, Involuntarily : *Val.*

DRINKING Water Agg : Ars;
Bad; Pho; Zing.

Ice-cold Agg : Calc-p;
Nux-m; Rhus-t.

Amel : Elap.

DROPSY, Ascites(See Dropsy)
: Acet-ac; Ap; Apo; Ars; Aur;
Hep;Lyc; Mur-ac; Scil; Terb.

Cirrhosis of liver, from :
Mur-ac.

Diarrhoea, frequent
attacks, with : Sil.

Menses, suppressed, from
: Senec.

Suffocation lying on left
side : Ap.

Urination, scanty, with : Scil.

With fold on pelvic region
: Colch.

EATING Amel: Anac; Bov;
Chel; Grap; Hep; Ign;
Kali-p; Lach; Mag-m; Med;
Petr; *Zin.*

Fruits Agg : Lyc.

Too much Agg : Ant-c; Cof;
Ip; Nux-v; *Pul.*

EMPTY : See Hollow.

ERUCTATION Amel : Amb;
Bar-c; Rat.

Not Amel from : *Chin;* Lyc.

EYE Symptoms,with : Arg-n.

FASTING Amel : Caus; Sil.

FAT : Am-m; *Chel.*

FATS Agg : Carb-v; *Pul.*

FIST Of a Child moving, as of
: Conval; *Nat-c; Sul;* THU.

FERMENTATION, In : Chin; Lyc.

FEVER, In Agg : Ip; Ver-a.

FLABBY : See Weak.

FLATUS Passing Agg : Aur;
Canth; Flu-ac; Scil.

Amel : Hep; Nat-m; Tarn.

FOOD, Stale Agg : Ars.

FORMICATION : Plat.

Voluptuous : Plat.

FULLNESS : *Carb-v; Chin;*
Dig; Grap; *Kali-c;* Kali-m;
LYC; NUX-V; Pho; Pho-ac;
SUL.

Food, small quantity :
Mur-ac.

FULL of *Water* as if : Crot-t;
Hell; Pho-ac.

GURGLING In : ALO; *Crot-t;* Old;
Pod; Pul; SUL.

Stools, gushing, then : Alo;
Crot-t; GAMB; Iris; Jat;
Nat-s; Pho; Pod; Sec; *Sul;*
Thu; Ver-a.

HAND, Placing on Agg : Psor;
Zinc-chr.

HANGING or falling down, as
if : Acet-ac; Laur; Nat-m;
Pho; Pod; *Sep.*

Walks bent, therefore :
Carb-v.

carefully : Nux-v.

Walking, when : Nat.m.

HARD : Bar-c; Bar-m; Calc;
Grap; Merc; Sil.

Body, moving in, as if :
Bor; *Lyc.*

HEART, with : Merc-i-f.

HEAVY : *Alo;* Am-m; Cup;

3

Grap; Kali-c; Lyc; *Nux-v;*
Pul; Sep; *Spig;* Stap.

Right : Tab.

Left : Lyc.

Menses, during : Kali-s.

HOLDS : Agn; Lil-t; Merc;
Rhus-t; Sep; Stap.

HOLLOW, Empty, sinking
sensation : Arg-n; Cocl; Ip;
Old; PHO; *Pod;* Pul; Sec; SEP;
Stan; Stap; Sul-ac; *Tab.*

Bowels, knotted feeling
with : Cham.

Gnawing : Ox-ac.

Stools, after : Petr; Pho; Pod;
Sul-ac.

Amel : Mur-ac.

HOT Food And Drink Amel :
Lyc; Mag-p; *Nux-v;* Sul-ac.

INACTIVE : See Paralysis.

INFLAMMATION, Peritonitis : Aco;
Ant-t; ARS; Bell; *Bry;* Colch;
Hyo; *Ip;* Lach; Laur; Lyc;
Nux-v; PHO; *Pul;* Pyro;
Rhus-t; Terb; Til.

Cold application Amel : Calc.

Tuberculous : Abro.

KNEADING By hand Amel :
Nat-s.

KNOTS, Lumps, felt in : Abro;
Ars; Bism; Ign; Plb; Saba;
Sec.

LAPAROTOMY, After : Bism; Hep;
Nux-v; Op; Raph; Stap.

LEGS, Extending, Amel : Phys.

LIFTING Agg : Bry.

LIME Boiling, as if, in : Caus.

LUMPS, Balls, as if, in : Anac;
Kre; *Nux-v; Rhus-t;* Sul; Thu;

Ust; Verb.

Moving rapidly in : Saba.

Rising, throat, to : ARG-N;
Raph.

coughing when : Kali-c.

LYING on back, with knees
drawn up Amel : Bry;
Lach; Rhus-t.

Left side, on, Amel : Scil.

Stomach, on, Amel : Rhus-t.

MILK Amel : Grap; Merc;
Mez; *Nux-v;* Rut; Ver-a.

Hot Amel : Crot-t.

MOTION Amel : Chin; Petr.

MOVING Up and Down,
something, in : Lyc.

Convulsions, after: Buf.

+ NAUSEA, In : Polyg.

NUMB : Aco; Bry; *Plat;* Pul;
Sars.

PAIN Boring, grinding : Flu-ac;
Plb; Polyg; Sars; Stan.

Cutting : Bell; *Bry;* Chin;
Colo; Dios; Ip; *Mag-c;*
Merc; Nit-ac; Nux-v;
Polyg; Pul; Rhe; *Sul;* Ver-a.

Flatus passing on : Con.

Gnawing, eating, ulcerative
: Bell; *Carb-v;* Colo; Lyc;
Pho; Sep.

Griping, Cramp, Colic :
Bell; Cham; Cocl; COLO;
Cup; *Dios;* Ign; Kre;
Mag-m; NUX-V; OP;
Plb; Polyg; Radm; Rat;
Sul; Val; *Ver-a; Zin.*

arms, raising Agg : Cup.

associated symptoms,

4

with : Plb.

backache, with : Sars.

+ coffee amel : Colo.

cold drinks agg : Manc.

coryza, stopped, after : Calc.

diarrhoea Agg : Phys.

eating amel : Psor.

+ after : Val.

eructations, with : Mag-p .

habitual, children, in : Bar-c.

nightly : Calc; Cham; Chin; Lyc.

riding in, carriage Agg : Carb-v.

stools, hard Amel : Ust.

trembling and chattering of teeth with: Bov; Meph.

yellow hands and blue nails, with : Sil.

Hysterical : Stan.

Indefinite, dull, aching : Ars; Colo; Cup; Lept; *Nux-v*; Plb; Pod; Pul; Rhus-t; Sep; Ver-a; Ver-v.

Menses, instead of : Spo.

Nausea, after: Latro.

Paralytic : Grat.

Pinching : Ran-b; Tell.

Radiating : Ip; *Mag-p;* Plb.

Smarting, rawness : *Ars;* Bell; Canth; Nux-v; Ran-b.

Sore spot in : Arg-n; Bar-c; Bism; *Kali-bi;* Pho; *Rhus-t.*

Menses, after : Pall.

with : Ham.

Spasmodic : Caus.

Stitching : *Bry;* Ip; *Sul.*

Tearing, shooting : Ars; Cham; Colo.

Uncovering Agg: Rhe.

PARALYSIS Of INTESTINES : Bry; Con; Lyc; Mag-m; Nux-v; OP; Pho; PLB; *Rhus*-t; Tab; Thu.

Laparotomy, after : Op.

PRESSURE Agg : Ars; Bry; Calc; Chel; Merc-c.

Amel : Arg-n; Castr; COLO; Cup; Plb; Stan.

Clothes, of Agg: Arg-n; Bov; Calc; *Lach; Lyc; Nux-v.*

Right hand on stomach, left on lumbar region Amel : Med.

PROTRUDES, Here and there : Thu.

PUSHING : Thu.

QUIVERING, In : Calc; Con; Iod; *Nux-v;* Sabi; *Sul-ac.*

RESTLESSNESS, Uneasiness : Ars; Calc; Ip; Pho; Sep.

RETRACTED, Sunken: Ap; *Calc-p;* Cup; *Hyd;* Kali-br; PLB; *Ver-a; Zin.*

Cholera, in : Kali-br.

Constipation, with : Carb-ac.

RETRACTION Agg : Ant-t; Asar; Nux-v; Zin.

Amel; Distending Agg : *Ign.*

Involuntary : Val.

Vomiting, during : Ver-a.

ROLLING Something, in : Lyc.

RUBBING Amel : Nat-s; Pall; Pho; *Pod.*

Gently, warm hand, with

Amel : Lil-t.

RUBS : Aran; Kali-c; Mag-c; Nat-c; *Pho*; Plb.

RUMBLING, In : See Flatus, noisy.

SHOCKS, In : *Agar*; Bry; Nux-v.

SINGING Agg : Pul.

SITTING, Crooked Amel : Sul.

SNEEZING Agg : Pul.

+ SQUEAKING, In: Kali-io.

SQUEEZING, In: Ant-t; Cocl; *Colo*; Scop; Stap.

STANDING Agg : Nat-p.
Amel: Thu.

STIFF : Lil-t; *Rhus-t.*

STONES As if, in : Ant-t; *Calc*; Cocl; Colo; Hyds; Nux-m; Osm; Pul; Scop; Sep.

Sharp : Cocl; Colo.

STOOLS Amel : Colch; *Colo*; *Gamb*; Mag-c; NUX-V; Stan; Ver-a.

After, Agg : Petr; Pho; Pod; Sul-ac; Ver-a.

Hard, Amel: Ust.

+ STREAM of Fire, passing through : Ascl.

STRETCHING, With : Plb.

STRING, About : Chel.

SUGAR AGG : *Arg-n;* Ign; Ox-ac; SUL.

SUMMER AGG : Guai.

SUNKEN : See Retracted.

SWASHING In, as if : Rhus-t.

SWEET Things Agg (See Sugar Agg) : Zin.

TALKING Unbearable : Caus; Hell; Kali-c; Laur.

TENSION: Ap; *Arn;* Bar-c; Calc; *Caps*; CARB-V; Chin; Colch; COLO; Cup; Hep; Lil-t; Lyc; Mos; Plb; *Rhus-t;* Scop; Sep; *Sil;* Sul.

Menses, during : Colo; Grap; *Nux-m.*

THREAD, Moving rapidly, in : Saba.

THROBBING, Pulsations : *Ant-t;* Calc; *Nux-v;* PUL; *Sele;* Sep.

Aneurism, from : Bar-m.

Deep in : Aesc.

Eating Agg : Sele.

Here and there : Cann.

Pregnancy, during : Sele.

Sleep, preventing : Sele.

TIGHT Clothes, Agg : Caus.
Amel : Flu-ac; Nat-m; Nit-ac

TOBACCO, Smoking Amel : Colo.

TREMBLING in : See Quivering.

TUMOUR : Con.

ULCER, Ulcerative feeling : Kali-bi; Pho; Ran-b.

UNCOVERING Amel : Cam; Med; Sec; Tab; Vip.

Arms or legs Agg : Rhe.

UNEASINESS : See Restlessness.

URINATING, While Agg : Cham; Colo; Ip; Merc.

URINATION, After Agg : Eup-pur.
Amel : Carb-an; Dios; *Sep*; Tarn.

URINE, Diminished secretion of, during pain : Am; Grap.

VOMITING Agg : Grap; Merc;

Stap; Ver-a.

Amel : Arg-n; Ars; Asar; Hyo; Plb; Tab; Tarn.

WATER, Cold, flowing through : Kali-c.

Full of, as if : Crot-t; Hell; Pho-ac.

Hot, flowing or pouring in : Chin; Sumb; Sang.

WEAK : Arg-n; *Ign; Merc; Pho;* Sul-ac.

Eructations Amel : Kali-m.

WEIGHT, Load, pressure: Agar; Arn; Ars; *Bry;* Calc; Cham; Chin; Hyo; Lyc; *Nux-v; Pul;* Sep; Sil; *Sul.*

YAWNING Agg : *Ars;* Phyt.

Amel : Lyc; Nat-m.

ABDOMEN EXTERNAL : Ap; Bry; Merc; Nux-v; Plb; Sele; Sul.

BROWN, Spots, on : Lyc.

BRUISED, Sore: Aco; *Ap;* Ars; *Bell;* Bry; Chin; *Lach;* Lyc; Merc-c; NUX-V; Ran-b; Stan; Sul; Terb.

COLD, Touch, to : Kali-s; Merc.

CRACKS, On skin : Sil.

HARD : Sil.

HOT: Sil.

Clothes, on, as from : Nit-ac.

MOTIONS, Spasmodic : Cup.

MUSCLES, Emaciation of : Plb.

Twitching : Sec.

PENDULOUS, enlarged : Alu; *Calc;* Carb-v; Caus; Colch; Sanic; *Sep;* Sil; Sul; Syph;

Tab; Vario.

Children, of : Alu; Bar-c; Calc; Sanic; Sil.

glands, swelling of, with : Mez.

Girls, puberty, at : Calc; *Grap;* Lach; Sul.

Mothers, of : *Iod;* Nat-c; *Sep.*

Navel : See Navel.

RED : Sang.

Spots on : Hyo.

SWEAT On : Amb; Anac; Cic.

YELLOW, Spots, on: Kob; Pho.

ABORTION : Ap; *Bell; Cham; Croc;* Erig; Gel; *Ip;* Nux-m; Pul; SABI; SEC; SEP; VIB.

AFTER, AGG : Helo; Kali-c; *Lil-t;* Murx; Pyro; Rut; Sabi; Sec; Sep.

Haemorrhage : Sabi.

Urinary, troubles : Rhe.

EXERTION, from : *Erig;* Rhus-t.

HABITUAL : Alet; Ap; Bacil; *Caul;* Fer; Lyc; *Plb; Syph;* Thu.

Second month : Ap; Cimi; Kali-c; Vib.

Third month : Bell; Plb; Sabi; Sep; Thu; Ust.

Fourth to Seventh month : Sep.

MENTAL Shock or Depression from : Bap.

PREVENTIVE : Rat; Vib.

SEXUAL Frequency, from : Cann.

+ TENDENCY : Fer.

TENESMUS Recti Agg : Bell; Calc; Cocl; Con; Ip; Lyc;

Merc; Nux-v; Rhus-t; Sep; Sul.

+ THREATENED : Asar.

+ Falls, from : Arn.

WEAKNESS, from sheer : Merc; Sil.

ABRUPT : Cham; Med; Nat-m; Plat; *Tarn.*

ABSCESS (Suppuration) : Arn; Ars-io; Bell; *Calc;* Calc-io; CALC-S; Calend; Cist; Echi; HEP; Kali-s; LACH; Lyc; MERC; Pho; Pul; Pyro; Rhus-t; SIL; Sul; Sul-ac; Sul-io; Syph; *Tarn.*

BLIND : Lyc.

BLOODY : Crot-h.

BLUISH : Tarn-c.

BONES, About : Asaf; *Aur:* Calc-f; Calc-hyp; Calc-p; Flu-ac; Guai; *Pho;* Pul; Sec; Sil; Stap; Symp.

In : Guai.

BURNING : ANTHX; ARS; *Pyro;* TARN-C.

CHILLY, Within : Merc.

CHRONIC : Calc-f; Iod; Merc; Sil; Stram; Sul.

COLD : Ol-j.

DEEP: Calc; Caps; Tarn.

EXERTION, Physical, from : Carb-ac.

FIBRINOUS Parts, of : Mez.

GLANDS Of : Bell; CALC; *Calc-s;* Carb-an; Dul; HEP; Kali-io; Lyc; MERC; Nit-ac; *Pyro; Rhus-t;* SIL; *Sul;* Syph; *Tub.*

IMPENDING, Suppressed : Ars; Bell; Calc; *Hep;* Kre; Lach;

Lyc; Merc; Sil.

JOINTS, About : Calc-hyp; Merc; Pho; Psor; Sil.

MENSES, At : Merc.

MULTIPLE, Fever, during : Ars; Hep; Sil.

PSOAS : Chin; Sul; Symp.

RECURRENT : Anthx; Calc-s; *Pyro; Syph.*

Fever, after : Pho-ac.

SLOW : Hep; *Merc;* Sil.

SUBMENTAL : Stap.

TO HASTEN : Guai; *Hep; Merc;* Phyt; Sil.

VESICLES, On : Rhus-t.

ABSENT MINDED, Absorbed, Buried in thought : Aco; *Ap;* Arn; *Asar;* Bov; Calc-p; Cann; CAUS; CHAM; Hell; *Lac-c;* Lach; *Laur;* Mez; Nat-m; *Nux-m; Old;* Pho; *Plat;* PUL; SEP; Sul; Ver-a.

As if, in Dream: Anac.

As to what will become of him : Nat-m.

MENSES, During : Mur-ac.

ABSENT PARTS of body were : Cocaine.

ABSORBENT *Action* : Arn; Kali-io; Merc-d; *Sul;* Sul-io.

ABUSIVE, Scolding, Quarrelsome : *Aur;* CHAM; Dul; Hyo; *Ign;* Kali-io; LYC; Merc; Mos; Nit-ac; *Nux-v;* Petr; Plat; Ran-b; Sep; Sil; Stap; Sul; *Tarn.*

+ ANGRY, When not : Dul.

CHILDREN and Family, to : Kali-io.

+ His pains, in : Cor-r.

Husband, To : Thu.

Menses, Before : Cham.

Mother, To : Thu.

+ Person, Absent : Lyc.

Somebody, On the road, to : Con.

Until the lips are blue, eyes stare, and she falls fainting : Mos.

ACHING : See under Pain.

ACIDITY : See Sour.

ACIDOSIS : Nat-p; Pho.

ACNE : See Eruptions,

ACRIDITY : See Discharges, acrid.

ACROMEGALY : Pit-ext; Thyr.

ACTINOMYCOSIS: Hecla; Kali-io; Nit-ac.

ACTIVE, Agile : Ap; Cof; Lach; Nux-v; Stram; Tarn; Val.

Mentally : COF; OP.

+ Restless, Hence : Chel.

When, Amel : Con; Cyc; Helo; Lil-t.

ACTIVITY FRUITLESS : Ap; Arg-n; Bor; Calc; Kali-br; Lil-t; Stan; Tarn; Ther.

ACTS, As If Born Tired : Onos.

ACUMINATE, Conical, growth, eruptions etc : Ant-c; Ant-t; *Ars;* Hyds; Pul; *Sil;* Syph.

ADDISON'S DISEASE : Calc; Calc-p; Iod; Nat-m; Pho; Sil.

ADENOIDS: Agrap; Calc; Calc-io; *Calc-p;* Iod; *Merc;* Tub.

Post Nasal : Mez.

Removal, After : Kali-s.

ADHERENT, INTERNAL sensation : Berb; *Bov; Bry;* Calc; *Colo;* Hep; Ign; Kali-bi; Kali-io; Merc-c; Nux-v; Ol-an; Osm; *Pho;* Plb; Pul; RHUS-T; Rum; SEP; Ust.

ADMONITION AGG: Bell; Kali-c; Nit-ac; Plat.

ADYNAMIA : See Weakness.

AEROPLANE Flying, In Agg : Ars; Bell; Bor; Coca; Petr.

AFFECTATION : Stram.

AFFECTIONS, Stifled : Sep.

AFTERPAINS: *Arn; Cham; Cimi;* Cup; Hypr; Kali-c; PUL; *Rhus-t; Sabi;* Sec; Vib; Xanth.

Child Nurses, When : Arn; Cham; *Sil.*

Fear of Death, with: Cof.

Frequent : Rhus-t.

Headache, With : Hypr.
   Intolerable : Cham; Cimi.

+ Lochia, With : Xanth.

Violent, Persistent : Vib.

Women, Who had borne many children, in : Cup.

AGILITY : See Active.

AGITATION: See Excitement.

AGONY, Anguish : *Aco; Ars; Aur;* Bell; Calc; Caus; Cann; Dig; Hep; Lach; Plat; Stram;Ver-a.

Can Not Rest, In Any Place : *Ars.*

AGORAPHOBIA : Aco; Arg-n; Arn; Calc; Hyd-ac; Nux-v; Sep.

AGUE : See Fever, Intermittent.

AIR Blowing On Part, Through Hole As If, or fanned as if : Aur; *Cam; Chel; Chin; Cor-r;* Croc; *Culex;* FLU-AC; Helod; HEP; Lac-d; Laur; Lil-t; Med; Mos; Naj; Nat-m; Nux-v; Petr; Sele; Sep; Sul; Syph; Ther; Thu; Thyr; Zin,

Clear, Dry or Cold Weather Agg : ACO; Ars-io; *Asar;* Bry; Carb-an; CAUS; Cham; *Hep;* Ip; Kali-ar; Kali-c; Med; NUX-V; Samb; Sep; Spo.

Close, Too, as if: Sars.

Cold, As if : Benz-ac; Chin; Lac-d; Laur; *Lyss;* Mez; Mos; Thyr.

Draft Agg : See Wind Agg.

Hot, As if : Ast-r; Bry; Kali-c; Pul; Sul; Ver-a.

Hunger : See Open Air Amel.

Flatulency, with : Kali-io; Zin.

Impurities, Full of, as if : Trifo.

Inspiring, Cold, AGG : Aesc; *Am-c;* Ars; CAUS; *Cimi;* Cist; Hep; Hyds; *Hyo; Ign;* Merc : *Nux-v; Psor; Rum; Saba;* Seneg; Sep; Syph.

Amel: Sele.

Feels, cold : Lith.

Night or Evening Agg: Aco; *Am-c; Carb-v;* MERC; Nat-s; Nit-ac; *Sul.*

Open Cool Agg : Am-c; Aran; Calc; Cal-p; Cam; Caps; Caus; Cham; *Chin;* Cist;

Cocl; Cof; Colch; Cyc; Dul; *Guai; Hep;* Ign; Kali-bi; Kali-c; Mag-p; Merc; Nat-c; Nit-ac; Nux-m; NUX-V; Petr; *Pho;* Rum; Saba; Seneg; SIL; *Sul;* Urt; Vio-o.

Amel : Bap; *Bry;* Nit-ac; Plat; Radm.

And in House, both Agg : Ars; Aur; Iod; Mez.

Open Amel, in room Agg, Air hunger etc. : Alu; *Ap;* Arg-n; Ars; Ars-io; AUR; Cann; Carb-v; Cep; CROC; Fer; Glo; Grap; *Iod; Kali-io;* LACH; Lil-t; *Lyc; Mag-c;* Mag-m; Med; Nat-s; Op;; Pru-sp; PUL; Radm; Rhus-t; *Saba; Sabi*: Seneg; *Sul;* Tab; Tarn; Tub.

Riding in carriage, Amel : Arg-n; Naj.

Penetrating, Too : Calc; Cimi; Colo.

Smoky, As if : Berb; Bro.

Thick And Heavy, As if : Agn.

Too Much Enters the Chest, as if : Chlor; Ther.

AIR Castles : Arg-n; *Cann;* Chin; Cof; Sul.

AIR HUNGER : See Air, Open, Amel.

AIR PASSAGES Burning : Ars-io; Sang; Seneg. Numb : Sil.

AIR-SICKNESS : See Aeroplane flying Agg.

ALBUMINOUS, GLAIRY: See Discharges.

ALBUMINURIA : Ant-c; *Ap;*
Ars; Aur; Bry;Calc-ar; *Canth;*
Fer; Glo; Hell; Kali-c; Lac-d;
Lach; Lyc; *Merc-c;* Nat-c;
Nat-p; *Pho;* Pho-ac; Phyt; *Plb;*
Pul; Rhus-t; *Sul;* Terb; Thu;
Val.

ALCOHOL, After abuse of: Ars;
Carb-v.

DIPHTHERIA, After : Phyt.

HEART Disease, from : Calc-ar.

PERIODICAL : Pho.

PREGNANCY, During : Ap;
Bur-p; Helo; *Merc-c;* Pho.

During and after Delivery
: Merc-c; Pyro.

SEPTIC : Carb-v.

ALCOHOLIC DRINKS AGG : See
under Food & Drinks.

+ ABOLISHES Taste, for: Strop.

ALCOHOLISM, ACUTE : Aco;
Bell; *Op.*

DELIRIUM TREMENS : Agar;
Ars; Caps; *Cimi;* HYO; Lach;
Nat-m; Nux-m; Nux-v; *Op;*
Stram; Stry.

LATER : Carb-v; Nux-v.

Recurrent : Anac; Aur; Bell;
Chin; Hyo; Nux-v; Op;
Stram; Thu.

ALIVE SENSATION, As if,
something in: Calc-p; *Cann;*
Caus; Cocl; CROC; Cyc; *Ign;*
Op; Pul; *Sabi;* Sil; *Sul;* Thu.

WALLS, Floor, etc, on : Cocl.

ALL-GONE Sensation : See
Empty.

ALONE, WHEN AGG : See
Company Amel.

ALTERNATE DAYS ON AGG :
See Day alternate Agg.

ALTERNATIONS MENTAL
: Alu: Aur; *Bell;* Croc; Con;
Fer; IGN; NUX-M; *Plat;*
Stram; Sul-ac; Val; *Ver-a;*
Zin.

NERVOUS, WITH PHYSICAL :
Saba.

WITH PHYSICAL : Arn; Cimi;
Croc; Ign; Lit-t; *Murx;* Plat.

ALTERNATING EFFECTS,

STATES, SIDES, METASTASIS :
Abro; Agar; Alo; *Amb;*
Ant-c; Arn; Ars; Bell; Berb;
Cann; Cimi; Cocl; Croc; Cup;
Fer-p; Glo; *Ign;* Iris; LAC-C;
Lach; LYC; *Pho;* Psor; *Pul;*
Sep; Stram; SUL; Sul-ac; Val;
Xanth; Zin.

CONTRADICTORY : *Ign;* Nat-m;
Pul.

+ DIGESTIVE and Skin : Grap.

RAPIDLY : Croc.

REACTION, Want of, with : *Val.*

AMAUROSIS See Vision.
Pa-ralysis of optic nerve

AMBITION, LOSS OF (See Indo
lence) : Arg-n; Caus.

DISAPPOINTMENT, From : Nux-v.

AMENORRHOEA: See Menses
absent.

AMMONIACAL ODOUR : See
Discharges.

AMOROUS AMATIVE, Erotic,
Lascivious: Agn; *Canth;* HYO;
Lach; Lil-t; Lyc; Murx; Orig;
Pho; Pic-ac; *Plat;* Scil;*Sele;*
Senec; Stan; Stap; Stram;
Ver-a.

MENSES, Before: Stram.

ANAEMIA: ARS; CALC; *Calc-p*; CHIN; FER; Fer-ar; *Grap*; *Kali-c*; Lac-d; Lyc; Mang; Med; Nat-c; NAT-M; *Nit-ac*; *Nux-v*; *Pho*; Pic-ac; Plat; Plb; *Pul*; Senec; Sep; SUL; Sul-ac.

GRIEF, From : Nat-m; Pho-ac.

HAEMORRHAGE, After : *Chin, Fer.*

PERNICIOUS : *Ars; Pho;* Pic-ac; Thyr.

ANALGESIA : See Numbness.

ANASARCA (See Dropsy) : Ant-c; Ap; Ars; Bell; Bry; Chin; Colch; Dig; Dul; Fer; Hell; Kali-c; Led; Lyc; Merc; Op; Pho; Pul; Rhus-t; Sabi; Samb; Sars; Scil; Sul.

SUDDEN : Kali-n.

ANEURISM : Aur; Bar-c; Cact; Calc-f; Carb-v; Kali-io; Lach; *Lyc;* Pul; Sul; Thu.

ANASTOMOSIS, From : Thu.

AORTA, Of : Spo.

PAINS, Of : Gal-ac; Sec.

SMALL, ALL over body : Plb.

+ **ANGEL WHEN WELL, DEVIL WHEN SICK** : Bell.

ANGER, VEXATION, Irritability, fretfulness, Bad temper : Aco; Anac; *Ant-c;* Ant-t; Aru-t; Aur; *Bry;* Calc; CHAM; *Cina;* Cocl; *Colo;* Hep; *Ign;* Iod; Ip; Kali-c; Kali-io, Kali-m; *Kre;* LYC; Mag-c; Nat-c; *Nat-m; Nit-ac;* NUX-V; Op; Petr; Pho; Rut; Saba; Samb; Senec; *Sep; Stap; Sul;* Sul-ac; Syph; Tarn;

Thu; Thyr; Tub; Val; Zin.

+ **ALWAYS** : Stap.

+ **BEATS**, anything in way : Stro-carb.

BRIGHT Light Agg : Colch.

CONSOLATION Agg : Ign; Nat-m; Sep; Sil.

+ **EASY** : Ab-c; Dros; Radm.

MENSES, Before : Cham.

ODOURS Agg : Colch.

PAIN, Agg : Ant-t.

+ **SELF**, About : Elap.

SYMPATHY Agg : Sabal.

TOUCHED, When : Ant-c; Sanic; Tarn.

TRIFLES, At : Dros; Kali-m; Pho; Sanic; Sep; Tub.

UNDERSTOOD, When not : Laur.

+ **VIOLENT** : Mos.

Fits of : Stro; Tub.

WAKING on: Kali-c; LYC; Pho; Sanic; Tub.

ANGINA PECTORIS : Agar, Am-c; *Amy-n;* Ap; *Arn;* ARS; Arg-n; *Cact;* Chin-ar; Cimi; Cup; Glo; Kalm; *Lach; Latro;* Lil-t; *Naj;* Nux-v; *Ox-ac;* Pho; Pru-s; Rhus-t; *Spig; Spo; Tab.*

+ **CONSTRICTION OF throat, with** : Tab.

HOT Drinks Amel : Spig.

LIES, Knees, on body, bent backwards, with : Nux-v.

PAIN, Excessive : Agar.

ANGLES : See Skin, Folds.

ANIMATION : See Cheerful.

ANKLES : Caus; Led; Lyc; Nat-m; Rhus-t; Rum; Sep; Sul.

BREAK : Pho.

BURNING : See Heat.

CALF, to : Meny.

CARIES, BONES, of; Guai; Pul.

COLD : Calc-f; Ign; Mag-m; Med.

CRACKING, in : *Canth*, Nit-ac.

CRAMP : Meny; Plat; Rum; Zin-io.

Feet pressed on floor Amel : Zin-io.

Toes, into : Nat-c.

ERUPTIONS, on : Calc; Chel; Nat-p; Psor.

FISTULOUS, Opening : Calc-p.

+ GIVE WAY, Afternoon : Cham.

HEAT : Kali-bi; Nat-c.

HEAVY : Ant-c; Crot-t; Cup; Led; Nit-ac; Sec; *Sul.*

Painful : Cup.

INFLAMMED : Mang.

ITCHING : Nat-p; Led; Sele.

JERKING : Calc.

LAMENESS : *Rut.*

NERVOUS : Mag-m.

NIGHT Agg : Mag-m.

NUMBNESS : Lac-c.

PARALYSIS : Abro.

Sensation of : Dros.

SPRAIN : Anac; *Led*; Nat-c; Rut; Stro.

As if : Pru-s.

STIFFNESS : Caus; Chel; Lathy; Sil; Sul.

SWEAT, on: Crot-h; Naj.

SWELLING : Ap; Arg-m; Arg-n; Asaf; Chel; Med; Stan; Stro.

+ Cold : Asaf.

Diabetes, in : Arg-m.

Evening : Kali-chl.

Foot, use, cannot : Asaf.

Painful : Led.

Sitting long, after : Rhus-t.

TENSION: Caus; Merc; Pho.

TOES, to : Nat- c.

TUMOURS : Cup-ar.

TURNED, Easily : Med.

ULCERS : Calc-p; Hyds; Syph.

UPWARDS : Guai.

WALKING Agg : Lith; Med; Nit-ac.

Amel : Caus.

WEAK : Calc; Carb-an; Mang; *Nat-c; Nat-s; Nit-ac; Pho-ac; Sec; Sil;* Stro.

Children, while learning to walk : *Carb-an;* Mang; Nat-s.

ANNOYED EASILY : Ant-t.

ANOREXIA : See Appetite Lost.

ANSWERS AVERSION to : See Aversion.

+ HASTILY : Rhus-t.

IMAGINARY Questions : Pho.

IRRELEVENTLY : Hyo; *Pho*; Stram; *Sil.*

MONOSYLLABLE : Pho-ac; Pul; Sep.

No Questions : Cam.

NODS, By : Pul.

REFUSES To : Pho; Sul.

+ RELUCTANTLY : Rhus-t.

REPEATS Question, then : Zin.

SLOWLY : Arn; Bapt; Cocl; Gel; Hyo; Lyc; *Merc; Pho; Pho-ac;* Rhus-t; Thu; Zin.

THEN Sleeps : Arn; *Bapt; Hyo;* Pho-ac.

ANTAGONISM WITH SELF : Anac; Bar-c; Cann; Kali-c.

ANTHRAX : Anthr; Ars; Echi; Lach; Sec.

ANTHROPOPHOBIA BASHFUL (See Shy) : Amb; Anac; BAR-C;Cocl; HYO; Iod; Kali-io; Kali-p; *Lyc;* Nat-c; Nat-m; PUL; *Rhus-t;* Sil.

ANTICIPATIONS, AND AGG From : *Arg-n;* Ars; Carb-v; *Gel;* Lyc; Med; Nat-m; Pho-ac; Plb; *Sil.*

DISEASED, Conditions of : Ap; *Ars;* Bry; *Chin;* Chin-s; Nat-m; Nux-v.

ANTISOCIAL : Syph.

ANUS : Aesc; Carb-v; Grap; Kali-c; Lach; Mur-ac; Nit-ac; *Nux-v;* Paeon; Pho; Saba; Sep; *Sil.*

APHTHOUS : Sul-ac.

BALL, Sensation of a : *Sep.*

BUBBLES : Colo; Nat-m.

BUG Crawling, as if : Aesc; Fer-io; Sul.

Stools, after : Kali-m.

BURNING : Scop; Sul-ac.

CONTRACTED, Painfully : Plb.

Prolapse, after : Mez.

CRAMPS, Sitting, when : Mang.

CRUSTS : Paeon; *Petr.*

DESIRE to draw in : Agar.

DISCHARGE Black, with or without stool : Merc-i-f.

DRAWN Up: Plb.

DRY : *Aesc;* Rat.

ERUPTIONS : Merc; NAT-M; *Nit-ac;* PETR; Polyg.

Eczema : Berb.

Hard, small : Caus.

EXCORIATED: Carb-v; Caus; Grap; Lyc; Sul.

FISSURE : Alu; Caus; Cham; GRAP; *Ign;* Led; Nat-m; NIT- AC; Paeon; *Rat;* Sep; Sil; Syph; *Thu.*

Bleeding : Grap.

Children, tall, in : Calc-p.

+ Deep : Arn.

Infants, in: Kali-io.

Ulcerate : Grap.

FISTULA : Aur-m; Berb; Calc; Calc-p; Carb-v; Kali-c; Nit-ac; Paeon; Sil.

Itching, with : Berb.

Palpitation, with : Cact.

Pulsating : Caus.

FLUID, Warm, escaping from : *Aco.*

FORMICATION : Calc; Calc-s; Kali-c; Kali-m; *Saba;* Sul.

Worm, as from : Cinb.

HAMMERING : Lach.

Menses, with : Lach.

ITCHING : Carb-v; *Caus;* Coll;

Flu-ac; Grap; *Lyc;* Mar-v;
Med; *Nit-ac; Saba; Sul;*
Vio-o.

Alternating with itching in
nose and ears : Saba.

Around : Petr; Sul.

Coition, after : Anac.

Eczematous: Nit-ac.

Menses, before : Grap.

Pain, ending in : Zin.

Pimples : Polyg.

+ Pinworms, from : Urt.

Sleep, preventing : Mar-v.

Stick, as if, with a : Rum.

Sticking and : *Aco.*

Stools, after : Kalm; Tell;
Zin.

Stooping, on : Arg-m.

LIVER, To : *Dios;* Lach.

LONG After stool : Nit-ac;
Paeon.

LOOSE : See Open.

MOISTURE, At : ANT-C; *Caps;*
Carb-an; Carb-v; *Caus;*
Grap; *Hep;* NIT-AC; *Op;*
PHO; *Sep; Sil; Sul;* Sul-io.

Bloody : Ap.

Constant : Sep.

Staining yellow : Ant-c.

Flatus, from : Ant-c; Carb-v.

Foul : *Ant-c;* Hep; Paeon;
Sul-io.

Menses, during : Lach.

Mucus, from, Urinating
when : Carb-ac.

bloody : Op.

foul : Hep.

Staining yellow : Ant-c.

NAVEL, To : Colo; Lach.

OPEN, Inactive, powerless :
Ail; ALO; Alu; Ap; Ign;
Kali-c; Op; PHO; Sec.

As if : Ap; Pho.

And stools pass right
through : Apoc.

+ PLUG In, as if : Kali-bi.

PRICKING : Cact.

POUTING, Swollen and :
Cham.

PUSTULES, Small, hard : Caus.

RAW : See Sore.

RED : Med; Petr; Sul.

Fiery : Med.

RETRACTED : Kali-bi; Nat-p;
op.

SORE : Kali-m; Lyc.

Menses, during : Mur-ac.

Stools, from : Kali-m.

Walking, when : Kali-m.

SWEAT : Sep.

TORN, as if : Erig.

Warm cloth, Amel : Pho.

TREMBLING, In : Con.

ULCER : *Carb-v;* Cham;
Kali-bi; Nit-ac; Sul.

+ WARTS, around : Aur.

WIPING Agg : Grap.

ANXIETY : See Fear.

OTHERS , For : Ars; Cocl; Pho;
Sul.

APATHETIC : See Inactive.

UNEQUAL STRUGGLING adverse
circumstances, with :
Pho-ac.

APATHY : See Indifference.

+ ALL PERVADING : Bry.

APHASIA : See SPEECH, Lost.

AMNESIC : Kali-br; Plb.

APHONIA : See *Voice*, Lost.

APOPLEXY : ACO; Ant-c; Ant-t; ARN; Ars; Aur; Bar-c; *Bell;* Calc; COCL; Cof; Fer; *Gel; Glo;* HYD-AC; Hyo; *Ip;* Kali-m; *Lach;* Lyc; Nux-v; OP; Pho-ac; Pul; Rhus-t; Samb; Sep; Stram; Thu; Ver-a; Ver-v.

PULSE, Irritable, with : Aco.

> Slow, full, face red,
> pupils small : Op.

> Small, weak, face
> bluish, pale : Lach.

SUBARACHNOID : Gel.

WAVES of congestion, burning, throbbing, holds head : Glo.

APPARITION : See Vision, Fan-tastic.

APPENDICITIS (IIeo-caecal re-gion) : ARS; Bapt; Bell; BRY; Carb.v; *Chin;* COLO; LACH; Lyc; *Merc-c;* Mur-ac; *Nux-v; Pho;* Pho-ac; Plb; Pul; RHUS-T; SEP; SUL; THU.

+ LYING, Back on Amel : Lach; Merc.

APPETITE, AFFECTED in general : Ant-c; Ars; *Calc;* CHIN; *Cina;* Grap; Iod; *Lyc;* Merc-cy; *Nat-m;*NUX-V; Petr; Pho; PUL; Sil; Strop; SUL; Ver-a.

CAPRICIOUS, Variable : Calc;

Cina; Coc-c; Fer; Grap; *Iod;* Lach; Merc; Nat-m: Petr; *Pho;* Syph.

EASY SATIETY : Chin; Cyc; Lyc; Plat.

INCREASED, HUNGER : Ab-c; Arg-m; Ars; *Calc; Chin;* CINA; *Grap;* Iod; *Lyc; Nat-m; Nux-v;* Old; Petr; Pho; Psor; Pul;*Saba;* Sep; Stan; Stap; *Sul;* Ver-a.

11 A.M. : Hyds; Pho; SUL; Zin.

Alternating with loss
> of appetite : Anac; Calc; Cina; *Fer;* Pho.

Attacks of sickness,
> before : Bry; Calc; Hyo; Nux- v; *Pho; Psor;* Sep.

Chill before : Cina.

> during : Ars; Sil.

> after : Ars.

Cough, during : Nux-v.

Diarrhoea, with : Nux-v; Petr.

Digestion, weak, with : Merc.

Eating, after : Chin-ar; CINA; Iod; Kali-p; *Lyc;* Murx; PHO; Phyt; Sars; Sil.

> no desire, for : Op.

Epilepsy, before : Calc; Hyo.

Fever, during : Chin; Cina; *Pho.*

> after : Ign.

Headache, with : Bry; Kali-c; Kali-s; *Pho*; PSOR; Sele; Sep.

before : Epip.

Nausea, with : Petr; Val; Ver-a.

Navel, from; : Val.

Nightly : Chin; Lyc; *Pho*; *Psor.*

Pain in stomach, with : *Lach*; Lyc; Sil.

Ravenous : Ars; *Calc*: Cann; CHIN; CINA; Grap; IOD; *Lyc*; Nat-m; *Nux-v*; Old; Petr; PHO; PSOR; Pul; Rum; *Saba*; *Sil*; Spig; SUL; *Ver-a*; Zin.

meals, 2 hours after: Calc-hyp.

more he eats, more he craves : Lyc.

Refuses to eat, but : Bar-c.

Relish, without : NAT-M; Old; *Op; Rhe; Rhus-t.*

Sleep, prevents : Chin; Ign; Lyc; Pho.

Spine, from : Lil-t.

Stomach, full, when : Stap.

Stool, after : Alo; Kali-p; *Petr.*

Sudden : Sul.

Sweat, after : Cina.

Sweets only, for : Kali-p.

Vanishes, attempting, to eat, on : Sil.

drinking water, after : Kali-m.

food, sight of : Caus; Pho; *Sul.*

smell or thought of pregnancy during : Caus.

Vomiting. during : Caus.

after : Cina.

KNOWS NOT, For What : Mag-m; Pul.

LOATHING, After first bite : Caus; Cyc: Lyc; Plat; Pru-s; Rhe.

LOST, DIMINISHED, Wanting: Alu; Ars; Calc; Cham; Chol; CHIN; Cocl; Cyc; Fer; Kali-bi; Lyc; Nat-m; *Nux-v*; Pho; Pic-ac; Psor; *Pul*; Rhus-t; Sep; Sil; Sul.

Brain troubles, in : Hell.

Coition, after: Agar.

Day, only in : Ars.

Drinking water, after : Kali-m.

Food, at the sight of : Colch; Kali-p; Pho; Sul.

pregnancy, during : Caus.

until it is tasted, then ravenous : Lyc.

Habitual : Kali-m.

Hunger, with : Chin; Cocl; Nat-m; Nux-v.

Illness, severe, after : Ant-c; Psor.

Lifting Agg : Sep.

Months, for : Syph.

Neither eats nor drinks for weeks : Ap.

Overwork, from: Calc.

Pregnancy, during : Saba.

Returns, eating

mouthful, after: Calc;
Chin; Saba.

thinking of food after :
Calc-p.

Sadness, from : Plat.

Suddenly, eating, when:
Bar-c.

Thirst, with : Psor; Rhus-t.

Tobacco, from : Sep.

When desired thing is
offered : Ign.

NIBBLING: *Aeth*; Calc; Mag-c;
Mag-m; Nat-c; Petr; Rhus-t.

ARMS (UPPER LIMBS) : Am-m;
Ars; Bell; *Calc; Caus;* Cocl;
Fer; Kali-c; Lyc; Merc; Nux-v;
Pho; Pul; RHUS-T; Sep; *Sil;*
SUL.

RIGHT : Bell; Bism; Bry; Calc;
Caus; Colo; Grap; Nat-c;
Ran-ac; Sars; Sec; Sil; Stro.

Dead : Scop.

Heart affections, in : Ars;
Kalm; Merc-i-f; Merc-i-r.

Holds, palpitation, during :
Aur.

Longer than body, as if :
Cup.

Motion, involuntary : Cocl.

Numb : Lach; Mur-ac.

aphasia, with : Mur-ac.

neuralgia, over left eye,
with : Mur-ac.

then left : Zin-io.

Writing Agg : Merc-i-f.

LEFT : Anac; Arn; Asaf; Cact;
Cimi; Kali-st; Nit-ac;
Rhus-t; Sabi; Scil; Stan;
Stram; Sul.

Bound, as if, to the side :
Cimi.

Jerking all day : Cic;
Cimi.

Numb : Cact.

Pinching : Kali-c.

Shakes, epilepsy, before :
Sil.

ALTERNATING Between : Aco;
Alu; *Calc;* Caus; Cham;
Chin; *Cocl;* Colch; *Lac*-c;
Lyc; Mag-m; Mang; Plat;
Sep; *Zin.*

Upper and Lower : Cocl;
Fago; Kali-bi; Kali-m;
Kalm; Nat-c; S*il; Val;*
Visc.

UPPER : Cocl; Fer; Nat-m.

Bone: See Humerus.

Burning : Ther.

Coldness : Ign.

Contraction : Nat-m

Cramps, writing while :
Val.

Drawing : Lyc.

Electric Shocks, as if :
Agar; Val.

Emaciated : Nit-ac.

Fluttering in while
resting on table : Phyt.

Heavy : Alu; Latro.

Numb : Cact; Latro;
Mag-m.

Raise, Cannot : Sang.

Singing Agg : Stan.

Thumping pain, in middle : Anac.

Weak : Stan.

Writing Agg : Val.

FORE : Calc; Caus; Merc; Phyt; Rhus-t; Stap.

Blue : Bism.

+ Bone, exostosis of : Dul.

Cold : *Grap*; Med; *Pho.*

icy : *Bro.*

menses, during : Arg-n.

Crushed, as if : Guai; Gymn.

Drauing; Calc; Card-m; caus; Rhus-t.

Heavy : Arg-n; Mur-ac; Pho-ac; Strop.

Hip, left, with : Merc-i-f.

Moving the fingers, Agg : Asaf.

Numb : Grap.

Paresis, contraction of fingers, with: Arg-m.

Pronated: Cup; Plb.

Trembling, coition after: Nat-p.

writing while: Caus; *Merc.*

Writing Agg : Merc-i-r; Ran-b.

BEND, Irresistible desire to : *Fer.*

BOILS : Bro; Petr.

BONES : Asaf; Chin; Rhus-t; Sil; Stap.

BREATHING Deep Agg : Cann.

BURNING : Ver-a.

Up : Ther.

CHEST, Keeping on, Agg : Psor.

CLAWING : Lach.

COLD : Bell; Kali-chl; Pho; Pul.

Diarrhoea, during : Pho.

COUGH Agg : Dig.

CRAMP : Am-c; Calc; Colo; Old.

EMACIATED : Iod; Lyc; Plb.

EXTENDED, As if he had intended to take hold of something : Dul; Pho.

Flexed, and alternately : Cic; Cup; *Lyc;* Tab.

FALL, Helpless: Colch.

FLOATING, As if : Pho-ac.

FORMICATION : Aco; Sec.

FUZZY *(R)* : Phyt.

GRASPING Amel : Lith.

HAIRY : Med.

HANGING Down Amel : Aco; Arn; Bar-c; CON; *Fer;* Led; Lyc; Mag-m; Pho; Rhus-t; *Sang;* Sil; Sul.

+ Forceless : Aco.

HAS Many, as if : Pyro.

HEAVINESS : Arg-n; Caus; Con; Gel; Kali-p; Nat-m; Plb; Pul; Strop.

Right : Am-c.

HOT, Water Flowing on, as if : Rhus.t.

ITCHING : Bov; Caus; Sul; Tell.

JERKING Up : Cic; Cina; Saba; Stram; Sul.

Outwards : Arg-n.

Towards each other : Ip.

Upwards : Arg-n.

LAMENESS : Bell; Calc; Sil.

Right : Fer; Sang.

Left : Bro.

LAUGHING Agg : Carb-v.

LIFTING Weight Amel : Spig.

LIGHT, As if : Pho-ac.

MOTION of Agg : Anac; Dig; Led; Nat-m; Ran-b; Rhus-t; Sep; *Spig;* Sul.

Behind him Agg : Fer; Ign; Kali-bi; Mar-v; Pul; *Sanic; Sep.*

Clutching : Hyo.

Constant, of one: Bry.

Involuntary, of arm and leg : Cocl.

To and Fro : Op.

NERVOUS : Rhus-t.

NUMB: Aco; Ap; Cocl; Grap; Kali-c; Kali-m; Lyc; Ox-ac; Plat; Rhus-t; Zin.

Right : Phyt; Scop.

then left : Zin-ars.

Left : Aco; Cact; Dig; Lach; Naj; Rhus-t; Spig; Sul.

heart diseases, in : Aco; Cact; Latro; Rhus-t.

Carrying anything, when : Amb.

Grasping, anything firmly : *Cham.*

Holding anything, in the hand : Ap.

Lain, on : Carb-v; Kali-c; Nat-m; *Pul; Rhus-t.*

not lain on : Flu-ac; Mag-m.

Lying Agg : Sul.

Raising them upright Amel : Ars; Pul.

Shoulder to fingertips : Ox-ac.

PARALYSIS, Left : Calc; *Dig.*

Right : Am-c; Cup; LYC; *Sul; Zin.*

Tongue, Paralysis of with : Caus.

+ Writing, from : Agar.

PRONATION, Agg : Petr.

PURRING : Sep.

RAISING Up AGG : Ap; Arg-n; Bar-c; Berb; Bry; Cocl; CON; Dig; Fer; Grap; Led; Mag-c; Nit-ac; Ran-b; Rhus-t; Sanic; *Sang; Spig; Sul;* Sul-ac; Tell.

Laterally Agg : Syph.

RAT, running upwards : *Bell;* Calc; Sul.

RED Spots on : Saba.

RESTLESS : Agar; Ant-t; Caus; Kali-br; Mur-ac; Samb; Tarn.

Sleep, during : Caus.

SEPARATED from body, as if : Bap; Daph; Psor.

SHOCKS : Cic.

SHORT, As if : Aeth; Alu.

SINKING Down: Nat-m.

SLEEPS Arms apart, with : *Cham;* Psor.

STICKY : Cam; Carb-v; Pic- ac.

STIFF, Become, convulsions, before : Buf.

STRETCHED, Palpitation, with : Cocl.

Right angle, at : Op.
Spasmodically, Clenched
  fingers, with : Chin.
SUPINATION Agg : Cinb.
SWEAT Amel : Thu.
SWINGING : Cina.
  To and fro Amel: Sang.
+ SWOLLEN : Ver-a.
TENSION : Dig.
  Writing, while : *Mag-p.*
THIGHS, Puts on, coughing,
  when : Nic.
THROWS wildly : Kali-br.
TINGLING : Grap; Pho; Sil.
TREMBLING : Merc; Nit-ac;
  Op; Plb.
  Concomitant, as a: Calc-p.
  Lain on : Cam.
  Taking hold of anything :
  Ver-a
  Urinary difficulty, with :
  Dul.
  Writing, while : *Merc.*
TURNING Agg : Sang.
  Amel : Spig.
TWISTING Sensation : Bell.
TWITCHING : Cic; Thu.
+ ULNAR Nerves, along, both
  : Pod.
VEINS : Nux-v; Plb; *Pul;* Thyr.
WEAKNESS : Aesc; Anac;
  Bell; Calc; *Cic;* Con; Dig;
  Elap; KALI-C; Stan; Sul;
  Val.
  One, of, apoplexy, after :
  Cadm; Pho.
  Right : Am-c.

Taking hold of something
  : *Ars.*
WIND Blowing, as if, shoulders
  to fingers : Flu-ac.
  Cold, blowing on as if :
  Ast-r.
WRITING Agg : Merc-i-f.
  Amel : Zin-ar.
ARROGANCE : See Pride.
ARTERIO SCLEROSIS : Sumb.
ARTHRALGIA(See Joints):
  Arg-m, Plb; Symp.
ARTHRITIS DEFORMANS : Arn;
  Ars; Aur; Caus; Cimi; Colch;
  Cup; Guai; Hep; Iod; Kali-io;
  Merc; *Pul;* Radm; *Sabi;* Sul.
ASCENDING AGG : Ars; Aur;
  Bor; *Bry; Calc;* Iod; Merc;
  Nat-m; Nit-ac; Nux-v; Pho;
  Pul; Sep; *Spo;* Sul.
  AMEL : Con; Fer; Rhod; Val.
  STEPS AGG : Stan.
ASCITES : See Abdomen,
  Dropsy.
ASKS FOR NOTHING : Bry; *Op;*
  Pul; Rhe.
ASLEEP SENSATION : See
  Numbness.
ASPHYXIA CHARCOAL FUMES,
  From : Bov.
  NEONATORUM : Ant-t; Cam;
  Laur.
  Loss of blood, in mother
  from : Chin.
ASSOCIATED EFFECTS : Ars;
  Cham; *Merc; Nux-v;* Pho;
  Pul; Sep; Sul; Tarn; Ver-a.
ASTHENOPIA : See under
  Vision.

ASTHMA (Bronchial) :
Aco; Amb; Arg-n; ARS; Ars-io;
Cup; *Ip*; Kali-ar; *Kali-c;*
Kali-n; *Lach; Lob;* Merc-i-r;
Nux-v; PUL; *Samb; Sil;* SPO;
Stan; Stram; Sul; Tab; Terb;
Thu; Tub; Visc.

BED, Turning in, Agg : Ars.

BENDING Head backwards
Amel : *Spo*; Ver-a.

Shoulders, backwards,
Amel : Calc-ac.

CARDIAC (See Respiration
Difficult) : Cact; Chin-ar;
Laur; Naj; Psor; Spo; Sumb.

CATARRHAL : Calad; Caps.

COITION, Agg : Amb; Asaf;
Kali-bi.

+ COLD, Preceded by: Sul.

CONSTITUTIONALLY : Calc; Iod;
Sul.

CONSUMPTIVES, Of: Meph.

CORYZA, With : Arg-n; Just;
Nat-s; Spo.

After : Just, Naj.

summer, in: Ars.

COUGH, With : Calad; Nat-m.

After : Pho.

DIARRHOEA, After : Kali-c.

Alternating, with : Kali-c.

Before : Nat-s.

DIGESTION Disturbed, after :
Sang.

DRUNKARDS, Of : Meph.

DUST, Inhalation of : Poth.

DYSURIA, Night at, with : Solid.

EATING Amel : Amb; *Grap.*

Satisfying Agg : Asaf.

ERUCTATION Amel : Carb-v;
Nux-v.

ERUPTIONS, Alternating with
: Calad; Hep; Kalm; Sul.

EXERTION, Excessive, from :
Sil.

EXPECTORATION Amel : Ant-t;
Calad; Hypr; Ip; Stan; Zin.

FOG Agg : Hypr.

FOOT Sweat, suppressed,
from : Ol-an.

FRIGHT, After: Samb.

+ FULL Moon: Spo.

GOITRE, In: Spo.

HAY FEVER, Of: Ars; Aru-t;
Chlor; *Iod; Naj;* Sep.

HIVES, From: Ap; Pul.

HUMID : Cann; Dul; Kali-bi;
Nat-s; Seneg; Sul.

Weather Agg : Bar-c;
Syph.

HYSTERICAL: Cocl; Ign; Lob;
Mos; Nux-m; Nux-v; *Pul.*

Tears, flow of, ending in :
Anac.

ICE WATER Agg: Meph.

INFANTILE : Med; Vib.

INJURY, Spine, to from : Hypr.

ITCHING, With: Calad; Cist;
Saba.

LAUGHING, Agg : Ars.

MENSES, Absent, with: Spo.

During, waking, from
sleep: Cup; *Iod; Lach;*
Spo.

Scanty, with: Arg-n.

MINER'S: Card-m; Nat-ar.

Coal: Sul.

NERVOUS : Cham; Kali-p;
Mag-p; Stram.

NIGHT, From 1A.M. to 4 A.M
: Syph.

ODOURS, From: Asar; Sang.

OLD PEOPLE, In : Amb; *Ars;*
Bar-c; Bar-m; Carb-v;
Coca; Con; Seneg.

OVERHEATED, Being, after : Sil.

RHEUMATISM, With : Benz-ac;
Visc.

ROCKING, Amel : Kali-c.

SAILORS, On shore: Bro.

SEXUAL, Excitation, with:
Nat-c.

SITTING, Up, Amel : Ip.

SKIN Disease, with : Naj.

SPASMODIC : Val.

STOOLS Amel : Poth.

SUMMER, During: Arg-n;
Syph.
Amel : Carb-v.

SUPPRESSIONS, From : Hep.

SYCOTIC : Med; Nat-s; Sil.

TALKING Agg : Dros.

THROAT, Choking of, with :
Hyd-ac.

THUNDER STORM, During :
Pho; Sep; *Sil*; Syph.

TOBACCO, Smoking, Amel :
Merc.

URAEMIC : Solid.

URINATING, When : Chel; Dul.

URTICARIA, Alternating with :
Calad.

VERTIGO, With : Cup.

VOMITING, alternating with :
Kali-c.

WEATHER, Cold, Agg : Arg-n.
Damp Cold Agg : Ver-a.
Damp Amel : Caus; Hep.
Dry Agg : Cham.

WEEKLY : Chin; Ign; Sul.

WINTER Agg : Carb-v; Nat-m;
Nux-v.

ASTIGMATISM : See Under
Vision.

ATHLETE'S FOOT : Grap;
Sanic.

ATHEROMA : See Calculi.

ATHETOSIS :Lathy; Stry; Ver-v.

ATONY : *Op;* Passif.

ATROPHY : See Emaciation.

ATTACKS ,RECURRENT : See
Relapses, Recurrences.

ATTENTION AGG : Ign.
AMEL : Cam; Gel; *Hell.*

ATTITUDE, BIZZARE : *Cina;*
Cocl; *Colo;* Gamb; Lyc; Merc;
Nux-v; *Plb*: Zin.
AMEL : Rhe.
As If in: Nat-s.

AURA : (See Different Sensations)

ABDOMEN, to Head : Ind.

ARMS, In : Calc; *Lach*; Sil; Sul.

BRAIN, Wavy sensation in :
Cimi.

GENERAL Nervous feeling:
Arg-n; *Nat-m.*

GENITALS : See Solar Plexus.

GLOW, From foot to head :
Visc.

HEELS to occiput : Stram.

HEART, From : *Calc-ar;* Lach; Naj.

KNEES, to hypogastrium : Cup-ac.

MOUSE Running : See Creeping.

SOLAR Plexus or Genitals from : Buf; Cic; *Nux-v; Sul.*

VARIOUS Symptoms : Buf.

AUTOMATIC ACTS, Motion : Bell; Calc; Hell; Hyo; Lyc; Mag-c; Nux-m; Pho; Sil; Stram; Zin.

Hand, Right, towards mouth : Nux-v.

ONE Arm and leg, head, etc. : Apo; Bry; Hell; Iodf; Myg; Pyro; Zin.

AUTUMN AGG : Chin; Colch; *Dul;* Lach; *Merc;* Merc-c; RHUS-T; Ver-a.

AVARICIOUS, Greedy, Mi-serly : *Ars;* Lyc; Med; Pul; Sep; Sul.

AVERSIONS, DISLIKES :

ACIDS, Sour things: Bell; Cocl; Dros; Fer; Saba; *Sul.*

ALCOHOLIC Sitimulants: Hyo; Ign; Rhus-t; Strop.

ALE : Nux-v.

AMUSEMENT : Bar-c; Hep; Lil-t; Old; Sul.

ANSWER, To : *Glo; Hyo; Nux-v;* Sul-ac.

APPLES : Lyss.

APPROACHED, or Being Touched : ANT-C; *Arn;* CHAM; Cina; Con; Cup; Ign; Kali-c: Lyc; Tarn; Thu.

BANANAS : Bar-c; Elap.

BATHING To : See Bathing.

BED : Cedr; Grap.

BEEF : Merc; Ptel.

BEER : Chin; Cyc; Fer; Lyc; Nux-v.

BLACK Things : Tarn.

BRANDY : Ign; Merc.

Brandy drinkers, in : Arn.

BREAD : Chin; Con; Cyc; Kali-c; Lil-t; Lyc; NAT-M; Nit-ac; Pul; Sul; Tarn.

Butter, and : Mag-c; Meny; Nat-p.

BRILLIANT Objects : Buf.

BUSINESS : See Work.

BUTTER : Ars; Chin; Cyc; Hep; *Pul;* Sang.

CHEESE : Arg-n; *Chel;* Old.

CHILDREN : Lyc; Plat.

CHOCOLATE : Osm; Tarn.

COCOA : Osm.

COFFEE : CALC; Cham; Chel; Flu-ac; Lil-t; Merc; Nat-m; NUX-V; Sul-ac.

Smell of : Sul-ac.

COITION, To : See Coition and Female Affections.

COLOURS, Black, red, yellow, green : Tarn.

Red : Alu.

COMPANY : See Company agg; Fer-p.

CONVERSATION : Chel.

COVERS, To : Aco; Cam; Iod; Pul; Sec; Sul.

DISTURBED, Being : Bry; Gel.

DRINKS, HOT : Kali-s.

Thirst, with : Hell.

EDUCATION : Sul.

EGGS : Fer; Kali-s.

Odour, of : Colch.

EVERYTHING, For : Ant-c;
Canth; Merc; Pul.

FARINACIOUS Food : Ars; Pho.

FATS : Ars; Chin; Cyc;
Kali-m; Merc; Nat-m; *Petr;*
Ptel; *Pul;*

FISH : Colch; *Grap;* Pho; Zin.

Salted : Pho.

+ FLUIDS, ALL : Stram.

FOOD : ARS; Chin; Cocl;
Colch; Fer;Ip; Lil-t; NUX-V;
Pul; Senec; Tub.

+ All : Kali-io; Tub.

Best and digestible : Carb-v.

Boiled : Calc.

Certain : Pul.

Every kind, of : Plat.

Fried : Plb.

Hot : *Chin;* Merc-c; Sil.

Hunger, with : Cocl;
Nat- m; Nux-v.

Diarrhoea, chronic, in :
Ant- c; Ars; Chin; Nux-m;
Pho; Pul.

Loathing, disgust, with :
Ant-c; Arn; Ars; Cham;
Colch; Cyc; Ip; *Kali-c;*
Nux-v; Op; Pul; Sep.

all : Cocl.

animal food : Sil.

convalescence, during :
Kre.

eating, when : Nux-m.

suddenly : Bar-c; Pul; Rut.

first bite, after : Rhe.

rich : Kali-m.

sadness, from : Plat.

salty : Sele.

seen, if : ARS; Colch;
Nux-v; Pho; Sil.

smell of : Ant-c; Ars;
Cocl; Colch; Ip; Nux.v;
Pho.

solid : Coca; Fer; Stap.

thinking, of : Ars; Carb-v;
Nux-m; Zin-ch.

warm : Chin; Grap; Ign;
Pho; Pul; Sil.

FRIENDS : Colo; Led.

Pregnancy, during : Con.

FRUITS : Bar-c; Ign.

Sour : Fer.

FUSS, To : Nat-m.

GARLIC : Saba.

GOING Out : Cyc.

GREEN Things: Mag-c.

GRUEL : Ars; Calc.

HERRING : Pho.

HERSELF : Lac-c.

ICE CREAM : Radm.

LIQUIDS, For : Grap; Hyo;
Nux-v.

LITERARY Persons : Sul.

MARRIAGE : See Marriage.

MEAT : Arn; Ars; Calc;
Calc-s; Chel; Chin; Cyc;
Fer; *Grap;* Hell; Manc;
Merc; *Mur-ac;* Nux-v; PETR;
PUL; *Sep; Sil;* SUL; Syph;
Tarn; Tub.

Fond of, was : Cact.

Fresh : Thu.

Salted : Card-m.

MEMBERS of the family : Crot-h; Flu-ac; Iod; Kali-p; Lyc; Pho; Plat; Senec; *Sep.*

Children, One's own : Lyc; Pho; Plat.

Husband : Glo; Nat-c; *Sep;* Thu.

Mother : Thu.

Talks, pleasantly to others : Flu-ac.

Wife : Ars; Nat-s; Plat; Stap.

MEN (Females): Nat-m; Sep.

MILK : Ant-t; Arn; Bry; Fer-p; Guai; *Ign;* Lac-d; Nat-c; Pul; Sep; *Sil.*

But relishes it : Bry.

Mothers's : Cina; *Sil.*

MUSIC (See Music Agg) : Nux-v; Sep; Vio-o.

Violin : Vio-o.

NIGHT, Of : Buf.

NOISE (See Noise, Sensitive to) : Asar; Bor; Con; Kali-c; Op.

+ NOURISHMENT, All kind of : Ant-t.

ONIONS : Saba.

OYSTERS : Pho.

PERSONS, To certain : Am-m; Calc; Hep; *Nat-c.*

Sight, of : Cic.

Who do not agree, with him : Calc-s.

PICKLES : Ab-c.

PLACES : Hep.

PLAY (Child) : Hep.

PLUMS : Bar-c.

PORK : Colch; Dros; Psor; Pul.

POTATOES : Alu; Cam; Thu.

PUDDINGS : Pho; Ptel.

RELIGIOUS, to opposite sex : Lyc; *Pul;* Sul.

RIDING in Carriage : Psor.

SALT FOOD : Carb-v; Cor-r; *Grap;* Nat-m; Sele; Sep.

SAURKRAUT : Hell.

SCHOOL, To : Calc-p; Nat-m.

SITTING : Iod; Lach.

SNUFF: Spig.

SOCIETY : Anac; Nat-c; Stan; Syph.

SOUP : Arn; Grap; Lyc; Rhus-t.

SOUR Things : See Acids.

SPOKEN To : Cham.

SWEETS : Ars; Bar-c; CAUS; *Grap;* Lac-c; Nit-ac; Radm; Sene; Sul.

TALK, To : See Taciturn.

TEA : Pho.

THINKING : Pho; Pho-ac.

TOBACCO : Arn; *Calc;* IGN; Lob; Nat-m; *Nux-v.*

To his accustomed cigar : Bro; Fer; *Ign.*

TOUCHED : See Approached.

VEAL : Zin.

VEGETABLES : Hell; Mag-c.

WATER (See Thirstless): Am-c; *Hyo; Nux-v; Stram.*

Cannot bear touch of it : Am-c.

Pregnancy, during : Pho.

Thinking of it Agg : Ham.

Thirst, with : Hell.

WINE : LACH; Manc; Merc; SABA; Sul.

WOMEN : Dios; Lach; Pul.

Men, to : Nat-m; Sep.

To her own sex: Raph.

WORK, For: Alo; Arg-n; Bap; Carb-v; Chel; *Chin;* CON; Cyc; GRAP; Ham; Lach; Meph; Mill; NAT-M; *Nux-v; Pho;* Pul; Psor; Rhod; Rhus-t; Sul; Zin-ch.

Customary : Sep.

WRITING, For: Hyds; Scil.

AWAKES, ANGER, In : Cham; *Lyc.*

ANXIOUS : *Lyc;* Spo.

BED Moving, as if from : Lac-c.

BRAIN, Shock in, with : Coca.

CALLED, As if : Rhod; Sep.

COLDNESS Of Hands & feet, from : *Carb-v.*

CONFUSION, In : Bov; Chin; Gel; Petr; Pho; Pul.

Children: Aesc.

COUGH, From : Hyo; Pul; Samb; Sul.

DREAMS, From : Bell; Lach; Sil; *Sul.*

ERECTION, with and desire to urinate : Hep.

EXACT Hour : Sele.

FALLING, As if : Guai.

FEVER From: Bar-c; Nit-ac; Pho.

FREQUENTLY (Cat naps) : Alu; Bar-c; *Calc; Hep*; Mur-ac; Op; *Pho; Pul;* Rut; *Sep; Sul.*

FRIGHT, Nightmare, etc; in :

Arn; Bell; Bor; Cact; Carb-v; *Cina;* Hyo; *Ign; Lach;* Lyc; Nat-m; Paeon; Sep; Sil; *Stram;* SUL; Thu; Tub; Zin.

Menses, before : Sul-ac.

HEART, Burning at, with : Benz-ac.

Tremors, with : Merc.

HUNGER, From : Lyc; Pho-ac; Psor.

JERK, With a : Bell.

NERVOUS : Rhus-t.

NOISE, From very slight : Asar; Calad; Nux-v; Sele.

PALPITATION, With : Benz-ac; Calc; Merc; Merc-c; Nat-c; Radm; Sep.

PANTING, With : Radm.

PERSPIRATION, From : Ars; *Con.*

PULSE, Slow, with, at 11 P.M. : Ther.

SAD : Lyc.

SCREAMING : Stram; Sul.

SHOCKS, through body, from : Dig; Mag-m.

SINGING : Sul.

SLEEP, Cannot again : Nux-v.

+ SOMEONE were in room, As if, from : Mag-p.

STUPOR, Then : Hyo.

SUFFOCATING : Kali-io; Samb; Spo; Val.

Menses, during : Spo.

TIRED (See Sleep unrefreshing) : *Nat-m;* Pul; Rhus-t; *Syph.*

TOO early : *Kali-c; Nat-c;* Nit-ac; *Nux-v;* Pic-ac;

Ran-b; Sul.

Late : *Calc;* Calc-p; *Grap; Nux-v; Sep;* Sul.

TREMBLING : Ign; Ver-a.

Heart, of with: Merc.

AWAKENING AGG (Mental symptoms) : Calc; LACH; *Lyc; Stram;* Zin.

AFTER **A**GG (General): Amb; Am-m; *Ap; Ars; Bell;* Calc; *Chin;* Caus; Hep; Hyo; Kali-bi; LACH; *Lyc;* Lycps; Nat-m; Nit-ac; *Nux-v;* Onos; *Op; Pho; Pul;* Sele; Sep; *Spo;* Stram; *Sul;* Tarn; Tub; Val.

AMEL : Pho; Radm; Sabal; Sep; Val.

AND **F**ALLING to sleep, both **A**GG : Stan.

AWKWARDNESS (Mental, Physical) drops things etc. : Aeth; *Agar; Amb;* Anac; AP; Bar-c ; *Bov;* Calc; Cam; CAPS; Caus; *Hell;* Ign; Ip; *Lach;* Lol-t; Mos; Nat-m; Tarn.

PREGNANCY, During : Calc.

AXILLAE : Carb-an; Carb-v; *Hep;* Pho; Sep; Sil; Sul.

ABSCESS : Hep; *Lyc;* Merc; Nit-ac; *Pho;* Rhus-t; Sil.

Delivery, after : Rhus-t.

ACHE, In: Latro.

ACNE : Carb-v.

ALTERNATELY : Colch.

BOILS : Lyc; Pho; Sep.

BUBBLING : Colch.

BURNING, Pressure : Grap.

CANCER : Ast-r.

ERUPTIONS, In : Elap; Lyc; Nat-m; Psor; Sep.

EXCORIATION : Carb-v; Grap; Mez; Sep; Sul.

GLANDS, enlarged : Ast-r; Bar-c; Hep; Lach; LYC; *Nit-ac; Pho-ac; Sil;* Sul.

Breast, pain in with: Lact-ac.

Hard : Ast-r; Carb-an; Iod; Sil.

HERPES : Carb-an.

ITCHING : Pho; Sang; *Sul.*

LUMP, Bluish, hard, in : Calc-p.

MENSES, Before, Agg : Sang.

SCURFS, Scabs, in : Nat-m.

STITCHES : Caus; Dros; Lyc; Sul.

Below, left : Stan.

SWEAT: Bry; Calc; Dul; Kali-c; *Lapp;* Nat-m; Petr; Rhod; Sele; *Sep;* Sil; Sul.

Brown : Lac-c.

Cold : Lapp .

Garlicky : Lach; Sul.

Offensive : Hep; Lapp; Lyc; Nat-s; Nit-ac; Petr; Sil; Sul.

Red : Lach; Nux-m.

TUMOURS : Ars-io; Bar-c.

ULCERS: Bor.

BACK : AGAR; Ars; Aur; *Bell;* CALC; Chin-s; *Cimi;* Cocl; Gel; Hypr; Kali-c; *Lach;* Nat-m; Nat-s; *Nux-v;* PHO; Pho-ac; *Pic-ac; Rhus-t;* Sec; SIL; *Sul;* Zin.

RIGHT : Calc; Cic; Flu-ac;

Sul; Zin.

To left : Calc-p; Cocl; Kali-p; Sul; Tell.

LEFT : Dros; Glo; Sil.

To right : Bell; Cund; Nat-c; Ox- ac.

ABDOMEN, To : Vario.

ALTERNATING, Sides: Agar; Bell; *Berb;* Calc; Calc-p; Kali-bi; Kalm.

Headache, with : Aco; Alo; Alu; Bro; Ign; Meli; Sep.

CHANGING, Here and There : Berb; Cimi; Kali-bi.

CHEST, Into : Arn; Berb; Cam; Kali-n; Laur; Petr; Samb; Sars.

Right : Aco; Calc-p; Kali-c; Lyc; Merc; Sep.

Left : Bar-c; *Bry;* Mez; Plat; Zin.

DOWNWARD : Agar; Pul; Stram.

FORWARD, Scapular region, from : Bry.

Left : Pho; Sul; Zin.

Lumbar region : *Berb;* Cham; *Kali-c;* Kre; SABI.

Pelvis, around : Sabi; Sep; Vib.

GENITALS, To : Kre; Sul.

STOMACH, To : Berb; Cup.

THIGHS, Down : Berb; Caus; Cimi; Hep; Kali-c; Vib.

Stools Agg : Rhus-t.

UPWARD : Ars; Gel; Lach; Lil-t; Nit-ac; Pho; Radm;

Sul; Zin-val.

Occiput, to from : Ol-j.

UTERUS, To : Sep; Vib.

ACHE : *Eup-p; Phyt;* Pic-ac; Sanic; Stap; Vario; Zin.

Chill, with : Caps.

Colic in abdomen, with : Sars.

Feet, to: Kob.

Leucorrhoea Amel : Eupi.

with : Alet.

Menses, before : Asar.

start, at : Jab.

with : Mag-m.

Palpitation, with : Tub.

Prostration, with : *Berb.*

Sexual excess, from : Symp.

Stools, hard, after : Fer.

Takes the breath away : Asar.

Work, cannot : Aesc; Asaf.

Wrestling, from : Symp.

ACNE : Carb-v; Rumx.

AIR, WARM, Streaming up to head, as if : Ars.

BANDAGED, As if : Pul.

BAR On, as though a : Ars; Lach.

BED, Early in, Agg : Nat-m; Stap.

BENDING Backward Agg: Calc-p; Chel; Cimi; PLAT.

Amel : Ign; Petr; Rhus-t.

Forward Agg : Pic-ac.

BLOOD BOILS : Carb-an; Caus; Grap; Thu.

29

BLOW or SUDDEN SHOCK : Bell;
Cic; *Sep*; Stan.

BOILING Water along : Ust.

BREAKING, Broken, as if, Pain :
Arn; *Bell*; *Eup-p*; Ham;
Kali-c; Lyc; Mag-s; Nat-m;
Pho; Senec.
Piles, with : Bell.

BREATHING Deep Agg : Colo.

BUBBLING Sensation : Lyc;
Petros; Tarx.

BURNING, Heat : Agar; Alu; *Ars*;
Bap; Carb-an; Mag-m; *Pho*;
Sec; Sil; *Sul*.
Coition, after : Mag-m; Merc.
Downward : Calc-p.
Upward : Bap; Pho.
Walking in open air Agg :
Sil.

CATCHING, In : Dios.

CHAIR, Leaning on, Agg : *Agar*;
Plb; *Ther*.
Amel : Eupi; Sarr.

CHILL, Coldness : Cact; Caps;
Eup-p; Gel; Lach; Merc;
Nat-m; Nat-s; Nux-v; *Pul*;
Sil; *Sul*; *Ver-a*.
Down : *Agar*; Canth; Eup-p;
Lac-c; Pho; *Pul*; Stram; Val.
Up : Arg-n; Calc-p; *Lach*;
Ol-j; Ox-ac; *Sul*.
and down : Eup-p; Gel; Ip;
Pul; Sul.
Itching,then : Am-m.
Sudden : Croc.
Urinating, after : Sars.

COITION, Emission Agg : Fer;
Kob; Mag-m; Nat-m; *Nit-ac*;
Sabal; Stap; Sul.

COLD Air spreading on :
Agar.
Water trickles down
or spurts : Caps; Lyc;
Pul; Vario.

COLIC, With : Sars.

CONTRACTION : Cimi; Hyd-ac;
Rhus-t.

COUGHING Agg: BELL; BRY;
Kali-bi; Nat-m; Sep.

CRAMPS : Arg-n; Caus; *Chin*;
Led; Mag-m; Mag-p.
Rising from sitting Agg :
Led.
Walking Agg : Mag-m.

CRAWLING : Euon; Lac-c;
Pho; *Sec*.
Cold : Ars; Lac-c.

CYST, On: *Pho*.

DRAFT of Air Agg: Sumb.

DRAWING: Card-m; Cimi;
Nux-v; Stram.

DRINKING Agg : Caps.

EATING Agg : Kali-c.
Amel : Kali-n.

EMACIATED : Nux-v; Plb;
Tab; Thu.

ERUCTATION Amel : Sep; Zin.

EVERYTHING Affects or Agg :
Kali-c; Lach; Sep.

+ FLATUS, Felt in : Rhod.
Passing Amel : Berb;
Pic-ac; Rut.

HEAVINESS: Bar-c; Cimi;
Kali-c.
Stooping, after : Bov.

ITCHING : Ant-c; Caus; Mez;
Nit-ac; Sul.

JARRING Agg: *Grap*; Thu.

KIDNEYS Agg : Cadm; Senec; Solid.

LAUGHING Agg: *Cam;* Con; Pho.

LIFTING Agg : Ant-t; *Grap*; Lyc.

LYING Abdomen on Amel: Acet-ac; Nit-ac; Sele.

Back on Agg : Colo; Pul.

Amel : Kali-c; Nat-m; Pho; Rut.

Hard surface, on Amel : Kali-c; *Nat-m; Rhus-t; Sep.*

Pillow, on Amel: *Carb-v;* Sep.

MENSES Amel : Senec.

During, Agg : Bry; Caus; Sul.

+ Start of : Jab.

MENTAL Exertion Agg : Cham; Con; Nat-c; *Pic-ac.*

MOTION, Walking Agg : Aesc; Agar; *Kali-c;* Mur-ac; Ran-b; Rut.

Amel : Arg-m; Arg-n; *Dul*; Pho-ac; Tab.

MOVE, Must, but no Amel : Lach; Pul.

MUSCLES Atrophy : See Ema ciation,

Paralysed : Cup; Gel; Led.

NIGHT Agg : Abro.

NUMBNESS: Aco; Agar; *Berb;* Bry; Kali-bi; *Ox-ac;* Plat; Sep.

Prickling : Ox-ac.

NURSING, While Agg : Cham;

Crot-t; Pul; Sul.

PAIN, Palpitation, with : Tab.

Spreads like a fan upwards : Lach; Nat-s.

Takes the breath : Asar.

PLUG, Lump, nail, etc sensatcon : Anac; *Arn*; Berb; *Carb-v;* Cinb; Pho.

PRESSURE Agg : Agar; *Bell; Chin-s;* Cry; *Dul*; KALI-C; *Nat-m*; Rhus-t; Rut; *Sep.*

By the end of stick Amel : Sep.

PULLING Agg : Dios.

RAISING Arm Agg : Grap; Nat-m; Rhus-t; Sanic.

RAT Running up, as if : Sul.

RIDING in Carriage Agg : Calc-f; *Nux-m;* Petr.

RISING, Sitting, from Agg : Led.

SHARP, Darting, shooting : Kali-c; Nat-m; Ox-ac.

SHORT, As if : Agar; Aur; Hyo; Lyc; Sul.

SIT Must, while turning in bed : Bry; *Nux-v.*

SITTING Agg : Agar; *Arg-m*; Arg-n; Calc; Kob; Rhus-t; *Sep*; Sul; Val; *Zin.*

Down, when, Agg : Zin.

Erect Agg : Kali-c; Lyc; Sul.

SPASMS : Sec.

SPOTS, In, Agg : Agar; *Alu;* Caus; Chel; Chin; Kali-bi; *Lach*; Nit-ac; Ox-ac; *Pho;* Pho-ac; Plb; Rhus-t; Thu; Zin.

SPRAINED, Easily, as if : Calc;

Grap; Lyc; Rhus-t.

STANDING Amel : Arg-n; Caus; Mur-ac; Sul.

STIFF: Agar; Berb; CAUS; Cimi; Dul; Kali-c;Led; Lyc; *Nux-v;* Pul; Rhus-t; Sanic; SEP; Sil; Stram; Sul.

Ascends : Ars.

Bend, backwards, cannot : Stram.

Menses, before: Mos.

Painful : Caus; Rhus-t; Sanic.

Side, One: Guai.

Stools Agg : Fer.

Amel : Asaf.

Turns whole body to look around : Sanic.

STOOPING Agg : Agar; Sep.

Inability : Bor.

Prolonged Agg : Nat-m.
Straightening, after Agg : Nat-m.

STRUCK, With Hammer, as if : See Blow, Sudden shock.

STUMBLING Agg : Sep.

SWALLOWING Agg : Caus; Kali-c; *Rhus-t.*

THREADS, Extending to limbs (arms, legs), as if : Lach.

THROBBING, Pulsating : Bar-c; Bell; Lyc; Nat-m; Pho; Sep; Sil; Thu.

THROWING shoulders backward Amel : Cyc.

TUMOUR, Peduncle, with : Con.

TURNING, Least, Agg : Sanic.

URINATION, Before Agg : Grap; *Lyc.*

Delayed Agg: Grap; Nat-s.

During Agg : Ant-c; Ip; Kali-bi; Sul.

After Agg : Caus; *Syph.*

Amel : *Lyc*; Med.

WEAK : Arg-n; Ars; Bar-c; Calc; *Cocl*; Grap; Kali-c; Nat-m; Nux-v; Pho; Pho-ac; Pic-ac; Sele; Sep; Sil; Zin.

Coition after : Nat-p.

Leucorrhoea, during: Con; Grap.

+ Ovarian pain, with : Abro.

Too, To hold body : Ox-ac.

whooping cough, in : Ver-a.

WRESTLING Agg : Symp.

WRITING, While or continuous Agg : Lyc; Mur-ac; Sep.

YAWNING Agg : Calc-p; Plat.

BAD FEELS Good and, by turns : Alu; Psor.

INHERITANCE : Buf.

NEWS, Ailments, from : Alum; Ap; *Calc;* Calc-p; Cic; *Gel;* Ign; Lyss; Med; Nat-m; Pall; Pho-ac; Pul;Sul; Tarn.

+ Fear of : Ast-r.

Tremors, nervous, from: Alum.

PART, Takes everything in : Anac; Bov; Caps; Cocl; Nat-m; Nux-v;Pul; Sanic; Stap; Ver-a.

BALDNESS : See Head.

BALL LUMP KNOT etc :

Arn; Asaf; *Bry;* Cham; Chin; Con;Gel; *Ign;* Kali-c; Kali-m; Kob; Lac-c; LACH; Lil-t; Lyc; Mar-v; Merc-d; Merc-i-r; Mos; Nat-m; Nat-s; Nit-ac; Nux-m; *Nux-v;* Plant; Pho; *Pul;* Rhus-t; Senec; SEP; Ust; *Val;* Zin.

COLD, Running through Bowels : Buf.

HARD : Nux-m.

HOT : Carb-ac; Lyc; Phyt; Raph.

Cold, alternating with : Lyc.

BAND : See Constriction.

BANDAGED FEELING : Pic-ac; Plat; Tril.

BANDAGING AMEL : *Arg-n;* Bry; Lac-d; *Mag-m;* Pic-ac; Tril.

BARBERS ITCH : See under Itch.

BARKING (like a dog) : Bell; Canth.

BAROMETER: Merc; *Pho; Rhod.*

BASHFUL : See Anthropophobia.

BATHING AVERSION, To, or from AGG : *Am-c; Ant-c;* Calc; Calc-s; Clem; Phys; Psor; Radm; Rhus-t; Sep; Sil; Spig; SUL.

AMEL: Aco; Ap; *Ars; Asar;* Buf; Bur-p; Calc-s;Caus; Cep; Euphr; *Pul;* Spig.

COLD AGG: *Ant-c;* Bels; Clem; Dul; Mag-p; Nux-m; *Rhus-t;* Sil; *Tub;* Urt.

AMEL : Ap; Asar; Bels; Bry; Buf; Coc-c; Flu-ac; Hypr;

Iod; Led; *Meph;* Nat-m; Phyt; Pul; Rat; Sep; Sul.

EYES Closes, when : Pho.

FACE AMEL : Asar; Calc-s; Pho.

HOT AMEL : Anac; Chel; Lyss; Mag-p; Mez; Pyro; Radm; Rat; Stro.

RIVERS, Summer, in Agg : Caus.

SEA, In, AGG: *Ars;* Bro; *Mag-m; Rhus-t;* Sep.

AMEL : Med.

STEAM AGG : Lyss.

BEADS, LIKE Swelling, etc : Aeth; Am-c; Ap; Iod; *Nat-m;* Pho.

GLANDS : See Glands.

BEARING DOWN : See Pressing Pain.

BECLOUDED : See Comprehension difficult.

BEAUTIFUL, THINGS Look : Sul.

BED, AVERSION, to: See Aversion.

DESIRE To remain in : Arg-n; Hyo.

FALLING, Out of, as if: Arg-n; Ars.

GETTING Out of AGG : Am-m; *Bry;* Calc; CARB-V; Cimi; Cocl; *Con;* Ign; *Lach; Pho; Pul; Rhus-t;* Sul.

AMEL : *Aur;* Dul; Ign; *Pul;* Sep.

HARD, Sensation : ARN; *Bapt;* Con; Dros; Gel; Kali-c; Nux-v; Pho; Plat; *Pyro; Rhus-t; Sil;* Til.

HEAT, Of AGG : Dros; *Merc*; Op; Psor; Pul; Sabi; Sec; *Sul*.

HOT, As if : Op.

LEAVES : Cham; Grap; Lac-c; Led; Merc; Ver-a.

LUMPS In : Arn; Mag-c.

LYING, In AGG: Alu; AMB; Calc; Carb-an; *Chel*; Chin; *Dros*; Fer; Hell; *Hep*; Hyo; *Iod*; Kali-c; LACH; *Lyc*; Merc; *Nit-ac*; PHO; PUL; Rum; Sang; SEP; SIL; SUL.

　AMEL : Am-m; *Bry*; Caus; Cic; Cocl; Kali-c; Hep; Mag-m; NUX-V; Pyro; Scil; Stan.

　+ All troubles : Mang.

MOVING, As If : Lac-c.

OCCUPIED By whole body, as if : Pyro.

+ REMAINS, In, trifle indisposition from : Arg-n.

RISING From *A*MEL : Pho-ac; Pul.

SINKING Under him as if : Bap; Bell; *Bry*; Calc-p; Chin-s; Kali-c; Lach; Lyc; Rhus-t.

SITTING Up in, AMEL : *Kali*-c; Samb.

SLIDING Down, in: Ap; Ars; *Bap*; Chin; Colch; Hell; *Hyo*; Mur-ac; Tab; Zin.

SMALL, Too, to hold him: Sul.

SORES, (See Ulcers) : Arn; Chin; *Flu-ac*; Grap; Lach; Petr; Sep; Sil; Sul-ac.

　Children, in : Cham; Sul.

　Early : Val.

TURNING Over in AGG: Bell; Cact; Calad; Carb-v; *Con*; Lac-c; NUX-V; *Pul*; Sang; Stap; *Sul*; Zin.

　AMEL : Nat-m.

　Rises for : Bry; NUX-V.

WETTING : Ap; Arg-n; Arn; Ars; BELL; *Calc; Caus*; Cina; Equi; Fer; Grap; Lac-c; Kre; Mag-p; *Merc*; Nat-m; Nit- ac; PUL; *Rhus-t*; Sabal; Sec; Sep; *Sil*; SUL; Syph; Tab; Tub;Verb; Vio-t.

　Adults, of : Kali-c.

　Catheterisation, from : Mag- p.

　Cause, without any, except habit : Equi.

　Children, weakly, in : Chin; Kali-p; Thyr.

+ Exertion, any, from : Sabal.

　Head, blow on, from : Sil.

　Menses, during : Hyo.

　Moon, Full, Agg : Cina; Psor.

　Morning : Carb-v.

　Old men : Apoc; Benz-ac; Kali-p; Sec.

　Pregnancy, in : Pod.

　Sleep, During first : *Caus*; Kre; Pho-ac; *Sep*.

　　later, part : Chlo-hyd.

+ Specific (for) : Lac-c.

　Waking difficult : Bell; Chlo- hyd; *Kre*

+ Worms, from : Sil.

BEES STINGING, As if : Ap; Gel.
AGG : Led; Urt.

BEHIND, As If someone, or desire to look : Anac; Bro; Crot-h; Led; Med; Sanic; Tub.

ABYSS : Kali-c.

WHISPERING : Med.

BENDING BACKWARDS, Stretching limbs **AGG** : Aco; *Calc*; CHAM; Chel; Cinb; COLCH; Iod; Kalm; Merc-c; PLAT; *Pul*; Radm; *Ran-b*; RHE; RHUS-T; *Sep*; STAP; *Sul*; *Thu.*

AMEL : *Alu;* ANT-T; Arn; Bell; *Calc;* Cham; Chel; Cocl; *Dios*; Flu-ac; *Guai*; Hep; Hypr; *Ign;* Lach; Lyss; *Nux-v;* Plb; *Pul;* Rhus-t; Sabi; Sec; Seneg.

FORWARDS, or Doubling up **AMEL** : Aco; *Calc;* Caps; Caus; Cham; Chin; Cimi; *Colo;* Grap; *Kali-c;* Lil-t; Lyc; Mag-m; *Mag-p;* Merc-c; Par-b; Plat; Pul; *Rhe;* *Rhus-t;* Sec; *Sep;* Sul; Thu; Tril.

FORWARD And **BACKWARDS** **AGG** : *Chel;* Cof.
AMEL : Tril.

PROLONGED, AMEL : Pul; Rhus-t; Scil.

SIDEWAYS AGG: Bell; Calc; Kali-c; Nat-m.

BEREAVEMENT : *Amb*; Plat.

BERI BERI : Ars; ELAT; Rhus-t.

BESIDES HIMSELF, Frantic

Madness, from pain etc :
ACO; Aur; Calc; CHAM; *Cof*; Hep; Hyo; Lyc; Nat-m; *Nux-v;* Stram; Ver-a.

WALKING, Someone : Calc.

BEWILDERED, Things look strange, loss of sense of location : Apoc; ARG-N; Bap; Bell; *Bry; Calc; Cann;* Carb-v; *Cocl;* Crot-h; Flu-ac; *Glo;* Grap; Hell; Hyo; *Lach;* Med; Merc; Nat-m; *Nux-m;* Onos; *Op;* PETR; PLAT; Rhus-t; *Sep; Sil;* Stram; Stry; Tub; Val.

+ **CHILDREN** : Aesc.

WASHING, Face, Amel : Ars; Pho.

BILATERAL : See Symmetrical.

BILE DUCTS : Am-m; Chel; Gel; Merc-d; Nat-p; Rhe.

BILHARZIASIS: Ant-t.

BILIOUS (See yellow) : Chio; Eup-p; Nat-s; Sang; Tarx.

BIRTHMARK, Naevi: Arn; Ars; Calc; Calc-f; Carb-an; Carb-v; Flu-ac; Lach; *Lyc;* Pho; Plat; Radm; *Sep; Sul;* Thu; Ust.

+ **FLAT** : Mur-ac.

SMOOTH, Mottled : Con; Pho; Sep; Thu.

SPIDERY: Carb-v; Lach; *Plat;* Sep; Thu.

Red : Med.

BITE, IMPULSE, to : Bell; Buf; Cup; Hyo; Lyss; Phyt; Pod; Sec; Stram.

BITES, CHEEKS, or Tongue

while chewing or talking : Buf; Caus; *Cic*; Hyo; *Ign*; *Nit-ac;* Ol-an.

When not : Dios.

FINGERS, Hands, etc : Aco; Aru-t; Med; Op; Plb.

Sleep, in : Elap.

NIGHT, Sleep in : Cic; Pho.

OBJECTS, Any: Buf.

PILLOW : Lyc; Pho.

SPASMS, In : Art-v; Buf; Caus; Cup; Oenan; Op.

SPOONS, Pots etc : Ars; Bell; Hell.

TONGUE, Tip of, sleep, during : Ther.

BITING CHEWING **A**GG : Alo; *Am-c*; Am-m; Bry; Chin; Euphr; Hep; Ign; Meny; *Merc; Mez;* Nat-m; Nit-ac; Pho; Pod; Pul; RHUS-T; *Sep; Stap; Verb*; Zin.

AMEL : Bry; Cocl; Cup-ac; Seneg; *Stap.*

BUG, Like: Kali-bi; Syph; Tell.

FLEAS, As of : Mez; Stap; Syph; Tab; Visc.

BLACK DARK (Discharges, Discolouration of skin, etc) : Ant-t; Arn; *Ars*; Bap; Carb-ac; Carb-v; *Chin*; Crot-h; Cyc; Elap; Fer; Gel; Hell; Kre; *Lach*; Mag-m; *Merc;* Merc-c; Nux-v; Op; Pho; Plb; *Sec;* Stap; Stram; Sul-ac; Ver-a.

BLUE : See Ecchymosis.

SPOTS : Ars; Crot-h; Lach; Vip.

Removes : Sul-ac.

BLACKWATER FEVER : *Ars;* Crot-h; Lyc.

BLADDER (Urinary) Affections in general : Aco; Ap; Bell; Benz-ac; *Canth; Caus*; Colo; *Dul*; Equi; *Hyo;* Lach; *Lyc; Merc-c; Nux-v;* **Pul;** *Ruta Sabal*; Sars; Sep; Stap; *Sul;* Uva-u.

ACHING : Caps; Terb.

Heavy : Sabal.

ATONY : Ars; CAUS; Mur-ac; Op; Plb; Stan.

+ Laparotomy after : Op.

Old age : Ars; Stram.

Retention, long, from : Canth.

BACK, to : Sars.

BLEEDING : Terb.

BURNING : Berb; CANTH; *Caps*; Cep; *Merc-c*; Pul; Rhe; Senec; Terb; Zin-ar.

Neck : Canth; Zin-ar.

BURSTING : Par-b; Sanic; Zin.

CALCULI : Benz-ac; Berb; Calc; Canth; Lyc; Sars; Sep.

CANCER : Crot-h.

CHILL, Spreads from : Sars.

COITION, After : Cep.

COLDS Agg : Caus; Dul; Pul; Sul.

COLD, Sensation, in : Lyss; Sabal.

Genitals, extending, to : Sabal.

COUGHING Agg : Caps; Ip.

CRAMP : Berb; Caps; Carb-v;
Mez; Nux-v; Pru-sp; Pul;
Sars.
Operations, after : Colo;
Hypr.

CRAWLING, In : Sep.
Urination, after: Lyc.

CUTTING : Aeth; Pall; Terb;
Thu.
Stools, Amel : Pall.

DESIRE for urination
postponed, if, Agg : Pul;
Sul-ac.

EMPTY, Sensation, in :
Stram.
Distended, when : Lycps.
Involuntary urination
after : Helo.
Pain, with : Calc-p.

FALLS To side lain on,
sensation : Pul; Sep.

FULLNESS, Sensation : Dig;
Equi; Pall; Rut.
Desire to urinate, without
: Ars; Caus.
Motion, up and down,
with : Rut.
Sensation, without : Lac-d.
Urination, after : Dig;
Eup-pur.
scanty, with : Pall.

GRIPING : Canth.

HEAVINESS : Canth; Lyc;
Nat-m; Pul; Sep.

INFLAMMED: Aco; Ap; Bell;
Canth; Cub; Equi; Lach;
Lyc; Polyg; Sars; Solid;
Terb.

+ Prostate hypertrophy :
Sabal.

INJURY, Operations, after :
Arn; Calend; *Stap.*

INSENSIBLE : Stan.

IRRITABLE : Bell; Buchu;
Nux-v; Sabal; Stap.

ITCHING in; with urging to
urinate, at night : Sep.

LUMP In : Kre; Lach.

LYING, Abdomen, on Amel : Chel.

NAVEL, Alternating, with :
Terb.

NECK, of : Bell Canth;
Merc-c.

PARALYSIS : *Ars;* Caus; Dul;
Gel; Hyo; Nux-v; Op; Plb;
Stram; Zin.
Hysterical : *Zin.*
Laparotomy, after : Op.
Old people : Ars.
Parturition after: Ars; Caus.

PELVIS and Thighs, to,
urination, after : Pul.

RECTUM, With : Amb.

RETENTION of Urine : See
Under Urine.

SITTING Agg : Card-m.
Amel : Con.

SORE : Ap; *Canth; Equi; Terb.*
Urination, profuse, with :
Stic.

SPERMATIC Cord, to : Lith.

STABBING, In region of : Chel.

STONE Rolling Sensation : Pul.

TENESMUS: Agar; Ars; Bell;
Cann; CANTH; *Dig;* Dul;
Equi; Lil-t; MERC-C; *Par-b;*

Plb; Pru-s; Sul; *Terb*; Thu.

Menses during : *Tarn*.

Rectum, with : Erig; Canth; Caps; Merc-c.

Stool, during : Caps; Nux-v. Vomiting, purging, micturition, with : *Crot-h*.

THICK : Dul.

THROBBING, Pulsating : Dig.

ULCERATION, Suppuration : Petr; *Pul;* Sep; *Sul*.

URGING To Urinate, when not attended, to Agg : Pul; Sul-ac.

WALKING Agg : Con; Pru-s; Pul. Amel : Ign; Terb.

Open air, in Amel : *Terb*.

WEAKNESS : Caus; Hep; Mag-m; Mur-ac; Op.

Parturition, after : Ars; Caus.

WORM Sensation, In : Bell; Sep.

BLAMES HIMSELF : Op.

BLAND : See Discharges.

BLEEDING AGG : *Chin;* Fer; Ip; Nat-m; Pho-ac; Stic; Sul-ac.

AMEL : Ars; Bov; Buf; Calad; Card-m; Fer; Fer-p; Ham; Lach; Meli; Sars; Sele.

NOSE, From AMEL : Bro.

PROLONGED AGG : Plat.

+ SEQUELAE, Chronic : Stro.

SLIGHT, Causes great AGG : Buf; Carb-an; *Chin*; Ham; Hyds; Sec.

SUPPRESSION, Of AGG : Bur-p.

BLINDNESS: See under Vision.

DAY : See under Day.

NIGHT : See Night Blindness.

BLISTERS : See Eruptions, Vesicles.

BLOATED : See Puffiness.

BLONDES : Bro; Calc; Pul.

BLOOD BOILS : Anthx; Arn; Crot-h; Lach; Pho; Pyro; Thu.

BLISTERS : Sec.

CAN NOT Look at : *Alu*; Nux-m; Plat.

CIRCULATION Stands still : Aco; Lyc; *Saba*; Sep; Zin.

CLOT, Would not and wound would not heal : Visc.

COLD, As if : Ver-a.

GUSHING, As if : Ox-ac.

HOT, As if : Med; Sec.

RESTLESSNESS In : Iod.

RUSHES, *Of* : Bell; Fer; Glo; Lach; Sang; Spo; Sul.

Downward : Aur; Meph; Thyr.

Upward : Aco; Arn; Bell; Bry; Fer; Glo; Kali-io; Meli; Pho; Sang; Stro.

STAGNATED, As if : Carb-v; Lyc.

STASIS : Carb-v; Ham; Pul; Sep; Sul.

STREAKED : See Discharges, Blood streaked.

+ TURMOIL, Constant, in : Am-m.

WATERY and Mixed with clots : See Haemorrhages.

BLOOD PRESSURE HIGH

: Aur; Bar-c; Bar-m; Cof; Con; Cratae; Glo; Iod; Lycps; Scop; Stro; Sumb; Tab; Uran-n; Ver-v; Visc.

Diastolic Low, and : Bar-m.

LOW : Cact; Gel; Naj; Radm; Ther.

SUDDEN Rise of : Cof.

BLOOD SEPSIS (Septic conditions, fevers etc) : Ail; Am-c; Anthx; *Arn*; ARS; *Bap*; *Bell*; Bry; Calc; *Carb-v*; *Chin*; Colch; Crot-c; *Crot-h*; Echi; Elap; *Fer*; Gel; Hyo; Kali-c; Kali-p; Kre; LACH; Lyc; *Merc*; Merc-cy; *Mur-ac*; Naj; *Nat-m*; Nit-ac; Nux-v; *Pho*; *Pul*; Pyro; *Rhus-t*; Sec; Stram; *Sul*; Sul-ac; Tarn-c; Vario; Ver-a; Ver-v; Zin.

ADYNAMIC : Elap; Pyro.

BLOOD VESSELS Affections in general : Aco; Amy-n; Ap; *Arn*; *Bell*; CARB-V; Fer; *Flu-ac*; Gel; Glo; *Ham*; *Hyo*; *Lach*; Lyc; Nat-m; *Pho*; PUL; Sang; *Sec*; Sep; Sul; Sul-ac; *Thu*; Vip; Zin.

BUBBLE Rolling through : See Shot rolling through.

CALCAREOUS, DEPOSIT, IN : Vario.

COLD Feeling, in : ACO; ARS; Pyro; RHUS-T; Sul-ac; *Ver-a*.

DISTENDED, Full Varicose (See Veins) : Arn; *Ars*; Bell; Calc; Calc-f; Carb-v; Card-m; *Flu-ac*; *Ham*; Lach; Lyc; Lycps; Plat; *Pul*;

Sang; Sec; *Sep*; Stap; Sul; Vip; Zin.

Fever, during : Chin; Hyo; Led; Pul.

Insanity, with : Arn; Ars; Flu-ac; Lach; Lyc; Sul; *Zin*.

followed, by : Anac; Ant-c; Arn; Ars; Bell; Caus; Hyo; Ign; Lach; Lyc; Nux-v; Pho; Sep; Sul; Ver-a.

Knots, and enlargements, in : Sabi.

Menses, Agg : Amb; Fer.

Pregnancy, during : Fer; Mill; Pul; Tril; Zin.

Tenderness, with : Ham; Merc-cy.

Ulceration : Card-m; Caus; Clem; Ham; Lach; Lyc; Pul; Sec; Vip.

HEAT, Burning, in : Ars; Bry; Calc; Med; *Rhus-t*; Syph.

INFLAMED, Phlebitis : Aco; Ap; *Ars*; Chin; Kali-c; Ham; *Lach*; PUL; SPIG: SUL; Vip.

Forceps delivery, after : Cep.

PAINFUL : *Ham*; *Pul*; Thu; Zin.

SHOT Rolling through the arteries, sensation : Nat-p.

SWELLED : Ap; Paeon; *Pul*.

VASCULAR : Lach; Lyc; Thu; Tril; Zin.

VIBRATE, As if : Phel.

WRITHING In : Bell; Hyd-ac.

BLOODY : See Discharges, Bloody.

BLOWING NOSE AGG : Arn; Aur : Calc; CHEL; Grap; HEP;

Iod; Kali-bi; Lach; *Merc;* Pho; Pho-ac; *Pul;* Spig; SUL; Zin.

AMEL : *Mang;* Merc; Sil.

INABILITY, Children, in : Am-c.

BLOWS, SHOCKS, Thrusts crash explosions, as from : Alo; Ap; Arg-m; Bell; CANN; Chin; Cic; Croc; Cup; Dig; *Glo;* Hell; *Naj;* Nat-m; Pho; Spig; Sul; Sul-ac; Tab; Tarn; Zin.

BLUISH, PURPLE (discharges, discolouration of skin), etc. : Aco; *Arn; Ars;* Bap; Cam; Carb-an; *Carb-v; Crot-h;* CUP; DIG; Elap; *Fer-p;* Kre; LACH; Laur; Mang; Merc-cy; *Mur-ac; Nux-v; Op;* Ox-ac; Rhus-t; Sec; Sil; Sul; *Tarn-c ;* Thu; *Ver-a;* VER-V.

AFFECTED Parts : Carb-an; Lach; Sec.

BURNING, With : Anthx; Ars; Lach.

INJURY, From : *Arn;* Bell; Con; Lach; Pul; Sul-ac.

SPOTS: Arn; Ars; Crot-h; Hell; Lach; Led; Nux-m; Nux-v; Op; Pho; Pho-ac; Sec; Sul-ac.

Red : Plb; Phyt.

+ Removes : Sul-ac.

BOARD LIKE Sensation or feel : Bap; Carb-an; Dul; Nux-m; Rhus-t; Tarn-c.

LYING, On, as if : Bap; Sanic.

BOILING, As if : Am-m; Led; Ust.

+ **T**EA Seems cold : Cam.

WATER, Side, lain on : Mag-m.

BOILS : Arn; *Bell;* Bels; *Hep; Lach; Lyc;* Merc; Petr; Psor;

Rhus-t; Sil; Sul.

BLIND : Fago; Lyc.

BLOOD : See; Blood.

BODY, All over: Bels; Vio-t.

CROPS, Of : Echi; Sil; Sul; Syph.

IMPOTENCY, With : Pic-ac.

INJURED, Places, on: Dul.

MATURE, Do not : Sanic.

MENSES, At : Merc.

PERIODICAL : Ars.

RECEDING : Lyc.

RECURRING : Calc.

Spring, every : Bell.

SCARS, Leave : Kali-io.

SMALL and SORE : *Arn;* Lapp; Pic-ac; Sec; Tub.

Green : Sec.

Menses, during : Med.

SUCCESSION Of : Anthx; Arn; Sul.

BOLDNESS DARING Courageous : *Ign; Op; Tub.*

BONES Affections, in general : Arg-m; ASAF; *Aur;* CALC; *Calc-f;* CALC-P; Chin; Cocl; Cup; Eup-p; Flu-ac; Hep; Kali-io; Lyc; MERC; Mez; *Nit-ac; Pho;* PHO-AC; Phyt; PUL; Pyro; Rhod; Rhus-t; *Rut; Sil;* Stap; *Sul;* Syph.

BAND Sensation : Con.

BARE, Become : Ars; Asaf; Aur; Calc; Chin; Con; Hep; Lach; Lyc; Merc; Mez; Nit-ac; Pho-ac; Pul; Rut; Sabi; Sep; Sil; Stap, Sul.

Necrosis, with : Bothr.

BREAKING, Bruised Pains : *Ars*; Cocl; *Eup-p*; Hep; Nit-ac; Pul; Rut; Thu; Val.

BRITTLE, Fractured, etc. : Asaf; Buf; *Calc*; Calc-f; Calc-p; *Lyc*; *Merc*; Par; Pho-ac; Rut; *Sil*; *Sul*; Symp; Thu.

BURNING : Euphor; Mez; Zin.

CARIES : Ang; Ars; *Asaf*; *Aur*; Calc; Calc-f; Con;*Flu-ac*; HEP; Kali-io; Lach; *Lyc*; Mang; MERC; Mez; Nit-ac; Pho; Pho-ac; Pul; Radm; SIL; Stap; Syph; Tell; *Ther*; Tub.

Sweat, profuse, with : Chin.

COLD, Chilly feeling : *Aran*; Berb; Calc; *Eup-p*; Kali-io; Pyro; Ver-a.

CONDYLES, Prominences : Arg-m; Cyc; Rhus-t; Sang; Ver-v.

CURVATURE, Soft, etc. : ASAF; CALC; Calc-io; CALC-P; Hep; *Lyc*; *Merc*; PHO; Pho-ac; Pul; Sep; *Sil*; *Sul.*

CUTTING : Anac; Aur; Dig; Kali-m; Lach; Osm; Saba.

DEEP, In, Long : Rut.

EXOSTOSES : Arg-m; *Aur*; Aur-m; Calc; CALC-P; Hecla; Merc; Mez; PHO; Pho-ac; *Sil*; Stap; Sul; Syph.

Injury, after : Calc-f.

Painful : Aur; Daph; Kali-io; Merc; Syph.

Suppression, itch, of, after : Sul.

Syphilitic : Flu-ac; Hep;

Merc.

FRACTURE : See Brittle.

Often : *Merc.*

Union delayed : Thyr.

GNAWING : *Bell*; Stro.

GROWTH, Defective : Agar; Calc; *Calc-p*; Fer; Pho-ac; Sil.

HEAVY : Sul.

INFLAMMATION : Sil.

INJURY To : See Under Injuries.

ITCHING : Caus; Cocl; Cyc; Kali-m; Pho; Ver-a.

JERK In : Asaf; Chin; Sil; Sul.

LARGE, As if : Mez.

MARROW : Am-c; Chel; Chin; Kali-c; *Lyc*; Mag-m; Naj; Ol-an; Op; Stro; Sul.

Pain in : Chin.

NIGHT Agg: Aur; Kali-io; *Lyc*; MERC; Nit-ac; Pho-ac; Sil; *Syph.*

NON UNION : *Calc*; *Calc*-p; Pho-ac; Sil; Symp.

OSSIFICATION Slow: Calc-p.

PAINFUL, In general: Asaf; *Eup-p*; Kob; *Merc*; Nit-ac; Pho-ac; *Phyt*; Pul; *Pyro*; Rut; Zin.

PERIOSTEUM : Asaf; Flu-ac; Kali-io; Kali-n; Mang; Merc; Mez; Pho; *Pho-ac*; Phyt; Rhod; Rut; Sul.

Inflammation : Ars; Asaf; Aur; Calc; Calc-f; Con; Hep; Lach; Merc; Mez; Nit-ac; Pho-ac; Pul; Sep; Sil; Stap; Sul; Tell.

Painful : *Merc*; Rhus-t.

PINCHING : Pho-ac; *Verb.*

PRICKING : Thu.

RENT Asunder, tearing, Shattered : Aur; Chin; Kali-c; Lach; Merc; Rhod; Spig.

SAWING : Pho; Sul; Syph; Tarn.

SCRAPING : *Chin; Pho-ac; Rhus-t;* Saba; Thu.

Night, at : Pho-ac.

SENSITIVE : Mang; Nit-ac.

SKIN, Near, pain : Cyc; Merc; Sang.

SPONGY : Guai.

+ SQUEEZED, As if : Alu.

STICKING, In: Arn; *Symp.*

SWASHING, like a wave: Bell.

TENSION *:* Bell.

TORN LOOSE, Flesh, from, as if : Ap; Bry; Dros; Lach; Nat-c; Ol-an; Pho-ac; *Rhus-t;* Rut.

Blow, from : Ign.

TUBERCULOSIS, Of : Dros; Pho; Pul; Stan.

+ ULCERATION, Deep : Asaf.

WALK, Must : Rut.

WEATHER Changes Agg : Am-c.

+ **BOOKWORMS** : Cocl.

BOOTS DRAWING, Of *Agg* : Calc; Grap.

BORBORYGMYS : See Flatus Noisy.

BORING, GRINDING **:** See Pain.

BORING Into Parts (nose, ears) AMEL : Aru-t; Chel; *Nat-c;*

Pho; Spig; Thu.

BORROWS TROUBLE : Acet-ac; Ap; Bar-c; Calc; Sang.

BOUNDING INTERNAL (See AliveSensation) : Croc; Ther; Thu.

BOWELS : See Abdomen, and Intestines.

BRAIN : Aco; Arg-n; Bell; Bov; Calc; Dul;Hyo; Lach; *Nux-v*; Pho; Pic-ac; Stram; Sul; Syph; Tub; Zin.

AIR, COLD, Blowing on,as if : Cimi.

BANDAGED, As if : Bry; Lac-c; Nat-m; Nit-ac; Sul.

BRUISED : Bap; *Chin;* Gel; Mur-ac; Phyt.

BURNING Heat : Aco; Bell; Canth; Glo; Med; *Pho*; Ver-a.

Boiling water, as if : Aco.

Fiery : Hyd-ac.

CLOTH, Cold, Around, as if: Glo; *Sanic.*

CLOUD *WAS* Going over : Hyd-ac.

COLDNESS : Mos; Pho.

CONCUSSION : *Arn; Cic;* Hell; Hyo; *Hypr*; Nat-s; Op; Sul-ac; Zin.

Headache, from : Kali-br.

Knocking foot against anything, when : Bar-c.

Mis-step, from : Led.

CONTRACTED, Hard, painful, as if : Laur.

+ Relaxed, and,as if : Lac-c.

CRAZY Feeling : Vario.

DEGENERATION, Softening of: *Arg-n;* Aur; Bar-c; Caus; *Pho;* Plb; *Sil; Stry;* Syph; Zin; *Zin-p.*

FAG, Weak, tired : Anac; Ap; Bar-c; Bell; Calc; *Caus;* Gel; Kali-p; *Lach;* Lyc; *Nat-c; Nux-v;* PHO-AC; *Pic-ac;* Plb; *PSOR;* Pul; Sil; Stap; Sul; *Zin;* Zin-p.

Grief, from : Kali-br.

+ Occiput, cold, with : Pho.

FALLS, Down : Laur.

Forehead from as if : Rat.

Side lain on : Amb; Phys.

+ FIRE On as if : Hyd-ac.

+ FOREHEAD And Empty space between, as if : Caus.

FORMICATION : Hyp.

FROZEN, As if : Ind.

FULL of Fluid, as if : Cur.

HAEMORRHAGE In: Aco; Bell; Calc; Gel; Ip; Lach; Op.

HEAVY : Form; Hypr; Mag-c.

HOT Vapour coming from below, as if : Ant-t; Sars; Sul.

Swallowing, when : Form.

HUMMING, Roaring in : Kre; Lach; Pho.

KNOCKING Against, skull, as if : Chin.

LARGE, As if: Cimi; Form; *Glo.*

LIQUID, As if : Mag-p.

LOOSE, As if: Aco; Amb; Am-c; Bar-c; *Bell; Chin;* Glo; Guai; Hyo; Hypr;

Kali-c; Kali-m; Laur; Nux-m; NUX-V; Rhus-t; *Spig;* Sul; Sul-ac; Tub.

Sitting quiet Amel : Sul-ac.

Stooping, on : Nat-s.

Walking, on : Cyc.

LUMP, As if, on right side : Con.

MARBLE, Feels as if changed to : Cann.

+ METAL Striking on, as if : Phel.

NEEDLES, At : Tarn.

NUMB : Ap; Buf; Calc; Con; Grap; Hell; Kali-br; Plat.

PARALYSIS Of, Incipient : Am-m; LYC; Zin.

Sensation of, emission after : Sil.

PARTS, Were changing, as if : Mag-p.

PRESSED Out of forehead, as if : Bell; Lach.

RAISED, Several times in succession, as if : Thu.

Stooping, on : Kob.

ROLLING Over : Plant.

SHATTERED, As if : Rhus-t.

SOFTENING, Of : See Degenera - tion.

SPOON, Stirred with, as if : Arg-n; Iod.

STITCHES, At : Alu.

SWASHING, To and fro, as if : Chin; Hell.

Water, as of : Hyo.

TORN, As if : Cof; Stap.

TUMOUR : Arn; *Barc-c;* Bell;

Calc; *Con;* Glo; Grap; *Kali-io; Plb;* Sep.

+ TURNED Over, as if : Plant.

WAVING In, as if : Cimi; Glo; Phys.

WRAPPED, As if : Cyc; Op.

BRANNY : See Dequammation.

BREAKFAST AGG : Carb-v; CHAM; Nat-m; *Nat-s;* NUX-V; PHO; Sep; Thu; Zin.

AMEL : Calc; Croc; Iod; Myr; Nat-s; Stap.

BREAKING, BROKEN : See Pain.

Things : Ap; Stram; Tub.

BREATH *Cold* : *Cam; Carb-v;* Chin; Cist; Pho; VER-A.

DESIRE, To take deep : See Respiration , Deep.

HOLDING *Agg*: Cact; *Kali-n;* Led; Merc; *Spig.*

HOLDING AMEL : *Bell.*

HOT : *Bell;* Cham; Cof; Med; Nat-m; Rhus-t;Saba; Stro; Zin.

As if : Radm.

Burns, nostrils : Ptel; Rhus-t.

LOSS of, Standing in water, when : Nux-m

OFFENSIVE : Ail; Anac; ARN; *Ars; Aru-t;* Aur; Bap; CARB-V; *Cham;* Crot-h; Hell; Kali-chl; Kali-p; Kre; *Lach;*Meph; MERC; Merc-cy; *Nit-ac;* NUX-V; Plb; Pod; Pul; Pyro; Rhe; Spig; Sul; Tub; Ver-v.

Cheese, like rotten : Mez.

Constipation, with : Carb-ac.

Ether, or Chloroform, like : Ver-v.

Garlicky : Petr; Tell.

Girls, Puberty at : Aur; Onion like : Asaf; Sinap.

Palpitation, With : Spig.

Sour : Grap.

Un-noticed, by himself : Bar-c.

Urine, like : Grap.

STOPS, Coughing or drinking on: Am-m; Anac.

Children, in, when they are lifted : Calc-p.

Swallowing when : Anac.

BREATHE, AGAIN, Cannot : Ap; Bell; Coca; Dros; Helo; Latro; Laur; Rum.

BREATHING DEEPLY AGG: *Aco;* Arn; Ascl; *Bor;* BRY; Calc; Caus; Grap; *Kali-c;* Lyc; Merc; *Pho;* Ran-b; Rhus-t; Rum; Sabi; Sang; Scil; Spig; Sul.

AMEL : Aco; Cann; *Colch;* Cup; *Ign;* Lach; Nat-m; Osm; Ox-ac; Seneg; Spig; *Stan;* Verb.

HOT Air, as if : *Trif.*

Takes the breath away : Arg-n.

IRREGULAR Agg : Cact; Rum.

SPONGE, Dry, through as if : Spo.

TUBE, Metallic, through, as if : Merc-c.

BREGMA : Ars; *Merc;* Zin-ch.

BRINY : See Salty, Fishy.

BRITTLE, BROKEN, Feeling : Chel; Cup; Flu-ac; Par;

Radm; Thu.

BRONCHIECTASIS
Bronchorrhoea : All-s; *Ars;*
Bacil; *Calc;* Cep; Cop; Eucal;
Grind; *Hep;* Kali-bi; Kali-c;
Lyc; Phel; *Pul;* Sil; STAN; Tub.

+ SENILE : Eucal.

BRONCHITIS : *Ant-t; Ars; Bry;*
Calc; Dros; *Fer-p;* Hep; Hyds;
Ip; Lyc; Nat-s; *Pho;* Pul;
Sang; Senec; Sil; Spo; Stan;
Stic; Sul.

CAPILLARY : *Ant-t;* Bell;
Carb-v; *Fer-p ; Ip;* Seneg;
Terb.

CHILDREN, Drowsiness, with
: Tub.

COLD, From every : Mang.

SENILE : Am-c; Ant-c; Ant-t;
Ars; Cep; Kre; Seneg.

BROWNISH, RUSTY (Dis-
charges, discolouration
of skin) etc. : *Ars;* Bap; Berb;
Bry; Carb-v; Chel; Hyo; Iod;
Kre; Lyc; Lycps; Manc; *Nit-ac;*
Op; Petr; Pho; *Rhus-t;* Sec;
SEP; Stap; *SUL;* Thu; Ver-a.

SPOTS : Crot-h; Iod; Lach;
Lyc; Merc; Petr; Pho; Sanic;
Sep; Sul; Thu.

BROWS : Bell; Caus; Kali-c;
Nat-m; Par; Sele.

ACHING : Stro.

DANDRUFF : Sanic.

HAIR FALLING : *Kali-c;* Med;
Plb; Sele.

KNITS : Vio-o.

OUTWARD, Along : Cinb; Echi;
Kali-bi; Mez; Vio-o.

QUIVERING Between : Ang.

SWELLING, Hard, over: Sang.

TWITCH : Cina; Echi.

WARTS, On : Caus.

BRUISED : See Pain, Sore.

BRUNETTES : Nit-ac; Plat.

+ FIRM-Fibered : Nux-v.

BUBBLES, Sensation of : *Berb;*
Nux-v; *Pul;* Rhe.

AIR, Suppuration, with: Sul.

BURSTING : Sul.

BUBO : Bad; Bell;; Carb-an;
Cinb; Hep; Kali-io; Merc-i-r;
Nit-ac; Phyt.

+ NEGLECTED : Carb-an.

SUPPURATION, Stubborn :
Merc-i-r.

BULLAE : Manc; Ran-sc; Syph.

BUNIONS : Agar; Benz-ac;
Grap; Paeon; Rhod; Sil.

+ PRESSURE, Amel : Grap.

BURNING (See Heat): ACO;
AP; ARS; *Aru-t;* BELL; BRY;
Buf; *Canth;* Caps; *Carb-v;*
Caus; Euphr; Grap; Iod; *Iris;*
Lyc; Mag-m; *Med;* Mez;
Nat-m; Nit-ac; Nux-v; PHO;
Pho-ac; Pic-ac; Pru-sp; PUL;
Rat; RHUS-T; Saba; *Sang;*
Sec; Sep; Sil; Spig; Spo;
Stan; SUL; *Terb;* Zin.

BATHING, Washing Agg :
Rhus-t; Sul.

COLD PARTS, In : Sec; Ver-v.

DRY, All Symptoms Agg : Bry.

FIERY : *Ap; Ars; Bell;*
Carb-an; Guai; Kali-c; Kre;
Mez; Pho; Radm; Spig;

Tarn-c; *Tub;* Vesp.

HEAT Agg : Rat; Zin-val.
Amel : Alu; *Ars;* Caps;
Carb- v; Lyc; Sec.

HOT Iron: See under Hot.

INTERNAL : Euphor; Merc-c;
Mez.
Coldness, external with :
Ars; Kali-n; Ver-a.
Itching, with : Mez.

INTOLERABLE : Sabi.

PAINFUL : Aco; ARS; Canth;
Carb-v; *Caus; Merc;* Pho;
Sul.

PARTS, Grasped with hand :
Caus.
Lain, on : Sul.

PEPPER, Like : Coc-c; Lach;
Mez; Nat-s; Xanth.

PRICKING : Ver-v.

PUNGENT, Glowing : Cep; Rut;
Tarn-c.

RAW, Smarting, biting : Am-c;
Aru-t; Berb; *Canth;* Caps;
Carb-v; Erig; Hyds; Lyc;
Manc; Ran-sc; Sinap; Sul;
Sul-io.

SHIVERING, With : Aco; Ars;
Bry; Chin; Ip; Samb; Ver-v.

SPOT, Local : Agar; Glo;
Ran-b; Sang; Sele; Sul;
Ver-v.

STEAM, Over, like : Pulex.

STINGING : Ant-c; AP; *Ars; Berb;*
Con; Dul; Glo; Iris; Lyc; Mez;
Nux-v; *Pho;* Pho-ac; Rhus-t;
Sil; Urt.

BURNS And SCALDS : Ars;
Canth; Carb-v; *Caus;* Ham;
Kali-m; Kre; Pic-ac; Stram; Urt.

GRANULATION, Unhealthy :
Petr; Plant.

ILL EFFECTS of : Carb-ac;
Caus.

RADIUM : Pho.

SUN : Bov; Cam; Canth;
Kali- c; Ver-a.

SUPPURATION, With : Calc-s.

VAPOUR, HOT, from : Kali-bi.

X-RAY : Calc-f; Pho; Radm;
X-ray.

BURNT, SCALDED, As if : ARS;
Canth; Cyc; *Hyds;* Hyo;
Iris; Lyc; *Mag-m;* Phyt;
Plat; PUL; Ran-b; Sang;
Sep; Ver-a; Ver-v.

BURROWING, Digging : See
Pain.

BURSAE : See Ganglia.

BURSTING : See Pain.

BUSINESS FAILURE : Amb;
Cimi; Kali-br.

WORRY : Amb; Acet-ac;
Caus; Kali-p; Lil-t; Nux-v;
Pod.

Though, prosperous : Psor.

BUSY, WHEN (See Occupa-
tion) *Amel :* Con; Cyc; Helo;
Ign; Iod; Lil-t; Nat-c; Nux-v;
Sep.

FORGETS, Everything, : Ant-c.

RESTLESSNESS : Ver-a.

BUTTOCKS : Grap; Pho-ac;
Stap; Sul.

ABSCESS : Sul.

BOILS : Pho-ac.

BURNING : Merc.

COLD : Agar; Daph.

Numb, And : Calc-p.

CRAMP : Grap.

   Leg, stretching, Agg : Sep.

EMACIATED : Lathy.

   Infants, in : Nat-m.

HOT : Colch.

JERKING Up : Cup.

LARGE : Am-m.

NODES, On : Ther.

NUMB : Alu.

PIMPLES On : Kob.

RED : Carb-v; Cham; Sul.

   Spots : Mag-c.

SITTING Agg : Stap.

SORE : Ars.

STITCHING : *Calc-p*; Guai.

SWELLING : Pho-ac.

UPWARDS,Lumbar region to : Stap.

WARTY Growth, small, flat : Con.

BUZZING : See Humming.

CALCULI: (urinary, biliary etc.) Formation, of in general : *Bell*; Benz-ac; *Berb; Bry; Calc; Chin;* Coc-c; *Colo;* Dios; Dul; Hyds; Lach; LYC; Merc; *Nux-v;* Oci-c; Par-b; Pod; Pul; *Sars*; Sep.

DEPOSITS : Vario.

OPERATIONS, After : Mill.

CALF : Alu; Arg-n; Ars; CALC; Cam; *Cham; Cup; Grap;* Ign; *Lyc;* Nit-ac; *Nux-v;* Pul; Rhus-t; Sep; Stan; Stap; SUL; Val; VER-A.

BOILS : Sil.

BRUISED, As if **:** EUP-P; Stap.

COLD : Con.

   Spots, On : Stro.

CORD, Bound by, as if : Lol-t.

CRAMPS : Arg-n; Ars; *Calc;* Cam; Caus; CHAM; Colo; CUP; Grap; Hep; *Ign; Lyc;* NUX-V; *Plat; Plb; Sec; Sep;* Sil; Stro; SUL; *Ver-a;* Vib; Vip; Zin-io.

   Bed, turning, over in : Mag-c.

   left, at night : Phys.

   Coition Agg : Cup; Grap.

   Colic, with : Colo; Plb.

   Crossing, legs on : Alu.

   Dysentery, in : Merc-c.

   Fear, from : Lach.

   Foot, turning, sitting, while : Nat-m.

   Heels, to : Val.

   Menses, before : Vib.

   Muscles become flat : Jat.

   Pressing foot on floor Amel : Zin-io.

   Soles, and : Stro.

   Standing Amel : Cup-ar.

   Stools, during : Ap; Pod; Sec; Ver-a.

   Stretching legs in bed : Calc; Sul.

    - Amel : *Cup*.

   Tailors : Anac; Mag-p.

   Walking, while : Anac; Calc-p; Cinb; Lyc; Sul.

   Amel : Ver-a.

CROSSING, Legs, Agg : Val.

DRAWING,Walking, when : Carb-an.

ITCHING : Caus.

JERKING : Op.

LUMPS, In : Merc; Nit-ac.

NUMB : Plat.

Aching, with: Lapp.

RIGID, Stiff : Arg-n; Mag-m.

RISING, Seat, from Agg : Anac.

SACRUM, To : Merc-i-r.

SHORT, As if : Arg-m; Sil.

SWELLING : Dul.

TENSE : See Rigid.

TWITCHING : Grap.

WEARINESS, Of : Bor.

Palpitation, with: Calc-p.

WIND, Cool up, from : Helo.

CALLOSITIES, *Corns* : ANT-C;
Bry; *Calc*; Cist; *Grap*; Ign; *Lyc*;
Pho; *Phyt*; Radm; Rhus-t;
SEP; SIL; Sul; Symp.

BURNING: Arg-m; Ign;
Ran- sc; Sep.

CRACKS, Deep in: Cist; Grap.

HANGING, Down, Agg : Ran-sc.

INFLAMMED : Sil; Sul.

PAINFUL : Ign; Lyc; Nat-m;
Ran-sc; Sul.

PRESSING : Lyc; Sul.

PRESSURE, Slight, from : Ant-c.

SHOOTING : Bov; Nat-m.

SOFT : *Sil.*

SORE : Carb-an; Flu-ac; Ign;
Lyc; Sil.

STINGING : Alu; Bry; Calc;Cal-s;
Nat-c; Nat-m; Rhus-t; Sul.

TEARING : Lyc; Sil; Sul.

CANCER : ARS; Ars-io; Ast-r;
Aur; Bels; *Bro*; Buf; *Calc*;
CARB-AN; Clem; CON;
Cund; GRAP; Hyds; Iod; *Kre*;
LYC; NIT-AC; Petr; Pho; *Phyt*;
Sec; Sep; SIL; *Sul*; Symph;
Thu.

CANCRUM ORIS, Noma : Ars;
Con; Kali-chl; Kali-p;
Tarn-c.

DEPOSITS, Removal after :
Kali-p; Maland.

ENCEPHALOMA : *Pho.*

EPITHELIOMA : *Ars*; Ars-io;
Con; Kali-s; Lyc; Ran-sc;
Sep; *Thu.*

Flat : Cund.

GLANDS, Of : *Aur-m*; CARB-
AN; CON.

LUPUS : *Ars; Calc; Grap; Lyc*;
Merc; Nat-m;Rhus-t; Sep;
Sil; Stap; Sul.

Hypertrophicus : Ars; *Grap.*

Vorax : Ars; Sep; Sil; *Stap*;
Sul

+ RELIEVES, Burning pain of :
Calc-ars.

+ RETARDS Progress of : Trifol.

SARCOMA (See Fungus
growths) : Ars; Bar-c;
Carb-an; Lach; Lap-al;
Pho; Sil; Symp; Thu.

Burning : Bar-c.

Lympho : Ars; Ars-io.

Osteo : Calc-f; Hekla; Syph.

SCIRRHUS : Bels; Carb-an;
Clem; *Con*; Petr; Sep;
Sil; Sul.

SMOKING, From : Con.

CANTHI (Eyes, of) : *Agar*;
Calc; Carb-v; Kali-n;

Nat-m; Nux-v; Pho; *Pul; Sil;*
SUL.

INNER : *Agar; Bell; Stap; Zin.*

Itching : Rut.

INNER Swelling, over : Kali-c;
Pul.

OUTER : Calc; Ran-b; Sul.

Lump, in : Sul-ac.

Polypus : Lyc.

Twitching, chewing,
while : Kali-n.

CRACKS : Ant-c; Caus; Grap;
Lyc.

GUM, In : *Agar; Ant-c;* Calc;
Grap; Lyc; Stap.

Sticky : Euphr; Kali-bi.

INFLAMED : Ant-c; ARG-N; Bor;
Calc; Euphr; GRAP.

ITCHING : Alu; Arg-m; Calc.

+ RAW : Ant-c.

RED, Dark : Rhus-t.

Pale : Ap.

CAP *SENSATION* : *Carb-v; Cyc;
Grap*; Lach.

Tight: Berb.

CAPRICIOUS : See Changing
Moods, and Appetite.

CARBUNCLE : Anthx; *Ars;
Bell*; Echi; Hep; Lach;Led;
Pyro; *Sil;* Sul-ac; Tarn-c.

BLUISH, Red: Lach.

BURNING : Tarn-c.

+ BURSTING : Vip.

IMPOTENCY, With : Pic-ac.

SCARLET : Ap; Bell.

STINGING : *Ap*; Nit-ac.

CARE AND WORRY : Acet-ac;

Ambr; Anac; Ars; Calc; Chin;
Con; *Ign*; Kali-br; Kali-p;
Mag-c; Pho; Pho-ac; Pul.

CAUSELESS : Petr.

TRIFLES, About : Ars.

CARESSES AGG : Bell; Calc;
Chin; Ign; Plat.

PROOFAgainst : Cina.

CARIES : See under Bones.

CARPHOLOGY, Picking at bed-
clothes, nervous picking :
Ars; Bell; Hell; HYO; Lyc;
Mur-ac; *Op*; Pho; Pho-ac;
Rhus-t; STRAM; Tarn;
Ver-v; Zin.

ONE SPOT, lips, fingers etc. :
Ars; *Aru-t;* Cham; Con;
Kali-br; Lach; Tarn; Thu.

Bleeds, until : Arg-m;
Aru- t; Cina; Con; Pho.

Sore, until : Aru-t; Pho-ac;
Zin.

CARRIED, *WANTS*, to be:
Acet-ac; Ant-t; Ars; Benz-ac;
CHAM; Cina; Kali-c; Lyc;
Rhus-t; Ver-a.

CARESSED, And : Kre; Pul.

+ DISLIKES : Bry.

+ ERECT, Wishes : Ant-t.

FAST : Aco; *Ars; Bro;* Ver-a.

SHOULDERS, Over : Cina; Pod;
Stan.

SLOWLY : Pul.

WILL NOT be laid down
(Children) : Benz-ac.

CARRIES THINGS, From one
place to another, and back
again : Mag-p.

CARRYING BURDENS AGG :

Cadm; Rut.

BACK, On AGG : Alu.

HEAD, On AGG : Calc; Rut; Tarn.

CAR SICKNESS, Sea sickness etc. : Ars; Bor; *Cocl;* Colch; Con; Glo; Kre; Lyss; PETR; Sanic; Sele; *Sep; Tub;* Ther.

RAILWAY: Kali-io.

RIDING *Amel* : Ars; *Grap; Nit-ac;* Tarn.

Air, open, in Amel : Naj.

Downhill Agg : Bor; Psor.

STOMACH, Felt in, nausea, without : Kali-p.

CARTILAGE : Arg-m; Calc-p; Nat-m; Rut; Sul; Symp.

ULCERATION : Merc-c; Merc-d.

CARUNCLE : See Urethra.

CATALEPSY : Cic; Cof; Gel; *Grap;* Hyo; Ign; Lach; Op; Pho-ac; Plat.

+ LIMBS Can be moved by others : Stram.

MENSES, During : Plat.

SEXUAL Excitement, from : Con; Plat.

CATARACT : See Lens.

CATHETERISM : Aco; Mag-p; Nux-v; Petros.

CAUTION : Calc; *Ign;* Nux-v; *Pul;* Ver-a.

CELIBACY : *Con;* Pho.

CELLARS, Vaulted places *Agg* : Aran; Ars; Calc; Dul; Nat-s; Pul.

CELLULAR TISSUE (Cellulitis, etc.) : Ap; Ars; Bry; Lach;

Merc; Rhus-t; Sil; Tarn-c; Vesp.

INDURATED : Anthx; Kali-io; Merc-i-r; Rhus-t.

SUBACUTE : Mang; Sil.

CENSORIOUS : *Aco;* ARS; NUX-V; Sul.

CEPHALHAEMATOMA : Calc-f; Merc; Sil.

CEREBRO-SPINAL Axis : Agar; Arg-n; Chin; Cocl; *Gel;* Ign; *Nux-v;* Pho.

FEVER (Meningitis) : *Ap;* Arn; *Bell;* Bry; Cup; *Gel;* Hell; Merc-d; Nat-s; Stram; Sul; Ver-v; Zin.

+ Basilar : *Ver-v.*

Suppressed discharges, from : Stram.

Tubercular : Bacil; Calc; Iod; Iodof; Lyc; Merc; Sil; Sul; Tub.

Urine, pale, clear with : Bell; Hyo; Lach; Pho.

CERVIX (UTERUS) CANCER (See Uterus) : Tarn.

CAULIFLOWER-LIKE, Growth : Kali-ar.

EROSION, of : Arg-m; Hyds; Kali-bi; Phyt; Sul-ac; Thu.

INDURATED : Aur; Carb-an; Con; Nat-c; Sep.

LOWER, Vagina, in : Calend.

OPEN, Dilated, as if : Lach; Sanic.

OS Rigid, contracted, labour during : Bell; *Caul; Cham; Cimi;* Gel; Ver-v.

PAINFUL : Goss.

Spongy : Arg-m; Ust.

Ulceration : Buf; Med; Mez.

+ Prolapse of uterus with :
Arg-n.

Warts, On : Calend.

CHAGRIN: See Mortification.

CHANCRE Hard : Carb-an;
Cinb; Kali-io; Merc; Merc-c;
Merc-i-f; Merc-i-r.

Soft : Cor-r; Merc; Nit-ac;
Thu.

CHANGE OF POSITION
Agg : *Caps*; Carb-v; Chel;
Con; *Euphor; Fer;* Lach; Lyc;
Pho; *Pul*; Samb.

Amel : Agar; Ars; Cham; IGN;
Meli; Nat-s; Pho-ac; Pul;
Pyro; RHUS-T; *Sep*; Syph;
Val; Zin.

Legs Drawn up, when : Hell.

Lying, Long, in one after, Agg
: Nat-s.

Temperature Or, Weather,
on-coming storms etc Agg
: Agar; *Ars;* Calc-p; Carb-v;
Dul; Gel; Hypr; Lach;
Mag-c; Mez; Nat-c; Nit-ac;
Nux-m; Petr; *Pho; Psor;* Pul;
Ran-b; *Rhod*; RHUS-T;
Rum; Sabi; Sep; *Sil;* Sul-io;
Tub; Verb.

Agg and *Amel* : Mang.

Rapid *Agg* : Sep.

Wants and *Amel* : Mang;
Sep; Tub.

CHANGING MOODS, Erratic,
fitful, capricious : Aco; ALU;
Amb; Bry; Cham; Cina; Croc;
FER; Grap; IGN; Ip; Kali-c;

LACH; *Nux-m*; PLAT; PUL;
Stap; Senec; *Stram;* SUL- AC;
Tarn; *Val;* ZIN.

Menses, Before : Cham.

Rapidly (Disposition or
Symptoms) : Asaf; Croc;
Rhod; Sep; Tab; Tarn;Tub;
Val.

Touch, on: Asaf.

CHAPS : See Cracks.

+ **CHARCOAL FUMES**, *Ill Effects*
: Am-c; Op.

CHEEKS : Bell; Caus; Ign;
Merc; *Rhus*-t; Stap.

Bites, Chewing or Talking
when : Carb-an; Caus; *Ign;*
Nit-ac; Ol-an.

Blisters Inside : Med.

Cold : Colo.

Contraction, Sudden : Eup-p.

Cyst : Grap; Thu.

Drawing, Bones, in : Caus;
Chel; Colch; Plat; Verb.

Eruptions : Ant-c; *Euphr;* Kre;
Rhus-t; Stap.

Herpes : Con.

Flapping, heavy breathing,
with : Cheno.

Hangs, Down : Ap.

Heat : Sang; Tab.

Affected side : Tub.

Toothache, with : Fer-p.

Induration, inside : Caus.

Numb: Caps; Mez; Nux-v;
Old; Plat.

Painful : Verb.

Splinters, as if : Agar.

+ Pale and Hot, one : Mos.

PURPLE (Centre) : Diph.

RED : *Aco;* Arn; Bell; CHAM; Chin; *Fer; Ign; Lyc;* Mos; Nux-v; Pho; *Pul;* Sang; Sul.

Colic, during : Cham.

Hot, air, open in : Val.

Left : Ver-a.

One : Sep.

and cold : Mos.

Spot : Rhus-t.

SCABS, Bran-like, covered with : Lith.

SWOLLEN : Arn Cham; *Merc.*

Hard : Am-c; Calc-f.

growth, over, with : Hep.

Inside : Am-c; Caus.

Menses, during : Ap; Grap.

TEARING, bones, in : Lyc; Merc.

TUBERCLES, Small, in : Asaf.

TWITCHING *(R)* : Mez.

CHEERFUL : Aur; Bell; CANN; COF; *Croc;* Hyo; Nat-m; *Op; Plat;* Spo; *Stram;* Tarn.

COITION, After : Nat-m.

CONVULSIONS, After : Sul.

FEARFUL, But : Nat-c.

HEART, Disease, with : Cact.

MENSES, Before : Coca; Flu-ac.

During : Flu-ac.

PAINS, During : Spig.

After : Form.

SAD, And alternately : Senec.

STOOL, After : Bor; Nat-s.

SUDDEN, Crying : Chin.

CHEESY, ODOUR : Pho; Sanic; Sep.

OLD : Bry; Hep; Sanic.

CHEST, AND LUNGS,

AFFECTIONS in General : *Aco;* ANT-T; Arn; ARS; BRY; Calc; Chel; Chin; Dul; *Fer-p;* Guai; Iod; Ip; *Kali-c; Lyc;* Op; Phel; PHO; PUL; *Ran-b;* Ran-sc; *Rhus-t;* Sang; Scil; Senec; Seneg; *Spig;* Stan; Sul; Tub; *Ver-v;* Verb.

RIGHT : Arn; Ars; *Bell; Bry;* Carb-an; Chel; *Colch;* Colo; Iod; *Kali-c;* Lach; *Lyc;* Mur-ac; Psor; Pul; Scil.

Into, right arm : Hyds; Kre; Lob; Pho; Phyt; Plb; Sang.

Nail, deep, in : Chel.

To left : Aco; Lach; Petr.

LEFT : Am-m; Arg-m; Calc; Con; Euphor; Flu-ac; Kali-c; Kali-n; Laur; Lyc; Nat-s; Nit-ac; *Nux-v; Pho;* Rhus-t; Seneg; Stan; Sul.

Lower epigastrium, to : Ox-ac.

Rumbling, audible : Cocl.

To right : Ap; Calc; Grap; Kre; Pho; Plb; Zin.

ALTERNATING Sides : *Agar;* Ap; Ars; *Calc; Cimi;* Dul; Grap; Hypr; Lyc; Mang; Mos; PHO; Plb; Ran-b; Rum; Thu.

Abdomen, with : Radm.

ARMS, Into : Bry; Dig; Dios; Latro.

Right : Pho.

BACKWARD, Extending : Ars; Bry; *Calc;* Caps; Carb-v; *Chel;* Con; Cup; Kali-bi;

Kali-io; Lil-t; *Merc*; Nat-m; Pho; Sep; Spig; *Sul*; Ther.

Right: Aco; Ars; *Carb-v*; *Chel*; Dul; Guai; Kali-bi; Nit-ac; Phel; Phyt; Sep; *Sul.*

Left : Bry; Kali-n; Lil-t; *Lyc*; Mur-ac; Nat-m; Phys; Rhus-t; Spig; Sul-ac; Ther.

CHANGING About : *Aco;* Alu; Arg-n; Bell; Cact; Caus; Colch; Fer; *Lyc*; Mag-m; Merc; Nat-c; Pho; *Pul;* Seneg.

Pressure Amel : Caus.

DEEP In : Arn; Bry; Cep; Dros; Eup-p; Kali-c; Kre.

DOWNWARD : Agn; Kali-bi.

Right : Dul; Nit-ac; Sang; Sep.

Left : *Kali-c*; Laur; Pho; Pul; Scil; Zin.

EPIGASTRIUM, To : Ox-ac.

FORWARD : Berb; Bor; BRY; Castr; *Kali-c*; Kali-n; Psor; Rat; *Sep*; Sul.

Right: Aco; Colo; Merc.

Left : Agar; Bar-c; *Bry*; Lac-c; Naj; Pho; *Sul*; Thu; Zin.

MIDDLE : Calc; Dul; Kali-bi; Phel; Sep.

UPPER : Calc; Iod; Mang; Pul; Stan.

UPWARD : Ars; Calc; Caus; Lach; Mang; Mur-ac; Thu.

Right : Arn; Plat; Thu.

to left : Petr.

Left : Am-m; Bov; *Coc-c*;

Kali-c; Laur; Med; *Scil;* Spig; Stan; Zin.

to right : Calc; Carb-v; Grap; Ign; Lil-t.

TRANSVERSELY : Caus; Thu.

Arms, to : *Alu.*

THROAT, Into : Ap; Bell; Calc; Laur; Pho; Sul; Thu; Zin.

ABSCESS, Lung, of : Calc; Hep; Pho; Sil.

AIR, IN, Too much enters or forced, as if : Chlor; Sabi; Ther.

ANXIETY Felt, in : Aco; Ars; Aur; Bry; Calc; Merc; Pho.

APICES, Pain in: Guai; Pul.

Left : Myr; Ther.

ARMS, Raising Agg : Tarn; Tell.

Using Agg : Rhus-t.

BAND, Sensation of a : Aeth; Cact; Helo; Ign; Lob; Pho; Sul.

Lower : Cocl; Cup; *Plat.*

BAR Across : Kali-bi.

BENDING, Backwards, Amel : Flu-ac.

Forwards, Amel : Ascl.

BLOWING Nose Agg : Chel; Sumb.

BOOTS, Putting, on, Agg : Arg-n.

BREATHING, Deep Agg: Nat-p.

Amel: Chel.

BROWN Spots on : Carb-v.

BUBBLES : Merc.

BURNING, Heat : *Aco*; Ap; *Ars*; Bell; Canth; *Carb-v;* Euphor;

Kali-m; Lyc; Naj; *Pho;* Sang; Spo; *Sul; Tub;*Ver-v.

Cold feeling in stomach, with : Polyg.

Coughing Agg : Iod; Pho; Seneg; Spo; Thu.

Epistaxis, with : Thu.

Expectoration, bloody, with : Psor.

Hands, icy cold, with : Thu.

Hot stream, as from : Kre; Merc; Sang.

Inspiration, on : Laur.

BURSTING : Bro.

CHLOASMAE : Card-m; Sep; Sul; Thu.

CLOTHING Agg : Ars; *Caus;* Chel; *Lach.*

+ Too tight : Chel.

Wet, as if : Ran-b.

COLD, Air, draft Agg : Act-sp; *Calc-p;* Petr; Pho-ac; Ran-b.

Amel : Fer.

Drinks Agg : Pho; Psor.

Pain, coughing, on : Med.

Water, washing, with Amel: Bor.

COLDNESS In : ARS; Bry; Carb-an; Kali-c; Lil-t; Med; Nat-c; *Old; Sul.*

Cold air, breathing, on: Cor-r; Lith; *Ran-b.*

Drinking, after : Elap.

Expectoration, after : Zin.

CONGESTION : *Aco; Bell;* Bry; *Cact;* Cam; Dig; Fer; Fer-p; Ip; Lach; *Nux-v; Pho;* Rhus-t; Seneg; Sep; Spo;

SUL; Terb; *Ver-v.*

Urination, desire for if not attended to : Lil-t.

+ CONSTRICTION, As from sulphur fumes : Kali-chl.

CONTRACTED, Asthma, with : Cadm.

COUGHING Agg: Bor; BRY; Caus; Elap; Lyc; *Pho;* Scil; Seneg; Spo; Stan; Sul.

CRAMP, Constriction, Spasm : Aeth; Asaf; Cact; Fer; Grap; Ign; Mos; Nux-m; Nux-v; Radm; Sul; Tab; Vip.

Bends, double : Hyo.

DANCING, Amel : Caus.

DESIRE To urinate if delayed Agg : Lil-t.

DIRECTION Of, Pain, various : Thu.

DISTENSION : Ars; *Lach;* Thu.

DRYNESS : Fer; Lach; Merc; Pho; Pul.

Coughing, with : Pho.

Left : Naj.

EMACIATION : Kali-io; Petr; Senec.

EMPHYSEMA : Am-c; Ant-t; Ars; Coca; Grind; Hep; Lach; Lob; Seneg.

Senile : Lob.

EMPTY, Hollow : Carb-an; Cocl; Med; Pho; Stan.

Coughing, when : Sep; Stan.

Eating, after : Nat-p; Old.

Expectoration, after : Rut;

Stan; Zin.

Left : Naj.

Singing, while : Stan.

EMPYEMA : Arn; Ars; Calc-s; Kali-s; Merc; Sil; Sul.

Pleurisy, after : Sil.

EPISTAXIS Amel : Bro; Carb-v.

ERUCTATION Amel : Amyl-n; Bar-c; Canth; Lach; Pho; Sep.

FASTING Agg : Iod.

FIXED, Immovable : Ox-ac; *Pho*; Stry.

FLUTTERING, In: Lil-t; Naj; Nat-m; Nat-s; Nux-m; Pho-ac; Spig.

FULLNESS : Aco; Ap; Glo; Lach; *Pho; Sul.*

Heart, weak or dilated with : Chlo-hyd.

GANGRENE, Lung, of : *Ars;* Caps; Carb-*v; Kre;* Lach.

HAEMORRHAGE (See Haemoptysis) : Chel; Stan.

Menses, before : Dig.

Parturition, after : Arn; Chin; Pul.

Pneumonia, results, of: Calc-s; *Sul-ac.*

Puerperal fever, in : Ham.

HAWKING Agg : Calc; Rum; Spig.

HEAVY : See Load.

HEPATISATION, Lung, of : Pho; Sul.

HICCOUGH Agg : Stro.

HOLD, Must : Arn; *Bry; Dros;* Eup-p; Nat-s.

HOLLOW : See Empty.

HOT Application, Amel : Pho.

Drops, as of : Hep.

HYDROTHORAX : Adon.

INJURY, After : Rut.

ITCHING : Ant-c; Sul.

Nose, up to : Con; *Ip.*

LAUGHING Agg : Bry.

LEGS, Hanging, Amel: Sul-ac.

LIFTING Agg: Alu; Psor; Sul.

LOAD, Heavy on, Pressure : Am-c; Ant-t; Aur; Cact; Fer; Lach; Lil-t; *Nux-v; Pho; Pul*; Seneg; Stro; *Sul;* Ver-v.

Motion Amel : Seneg.

LUMP, Plug, Sensation : *Amb;* Am-m; *Anac;* Bur-p; Cup; *Kali-m; Pho; Ram-sc*; Stic; Sul; Tarx; Zin.

+ Behind : Gel.

Moving up and down, swallowing, empty, on : Lil-t.

LUNG, Apex (R) : Elap.

Bubbling in (R) : Tell.

Burning like fire : Buf.

+ Constricted by wire, as if : Asar.

Distend, can not : Asaf; Crot-t.

Down, coated, with as if : Bro.

Hard and small, as if (R) : Ab-c.

+ Hot, feel : *Aco.*

Moving , waves, in, as if : Dul.

+ Rivet, as of (L) : Sul.

Seperated forcibly, as if : Elap.

Smoke, full of, as if : Bar-c.

Sticking, ribs to, as if : Kali-c.

Stuffed up cotton with, as if : Kali-bi; Med.

LYING, Abdomen, on Agg : Ascl.

Amel : Bry.

Back, on Amel: Bor; *Cact;* Pho; Sul.

Painful, side, on Amel : Amb; *Bry;* Nux-v.

With, arms, near chest Amel : Lac-ac.

MORNING Agg : Calc; *Carb-v;* Sep.

MOTION Amel : Seneg.

NARROW, As if : Agar; Seneg.

NUMB : Glo; Stic.

Left arm, down : Glo.

OEDEMA, Pulmonary : Ant-t; Ars; Lach; Merc; Sul.

Sudden : Rhus-t.

OPERATION For fistula after : Berb; Calc-p; Sil.

Upon, chest after : Abro.

PARALYSIS Of Lungs : ANT-T; Ars; *Bar-c; Carb-v; Chin;* Ip; Kali-io; *Lach; Lyc;* Op; *Pho.*

Old people, in : Bar-c; Chin.

PLEURISY : Aco; Arn; Ascl; Bry; Carb-an; Guai; Kali-c; Merc-d; Pho; Seneg; Sul.

Adhesions, after : Ran-b.

Breathing, deep Agg : Guai.

Debility, paralytic, with : Saba.

Exudation : Abro; Fer; Iod; Kali-iod; Seneg.

Neglected : Ars; Sul.

Recurrent : Guai.

Stitch, after : Carb-an.

PNEMONIA : ACO; *Ant -t;* Ars; *Bry;* Carb-v; Chel; *Fer-p;* Hep; Iod; Kali-bi; Lob; *Lyc; Merc;* PHO; *Pul; Rhus-t;* Sang; Seneg; *Sep; Sul;* Tub; Ver-v.

Catarrhal : *Ant-t.*

Cerebral type : Aco; Arn; Bell; Bry; Cann; Canth; Hyo; Lach; Merc; Nux-v; Pho; Pul; Rhus-t; Stram; Sul.

Haemorrhage, after : Chin; Pho-ac.

Infants : *Ip.*

+ Influenza, after : Tub.

Neglected, unresolved : Ars-io; *Lyc;* Pho; Pyro; *Sil; Sul;* Sul-io.

Secondary: Fer-p; Pho.

PRESSURE Amel : *Arn;* Bor; BRY; Caus; *Dros;* Eup-p; Nat-s.

Clothes, of Agg : Benz-ac.

Hands, of Amel : Sep.

Spine, on Agg: Sec; Tarn.

PULSATION : Asaf; Bell; Cact; Seneg; *Sul.*

Night : Pul.

Right : Asar; Crot-t; *Dig;* Ign; Ind; Paeon; Pho.

Left : Am-m; Cann; Gel; *Meny.*

PURRING : Caus; Glo; Spig.

Rattling (See Respiration rattling) : Hep; Lob; Pho; Sil; Sul; Tub.

Coarse : Ant-t; Cup; Kali-s.

Expectoration, without : Am-c; *Ant-t;* Carb-v; Caus; Con; Hep; Ip; Kali-s; Lob; Pho; Sep; Sul; Tub; Ver-a.

Fine : Ip.

Loose : Seneg.

Rushes of blood : Kali-n; Pho; Seneg; Sul.

Scraping : Seneg.

Talking Agg : Seneg.

Shocks, Jerks : Agar; *Con;* Grap; *Lyc;* Plat; Sul.

Coughing, when : Lyc; Seneg.

Shoulders, Throwing back Amel : Calc.

Shuddering In : Agar; Aur.

Singing Agg : Am-c.

Small, Too, as if : Ign.

Sneezing Agg : Bry; Caus; Dros; Merc; Mez; Seneg.

Soreness : Alu; Calc; Chel; Chin; Kali-bi; *Pho;* Rhod; Seneg; *Stan.*

Cold air Agg : Pho-ac.

Expectoration, after : Cist.

Scapulae, between, with : Chin.

Touch Agg : Chin.

Spot, In : Agar; Anac; Buf; Nat-m; Ol-j; Seneg; Thu; Tub.

Brown : Lyc; Sul.

Red : Guai; Saba; Sul.

Yellow : Ars; Pho.

Sprain : Lyc; Rhod; Tell.

Squatting Agg : Cadm.

+ Squeezed, By hand, as if: Colch.

Stabbing : Kali-c; Nat-m.

Stitching : *Aco; Bry;* Kali-c; Myr; Ol-j; *Pho; Ran-b;* Rhus-t; Scil; Spig; Sul.

Right : Bor.

Left : Pho.

Bilateral : Ran-b.

Breathing, impending: Arg-m.

Burning : Sang.

Coughing Agg : Merc.

+ Flying : Fer.

Pleurisy, after : Carb-an.

Pressure Amel : Arn; Bor.

Sneezing Agg : Merc.

Stooping Agg : Mez. Seneg.

Stuffed Up, as if : Amb; Lach; Med; Radm.

Talking Agg : Alu.

Tickling : Rhus-t; *Rum*

Tight: Ars; Asaf; *Aur;* Cact; Caus; Fer; Ign; Ip; Nat-m; *Nux-v;* PHO; Pul; Sul; Tab; Terb.

Right : Am-m; Cocl; Sul.

Left : Grap; Lyc; Sul-ac; Sumb.

Coition, close of, at : Stap.

Coughing Amel : Con.

Motion, least Agg : Ip.

Stooping Agg : Mez.

TREMBLING, In : Lapp; Spig.

ULCERATIVE, Pain : Ran-b.

UNCOVERING Amel : Fer; Sars.

UTERINE, Symptoms, with : Stan.

VAPOUR, As if, in : Merc.

VELVETY, Feeling : Ant-t.

VOMITING, Green Amel : Cocl.

WEAKNESS : Ant-t; Arg-m; *Calc; Carb-v; Kali-c;* LAUR; *Nit-ac;* Ran-sc; *Seneg;* STAN; SUL.

Coughing, when : Pho-ac.

Exertion, after : Spo.

Expectoration, after : Stan.

Singing, when : Stan.

Sitting, when : Pho-ac.

Talking, while : Pho-ac; *Stan;* Sul.

Waking, after: Carb-v.

Amel : Pho-ac.

WANDERING Pain : Seneg.

WATER, In, as if : Hep.

WINE Agg : Bor.

YAWNING Agg : Bor; Grap; Nat-s; Sul.

CHEWING : See Biting.

CONSTANT, Frothy saliva, with : Asaf.

FOOD, Escapes from mouth, during : Arg-n.

MOTIONS : Aco; Amy-n; Bell; BRY; Calc; *Cham;* Cup; *Hell; Lach; Lyc;* Mos; *Ver-v.*

Brain affections, in : Bry.

Chorea, in : Asaf.

Sleep, in : Calc; Ign.

+ Spasms, before : Calc.

SWALLOWING, And, sleep, in : Calc; Cina; Ign.

CHICKEN POX : Aco; Ant-c; Ant-t; Bell; *Led;* Pul; *Rhus-t;* Sul.

CHILBLAINS, FROSTBITE : Abro; AGAR; Ars; Carb-v; Hep; *Nit-ac;* Nux-v; *Petr;* *Pul;* Sul.

+ UNBROKEN : Terb.

CHILDBED : See Pregnancy.

CHILDISH, FOOLISH : Aeth; *Alo;* Amb; ANAC; BAR-C; BELL; *Buf;* Cic; Con; *Hell;* HYO; Lach; Lyc; *Nat-c;* Nux-m; Nux-v; *Op; Pho-ac;* Pic-ac; Plb; Sep; Sil; *Stram;* Sul; Thyr; Ver-a.

BODY Grows, but : Buf.

EPILEPSY, Before : Caus.

After : Tab.

+ FUROR, Alternate, with : Aeth.

PARTURITION, After : Ap.

CHILDREN INFANTS : *Aco;* Ant-t; *Bell; Bor;* CALC; CALC-P; *Cham; Cina;* Cof; Ip; *Merc;* Phyt; Pod; Pul; Rhe; Sep; SIL; *Sul.*

AFRAID, Everything, of : Calc.

BOILS, Disposition, to : Mag-c.

BREATH, Loses, angry, when : Arn.

CHOKE, Liquids, swallowing, on : Kali-br.

+ CLUMSY : Asaf.

CRAWL, Nervously : Sil.

CYANOTIC, Birth, from : Bor;
Cact; Dig; Lach; Laur.

DRAGGED, Mother's arms on :
Sil.

EMOTIONAL, Chat and laugh : Alo.

FAT, Chubby : Bell; Seneg.

FED, Improperly : Aeth.

FONTANELLES, Depressed : *Ap*;
Calc.
Occipital bone, sinking :
Mag-c.
Open: *Ap*; CALC; CALC-P;
Ip; Merc; Pul; Sep; SIL;
Sul; Syph.
Pulsate strongly : Gel.
Reopening, of : Calc-p.

+ FUSS, Likes : Pul.

HOLD, On to mother's hand :
Bism.

JUMP, Start, scream fearfully
: Nat-c; Sul.

LIFTING Agg : Bor; Calc-p.

NOSE, Red, raw, dirty with :
Merc.

NURSE, Daytime only : Ap.
All the time : Calc-p.

PALE, Running, on : Sil.

+ SCHOOL, Overtaxed with : Zin.

SCREAM And cry, always :
Lac-c; Psor; Rhe.

+ SLEEP, All day, cry all night
: Lyc.

+ SOUR Smelling : Med.

STAMMERING : Bov.

SUCKLING : Bor; Calc; Calc-p;
Kali-bi; Mag-c; Pho-ac;
Pul; Sul.
Die, early, birth after :
Arg-n.

Few weeks old, shrivelled
and old looking : Op.

TALK Late : Agar; Bar-c;
Calc-p; *Nat-m*; Sanic.

+ TALL, Thin : Calc-p.

+ UNHEALTHY : Psor.

WALK Late : Agar; Calc;
Calc-p; Caus; *Sil*; Sul.
Unable to, from ankle
affections, : Mang.

WANT To be nursed in arms,
will not be laid down :
Benz-ac.

WEAK, Cause, without :
Sul-ac.

WEEP, Cry continuously,
infants, new born : Syph;
Thu.

CHILL : Ant-c; Ant-t; *Aran;
Arn; Ars;* Aur; CAM; Canth;
Carb-v; Caus; Chel; *Chin;
Chin-s; Eup-p;* Gel; Grap;
Hep; Ign; *Ip;* Lac-d; LYC;
Meny; Mez; MOS; NAT-M;
Nit-ac; *Nux-m;* Nux-v; PUL;
Rhus-t; *Saba;* Sep; *Sil; Stap;*
Symp; Thyr; VER-A.

ABDOMEN, Begins, in : Amb;
Ap; *Ars;* Ign; Pho; Sep; *Ver-a*

AIR, Craves : Alu; Sep; Tub.

ALTERNATING, Fever, with :
Am-m; *Ars; Bell;* Bry; *Calc;*
Cham; *Chin;* Cocl; Eup-p;
GEL; *Hep;* Hyds; Ip;
Kali-io; Lach; *Merc;* Nux-m;
NUX-V; Ol-an; *Rhus-t;*
Samb.

ANTICIPATES : Ap; ARS; *Bry;
Chin;* Chin-s; *Nat-m;*
NUX-V.

Postponing, or : Bry; Ign.

BACK, Starts, in : Bell; *Caps*; Caus; Cocl; Dul; *Eup-p; Gel*; Hyo; *Lach*; Lyc; *Nat-m*; Pul; *Rhus-t*; Sec; Sep; Stap; Stro; Sul.

BED, Putting hand out of : *Bar-c*; *Hep*; NUX-V; *Rhus-t*; Tarn; TUB.
Turning over in : Nux-v; Pul.

BLADDER, Starts in : Sars.

BONES, Felt, in : Pyro.

CHANGING, Type : Ign; Pul.

CHEST, Starts in: *Ap*; Carb-an; Sep.

COITIÓN, After : Nat-m.

COLD WATER, were dashed over him as if : Arn; Rhus-t.
Were poured over him, as if : Canth; Led; Merc; Pul.

CONCOMITANT, As a : Saba.

CONGESTIVE : Aco; Arn; Gel; Nux-v; Psor; Ver-a.

CONVULSIONS, After : *Cup*.

CORYZA, With : Mag-c.

COUGHING Agg : Ap; Eup-p; Pul; Rhus-t; Thu.

COVERS Agg : *Ap*; Calc-s; Cam; Ip; Led; *Pul*; *Sec*; *Sep*.
Did not Amel : Lyc.

CREEPING : Merc.

DESIRES, To be held down : Gel; Lach.
Talk, to : Pod.

DRINKS Agg : *Ars*; Asar; Calc; *Caps*; Chel; *Chin*; *Eup-p*; Lach; *Nux-v*; Ver-a.
Amel : *Caus*; *Cup*; Manc.

Cold Agg : Rhus-t.
Warm Agg: Alu; Bell; *Pul*.

DROWSINESS, With : Ant-t; Cam; Chel; Gel; Nux-m; OP; Ver-a.

DYSPNOEA, With : Ap.

EATING, After : Ars; Asar; Bell; Carb-an; Kali-c; Ran-b; Tarx.

EXERTION, After : Zin-val.

EXTREMITIES, Starts, in : Arn; Bell; *Carb-v*; Caus; Sec; Sul.

FEVER, With : Aco; Ars; Bell; Cham; *Gel*; Hell; Ign; Nit-ac; Nux-v; Rhus-t; Sul.
For a long time : Pod; Pyro.

FINGER-TIPS, Numb, with : Stan.

FIRE, Besides, Agg : Pulex.

FLOWER, Smell of, from : Lac-c.

FRIGHT, From : Gel.

GRIEF, From : Gel; Ign.

HEAD, To : Glo.

HEATED, Overheated, when : *Carb-v; Pul*; Samb; *Sil*; Ver-a.

HOLDING Cold things in hand : Zin.

IRREGULAR : Ars; Nux-v; Psor; Pul; Sep.

ITCHING, With : Mez.

LIPS, Begins in : *Bry*.

LYING, On : Pul.
Back, on : Tell.

MENSES, Before : Lyc; Mag-c;

Pul; Sil.

During : Pul; Sep; Sil; Sul.

Start, at : Jab.

MENTAL Exertion, after : Nux-v; Zin-val.

MOTION, Arms, of Agg : Rhus-t.

Slight, after : Ars; *Nux-v; Spig.*

MOVING Bed-clothes slightly, on : Arn; Nux-v.

NERVOUS : Gel; Zin-val.

NIGHTLY : Pyro.

NOISE, From : Ther.

NOSEBLEED, with : Thu.

PAIN, With: *Agar;* Ars; Bov; Calc-p; *Cam; Colo;* Dul; Kali-n; *Mez; Pul;* SEP.

PALM and SOLE, starts from : Dig.

PARTIAL : See Coldness.

POSTPONING : Chin; GAMB; Ign; *Ip.*

PRESSURE Amel : *Bry;* Pho.

RIGOURS, Shaking : Chin; Chin-s; Ign; Nat-m; Pyro.

Inspiring, on : *Bro.*

Skin, cold, with : Cam.

Urination Agg : Stram; Thu.

Yawning, with : Thu.

SCAPULAE, Between, starts : Pyro.

SCRATCHING Agg : Agar; Mez; Petr.

SINGLE Parts, in: See Coldness, partial.

SITTING Amel : Ign; Nux-v.

SLEEP, First, after : Lyc.

In : Bor.

SPINE, To arms : Lept.

STONE, Abdomen, in, as if : Aran.

STOOLS, After : Canth; Med; Merc; Merc-c; Plat; Rhe.

Urging, with : Dul.

SUFFOCATED, As if : Arg-n; Mag-p.

SUMMER, In : Psor.

SUNSET, After : Ars; Ign; Pul.

SUNSHINE Agg : Nat-m.

Amel : Anac; Con.

SWEAT, With : Cham; Eup-p; Lach; Nux-v; Pul; Pyro; Tub.

Alternating, with chill : Ars; Chin; Mez; Nux-v; Spig.

THEN Heat, Then Chill : Thu.

THROAT, Sore, with : Mag-c.

THROUGH And THROUGH : Am-c; Aran; Calc; Cinb; Elap; Kali-bi; Mos.

TOOTHACHE, With : Mag-c.

TOUCH Agg : *Aco; Chin;* Lyc; *Nux-c;* Spig.

TREMBLING And Shivering with : Anac; Ant-t; Plat; Sil.

UNCOVERING, Least : Hep; Nux-v; Rhus-t; Sil.

Hands : Mag-c.

URINATING, On: Gel; Nit-ac; Plat; Thu.

Urging, with : Dul.

URTICARIA, With : Ap.

VOMITING, With : Dul.

WAKING, On : Alu; Arn.

As often as he wakes :

Am-m.

WALKING, While : Chin.

WARM Covering, in spite of : Asar.

Room, in : Pho.

WAVES, In : Carb-an.

WET. From : Lapp; Led; *Rhus-t;* Thu.

WIND, In : Sanic.

WRITING, While : Agar.

YAWNING, With : Carb-an; Kre; Meny; Thu.

CHILLED FROM Exposure to Cold *Agg* : ACO; Ars; *Bell;* Bry; Cham; Clem; Cof; *Colch;* *Dul;* Hyo; *Ip;* MERC; NUX-V; PH**O**; *Pul;* RHUS-T; Sep; *Sil;* *Spig; Sul;* Ver-a.

WHILE HOT, SWEATING, by ices, exposure to cold of single parts *Agg* : *Aco;* Ars; Bell; Bels; Bro; Bry; Dul; Fer-p; *Hep;* Kali-c; Merc-i-f; *Nux-v;* Pho; Psor; Pul; Rhod; RHUS-T; Sep; SIL; Zin.

CHIN : Caus; Plat; Sil.

COLD : Aeth; Kali-n.

DRAWN, Sternum, to : Phyt.

ERUPTION : Nat-m; Rhus-t; Sep; Sil; Sul.

Between, lips and : Kali-chl.

Eczema : Merc-i-r.

Granular, honey coloured : Ant-c.

GLAND, Under : Led; Stap.

+ HAIR, Falling: Grap.

HAIR, On, women, in : Ol-j.

NUMB : Spo.

SWEAT : Con.

TOO Long, as if : Glo.

TWITCHES, Trembles : Agar; *Ant-t;* Gel.

ULCER : Cund.

CHLOASMAE : Card-m; Caul; *Lyc;* Rob; *Sep.*

SUN, Exposure, from: Cadm.

CHLOROFORM *Agg* : Pho.

CHOKING(See Throat, Difficult respiration) : Con; Grap; Lycps; *Meph; Mos;* *Tarn;* Terb; Thyr; Val.

COUGHING Agg : Tarn.

DRINKING Agg : Meph.

EATING, when : Zin-val.

GOITRE, In: Meph.

HEAD, Bending backward, Amel : Hep; Lach.

NERVOUS : Mos.

SLEEP Agg : *Lach;* Spo; Val.

SPEAKING Agg : Meph.

SUDDEN : Samb.

WATER Agg : Stram.

CHOLERA : Ars; *Cam;* Carb-v; *Cup;* Cup-ars; Hyd-ac; Sec; *Ver-a.*

DIARRHOEA Epidemic, during : *Ip;* Pho.

INFANTUM : Aeth; Guai; Med; Psor; Stram; Tab; Zin.

Body remains warm : Bism.

Opisthotonos, with : Med.

MORBUS : Ant-t; Crot-h; Guai; Iris; *Pod;* Ver-a.

CHORDEE : See Erections, Painful.

CHOREA : Abs; *Agar*; Art-v;
Bell; Calc; CAUS; Chin; Cic;
Cimi; Cina; *Cup*; Ign; LACH;
Mag-p; Myg; Nux-v; *Stram*;
Tarn; Ver-v.

CHILDREN, Who have grown,
too fast : Pho.

COITION, After (women) :
Agar; Ced.

COLOUR, Bright, sight of Amel
: Tarn.

CORDIS : Cimi; Tarn.

DANCING, Excessive : Bell;
Hyo; Stram.

EAR, Piercing, from : Lach.

EATING Agg : Ign.

EMISSION, Seminal, with :
Dios.

EMOTIONS, From : Laur; Mag-p.

EXERTION Amel : Zin.

FACE, Of : *Caus*; Cic; Cina;
Cup; Hyo; *Myg*; Nat-m; Zin.
Cold, clammy, up to knee
with : Laur.

FOOT, Sweat, suppressed,
from : Form.

FRIGHT or Shock : *Caus* : Cup;
Cup-ar; Nat-m; Visc; Zin.

HAEMORRHAGES, After : Stic.

HANDS, Of : Cina.

HOLDING Amel : Asaf.

+ HYSTERIA, And : Croc.

IMITATION, From : Caus; Cup;
Tarn.

JERKS, Constant, cannot
keep still : Laur.

LEFT Arm, right leg : Agar;
Cimi.

LONG STANDING, Obstinate :
Chlo-hyd.

LYING, Back, on Amel: *Cup;*
Ign.

MENSES, Absent or difficult,
with : *Pul.*
During : *Zin.*

MISSES, Laying hold on
anything : Asaf.

MUSCLES, Local, of : Hyo.

MUSIC Amel : Tarn.

+ OLD Age : Aeth.

POCKET, Keeping hand in :
Ast-r.

PREGNANCY During : Bell;
Caus; Cup; Gel.

PUBERTY, At: Asaf; Caul; *Cimi*;
Ign; Pul.

RHEUMATIC : *Caus*; Cimi;
Rhus-t; Spig.

RETURN At the same hour:
Ign.

RIGHT Arm, left leg : Tarn.

RUN or Jump, must, cannot
walk : Buf; Kali-br; Nat-m.
Better than walking : Tarn.

SIDE, One : Calc; Cocl; Cup.
Lain, on : Cimi.

SLEEP Agg : Tarn; Ver-v; Zin.
Amel : *Agar*; Cup; Hell;
Mag-p; Myg.

STOOLS, At Agg : Mag-p.

SWALLOW, Can not : Art-v.

SYMPATHETIC : Caus.

THUNDERSTORM, Approaching
Agg : Agar; Rhod.

TONGUE, Protrusion of, with :
Sumb.

WEEKLY : Croc.

WET, After getting : Rhus-t.

WINE Agg : Zin.

CHOROID : Pho.

CHRONICITY : *Alu*; Arg-n; *Ars*; *Calc; Caus*; *Con;* Kali-bi; Kali-io; *Lyc*; Mang; Pho; Plb; Psor; *Sep; Sul*; Syph; Tub.

STUBBORN : Kali-io.

CICATRICES : Calc-f; Caus; Flu-ac; *Grap*; Hypr; *Merc*; Naj; Petr; Phyt; Sil; Syph; Thiosin.

+ **A**BSORPTION, Aids : Grap.

BLUE, Become : Sul-ac.

BURN : Carb-an; Grap; Tell.

+ **C**ANCEROUS Diathesis : Grap.

DEPRESSED, Round : Kali-bi; Syph.

DESCOLOURED, Raised : Bad.

GREEN, Become : Led.

ITCH : Flu-ac; Iod; Led; Naj. Pimples, with : Iod.

PAINFUL : Hypr; Nat-m; *Sil*. Weather, change of, during : Nit-ac.

PURPLE, Become : Asaf.

+ Ulcerate, and : Asaf.

RED, Become : Lach; Nat-m; Sul-ac.

RE-OPEN: Carb-v; *Caus;* Croc; Crot-h; Flu-ac; Glo; *Graph;* Iod; Lach; Nat-m; PHO; SIL. Cracks and Burns : Sars. suppurate : Croc. turn black : Asaf.

SHINY : Sil.

TENSION, In : Kali-c.

THICK : *Grap.*

ULCERATE : Asaf; Calc-p.

VESICLES, Around : Flu-ac.

WHITE : Radm; Syph.

CIRCULATION : See Blood.

CLAIRVOYANCE : Aco; Lach; Lyss; Med; Nux-m; Op; Pho.

CLAUSTROPHOBIA : See Fear of narrow places.

CLAVICLE, AIR : Chlor; Rum.

COLD **W**ATER running from, down to toes, along a narrow line, as if : Caus.

EMACIATION, About : Lyc; Nat-m.

HAWKING Agg: Rum.

PAINFUL : Lac-c; Tell; Pul.

SKIN Blue : Thu.

STITCH : Ol-an; Pul.

TENSION : Lyc; Zin.

UNDER : Calc-p; Cratae; Rum.

CLAVUS : See Plug.

CLIMAXIS : Aco; Amyl-n; Cimi; Con; Fer; Gel; Grap; LACH; Mang; Meli; Murx; Psor; Pul; Sabi; *Sang; Sep;* Stro; *Sul;* Sul-ac; Sumb; Vip; Xanth.

HYPERTROPHY (Body) one side : Lyc.

PREMATURE : Abs.

WOMEN, Fat : Calc-ar.

CLITORIS : Am-c; Coll.

ERECT, Urination, after, sexual desire, with: Calc-p.

STITCHING, Stinging (night) : Bor.

SWOLLEN, As if : Colch; Coll.

64

CLOTHES COLD, As if : Ars-io.

DAMP, As if : Calc; Guai;
Lac-d; Lyc; Pho; Ran-b;
Sanic; Sep; Tub; Ver-v.

FIRE, On, as if : Ars-io.

FIT, HIM, would not: Ver-v.

HEAVY, Too : Con; Euphor.

LARGE, Too : Psor; Thu.

PACKS and UNPACKS without
consciousness : Mag-c.

PRESSURE Of *Agg* : Arg-n; Bov;
Bry; *Calc*; Carb-v; Caus;
Con; Glo; Hep; LACH;
Lil-t; LYC; Nit-ac; *Nux-v;*
Onos; Psor; Sec; Sep; Spo;
Sul; *Tub.*

AMEL : Psor; Saba.

Chest, on Agg : Benz-ac.

Groins, about Agg : Hyds.

Neck, about Agg : Agar; *Ap;*
Caus; Chel; Con; Glo;
Kali-c; LACH; Merc; *Sep.*

+ Pit of stomach : Lith.

Waist about, Agg : Ap; Bro;
Carbo-v; Grap; Lach.

+ TEARS : Cam.

TIGHT, As if : Arg-m; Caus;
Chel; Glo; Nux-v; Rum.

Abdomen, about : Mos.

Chest, about : Meli.

UNCOMFORTABLE : Spo.

Groins, about : Hyds.

WEAR His best : Con.

CLOUDY WEATHER AGG : Alo;
Am-c; Arn; Ars-io; Aur;
Bar-c; Cham; Chin; Hypr;
Lach; Mang; Merc; Nux-m;
Pul; *Rhus-t;* Sabal; Sabi;

Sep; Stram; Vio-o.

AMEL : Bry; Kalm; Lapp.

MENTAL EFFECTS Agg : Alo;
Pho.

CLUTCHING Sensation :
Bell; Cact; Lil-t; Thyr.

COAL GAS *AGG* : Am-c; Arn;
Bell; Bov; Carb-s; Cof; Op;
Sec.

COAT, Wears in summer, hot
weather : Hep; Hyo; Kali-ar;
Merc; Psor.

COATED or FURRED As if :
Alu; Caus; Chin; *Cocl*; Colch;
Dig; *Dros; Iris*; Kali-c; *Merc;*
Nux-m; PHO; Pho-ac; PUL;
Rhod; Ver-a.

COBWEB Sensation : Alu;
Bar-c; BOR; Bro; Calc; Con;
GRAP; Ran-sc; Sumb.

COCCYX : *Ap*; Arn; Bels; *Caus;*
Hypr; Kre; Rut; Sil; Zin.

ABSCESS Just below : Paeon.

BENT, Back, as if : Mag-p.

BRUISED, As if, sitting,
preventing : Am-m; Cist.

BURNING : Pho.

Sitting, on : Ap; Cist.

Touched, when : Carb-an;
Cist.

COITION Agg : Kali-br.

DRAWING : Caus.

ELONGATED, As if : Xanth.

HEAVY : Ant-c; Ant-t; Arg-n.

INJURY : Bels; Carb-an; *Hypr;*
Mez; Sil.

ITCHING : Bov; Grap.

JERKS, Menses, during : Cic.

MOTION, Slight Agg : Tarn.

NUMB : Plat.

PAINFUL: Carb-an; Cast-eq; Caus; Con; Grat; *Hypr;* Petr; Sil; Tarn; Thu; Xanth.

Abdomen, pressing on Amel : Merc.

Fall, as from : Kali-io.

+ Menses, during : Cic.

+ Soles, tender, with : Thu.

Stool, during : Pho; Sul.

after : Euphor; Grat.

+ Urination, before : Kali-bi.

PARTURITION, After : Tarn.

PULLING, Up, from : Lil-t.

RIDING, Carriage, in Agg : Nux-m.

RISING From a seat Agg : Euphor; *Lach; Sil*; Sul.

Amel : Kre.

SITTING Agg : Am-m; Ap; Kali-bi; Par; Petr.

On something sharp,as if : Lach.

SLEEP, During Agg : Am-m.

STANDING Amel : Arg-n; Tarn.

STITCHES : Pho-ac.

SWELLED, As if : Syph.

THIGHS, To : Rhus-t.

ULCER : Paeon.

+ UP and DOWN : Kali-bi.

UP, Spine to occiput : Pho.

Stools, after : Euphor.

during : Pho.

To, arms : Hypr.

URINATION Agg : Grap; Kali-bi.

WEIGHT : See Heavy.

COITION, AVERSION, to (males) : Arn; Clem; *Grap; Lyc;* Rhod; Psor.

AGG : AGAR; Buf; Calad; *Calc;* Canth; *Chin; Grap;* KALI-C; Kali-p; Kre; Lyc; *Nat-c; Nat-m;* Nat-p; Pho-ac; Sele; *Sep; Sil;* Spig; Stan; Stap; Sul.

AMEL : CON; Merc; *Stap.*

FRIGHT, During Agg : Lyc.

+ INCOMPLETE : Nat-c.

INTERRUPTED Agg: Bell.

MOTIONS, As of : Caus; Pho.

PAINFUL (males) : Arg-n; Calc; Sabal.

COLD AGG (Easily chilled, Lack of vital heat): *Agar;* Am-c; Ant-t; Aran; ARS; *Aur;* Bar-c; CALC; Calc-f; *Calc-p; Cam; Caps;* CAUS; *Chin;* Cimi; *Cist;* Cocl; Colch; *Dul; Eup-p;* Fer; *Grap; Hell;* Hep; Hypr; *Kali-bi;* KALI-C; Lac-d; *Lyc; Mag-c; Mag-p;* Merc; Mez; MOS; *Nit-ac; Nux-m; Nux-v;* Pho; Pho-ac; *Psor;* Pyro; Ran-b; *Rhod;* RHUS-T; *Rum;* SABA; *Sep;* SIL; Spig; *Stan;* STRO; Sul; VER-A.

AMEL (Uncovering or cold application amel): *Aco; Ap;* Arg-n; Asar; *Aur;* Calc; Cam; *Cham;* Dros; Fer; Flu-ac; Guai; IOD; Kali-i; Kali-s; *Led; Lyc;* Merc; Mur-ac; *Op;* Psor; PUL; Rhus-t; Sabi; *Sec;* Spig; SUL; Syph; Tab; Thu.

HEAD, To Agg : Ant-c; Bar-c.

HEAT, AND BOTH AGG : Ant-c; Calc; *Caus;* Fer; *Flu-ac;* Grap; Hell; Kali-c; Lach; MERC; *Nat-m; Pho-ac;* Sep; Sil; Sul; Sul-ac; Syph; Tab; Thu.

NEEDLES, as if : *Agar;* Ars.

NIGHT, HOT DAYS With AGG : Aco; Dul; Merc-c; Rum.

PAINFUL Is : Cist; Mez; Mos.

PAINS : Arn; Med; Syph.

PLACE, ENTERING AGG : *Ars;* Bell; *Ip;* Kali-ar; Nux-v; *Ran-b; Sep.*

SINGLE PART Of, as hands in cold water, head, feet AGG : Agar; Am-c; Bell; *Calc;* HEP; *Nux-v; Pho;* Psor; RHUS-T; *Sep;* SIL; Tarn; Thu; Zin.

SITTING, Lying on ground or a moist floor Agg : Ars; Calc; Caus; Dul; *Nux-v;* Rhod; Sil.

SORES : *Ars;* Hep; NAT-M; Pho; *Rhus-t;* Sep.

TENDENCY To Take : Aco; Alu; *Ars; Ars-io;* Bacil; Bar-c; Bry; CALC; *Calc-p; Cham;* Dul; Hep; KALI-C; Kali-p; Lyc; Mag-c; Merc; *Nat-m; Nit-ac;* NUX-V; Ol-j; Pho; Pho-ac; *Psor;* Rhus-t; *Sep;* SIL; *Sul; Tub.*

Draft, chest on Agg : Pho-ac.

Menses, first *A*gg : Calc-p.

Overheated, being, after : Kali-c.

Sweating, after : Nit-ac.

WEATHER Agg : See Air open or cool, Change of agg.

COLDNESS: *Aco;* Am-c; Aran; ARN; *Ars;* Aur; Bell; *Bry; Calc; Cam;* Caps; Caus; *Chin;* Dul; *Eup-p;* Fer; *Gel;* Grap; *Hep;* Ign; Ip; Kali-c; Kali-p; *Laur; Led; Lyc;* Mag-p; Merc; *Mos; Nat-m;* Nux-m; NUX-V; *Pho; Pho-ac; Psor;* Pul; *Pyro;* Rhus-t; Saba; *Sep; Sil;* Symp; VER-A.

AFFECTED PARTS, Of : Ars; Bry; Calc; Caps; Caus; Cocl; Colch; Lach; Led; *Meny; Mez; Rhus-t; Sec;* Sil.

ALTERNATING Or Coinciding, heat in other parts, with : Polyg.

BED, In : Pho; Sil.

Early *A.M,* : Mur-ac.

BEARING, Down, with : Castr; Sec; Sil.

COLD Water, as if in : Led.

COUGHING Agg : Lyc.

COVERS Agg : *Ap;* Calc-s; Cann; Ip; Led; *Pul;* Sec; Sep.

EXERTION, From : Plb; Sil; Zin-val.

EXTERNAL : Am-m; Ars; Cam; Ign; Kali-n; Nit-ac; *Nux-v;* Old; *Ver-a; Zin.*

+ Internal burning, with : Sec.

EXTREMITIES, Of : Amb; Ant-t; Ars; *Bell;* Calc; Cam; *Carb-v;* Caus; Pul; Sec; Sil; Stram;

Ver-a.

FANNING, Wants : *Carb-v*.

FLUSHES, Of : Lach.

+ HOT Weather, In : Asar.

+ Icy : Agar; *Ap*; Cact; *Carb-v*; Elap; *Helod*; Hyd- ac; *Lyc*; Med; Meny; Nit-ac; Ol-an; Pho; *Sec*; *Sil*; Ver-a.

+ Body, of : Bar-m; Jat.

Cramps, colic, with : Cup-ac.

Fire, even near : Cadm.

Menses, with : Sil.

Nausea, vomiting, with: Val.

Pain, with : Dul.

INTERNAL : Anac; *Ap; Ars; Calc*; Caus; Cocl; Dig; Elap; Hep; *Laur*; Merc; Nux-v; Pho; Pul; *Sul*; Ther.

MENSES, At the start of : Jab.

During : Led; Sil.

NIGHT Agg : Meny; Pho.

OF ONE PART, other Part hot : Ap; Bry; Cham; *Polyg*; Zin.

ONE SIDED: *Bry*; Carb-v; *Caus*; Con; *Dros*; Lyc; *Mos*; Nux-v; Par; *Pul*; Sil; Thu.

Convulsion, during : Sil.

Right : Bar-c; Bry; Chel; Rhus-t; Saba.

Left hot, as if : Par.

epilepsy, before : Sil.

Left : Carb-v; Caus; Dros; Lyc; Sul; Thu.

PAIN, During: Agar; Alu-sil; Ars; Caus; Dul; Led; Mos; Sil.

Nerve, along: Terb.

PARTIAL, of Single parts : Ars;

Berb; Calc; Carb-v; Chel; Chin;Cist; *Dul; Ign;* Kali-c; Kali-chl; Lyc; Meny; Nat-m; Pho-ac; Plat; PUL; *Rhus-t;* Sec; *Sep;* Sil; *Spig;* Sul; VER-A.

Burn, when become warm : Zin-val.

PARTS Lain, on : Arn; Mur-ac.

RISING From Stooping, on : Merc-c.

ROOM, Warm, in : Sep.

SCRATCHING, After : Agar; Mez; Petr.

SPOTS, In : Agar; Calc-p; Petr; Sep; Stro; Tarn; *Ver-a*.

UPPER, Parts : Ip.

COLDS : See Coryza.

TAKING AGG : Bell; Bry; Calc; *Cam;* Carb-an; Cham; Cist; Colo; Kali-n; Merc.

Menses, first, during Agg : Calc-p.

COLIC : See Pain, Cramping, and Flatulence.

COLITIS MUCOUS : Asar; Colch; Cop; Kali-p; Rhus-t; Zin-val.

COLLAPSE (Rapid, prostration) : *Aco*; Aeth; *Am-c;* Ant-t; Arn; ARS; *Cam;* Carb-s; CARB-V; Colch; Con; Cup; Hyd-ac; Ip; Laur; Merc-cy; Naj; Pho; Sec; Sep; Tab; Sul; VER-A; Ver-v.

DIARRHOEA, After : *Ars;* Cam; *Carb-v;* Sec; *Ver-a*.

DRY : Am-c; Cam; Phys.

HEART, Of : Am-c.

INJURY, From : Acet-ac; Sul-ac.

MOIST : Colch.

NERVOUS : Am-c; Laur.

PARALYSIS, Before : Con.

PHOTOPSIES, After : Sep.

SUDDEN : Ars; Crot-h; Grap; Hyd-ac; Pho; Sep.

VOMITING, After : *Ars*; Ver-a. During : Ars.

COLLAR (See pressure of clothes around neck) *Agg*.: Ant-c; Cench; Lach; Merc-c.

-TIGHT, Too, as if: Amy-n; Sep.

+ **COLLIQUATIVE** STATES : *Jab.*

COLOURS BRIGHT AGG : Sil.

AMEL : *Stram; Tarn.*

COMA : See Unconsciousness.

VIGIL : Aco; Hyd-ac; *Hyo;* Laur; Mur-ac; Op; Pho.

COME And GO: See Pain, Fleeting.

COMPANY CROWD *Agg* : Aco; *Amb*; Anac; Ant-c; Aur; BAR-C; Bell; *Carb-an; Cham; Cic;* GEL; IGN; Lyc; *Nat-c; Nat-m; Nux-v; Sep;* Thu.

Menses, during Agg : Con.

AMEL (Desire for) : Arg-n; *Ars*; Bism; Bov; Dros; Hep; Hyo; Kali-c; Lac-c; Lyc; *Pho*; Radm; STRAM.

COMPLAINING, LAMENTING : Aur; *Cof*; Lyc; *Ver-a*; Ver-v.

PLAINTIVE, Sleep, in : Stan.

COMPLAINTS, DESCRIBE,

Cannot properly: Pul.

BROODS Over imaginary : Naj.

+ **COMPLEXION** CLEARS : Sars.

COMPREHENSION, DIFFICULT : See Dull.

WHAT he reads or hears about : Sele.

COMPRESSION : See Pain, Squeezing.

CONCENTRATION, DIFFICULT : See Dull and Distraction.

CONCUSSIONS : Arn; Bry; Cic; Con; *Rhus-t*; Sul.

CONDIMENTS : See Food.

CONDYLES : See under Bones.

CONDYLOMATA (See Fungus Growth) : *Med; Nit-ac;* Psor; *Thu.*

CONFIDENCE, WANT of Self : *Anac;* Arg-n; Ars; *Lyc; Old;* Pic-ac; *Sil;* Ther.

CONFUSION, Incoherence, muddled : BELL; *Bry; Calc;* Caps; *Carb-v; Gel;* HYO; Lyc; *Nux-v;* PHO; PHO-AC; RHUS-T; Sep; STRAM; Tab; Tub; *Ver-a;* Zin.

DAILY *Affairs,* About : Lyc.

LOCATION, About : Cic; *Glo; Nux-m; Petr.*

ONE'S Own indentity : *Alu.*

PRESENT, For the past : Cic.

WAKING, On : Bov; Chin; Gel.

CONGESTION : *Aco; Alo;* Amyl-n; Ap; *Arn;* Aur; BELL; Bry; Cact; *Calc ; Chin;* Cup; *Fer-p;* Gel; *Glo;* Lach; Lil-t; Meli;Mill; Nat-s; Nux-v; Op;

Pho; *Pul;* Rhus-t; Sang; Sep; *Sul;* Terb; *Ver-v;* Vip.

SUDDEN : Aco; Bell; Glo; Ver-v.

CONICAL FORMATION : See Acuminate.

CONJUNCTIVA : *Aco;* Ap; ARG-N; Ars; *Bell; Cep;* EUPHR; Merc; PUL; Rhus-t; *Sul.*

GRANULAR : Ap; Arg-n; Ars; Kali-bi.

INFLAMED (Conjunctivitis): *Aco; Ap; Arg-n;* Arn; *Ars;* BELL; Calc; Calc-s; CEP; EUPHR; *Merc;* PUL; *Rhus-t;* SUL.

Gonorrhoel : Arg-n; Kali-bi; Nit-ac; *Pul.*

Menses absent, with : Euphr.

PHLYCTAENAE : Ars; Grap.

POUTING : Nit-ac.

RAW : Kali-io; Lyc.

SACCULAR : Ap; Ars.

SPOTS, Yellow: Pho-ac.

SPRING, In : Kob; Nux-v.

ULCER : Alu; Caus.

CONSCIENCE, + TERROR Of, ill effects of : Cyc.

+ TROUBLED, From, (anxiety) : Dig.

CONSOLATION *Agg* : Arg-n; Cact; Hell; *Ign;* Kali-s; Lil-t; *Nar-m; Sep; Sil;* Sul; Syph.

AMEL : Asaf; *Pul.*

REFUSES, For one's own misfortune : Nit-ac.

CONSPIRACIES, Suspects *Against Him,* there were :

Ars; Lach; Plb; Pul.

CONSTIPATION *Agg* : Alo; Arg-n.

AMEL: *Calc;* Merc; *Psor;* Ust.

CONSTIPATION (Remedies in general) : ALU; Alum; Anac; BRY; *Calc;* Caus; *Cocl;* Coll; Con; GRAP; *Hep;* Hydr; *Kali-c;* Lac-d; Lach; *Lyc;* Mag-m; *Nat-m;* Nux-m; NUX-V; *Op; Pho;* Plat; *Plb;* Rut; *Sanic;* Sep; SIL; *Stap; Sul;* Thu; Ver-a; Zin.

ABSOLUTE : Op.

ALTERNATE *Days, On* : Calc; Cocl; Con; Kali-c; Lyc; Nat-m.

BOWELS, Action lost, as if : Aeth.

Rectal atony : Alet.

CHRONIC : Bry; Grap; Lac-d; *Nux-v;* Op; Plb; Sul; Sul-io; Ver-a.

CLOUDY Weather Agg : Alo.

COLDS Agg : Ign.

+ DAYS, For, no desire : Alum; Grap.

+ DEBILITATED, Literary persons : Nicc.

DIARRHOEA, Alternating with : ANT-C; Calc; *Chel;* Fer; Kali-c; Lyc; Nat-s; Nit-ac; *Nux-v;* Op; Pho; *Pod;* Pul; Sul.

Old People, in : Ant-c; Pho.

+ HABITUAL : Sul; Tab.

HARD FAECES, from : Alu; *Bry; Grap;* Mag-m; Nat-m;

Nit-ac; Nux-v; Op; Plb; Sil;
Sul; Verb.

HEART, Weakness of, with :
Phyt.

HEAT Of body, with : Cup.

HOME, Away from, when :
Lyc.

INACTIVITY, From, difficult
stools : *Alu;* Alum; *Bry;*
Chin; Grap; *Hep;* Kali-c;
Mag-m; *Nat-m;* Nux-m;
Nux-v; Op; Plb; Pyro; Psor;
Rut; Sanic; Sele; Sil.

INFANTS. Of : Aesc; Alu; Bry;
Coll; Lyc; Mag-m; Nux-v;
Plb; Psor; Sele; Sep;
Ver-a.

Bottlefed, artificial food
: Alu; Nux-v; Op.

Newborn : Zin.

LEAN FAR BACK, must, to pass
stool : Med.

MENSES, After : Kali-c.

Amel : Aur.

Instead of : Grap.

MENTAL, SHOCK, Nervous
strain, from : Mag-c.

+ MILK, Cold, Amel : Iod.

MONDAY, Every : Stan.

NEURASTHENIA, With : Ign.

OBSTINATE : Aeth; Ascl; Hydr;
Sul-io; Syph.

+ Infants, in : Croc.

+ nursing : Ver-a.

. Old people : Phyt.

PAINFUL : Nit-ac; Tub.

PREGNANCY, During : Hyds;
Lach; Lyc; Nat-s; Nux-v;

Plat; Plb; Sep.

PURGATIVES Or Enema Amel
: Lac-d.

No relief from : Tarn.

RIDING, Carriage, in from :
Ign.

SEA, Going to, from : Bry;
Lyc.

STANDING Amel : Alu; CAUS.

STOOL, Difficult, from : Bry;
Chin; Mag-m; Nat-m;
Nux-v.

Though soft : *Alu;* Anac;
Chin; *Hep;* Ign; *Nux-m;*
Plat; Psor; Pul; *Sep;* Sil;
Stap.

STOOL Recede : Mag-m; *Op;*
Sanic; *Sil;* Thu.

menses during : Sil.

Removed must be : Lyc;
Nat-m; Plat; Sanic; Sele;
Sep; Sil.

Scanty, with profuse
urination at night : Alu;
Bry; Caus; Grap; Hep;
Kali-c; Kre; Lyc; Nat-c;
Nux-v; Rhus-t; Sabi;
Samb; Scil; Sep; Spig;
Sul.

STRAIN, Must : Alu; Chin; Coll;
Nat-m; *Nux-v;* Rat;Sep; Sil.

TRAVELLING, While : Alu; Lyc;
Nux-v; Op; *Plat.*

UNABLE To pass the stool in
presence of others : AMB.

UNSATISFACTORY, Insufficient
stools, from : Alo; *Alu;* Arn;
Caps;Card-m; Cham; *Grap;*
Kali-c; LYC; *Mag-m:*

MERC-C; NAT-C; Nat-m; Nit-ac; NUX-V; Sele; *Sep; Sul.*

URGING, Abortive : Anac; Con; Lyc; Mag-m; Nat-m; *Nux-v;* Pul; Sep; Sil; Sul.

Absence, of : Alu; *Bry;* Grap; Hydr; *Op.*

Coition, after : Nat-p.

Constant, not for stools : Lach.

   urination Amel : Lil-t.

Crampy : Plb.

Eating, on : Sanic.

Erection, with : Ign; Thu.

Ineffectual : Caps; Lac-d; Merc; *Merc-c*; Rhe; Rhus- t; *Sul.*

Irresistible : Alo; Nat-c.

Neuralgia, with : Iris.

Passes flatus only : ALO; Carb-v; Mag-m; Myr; Nat- c; *Nat-s*; Pho; Rut; Sep.

Rectum, prolapse of, with : Rut.

Sleep, in : Phyt.

Stool, after : Merc.

Urination, Amel : Lil-t.

Walking Agg : Kob.

URINE, Frequent, with : Sars.

   Retention of, with : Canth.

WEATHER Cold : Ver-a.

WORKING, Days, after : See Monday.

CONSTRICTION, BAND, Gathered together etc : Anac; Arg-n; Ars; Asar; BELL; CACT; Carb-ac; Carb-v; Chel; *Chin;* Cimi;Cocl; Con; Grap; Hyo; *Ign; Lach;* Lyc; Merc; Merc-c; *Naj;* NIT-AC; Nux- v; *Plat; Plb; Pul;* Radm; Rat; Rhus-t; Sil; Stan; Stram; Sul.

+ HOLLOW Organs : Tab.

+ IRON BAND encircled with, as if : Colo.

PAIN, During: Colo; Ign; Lyc.

PARALYTIC, States, in : Alum.

CONSUMPTION, TUBERCU *Losis* : Agar; Ars; CALC; CALC-P; Dros; *Hep; Iod;* KALI-C; Kali-s; Kre; Lach; LYC; Nit-ac; Ol-j; Phel; PHO; Psor; PUL; Sang; Senec; *Sep; Sil; Spo;* STAN; *Sul; Ther;* TUB; Zin.

FEVER, In : Bap; Chin-ar; Fer-p.

INCIPIENT : *Iod; Tub.*

INJURY To chest, after : Mill; Rut.

+ NEGLECTED : Kre.

RECURRING : Fer-p; Kali-n.

STONE-CUTTERS' : *Calc*; Lyc; Pul; *Sil.*

WEAKNESS, In : Ars-io; Chin-ar.

+ CONTEMPT, HOLDS Every thing in: Ip.

CONTEMPTUOUS SCORNFUL : Bry; Cham; Chin; Cic; Guai; Nux-v; Plat.

CONTINENCE AGG: Ap; Calc; *Con;* Flu-ac; Lyc; Plat.

CONTORTION, DISTORTIONS : Agar; Bell; Caus; Cic; Guai;

Hyo; Plat; Rut; Sec; Sil; Stram; Tarn.

CONTRACTION : *Am-m;* Anac; Calc; Caus; Colo; Grap; Guai; *Ign;* Lyc; Nat-c; Nat-m; *Plb;* Rut; Sec.

PAIN, After: Abro.

RELAXATION, And : See Opening and shutting.

SENSE Of GENERAL : Am-m; Cact; Guai; Kali-m; Nux-v; Pho.

STIFF, Pain, after : Pho.

CONTRACTURES : See Strictures.

CONTRADICT, Disposition, to : Hep; Rut.

CONTRADICTIONS, INTOLERANT of AGG : Ast-r; Aur; Calc-s; Cocl; Echi; Fer; Helo; *Ign; Lyc;* Nux-v; *Sep;* Thyr.

CONTRADICTORY And ALTERNATING states : Anac; *Ign;* Nat-m; *Pul;* Tub.

CONTRARINESS : Alu; Anac; *Ant-c; Ant-t;* Arg-n; Ars; Bry; *Cham;* Kali-c; Nux-v; Tarn.

CONTROL LACKS: Anac; Arg-m; Arg-n; Caus; Old; Stap; Tarn.

CONVERSATION AGG: Amb; Helo; Ign; Nat-m; Sil; Stap.

AMEL : Aeth; Eup-p; Lac-d.

IMAGINARY Beings, with : Chlo-hyd.

CONVULSIONS, SPASMS : Agar; Amb; *Ars;* Art-v; *Bell;* Buf; *Calc;* Cam; Castr; Caus; Cham; Chin; *Cic;* Cimi; Cina; *Cup; Gel; Hyo;* Hypr;

Ign; Ip; KALI-C; LACH; Med; Mez; Nux-m; *Nux-v;* Op; Plat; Plb; Pul; STAN; STRAM; Sul; Tarn; Thu; Ver-v; ZIN; Zin-val.

RIGHT Side : Bell; *Lyc;* Nux-v.

Left paralysed : Art-v.

LEFT Side : Calc-p; Ip; Sul.

BRAIN Tumour, from : Plb.

CEREBRAL Softening, from: Caus.

CHILDREN, In : Art-v; Bell; Cina; Cof; Hell; Ip; Meli; Op; Stram; Ver-a; Zin.

+ Attention thrust on them, from : Ant-t.

Dentition, during : *Calc; Cham;* Gel; Ign; Terb; Passi; Zin.

Diarrhoea, with : Nux-m.

+ Fear or Fright : Ign.

Holding, when Amel : Nic.

+ Hour, same, daily : Ign.

Nursing angry or frightened mother : Buf.

Playing or laughing, excessively, from : Cof.

Strangers, approach from : Op.

CHOREIC : Stic.

CLONIC and TONIC, alternately : Ign; Mos; Stram.

COITION, During, Agg : Agar; Buf.

After : Agar.

COLDNESS of body, with : Cam; Hell; *Oenan;* Ver-a.

COLIC, During : Bell; Cic; Plb.

CONSCIOUSNESS, with: Cina; Hell; *Ign;* Nux-m; *Nux-v;* Plat; *Stram; Stry.*

without : Arg-n; Buf; *Calc; Canth; Cic;* HYO; Oenan; *Plb;* Visc.

COUGHING, With, after: Cina; Cup; Ip; Just.

DEGENERATIVE : Aur-m; *Pho;* Zin-ph.

DIARRHOEA, After : Mag-p; Zin. with : Nux-m.

DYSMENORRHOEA, With : Caul; Nat-m.

DYSPNOEA, Alternating, with : Plat.

ELBOW, Bending or stretching Amel: Nux-v.

EMISSION, During : Art-v; Grat; *Nat-p.*

EMOTIONAL Excitement, from : Cham; Cup; Nux-v; Op.

EPILEPTIC : See Epilepsy.

ERUCTATION, Amel : Kali-c.

ERUPTIONS Fail to break out, when : Ant-t; *Cup; Zin.*

Suppressed, from : Caus.

FALLING, With : Bell; Cham; Cup; Hyo; Oenan.

FEAR, From : Art-v; Calc; Hyo; Ign; Ind; Op.

FEVER, During : Ars; Bell; Cam; Carb-v; Cina; Hyo; Nux-v; Op; Sep; Stram; Ver-a.

GOITRE Suppression, afte r: Iod.

GRASPING Tight Amel : Mez; Nux-v.

GRIEF, From: Art-v; *Hyo; Op.*

HAEMORRHAGE, After : Ars; Bell; Bry; Calc; Cina; Con; Ign; Lyc; Nux-v; Pul; Sul; Ver-a.

During : Chin; Plb; Plat; Sec.

+ Suppression, from : Mill.

+ HEAD Drawn back : Tab.

HEART Disease, from : Calc-ar.

HYSTERICAL : Asaf; Cimi; Con; Ign; Mos; Stan; Zin-val.

INJURIES, After : Cic; Hep; Hypr; Nat-s; Op; Rhus-t; Val.

Head, to : Art-v.

Slight : Val.

Spinal : Zin.

INTERNAL : Caus; *Cocl; Hyo;* Ign; Ip; Mag-m; Nux-v; Pul; Stan.

KNOCKING Body, from : Hypr.

LAUGHING, While: Cof; Grap.

LIGHT, Glare, of Agg : Op; *Psor;* Pul; *Pyro;* Rhus-t; Saba; *Sep;*

LIMBS, Attempting to use, on : Cocl; PIC-AC.

MASTURBATION, After : Buf; Calc; Lach; *Plat;* Stram; Sul.

MENSES, Before : Buf; Caus; Cup; Hyo; Kali-br; Pul; Ver-v.

During : Art-v; Cedr; Cup; Gel; Oenan; Plat.

After : Syph; Ver-v.

Instead, of : Cic; Oenan; Pul.

Suppressed, from : Buf; Calc- p; Cocl; Gel; Glo; Mill; Pul.

MILK, Suppressed, from : Agar.

MISCARRAIGE, After : Rut.

NIGHT, At : *Cup*; Nit-ac.

Vertigo, during day time : Nit-ac.

NOISE Amel : Hell.

ONE SIDE : Art-v; Calc-p; Ip; Plb.

Paralysis of other : Art-v.

Speechlessness, with : Dul.

OPISTHOTONOS, With : Ver-v.

PAINS, During: *Bell*; Colo; Ign; Kali-c; Lyc; Nux-v.

After : Chin; Plat.

PARALYSIS,With : *Caus*; Nux-m.

PREGNANCY, During : See Eclampsia.

PRESSURE on spine Agg : Tarn.

PRODROME, As a : Ver-v.

PUBERTY, At in girls : Art-v; Caul; Caus.

PUERPERAL : See Eclampsia.

PUNISHMENT, From : Agar; Cham; Cina; *Ign.*

RELIGIOUS, Excitement, from : Ver-a.

RUBBING, Amel : Pho; Sec.

RUNS, In Circle, before : Caus.

SLEEP, During : *Ars*; BELL; Kali-c; Lach; Sep; *Sil; Sul.*

+ SLEEPLESS, And : Alu; Bell;

Bry; Calc; Carb-an; Cup; Hep; Hyo; Ign; Ip; Kali-c; Merc; Mos; *Nux-v;* Pho; Pho-ac; Pul; Rhe; Rhus-t; Sele; Sep; Sil; Stro; Thu.

STOMACH, pressure Slight on, from : Canth.

STOOLS, During : Nux-v.

STRANGE PERSON approach or sight of : Lyss; Op.

SUDDEN : Hyd-ac.

SUPPRESSION From : Abs; Caus; Mill.

SUPPURATIVE Conditons from : Ars; Buf; Tarn.

TEARS and/or Laughter with : Alu.

TOBACCO Swallowing, from : Ip.

TONIC : *Bell;* Buf; Cam; *Cic; Ign; Ip; Op;* Petr; Plat; *Sec;* Sep.

Single parts, of : Ign.

TOUCHED, When : *Cic.*

TWITCHING, With : Ver-v.

URAEMIC : Ap; Ars; Oenan; *Ver-v.*

VACCINATION, Afte r: *Sil.*

VERTIGO, After : Hyo; Tarn.

VOMITING Amel : Agar.

with : Ant-c.

WETTING, From : Cup.

WHOOPING Cough, with : Hyd-ac.

WORMS, From : Cic; *Cina;* Ign; Stan.

YAWNING, While : Grap.

CO-ORDINATION DISTURBED
: *Agar;* *Alu;* Arg-n; Bar-c;
Bell; Caus; *Cimi; Cocl;* Con;
Echi; Fer; Gel; Glo; Grap;
Hyo; Ign; Kali-p; Lach; Merc;
Nux-v; Onos; Pho; Plat;
Rhus-t; Sul.

COPPER COLOUR (Discharge,
skin, etc.) : Carb-an; Cor-r;
Merc; Mez; Nit-ac; *Rhus-t;*
Syph.

ERUPTIONS : Hydroc; Merc-d;
Sars.

FUMES AGG : Ip; Merc; Pul.

SPOTS : Benz-ac; Lach; Med;
Nit-ac.

Remaining, eruptions after
: Med.

CORNEA, Affections, in
General : CALC; *Cann;* Con;
Euphr; Hep; Merc; Merc-i-f;
Pul; Sul.

HERPES On: Ran-b.

INFLAMED (Keratitis) : Calc;
Merc; Merc-c; Sul; Syph;
Thu.

Bathing cold Amel : Syph.

Recurrent : Grap.

INJECTED : *Aur;* Grap; Ign;
Merc.

OPACITY : *Ap;* Arg-n; Cadm;
Calc; CANN; Con; LACH;
Pul; Sil; SUL; ZIN-S.

Dense : Kali-bi.

Injury, from : Euphr.

Old age, in (Arcus senilis) :
Calc; Kali-c; Merc; Pho;
Pul; Sul; Vario.

Small-pox vaccination ,

after : Sil.

Spots, in : Calc-f.

PUSTULES, On : Kali-m.

ROUGH : Sil

+ SCRATCHED or Chipped, as
if : Merc-i-f.

SPOTS, On : Ap; Calc; Con;
Nit-ac.

Yellow, with network of
blood vessels around :
Aur.

+ SUNKEN : Aeth.

ULCERS : Arg-n; *Ars;* Calc;
Euphr; Hep; *Kali-bi;*
Merc-c; Sil; Sul.

Pain and photophobia,
without : Kali-bi.

Perforating : Ap.

CORNS : See Callosities.

CORPULENCE : See Obesity.

CORRODING : See Discharges
acrid.

CORYZA : *Aco;* Amb; ARS;
Bell; Calc; *Cam;* Carb-v;
CEP; *Cham;* Chel; *Euphr;*
Eup-p; *Fer-p;* GEL; *Hep;* Ign;
Kali-io; Lac-c; Lach; MERC;
Merc-c; Nat-m; Nit-ac;
Nux-v; Pho; PUL; *Rhus-*t;
Saba; Sele; Stap;*Sul;* Tell;
Thu.

AGED, of : Am-c; Ant-c;
Cam.

Palpitation, with : Anac.

AIR, Open, Amel : Calc-p;
Calc-s; Cep; Nux-v; Stic.

And Agg : Tell.

ALTERNATE Days : Nat-c.

ANNUAL (Hayfever) : Ars;

76

Ambro; Cep; Gel; KALI-IO;
Kali-p; Nat-m; *Nux-v;* Pho;
PSOR; Saba; Senec; Sep;
SIL; Sinap; SUL.

ASCENDING : Aru-t; *Bro;*
Lac-c; Merc; Sep.

AUTUMN, In : Merc.

BLOODY, Infants, in : Calc-s.

CHANGEABLE : Stap.

CHANGE of Season, tempera
ture : Cep; Gel.

CHILDREN, In : Merc-i-r.

+ Discharge, bluish : Am-m.

CHILL, With : Merc; Nux-v.

CHILLED By snow or ice, from
: Ant-c; Dros; Iod; Laur;
Pul; Seneg; Ver-a; Verb.

CHRONIC : Bro; Cist; Hep;
Kali-bi; Sil; Sul.

Asthma, causing : Sil.

COLD Bathing Amel : Calc-s.

COUGHING Agg : Agar; Bell;
Euphr; Ip; *Lach*; Nit-ac;
Scil; Sul; Thu.

DAY, By : Nux-v.

Damp Agg : Kali-io.

DESCENDING : Ars; Bry;
Carb-v; Iod; Kali-c; Lyc;
Pho; Stic; Sul; Tub.

DIPHTHERIA, In : Aru-t; Kali-
bi; Nit-ac.

DIARRHOEA, Then: Alu; Calc;
Sang; Sele; Tub.

DRAFT, Least Agg : Nat-c.

DRY: Calc; Caus; Chin;
Mag- c; Nux-v; Pho; Samb;
Stic.

Indoors : Thyr.

Nose, obstruction with :
Mang.

DYSPNOEA, With : Ars-io;
Kali-io; Nit-ac.

EATING Agg : Carb-an; Nux-v;
Sanic; Tromb.

EPISTAXIS, With : Senec; Sil.

EXHAUSTING : Arg-m.

FEVER, In : Bry; Merc.

FLOWERS, Odour of Agg : Saba;
Sang.

FLUENT, Indoors : Calc-p; Cep;
Nux-v.

Dry and alternately :
Nat-m.

Thick and alternately :
Stap.

HAIR-CUT, After : Bell; *Nux-v;*
Sep.

HEADACHE, Then : Ant-c.

HOARSENESS, With : Ars-io;
Caus; Tell.

HOT : Cham; Iod.

HUNGER, With : Ars-io.

+ KNEES, Hot, with : Ign.

LYING Agg : Euphr; Spig.

Amel : Merc.

MENSES, At : Am-c; Bar-c;
Grap; Kali-c; *Lach;* Mag-c;
Pho; Senec; Sep; Zin.

MILK Agg : Lac-d.

NEWBORN : Dul.

NOSE, Stopped, with : Ars.

ONE SIDE : Nux-v; Pho; Phyt.

PEACHES, Odour of Agg : Cep.

PERIODICAL Attacks : *Bro;*
Grap; Sil.

77

POLYURIA, With : Calc.

SALIVATION, With: Calc-p; Kali-io.

SEA-BATHING Amel : Med.

SINGER'S : Cep.

SLEEP, In : Flu-ac; Lac-c.

SMELL, Acute, with : Kalm.

SNEEZING, Then : Naj.

With : Carb-an.

STOOPING Agg : Laur.

STOPPED, Suppressed : Ars; *Aru-t*; Bell; Bro; Bry; Calc; Chin; LACH; *Lyc*; Mar-v; *Nit-ac;* NUX-V; Pul; Sil.

As if : Osm.

+ STUBBORN, Lingering : Saba.

SUDDEN Attacks : Iod; Plant; Syph; Thu; Zin.

SUMMER, In : Dul; Gel.

Diarrhoea, with : Ind.

SWALLOWING Agg : Carb-an.

TENDENCY To recur : See under COLD, Tendency to take.

THROAT, Sore, with : Merc; Nit-ac; Nux-v; Pho.

URINATION, Burning, with: Ran-sc.

VIOLENT, Attacks: Ars; Aru-t; Lyc.

+ Palpitation, with(aged) : Anac.

WARM Room Amel : Ars; Dul; Saba.

YAWNING Agg : Carb-an; Cup; Lyc.

COTTONY FEELING : Onos.

COUGH, Remedies in general : Aco; Amb; *Ars; Bell;* Bry;

Carb-v; Caus; Cham; Chin; Cina; Coc-c; Con; DROS; HEP; *Hyo; Ign;* Ip; *Kali-c; Lach;* Lyc; Merc; Nat-m; NUX-V; PHO; PUL; *Rum; Sang;* SEP; *Spo; Stan; Sul.*

ABDOMEN, Stomach or epigastrium, from : *Ant-c;* Arg-n; Bell; BRY; Dros; Ign; Kali-bi; *Kali-m;* Lach; Nat-m; *Nit-ac; Pho;* Pho-ac; Pul; Rum; Sang; SEP.

AIR, Open Agg : Ars; Kali-n; Pho; Rum.

Amel : Bry; Coc-c; Iod; Mag-p; Pul; Radm.

ALTERNATE Days Agg : Lyc.

ANGER, From : Ant-t; *Cham;* Saba.

Children : Anac; Ant-t.

ARMS, Raising Agg : Bry; Fer; Tub.

Stretching Agg : Lyc.

ASCENDING, Stairs, when : Arg-n.

AUDITORY Canal, touching Agg : Kali-c; Lach; Mang; Sil.

BARKING : Aco; Amb; *Bell; Dros;* Hep; Lyss; Rum; *Spo;* Stic; Stram.

+ Dry : Clem.

Eructations, with : Ver-a.

BED, Turning in Agg : Kre.

Warmth of Agg : *Caus;* Nux-m; *Pul.*

Amel : Arg-n; Cham; Kali-bi.

+ BENDS, Backwards, child :

Ant-t.

BLOODY, Taste, with : Ham.

BOUTS One : Calc.

Two or Three : *Merc;* Pho; Plb; Pul; Stan; *Sul;* Thu.

Three or Four: *Bell;* Carb-v; Cup.

First, More Violent, but succeeding weaker and weaker : Ant-c.

Isolated : Cor-r.

BRAIN Complaint, in : Glo.

BREAST, left, coldness of, with : Nat-c.

BREATHING, Interrupts : See Suffocating.

CANNOT, Deep enough : Caus; Rum.

CARDIAC : See Heart Com plaints, with.

CAUSES, Distant pain : Caps.

CHANGE of Position Agg : Kre.

CHEST, Holds, during : Arn; *Bry; Dros;* Eup-p; Nat-s; Pho; Sep.

Wetting Amel : Bor.

CHILL, Before : *Rhus-t;* Samb; Tub.

During : Pho; Rhus-t; Saba.

COITION, After : Tarn.

COLD Air, inspiring Agg : Cep; *Rum;* Sang.

Drinks Agg : *Ars;* Calc; Carb-v; Coc-c; Hep; Manc; *Psor;* Rhus-t; Scil; Sil; Spo; Ver-a.

Amel: Caps; *Caus;* Coc-c; *Cup;* Ip; Onos; Tab.

warm Agg : Stan.

From, every : Mang; Sang.

Milk Agg : Ant-t; Spo.

Water, standing in Agg : Nux-m.

Wind on chest Agg : Pho; Rum.

COMPANY Agg : *Amb;* Ars; Bar-c.

CONDIMENTS Agg : Alu.

CONSCIOUSNESS, Loss of, with: Cup.

CONSOLATION, Agg : Ars.

CONSTIPATION Agg : Con; Grap; Sep.

CONVULSIONS, With : Cina; *Cup;* Lach; Meph; Stram.

CORYZA, With : See Coryza.

COUGHING Agg : Bell; *Ign;* Hep; Mar-v; Stic; Thyr.

CRIES, Before: Arn; *Bell; Bry;* Cina; Hep; *Pho.*

DANCING Agg : Pul.

DAYTIME only : Rum; Thu.

Long spells, with : Vio-o.

DEEP : Dros; *Hep;* Lyc; Spo; Stan; Ver-a;Verb.

Breathing Agg: Bell; Bro; Con; Cup; Grap; Lyc; Stic.

Amel : Pul; Verb.

DESCENDING Agg: Lyc.

DIARRHOEA, Amel : Buf.

DRINKING Agg : Ars; Bry; Dros; Hyo; Meph; Psor.

Amel : Op; Spo.

DRUNKARDS, Of : Coc-c; Stram.

DRY Expectoration, without:

Aco; Alu; Ars; Bell; Bry; Calc; Hyo; Ign; *Ip*; Kali-c; Laur; Nat-m; Nat-s; *Nux-v*; Petr; *Pho*; Pho-ac; Pul; Rum; Sele; *Spo*; Stic; *Sul*; Tub.

Day and night : Xanth.

Diarrhoea, after : Abro.

Emaciation, with : Lyc.

Evening : Pul.

Hand, laying, on pit of stomach Amel : Arg-n; Croc.

Loose, dry, and, alternately : Ars.

Menses, at : Zin.

Night : Cimi; Hyo; Merc; Stic.

loose by day : Ars; Hep; Merc; Pul; Sil; Sul.

Pining children, in : Lyc.

+ Smoking, from : Hell.

+ Speaking : Cimi.

Spot, in larynx, from : Con; Hyo; Nat-m.

Vomits, until: Mez; Stic.

DUST, Feathers, as from : Chel; Ign; Rum.

EATING Agg : Bry; Chin; Cor-r; *Hyo;* Kali-bi; *Nux-v.*

Amel : Euphr; Radm; Spo.

Fatty food, from: Mag-m; Pul.

Fish Agg : Lach.

Fruits Agg : Arg-m; Mag- m.

Hastily Agg : Sil.

Irritating things Agg : Alu.

Meat Agg : Stap.

Warm food Agg: Bar-c.

EMACIATION, with : *Acet-ac;* Amb; Lyc; *Nit-ac.*

EMOTIONS, From : Amb; Caps; Ign; Spo; Verb.

Evening to sunrise : Aur.

EMPTY Tube, as if from : Osm.

ERUCTATION Agg : *Amb;* Bar-c; Carb-v; Lob; Stap.

Amel : Sang.

With : Kali-bi.

ERUPTIONS Receding, when : Dul; Led; Pul.

EVENING Agg : Bry; Calc; Nux-v; Rhus-t; Sep; Tub.

Midnight, to : Hep.

EXERTION Agg : Dul; Stan; Pho.

Amel : Radm; Stro.

EXHAUSTING : Ars; Bell; *Carb-v;* Caus; Hyo; *Pho;* Sep; Stan; Ver-a.

Sweat, with : Hyo.

EXPECTORATION Agg : Coc-c; Tarn.

Amel : *Ant-t; Ap*; Aral; Cist; *Coc-c*; Grind; Kali-bi; Sep; *Stan; Zin.*

EYES, Closing, for sleep at night Agg : Hep.

Complaints, with : Nat-m.

FALLS Down : Nux-v; Pho.

FATTY Food, from : Mag-m; Pul.

FEVER, During : *Aco;* Ars; Calc; Con; Ip; Kali-c; Nat-m; Nux-v; Pho; Saba.

Before : Samb.

FLATUS Passing Amel : Sang.

FLUID Gone wrong way, as if from : Lach.

FOG Agg : Sep.

FOUL AIR, Raises up : Calc; *Caps*; Culx; Dros; Guai; *Lach;* Mez; *Sang*; Sep; Sul.

FRIGHT, From : Samb.

FUTILE : Kali-c.

HABITUAL : Calc.

HAIR Sensation, in trachea, from : Sil.

HANDS, Puts, on thighs, during : Nicc.

HAWKING Agg : Am-m; Coc-c.

HEADACHE, With : Carb-v; Sul.

HEART Complaints, with : Adon; Arn; Lach; Laur; Lycps; Naj; Nux-v; Spo.

HOLLOW : Amb; Bell; Carb-v; Caus; Lyc; *Spo;* Ver-a.

HOT, Applications Amel : Ars; Hep; Lyc; Nux-v; Pho; Rhus-t; Rum; Sil.

Abdomen, to Amel: Sil.

Things Agg : Mez.

HOUR, Same : Lyc; Saba.

INCESSANT : *Aco;* ALU; *Caus;* Cham; Chin; *Cof;* Crot-h; Cup; DROS; HYO; Ip; Kali-c; Lach; Lyc; *NUX-V;* Pho-ac; Pul; *Rhus-t;* RUM; Scil; Sep; SPO; Ver-a.

Sleep, preventing : Stic.

INFLUENZA, After : Am-c; Sang.

INSPIRATION, Every Agg : Aco; Stic.

JERKING Lower limbs : Stram.

The body together : Agar; Ther.

+ LACHRYMATION, With : Scil.

LACTATION, During : Fer.

+ LAMENTING : Arn.

LARYNX, Pressure on Agg : See Pressure.

+ Spot, dry, in, from : Nit-ac.

LAUGHING Agg : Arg-n; Chin; Con; Mang; Pho.

LIFTING Agg : Amb.

+ LIVER, Symptoms, with : Am-m.

LOOKING, Fire, at Agg : Ant-c; Stram.

Light, at : Stram.

LOOSE, Expectoration, with : Ars; *Calc; Led;* Lyc; Nat-c; Pho; *Pul; Sep;* Stan.

By day : *Ars;* Calc; *Cham; Hep; Merc; Pul;Sil; Sul.*

Morning : *Bry; Carb-v; Hep; Par; Pho; Pul; Scil; Sep;* Sil; Stan; Sul; Sul-ac.

9 to 11 A.M : Nat-c.

Night, at : Sep.

LYING Agg : *Ap; Ars;* Caus; Con; Dros; *Hyo;* Kre; Psor; *Pul;* Radm; Rum; Sang; Sep.

Amel : Calc-p; *Euphr;* Fer; *Mang.*

Abdomen, on, Amel : Eup-p; *Med.*

+ Back, on Agg : Am-m.

Head, high pillow, on Amel : Carb-v; *Chin.*

Knees, on, with head on pillow Amel : Eup-p.

Right side, on Agg : Am-m;
Merc; Seneg; *Stan*; Stap;
Syph.

Left side on Agg : Sep.

MEASLES, In: Dros; Ip; Pul.

After : Cof; Stic.

+ MEAT Agg : Stap.

MENSES Amel : Senec.

Before : Arg-n; Grap.

During : Calc-p; Grap; Sep;
Zin.

Suppressed, Agg : Dig.

METALLIC : Kali-bi.

MIDNIGHT, At : Aral; Dros; Lach.
To morning : Rhus-t.

MILK, Cold Agg : Ant-t; Spo.

MORNING Agg : Ars; Euphr; Hep;
Lyc; Mos; Pul;Rum; Sele.

And Evening Agg : *Aco;* Bor;
Calc; Carb-v; Caus; Cina;
Fer; Fer-p; Ign; *Lyc*; Merc;
Nat-m; Pho; *Rhus-t*; Sil;
Ver-a.

MOUTH, Covering Amel : Rum.

Rinsing, when : Coc-c.

Rinsing, Cold water, with
Amel: Coc-c.

MUFFLED : Saba.

MUSIC Agg : *Amb;* Calc.

NECK, Touch of Agg : Bell; Bro;
Lach.

NERVOUS: Amb; Caps; Cimi;
Ign; Verb.

NIGHT Agg : Bar-c; Bell; Calc;
Cimi; Con; Dros; Hyo; Laur;
Nux-v; Petr; Pho; Pul; Stic.

Only : Amb; Caus; Petr.

Urine, spurting, with :
Colch.

+ NOISE Agg : Arn; Pho-ac;
Tarn.

+ OCCIPUT, Pain in, with : Anac.

ODOURS, Strong, Agg :
Merc-i-f; Pho; Sul-ac.

+ PAIN, Distant parts, in : Caps.

PAINFUL : *Aco;* Arn; BELL;
BRY; *Caps; Caus;* Dros;
Elap; Eup-p; Kali-c;
Nat-m; NUX-V; *Pho;*
Rhus-t; Scil; Seneg; Spo;
Stan; Stic; Sul.

PEOPLE Coming and Going
Agg : Carb-v.

PIANO Playing Agg : Calc.

PREGNANCY, During : Apoc;
Cham; Con; Kali-br;
Nux-m; *Pul.*

Early, Causing abortion :
Rum.

+ Reflex, from : Kali-br.

PRESSURE, Abdomen, on
Amel : Con.

Epigastrium, on Amel :
Croc; Dros.

Larynx, on Agg : Cina;
Lach; Rum.

Temples, on Amel : Petr.

Throat pit on, Agg : Rum.

PRODROME, As a : Bry;
Rhus-t; Saba; Samb; Tub.

READING Loudly Agg : Amb;
Mang; Nux-v; Pho.

Mind, in Agg : Cina.

REPOSE Amel : Ip.

RETCHING, Gagging, with : Pho.

Amel : Lach.

REVERBERATING : Cor-r; Kali-bi; *Stram;* Verb.

ROOM, Entering or leaving Agg : *Pho;* Rum.

Warm, entering, on : Bry; Nat-c; Thyr; Ver-a.

RUBS, Face and eyes, hands, with, during (child) : Caus; Pul; Scil.

SALIVA Runs : Am-m; Lach; Thu; Ver-a.

SALTY Things Agg : Alu; Con; *Lach.*

SAWING : Spo.

SCIATICA, Alternating with, in summer : Stap.

SHATTERING: Bry; Carb-v; Ign; Kali-c; *Mang; Nit-ac;* Nux-v; *Pho-ac;* Rum; Stan.

SHORT : *Aco;* Ars; *Caus; Cof;* Ign; Lach; Laur; *Merc;* Nat-m; Pho; *Rhus-t;* Sang; *Sep;* Stan; Tub.

SINGING Agg : Alu; Arg-n; Dros; Hyo; Kali-bi; Pho; Stan.

SIT Up, must: Con; Hyo; Phel; *Pho; Pul.*

+ SITTING, Agg : Nat-p. Bent Amel : Iod.

SLEEP, First, after : Aral.

+ In, without waking : Cham; Nit-ac.

SMALLPOX, After : Calc. During : Plat.

SMOKING Agg : Arg-n; Ars; Colo; Dros; Euphr; Hell; Merc; Radm; Stap.

Amel : *Arg-n;* Euphr; Hep; Ign; Merc; Sep; Tarn.

SNEEZING, Then : *Agar;* Scil; Seneg; Sul.

Amel : Osm.

With: Agar; Alu; Bell; Bry; Cina; Lob; Psor; *Scil; Seneg.*

SOUR Things Agg : Alu; Con; Sul.

SPEAKER'S : Coll.

SPINE, From: *Agar;* Nux-m; Tell.

SPLEEN, Enlarged or Pain with : Scil.

STANDING, While walking Agg : Ign.

Sitting, after : Alo.

+ STERNUM, Tickling behind with :Rhus-t.

STOMACH, Pain in, with : Lob.

STOOPING, Agg : Arg-n; Caus; Hep; Spig.

STRANGER, At the sight of : *Ars;* Bar-c; Pho.

STUDENT'S: Nux-v.

SUFFOCATING : Alu; *Ant-t; Bor;* Bro; Carb-*v; Chin;* Cina; *Cup; Dros;* Hep; Hyo; Ip; Kali-c; *Lach; Meph;* Nux-v; *Op; Samb; Sang;* Seneg; *Spo; Stram;* SUL.

Gurgling down in throat, then : Cina.

SULPHUR, Fumes, as from: Ign; Lyc.

SUN, In : Ant-t.

+ SUNSET To Sunrise : Aur.

SURPRISE, Happy Agg : Aco; Merc.

SWALLOWING Agg : Aesc; *Bro;* Cup; Nat-m.

Ame l: Ap; Spo.

Empty Agg : Lyc; Nat-m.

Amel : Bell.

SWEET Things Agg : Bad; Med; Spo; Zin.

Amel : Sul.

TALKING Agg : Alu; Amb; Anac; Con; Dros; Hyo; Meph; Rum; Sanic; Sil; Stan.

Loudly Agg : Coc-c.

TASTE, Bloody with : Ham; Rhus-t.

TEA Agg : Spo.

TEARING : Rhus-t.

TEETH Ache with: Lyc; Sep. Cleaning Agg : Carb-v; Coc-c; Dig; Euphr; Sep; Stap.

TEMPERATURE, Change of Agg : Kali-c; *Pho;* Rum; Sep; Verb.

THROAT or Larynx, from : *Aco;* Amb; Calc; CHAM; *Con;* Hep; IP; Kali-c; *Lach;* Nat-m; Nux-v; Pho; *Rum; Sang;* Sep.

Right, Side, from: Agar; Dros; Stan; Stic.

Left, Side, from : Caus; Hep; Lach; Lith; *Rhus-t;* Tell.

Back of, from : Dul.

Dry, with : Thu.

Stretching Agg : Lyc.

TICKLING : *Aco;* Ars; *Arn;* Bell; *Chcm; Con;* DROS; Hyo; *Iod; Ip;* Kali-c; LACH; *Lyc;* Nat-m; NUX-V; PHO; Pho-ac; Pul; *Rhus-t;* RUM; Sang; Sep; Spo; *Stan;* Sul.

Constant: Nat-c; Op.

Dry, with fever but no thirst : Ars; Con; Pho; Pul; Saba; Scil.

TIGHT : Pho; Stan.

Clothes Agg : Stan.

TIRED, When Agg : Stic.

TONGUE, Protruding Agg : Lyc.

TONSILS, Enlarged : Bar-c; Lach.

TREMBLING, With : Pho.

TUBE, Empty, as if from : Osm.

UNCOVERING, Agg: Hep; Nux-v; Rhus-t; Rum.

+ URINATION, Involuntary, with : Ver-a.

+ URINE Spurting, with: Scil.

+ UVULA Elongated : Alu; Merc-i-r.

VAPOUR, As from : Bro; Lyc.

VIOLENT : See Whooping.

VIOLIN, Playing, on : Kali-c.

VOICE, Excessive use of, from : Coll.

VOMITING, Before : Sul-ac. With : *Alu;* ANT-T; *Bry;* Carb-v; Coc-c; Cor-r; *Dros;* Fer; Hep; IP; Kali-c; Laur; Nux-v; Pul; Rhus-t.

Amel : Mez.

WAKES : Caus; Hyo; Pho; Pul; Samb; Spo; Sul.

Does Not : Arn; Bacil; Cham; Cyc; Lach; Lycps; Nit-ac; Verb.

Midnight, after : Samb.

WALK, Cannot, without : Stan.

WALKING, Fast Agg : Sep.

Amel : Canc-fl; Dros.

WARMTH Amel : Hep; Ip; Lyss; Pho; Rum.

Bed, of Amel: See under Bed.

WEATHER Change : See Temperature.

Cold, foggy Amel : Spo.

warm, to,and vice versa Agg : Rum.

WEEPING, Crying Agg: Arn; Bell; Hep; Ver-a.

WETTING The Chest Amel : Bor.

WHOOPING, Violent, Spas modic : Agar; BELL; CARB-V; Caus; Cham; *Cina; Coc-c;* Con; *Cor-r; Cup; Dros;* Hep; Ign; *Ip; Kali-c;* Kali-s; Lach; *Meph;* Mez; NUX-V; Pho; Pho-ac; *Pul;* Scil; Sep; Stan; Stic; *Stram;* Tub; *Ver-a;* Ver-v.

+ Air, cool Amel : Mag-p.

Catarrhal phase : Aco; Dul; Ip; Nux-v; Pul.

Defervescent stage : Ant-t; Pho; Pul.

+ Drags on : Sep.

Facial herpes, with : Arn.

+ Lachrymation, with : Nat-m.

Neglected, complications, with : Ver-a.

Obstinate : Calc-p.

Spasmodic phase : Carb-v; Cina; Coc-c; Dros; Kali-c; *Nux-v;* Pul; *Ver-a.*

+ Throws him down : Nux-v.

Torn loose feeling, with : Osm.

WINTER Agg : Ant-t; Cham; Kali-m; Nat-m; Nit-ac; Psor.

Old people, in, during entire season : Ant-c; Kre.

WRITING, While : Cina.

YAWNING, And, consecutively : Ant-t; Nat-m.

Agg : Arn; Asaf; Bell; Mur-ac.

+ YAWNS And sleeps : Anac.

COUGHING AGG : Aco; Ars; *Bell;* BRY; Calc; Caps; Carb-v; Cina; *Dros; Ip;* Merc; NUX-V; *Pho; Pul; Rhus-t; Sep;* Spo; Stan; Sul; Tell.

AMEL : Ap; Stan.

DISTANT Parts, pain in, when : Caps.

COUNTS CONTINUOUSLY : Phys; Sil.

COURAGEOUS : See Bold ness.

COVERS AGG (See also Heat Agg) Cold application, Amel : Aco; *Ap;* Calc; *Iod;* Kali-io; Kali-s; *Lach;* Led; Lil-t; LYC; Op; Pul; Sanic; *Sec;* Spig; *Sul.*

WANTS : Tub.

COWARDLY (See Anthropophobia)
: Amb; Anac; Bar-c; *Gel;* Kre;
Lach; *Lyc;* Nux-m; Ol-an;
Pul; Sil; STRAM;

CRACKING JOINTS In : See
Joints.

CRACKLING Like tinsel : Aco;
Calc; Cof; Hep; Rhe; Sep.

CRACKS, FISSURES**,** Chaps (See
also Skin) : Ant-c; Ant-t; Calc;
Calc-f; Caus; Cist; *Fer; Grap;*
Flu-ac; Hep; *Ign;* Lyc; *Merc;*
Merc-c; Mez; Mur-ac; Nat-m;
NIT-AC; PETR; Pho; Pul; Rat;
Rhus-t; Sars; *Sep; Sil; Sul.*

SMALL : Merc-i-r.

CRAFTY (See Deceitful): Tarn.

CRAMP : See Pain Crampy.

WRITER'S (See fingersworking
Agg) : Arg-m; Arn; Dros;
Gel; Mag-p; Pic-ac; Sul-ac.

CRASH : See Blows.

CRAVING (See also Desires),
ALCOHOLIC Drinks, for : Arn;
ARS; Asar; *Calc;* Caps;
Crot-h; *Lach;* Nux-v; *Op;*
Sele; Stan; Sul; Syph.

Beer : Aco; Mos; Nat-p; Petr;
Psor; Stro; *Sul.*

+ Brandy : Mos; Sul-ac.

Menses, before : Sele.

Which she disliked : Med.

+ Wine : Hypr; Mez; Ther.

ALMONDS : Cub.

APPETITE, Without : Op.

APPLES : Alo; Ant-t; Guai;

Sul; Tell.

ASHES : Tarn.

BACON : Calc; Calc-p; Mez;
Radm; Sanic; Tub.

BANANAS : Ther.

BITTER, Drinks : Aco.

Things : Dig; Nat-m.

BREAD : Fer; Grat; Stro.

Butter and : Merc.

Rye : Ign.

*B*UTTER : All-s; Fer; Merc.

Milk: Ant-t; Bur-p;
Chin-s; Elap; Sabal.

CABBAGES : Cic.

CHALK : See Lime.

CHARCOAL : Alu; Calc; Cic;
Psor.

CHEESE : Arg-n; Cist; Pul.

CHERRIES : Chin.

CLOVES : Alu; Chlor.

COARSE, Raw food : Ab-c;
Alu; Ant-c; Calc; Calc-p;
Ign; Sil; Sul; Tarn.

COFFEE : Ars; Aur; Bry;
Caps; Con; Lach; Mez;
Mos; Nux-v; Strop.

Black : Mez.

COLD Things, for : Aco; ARS;
Bism; *Bry;* Cadm; Cham;
Chin; Cina; Diph; Eup-p;
Flu-ac; Lept; Manc; Merc;
Merc-c; Nat-s; Onos; PHO;
Rhus-t; Thu; VER-A.

+ Water : Old.

CONDIMENTS, Spices, pickles
: Ant-c; *Ars;* Calc-p; Caps;
Chel; *Chin;* Cist; Flu-ac;
Hep; Lac-c; Nux-m; Nux-v;

Pho; Pul; Sang; Stap; *Sul*; Tarn.

CUCUMBER : Ant-c; Ver-a.

DELICACIES, Dainties : Aur; *Chin; Ip;* Lil-t; Mag-m; Petr; Rhus-t; Saba; Spo; *Tub.*

Sexual desire, with : Chin.

DIFFERENT, Kinds : Rhe.

DRY : Alu.

EFFERVESCENT Drinks: Colch; Pho-ac.

EGGS : *Calc*; Nat-p.

FARINACIOUS Food : Lach; *Nat-m;* Saba; Sumb.

FATS, Fatty things : Calc-p; Mez; *Nit-ac*; Nux-v; Sul.

FINERY, Beautiful things : Aeth; Lil-t; Sul.

FISH : Nat-m; Sul-ac.

Fried : Nat-p.

FRIED Things: Plb.

FRUITS: Alu; Ant-t; Mag-c; Pho-ac; Sul-ac; Ver-a.

Acid : Ars; Cist; Ther; *Ver-a.*

Juicy : Ant-t; Pho-ac; Stap; Ver-a.

Oranges : Cub; Med; Ther.

GREEN Things: Calc-s; *Med.*

+ HAM : Mez.

HERRING: *Nit-ac*; Pul; Ver-a.

HONEY : Saba.

HOT Things: *Ars; Bry;* Chel; Fer; Lac-c; Lyc; Saba.

ICE : Ars; Elap; Lept; Med; Ver-a.

Cream : Calc; Eup-p; *Pho*; Sil.

Pain, during : Med.

Water : Aco; Ars; Lept; Onos; Pho; Sil; Ver-a.

INDEFINITE Things (knows not what) : *Bry;* Chin; *Ign; Ip;* Pul; Ther; Zin-ch.

INDIGESTIBLE Things : Alu; Calc; Calc-p; Cyc.

JUICY Things : See Fruits, juicy.

LEMONADE : *Bell;* Cyc; Nit-ac; Pul; Sabi; Sec; Sul-io.

LIME, Chalk, Clay, Earth: Alu; Ant-c; *Calc;* Cic; Ign; *Nit-ac; Nux-v;* Psor; SIL; Sul; *Tarn.*

LIQUIDS : Stap; Sul.

MANY Things : Cic; *Cina*; Stap.

Pleased, with nothing : All-s.

Refuses, when given: Stap.

to eat them : Rhe.

MEAT : Kre; Lil-t; Mag-c; Vio-o.

MENSES, Before : Spo.

MILK : *Ap;* Ars; Aur; Chel; Cist; Lac-c; Merc; Nat-m; *Pho-ac; Rhus-t;* Saba; Sabal; Sanic; Stap; Sul.

Boiled : Abro; Nat-s.

Cold : Rhus-t; Pho; Pho-ac; Tub.

ice : Sanic.

Sour : Ant-t; Mang.

Warm : Bry; Calc; Chel.

+ Which Amel : Ap.

Which he disliked : Sabal.
he drinks much : Lac-c.
MORE Than he wants : Ars.
MUSTARD : Cocl.
NUTS : Cub.
ONIONS : Bels; Cep; Cub.
OYSTERS : Lach; Nat-m; Rhus-t.
PARTICULAR Thing : Rhe.
PEPPER : Lac-c.
Cayenne : Merc-c.
PICKLES : See Condiments.
PORK : Crot-h; Radm; Tub.
POTATOES : Nat-c; Ol-an.
Raw : Calc.
PREGNANCY, During : Calc-p; Chel; Sep.
Strange things : Chel; Lyss; Mag-c; Sep.
RAGS, Clean: Alu.
REFRESHING Things : Med; Pho-ac; *Pul;* Ver-a.
RELISH, What cannot : Bry; Ign; Mag-m; Pul.
SALTY Things : Alo; Arg-n; Calc-p; *Carb-v;* Caus; Con; Lac-c; Med; Merc-i-r; NAT-M; Nit-ac; *Pho;* Thu; Ver-a.
SAND : Sil; Tarn.
SARDINESS : Cyc.
SMOKED Things : *Caus;* Kre; *Tub.*
SNUFF : Bell.
SOUR Things : *Aco;* Ant-t; *Arn;* Ars; Bell; Cham; Con; Cor-r; *Hep;* Mag-c; Med; Myr; Pod; Pul; Radm; Sec; Sep; *Sul;* Ther; Ver-a.

SPICY Things : See Condiments.
STIMULANTS : Carb-ac; Crot-h; Sele.
+ Agg : Naj.
STRANGE Things : Bry; Calc; Calc-p; Chel; Hep.
Many from inability to distinguish, edible from nonedible : Cic.
SWEET Things : *Arg-n;* Calc; Carb-v; CHIN; Cina; Ip; *Kali-c;* Kali-p; *Lyc;* Mag-m; Med; Merc; Saba; *Sul;* Thyr; Tub.
Drinks: Buf.
Weakness, with : Thyr.
TEA : Alu; Hep; Sele.
THINGS That are refused, when offered : Bry; *Cham;* Dul; Hep; Kre; Pho; Phys; Stap.
That disagree : Pul.
TOBACCO : Asar; Carb-v; Daph; Stap; *Tab.*
Smoking : Calc-p; Carb-ac; Glo; Med; Ther.
TOMATOES : Fer.
VEGETABLES : Alu; Mag-c; Mag-m.
VINEGAR : Arn; Hep; Kali-p.
WINE : See Alcoholic drinks.
CRAWLING As of Insects, Bugs, Flies etc. : Calad; Carb-an; Dul; Lac-c; Myr; Nat-c; Oenan; Osm; Pho-ac; Pic-ac; Stram; Tab; Tarn.
BAD, News, after : Calc-p.
BODY, All over : Cist.

FLOOR, On : Abs; Lach.

OUTWARD : Chel.

SPIDER, As of a : Visc.

WAIST, Around : Oenan.

CRAZY: See Insanity.

FEELS Like going : Syph.

CREEPING, Running as of a mouse, etc. : *Bell; Calc*; Cimi; Lyc; Nit-ac; Pho; Rhod; Sep; Stap; *Sil; Sul.*

COLD : Frax; Lac-c.

Menses before : Ant-t.

LEFT Side : Nit-ac.

NERVOUS : Canc-fl.

CREPITATION : Aco; Calc; Cof; Rhe.

SKIN, Under : Carb-v.

SYNOVIAL : Nat-p.

CRETINISM : Aeth; Anac; Bar-c; Buf; Thu; Thyr.

AGILE : Calc-p.

CRIES, Shrieks, screams (See also Weeps, Sorrows) : *Aco*; AP; BELL; Bor; Calc; *Cam; Cham;* Cic; Cina; *Cup*; Glo; Hyd-ac; Ign; Jal; Kali-c; *Lyc;* Mag-p; Pho; *Plat;* Pul; Rhe; *Stram*; Syph; Ver-a; Ver-v; *Zin.*

ANGER, From : Nux-v; Zin.

CALLS Someone, as if: Aloe; Anac.

CEPHALIC : Ap; Bell; Hell; Lyc; Rhus-t; Zin.

CHILDREN : Bor; Lac-c; Rhe.

Fist in mouth, with : Ip.

Moved, when : Zin.

Sob, and, in sleep : Hyo.

Stools, before : Bor; Kre.

during : Val.

+ Sycotic taint : Thu.

Touched, when : Ant-t.

Waking, on, trembling, with : Ign.

CONVULSIONS Before : Cic; Cup; Hyd-ac; Ver-v.

COUGH Agg : *Arn; Bell*; BRY; Cina; *Hep.*

CRAMPS In abdomen, during : Cup.

+ DESIRE, But can not : Am-m.

FEELS As though, she must cry : Anac; Calc; Elap; Lil-t; Sep.

Reason, without : Chel.

GENITALS, Grasping, with : Aco.

HARD To please: Ip.

HELP, For : Cam; Ign; Plat.

HERNIA, Inguinal, congenital : Thu.

HICCOUGH, With : Cic.

HOLDS On to something, unless she : SEP.

INVOLUNTARY : Hyd-ac.

KINDLY, Spoken to, when : Sil.

LOUDLY : Hyd-ac.

As if to call someone: Anac.

NIGHT, At : Kre.

NURSING, When, (children): Bor.

PAINS, With : Aco; Ap; Bell; Cact; Cham; Cof; Cup; Mag-p; Plb; Sep; Zin.

PLAINTIVELY, Stupor, in, touch

Agg : Hyo.

SLEEP, During: *Ap*; Bor; Cina; Hell; Hyo; Ign; *Lyc*; Pul; Rhe; Tub; *Zin*.

Eyes fixed and trembling, with : Ant-t.

SUDDENLY : Chin; Plb.

TOUCH, On : Ant-c; Kali-c; Rut; Stram.

TRIFLES, At : *Kali-c*.

URINATION, Before : Aco; *Bor*; *Lyc*; Sanic; Sars.

WANTS, But Cannot : Am-m.

WAKING, On : Zin.

Without : Hyo.

+ **CRIME** Committed, As if : Caus.

CRITICAL, EXACTING: *Ars*; Lyc; Sil; Sul.

+ **CRITICISE**, Everything, Wants to : Guai.

CROSSING LIMBS AGG : Agar; Alu; *Asaf*; Aur; Bell; *Dig*; Lyc; Pho; *Rhus-t*; Val.

AMEL: Ant-t; Lil-t; Murx; Rhod; *Sep*; Thu.

CROSSNESS (See Anger) : Ant-c; Ant-t; Aru-t; *Cham*; Cina; Cratae; Hep; Iod; Kre; Nat-c; Radm; Sanic; Syph.

+ DAY, During, merry at night : Med.

+ FLATULENCE, With : Cic.

CROUP : *Aco; Hep*; Kali-bi; Kali-io; Kali-s; Merc-cy; Pho; *Spo*.

DIPHTHERITIC : Iod; *Lach;* Spo.

CROWD : See Company.

FEAR Of : See under Fear.

ROOM, In AGG : Lyc; Pho; Sep.

CRUELTY : Abro; *Anac*; Kali-io; Med; Plat.

HEARING AGG: *Calc*.

CRUSHING : See Pain, Squeezing.

CRUSTA LACTEA : See Eruptions on head.

CRUSTS, SCABS : Ars; CALC; *Dul; Grap; Lyc;* Mag-m; Manc; *Merc; Mez;* Nat-m; Nit-ac; Petr; Psor; Radm; *Rhus-t;* Sil; SUL.

ADHERENT : Arg-n; Lyc.

BENEATH, Pus : Bov; Lyc; Mez; Thu.

BODY, Over whole : *Dul;* Psor.

BROWN : Manc; Old.

Yellow : Dul.

BURNING : Ant-c.

CONICAL : Sil; Syph.

CRACKED : Vio-t.

DIRTY : Psor.

FALLING : Nit-ac.

GUMMY : Vio-t.

HORNY : Ran-b.

HUMID : Merc; Nit-ac; *Stap;* Vinc; Viot.

SHINY : Old.

TENACIOUS Fluid : Vio-t.

THICK : Bov; *Calc;* Clem; Dul; Kali-bi; Mez; Petr.

Foul : Vinc.

WHITE : Ars.

YELLOW : Grap.

CUNNING (See Deceitful) : Tarn.

CUPPED : Thu; Vario.

CURDY : See Discharges.

CURSING : Anac; Lil-t; Nit-ac; Stram; Tub; Ver-a.

CURVATURE : See Bones, Spine.

CUTTING : See under Pain.

CYANOSIS : See Bluish.

INFANTS, In : See Children, Cyanotic.

CYNICAL : Lyc; Nit-ac; Tarn.

CYSTITIS : See Bladder, In flamed.

CYSTS : Ap; Ars; BAR-C; CALC; GRAP; *Lyc*; Nit-ac; PHO; Sabi; SIL; *Sul*; Thu.

DAMP, COLD **A**GG: Bar-c; CALC; Carb-v; Cimi; DUL; Lach; *Merc*; Nat-s; Nux-m; *Rhod*; RHUS-T; Ver-a; Zin.

GROUND AGG : Dul; Rhus-t.

NIGHT AGG : Merc; Phyt; Rhus-t.

SHEETS, were, as if: Lac-d.

DAMPNESS, WET **W**EATHER, Working in water **A**GG : Alu; *Am-c; Ant-c*; Ant-t; *Aran; Ars*; Bry; Cact; CALC; Calc-p; Card-m; Caus; Cham; Cimi; *Clem;* Colch; DUL; Gel; Kalm; Lyc; Mag-p; Med; Merc; *Nat-s*; Nit-ac; Nux-m; Pho; Phyt; *Pul*; Pyro; *Rhod*; RHUS-T; Sabal; Sabi; Senec; *Sep; Sil*; Sul; Terb; Tub.

AMEL : See Air, Cold, Dry Agg.

DANCING : Agar; Bell; Cic; Cocl; Croc; Hyo; Stic; *Tarn*.

AGG : Bor; Spo.

AMEL : *Ign;* SEP; Sil.

DANDRUFF : Ars; Canth; *Grap*; Lyc; Nat-m; *Pho;* Stap; Sul; Thu.

ITCHING : Med.

SCALY, Profuse : Sanic.

WHITE : Ars; Kali-m; Mez; *Nat-m; Thu.*

YELLOW : Calc; *Kali-s.*

DARK : See Black.

DARKNESS AGG : See Light Amel.

AMEL : Con; *Euph;* Grap; Pho; *Sang.*

DARTING : See Pain, Darting.

DAY ALTERNATE on **A**GG : *Ars*; Canth; CHIN; Clem; *Ip*; Lyc; *Nat-m*; Nux-v; Pul; Rhus-t.

AMEL: Alu.

EVERY FOURTH AGG : Ars; Lyc; Pul; Saba.

EVERY SEVENTH (Weekly) AGG : Ars; Canth; Chin; Gel; *Iris;* Lac-d; Lyc; Pho; *Sang;* Sil; *Sul;* Tell.

EVERY TENTH AGG : Lach; Pho.

EVERY FOURTEENTH AGG : *Ars;* Calc; Chin; Con; *Lach*; Nic; Pul; Sang; Sul.

AMEL : Mag-m.

EVERY TWENTYONE (3rd week) AGG : Aur; Chin-s; Mag-c; Tarn; Tub.

EVERY TWENTYEIGHTH (Monthly 4th Week) AGG : *Nux-m;*

NUX-V; Pul; SEP; Tub.

EVERY FORTYTWO, (6th Week)
AGG : Ant-c; Mag-m.

EVERY NINETY AGG: Chin.

TWICE A DAY : Verb.

DAY-BLINDNESS : Both; Castr;
Lyc; Pho; Ran-b; Sil;Stram.

BREAK AMEL : Colch; Syph.

HOT with COLD nights AGG :
Aco; Dul; Merc; Rum.

TIME Only AGG : Agar; Euphor;
Med; *Nat-m; Pul*; Rhus-t;
SEP; STAN; SUL.

AMEL : Kali-c; Syph.

Pain : Ham.

DAZED : See Bewildered, Dull.

DEAD LOOK : Thu.

DEADNESS : Aco; Agar; Bar-c;
Grap; Lyc; Rhus-t; Sec.

DEAD THINKS, He is : Agn; Ap;
Ars; Grap; *Lach*; Mos; *Op;* Pho;
Plat.

Everything is : Mez.

DEAFNESS : See Hearing.

DEATH AGONY : Ant-t; *Ars;*
Carb-v; Tarn-c.

APPARENT : Aco; Ant-t; Carb-v;
Cof; Op; Petr; Plat.

BELIEVES, That she is going to
die soon and that she can
not be helped : Agn.

Certain day on : Aco; Hell.

CERTAIN, Is : Hyds.

DESIRES : *Aur;* Caus; Hyds; Kre;
Lac-c; Lach; Ran-b; Sep;
Sul.

FEAR, Of : See under Fear.

+ LONGS, For : Aran.

NEAR, Seems, must settle his
affairs : Petr.

+ PREMONITION : Ap.

THOUGHTS, Of : Aco; Grap.
Calmly: Zin.

DEBAUCHERY: Agar; Ant-c;
Carb-v; Lach; *Nux-v;* Sele;
Stram; Sul-ac.

DEBILITY : See Weakness.

DECEITFUL, TRICKY, Duplicity
: Arg-m; Buf; Cup; Merc; *Op;*
Plb; Tarn; *Ver-a.*

DECEIVED, Always being
: Rut.

DECOMPOSITION : Mur-ac;
Pho; Pyro; Sec.

RAPID : Crot-h.

DECUBITUS : See Bed Sores.

DEEDS He Could do great
: Hell.

DEFIANT : Arn; Lyc.

+ **DEGENERATION,**
CALCAREOUS : Flu-ac.

FATTY : See under Fatty.

DEJECTED : See Despair, Sad
ness and Sorrow.

DELICATE, TENDER, Sickly,
easily enervated : Ars;
Calc; Calc-p; Caus; Cimi;
Colch; Con; Croc; Cup; *Ign;*
Kali-p; Lyc; Mar-v; Nat-c;
Nux-m; Pho; Pic-ac; Psor;
Sep; Sil; Stro; Sul; Tab;
Ver-a; Zin.

DELIRIUM : *Aco; Agar;* Ars;
Aru-t; BELL; Bry; Cann;
Chel; *Cup; Dul;* HYO; *Lach;*

Lyc; Nit-ac; Nux-v; *Op;* Rhus-t; Sec; *Stram;* Syph; VER-A; Ver-v.

ABORTION, After : Rut.

ANXIOUS: Aco; Ap; *Stram.*

COLIC, Alternating with : Plb.

EASY : Agar; Dul; Ver-a.

EYES, Brilliant, with : Ail.

FOOLISH : Bell; Op; Stram; Sul.

FRIGHTFUL, Visions with : Bell; Calc; Stram.

HAEMORRHAGE, After : Arn; Ars; Bell; Ign; Lach; Lyc; Pho; Pho-ac; Sep; Scil; Sul; Ver-a.

LOQUACIOUS : See Loquacity.

MANIACAL, Furibund, wild, raving : *Aco;* Agar; Ail; *Ars;* BELL; *Bry;* Canth; HYO; Lyc; Nit-ac; Op; Sec; STRAM; VER-A.

+ Trifles, over : Thu.

MENTAL or PHYSICAL exertion, from : Lach.

MUSIC, Hearing, from : Plb.

MUTTERING : Ail; Ant-t; Bry; *Hyo;* Lach; *Mur-ac;* Pho; STRAM.
Himself, to : Tarx.

+ Incessant : Ver-v.

NIGHT, At : Plb; Syph.

PAINS, With: Dul; *Ver-a.*
Limbs, alternating with : Plb.

PICKING Lips, fingers, nose : See Carphology.

QUARRELSOME : Nit-ac.

ROLLS On floor : Calc; OP.

SAME SUBJECT all the time, Talks : Petr.

SLEEP, In : Ap; Bell.

SLEEPINESS, With: Bry; Pul.

SLEEPLESSNESS, And : *Aur;* Bell; Bry; Calc; Chin; Colo; Dig; Dul; Hyo; Ign; Lyc; Nat-c; Nux-v; Op; Pho; Pho-ac; Plat; Pul; Rhus-t; Saba; Samb; Sele; Spo; Sul; Ver-a.

SPEAKS In foreign language : Lach; Nit-ac; Stram.

STARES At one fixed point : Ign.

+ Wild : Ver-v.

TREMENS, Dipsomania: Agar; Ars; Caps; *Cimi;* HYO; Lach; Nat-m; Nux-m; Nux-v; *Op;* STRAM.

+ Hiccough, with : Ran-b.

VARIABLE : Lach; Stram.

WAKING, On : HYO; Lach; Zin.

DELTOID : Bar-c; Fer; Fer-p; Syph; Urt; Vio-o.

RIGHT: Colo; Kalm; Lycoper; Mag-c; Phyt; Sang; Stap.

LEFT : Fer.

ARMS, Raising up Agg : Zin.
Rotating inwards Agg : Urt.
Turning Agg : Sang.

MOTION, Violent Amel : Phys.

PARALYSIS : Caus.

READING Agg : Stan.

RELAXED, As if : Merc-c.

93

DELUSIONS : See Imaginations, Perception changed.

DEMENTIA : Anac; Bell; Lyc; *Nux-v; Pho.*

BUSINESS Worry, from : Lil-t.

SEXUAL Excess, from : Lil-t.

DENTITION : Calc; Calc-p; Cham; Cof; Kre; Mag-p; Rhe; Sil; Stap; Sul; Tub.

DELAYED: *Tub.*

DEPRAVITY (See Moral perversion) : *Buf;* Tarn.

DEPRESSION : See Sadness.

DERMATALGIA : See Skin, Painful.

DERMOID : Calc; Nat-c; Nat-m; Nit-ac.

DESCENDING *A*GG : Arg-m; *Bor;* Con; Fer; *Gel;* Phys; Rhod; RUTA; STAN; Ver-a.

AMEL : Bry; Spo.

MISSES, Steps of stairs while : Stram.

DESIRES (See also Craving)

BEAUTIFUL Things, Finery : Lil-t; Sul.

CERTAIN Things, but opposes it if proposed, by others : Caps.

CHANGE, Always : Tub.

DEATH : See Death, Desires.

FRIEND, But treats him outrageously : Kali-c.

MORE, Than she needs: Ars.

RESPECT Due to him, shown : Ham.

THINGS, Then throws them away : Sec.

TO BEAT Children : Chel; Ox-ac.

TO BE Read, to : Chin; Clem.

TO CUT Others: Lyss.

TO DO Mental Work : Aur; Tarn.

Something great : Cocain.

+ TO GET DRUNK : Sele.

TO GET into country, away from people : Calc; Elap; Merc; Sep.

Solitude in, to practise masturbation : Buf; Ust.

TO GO HOME (Thinking he is not there) : *Bry;* Calc; Lach; Op.

Place to place : Sanic.

TO KILL : See Kill.

TO PULL her Hair : *Ars; Bell; Cup;* Dig; Lil-t; Med; Tarn; Tub; Xanth.

Nose of strangers : Merc.

TO REMAIN, Bed, in : Arg-n; Hyo.

TO SCRATCH : Arn!

TO SET THINGS on Fire : Hep.

TO SING : Spo.

TO TALK : Arg-m; Arg-n; Stic.

TO TRAVEL : *Calc-p;* Cimi; Iod; Merc; Tub.

TO WEAR His best clothes : Con.

DESPAIR HOPELESSNESS : Aco; Anac; Arn; *Ars; Aur;*Calc; Caus; Cof; Hell; *Ign;* Iod; Kali-io; Lept; Lyc; Nit-ac; Pho-ac; PSOR; STAN; Syph; Tab; *Ver-a.*

ANGER, With : Tarn.

+ CURE, Of : Bry.

HEART Disease, in : Aur.

LIVER Affections, with : Lept.

POSITION in Society, about : Ver-a.

RECOVERY, Of : Aco; Ars; Bry; Calc; Psor; Syph.

+ SALVATION, Of : Ver-a.

TRIFLES, Over : Grap.

DESQUAMATION, Branny, Scaly, etc. : Am-c; *Ars*; Ars-io; Bell; Calc;Canth; Dul; *Grap*; Hep; KALI-C; Kali-m; Merc; Mez; Nat-m; Nit-ac; PHO; Pul; Rhus-t; Sars; Sele; Sep; Stap; SUL.

BRANNY : Radm; Tub.

BROWN : Am-m.

+ **DESPERATE**: Med.

+ **DESPONDENT** : Caus; Lac-c; Lac-d.

CONVERSATION Amel : Lac-d.

DESTRUCTIVE : Ap; Flu-ac; Pho; Stram; Tarn; Tub.

DETERMINED : See Stubborn.

DEVELOPMENT : See Growth.

DIABETES, INSIPIDUS : See Urine Profuse.

MELLITUS : Arg-m; Ars; BOV; *Carb-v;* Chio; Colo; HELO; *Iris;* Kre; LYC; *Nat-m;* PHO; PHO-AC; PLB; Ran-b; Sep; Scil; *Sul;* TARN; TERB; Thu; URAN-N.

Boils, successive,with : Nat-p.

Children, in : Cratae.

Lung affections, with : Calc-p.

DIAPHRAGM : Bry; Cact; Cimi; Cup; Ign; Stan; Stry.

CONTRACTED : Mez.

CORD, Bound, tightly by taking the breath away : Cact.

HIGH : Card-m.

INFLAMMATION : Cact; Nux-v.

NEURALGIA : Stan.

VISCERA, Drawn up against: Spo.

DIARRHOEA : Agar; *Alo;* Ant-c; Ant-t; *Ars;* Bap; Bar-c; Bry; Calc; Canth; Carb-v; *Cham; Chin; Cina;* Colo; Con; *Crot-t;* Dul; Fer; Gamb; Hell; Hep; Iod; Ip; *Iris;* Kali-bi; Lyc; *Merc;* Merc-c; Nat-m; *Nat-s;* Nit-ac; *Pho; Pho-ac;* POD; *Psor; Pul; Rhe; Rhus-t;* Sec; Sil; *Sul;* Thu; VER-A.

ACUTE Disease, after : Carb-v; Chin; Psor; Sul.

ALTERNATING, Other com plaints with: Pod.

AMEL : Abro; Nat-s; Pho-ac; *Zin.*

ASTHMA, Then : Kali-c.

BATHING Agg : Pod.

BEER Agg : Alo; Chin.

BLOODY, Infants, in: Calc-s.

BREAKFAST, After : Nat-s; Thu. Amel : Bov; Nat-s.

BURNS, After : Ars; Calc.

BUTTERMILK Agg : Pod.

CANCER Of rectum, from : Card-m.

CARE, Domestic Agg : Cof.

CHILDREN, Emaciated, of : Acet-ac; Tub.

+ Summer, in : Cup.

CHOCOLATE Agg : Lith.

CHOLERIC : See Cholera.

CHRONIC : Ars; Calc; Nat-m; Petr; Pho; Psor; Sil; *Sul*; Tub.

COFFEE Agg : Cist; Cyc; Ox-ac.

COLDNESS With : Grat.

Children : Chin.

Old people : Bov.

CONSTIPATION, Alternating with : See Constipation.

COLD Drinks Agg : Caus; Chin; Hep; Lyc; Stap.

Amel : Pho.

+ Cold Water, in hot days : Ver-a.

COLDS Agg : Calc; Dul; Nux-m; Rum; Tub.

CUCUMBER Agg : Ver-a.

DAY Only : Kali-c; Nat-m; Petr; Phyt.

DEBILITY, With : Ars; Ver-a.

Without : Ap; Calc; Grap; *Pho-ac*; Pul; Rhod; Sul; Tub.

DIURESIS, With : Mag-s.

DRINKING Agg: *Arg-n*; ARS; Caps; Cina; CROT-T; Fer; Nux-v; Pho; Rhus-t.

DROPSY, In : Acet-ac; *Ap*; Apoc; Hell.

EATING Agg : *Alo*; *Ars*; Calc; Calc-p; CHIN; Chin-ar; Cina; *Colo*; *Cort-t*; *Fer*; Grap; Iod; Kre; Lyc; Mag-c; *Nux-v*;

Pod; Pul; Tromb.

EGG , From : Chin-ar.

EXANTHEMATA, In : Ant-t.

FATIGUE Agg : Fer.

FEVER, Intermittent, during: Bap; *Cina*; Nux-v; Rhus-t.

Puerperal : Pyro.

FISH Agg : Chin-ar.

FLATUS, Passing, after : Kali-ar.

FRIGHT, From : Pho; Pul.

FRUITS Agg : Calc-p; Cist; Chin; Lach; Lith; Lyc; Rhod.

Acid, Sour : Pod.

Canned : Pod.

Unripe : Pho-ac; Rhe; Sul-ac.

GOITRE, With : Cist.

HAIR, Washing Agg : Tarn.

HOT Bath Amel : Sec.

+ Season Agg : Aco.

HOUSEWIFE, In : Cof.

INDISCRETION, Of food, slightest, after : Grap; Pho; Pul; Sul-ac.

INFANTS : Sul.

JAUNDICE, With : *Chio*; Dig; Lycps; Nux-v; Pul; Rhe.

LEMONADE Agg : Phyt.

LIENTERIC : See Eating Agg.

LUMBARACHE, with : Bar-c; Kali-io.

MENSES Agg : Am-m; *Bov*; Caus; Colo; Kre; Lach; Nat-s; *Pho*; Pho-ac; Pul; Sec; Sul; Ver-a; Vib.

+ Appear, would, as if : Kali-io.

Suppressed, from : Glo.

MENTAL Exertion Agg : Pic-ac.

MILK Agg : Calc; Chin; Mag-m; Nat-c; Pod; Sep; Sul.

Boiled Agg : Nux-m; Sep.

MORNING Agg : *Alo;* Bov; Bry; *Kali-bi;* Lil-t; Mag-c; Mag-c; *Nat-s;* Onos; Pho; Pod; Psor; Rum; SUL; Tub.

Bed, driving out of : Dios; Nat-s; Psor; *Sul;* Syph; Tub.

Children, of : Cimi; Iod.

Frothy : Stic.

Muddy water : Lept.

Offensive : Grap.

Rising, after : *Bry;* Lil-t; *Nat-s;* Rum.

+ Wait, cannot : Lil-t.

Watery : Colo.

Weakness, with : Dios.

MOTION Agg : Ap; Bry; Fer; Ver-a.

MUCUS, Then Weakness : Bor.

NERVOUS, Emotions Agg : Aco; ARG-N; *Cham; Cof;* Fer; GEL; Hyo; Ign; *Op;* Pho; Pod; *Pul; Ver-a;* Zin.

NIGHTLY : *Chin; Fer;* Psor; Rhus-t; Stro.

OLD Age : Ant-c; Ars; Bov; Gamb; Nit-ac.

Painful : Carb-v.

OPIUM, After : Nat-m.

OYSTERS Agg : Alo; Bro;

Sul-ac.

PAINFUL : Ars; Bry; Cham; Colo; Merc; Merc-c; Rhe; Rhus-t; Sul.

PAINLESS : *Ars;* Bap; Bism; Bor; *Chin;* FER; Hep; *HYO;* Iris; Kali-p; *Lyc;* Nat-m; PHO; PHO-AC; POD; *Pul;* Scil; *Stram; Sul;* Tub; VER-A.

Urination, frequent, with : Bism.

PARTURITION, After : Coll; Hyo; Rhe.

PERIODICAL : Stro.

Alternate days : Alu; *Chin;* Iris.

Fourth day, every : Saba.

Summer : Kali-bi.

Weeks, every three : Mag-c.

+ PERSISTENT : Kali-bi.

PHTHISIS Of : *Ars;* Bry; Carb-v; Chin; Fer; Hep; Nit-ac; Pho; Pho-ac; Pul; Rum; Sul.

Early : Fer; Kali-io.

PREGNANCY, During : Ant-c; Chin; Dul; Lyc; Merc; Petr; Pho; Pul; Rhe; Sep; Sul; Thu.

RHEUMATISM, Then : Cimi; Kali-bi; Dul.

With : Stro.

SEASHORE Agg : Syph.

SCHOCLGIRLS : Calc-p; Pho-ac.

SENSE Of : Dul; *Nux-v;* Pul.

SLEEP, During : Sul; Tub.

Amel : Pho.

SMALL POX, During : Ars; *Chin.*

SMOKING Agg : Bor.

SOUR Things, Agg : Bro; Lach. Amel : Arg-n.

SPASMS, Tonic, with : Terb.

STANDING Amel : Merc.

STARCHES, From : Nat-c.

STOPPAGE, Suddenly from Agg : Mag-p; Zin.

SUDDEN, Fever, with : Bap.

SUMMER : See Weather, hot.

THIN Persons, in : Calc; *Sil;* Sul-ac.

TYPHOID, In : Hyo; Pho.

ULCERS, In intestines, from : Kali-bi; Merc-c.

URINATING Agg : Alo; *Alu;*.Hyo.

VEGETABLES Agg : Lyc.

VOMITING, After : Manc.

WALKING, When, only : Rhe.

WARM Drinks Agg : Flu-ac.

+ WEAKNESS, Absent : Rhod.

WEANING, After: Arg-n; CHIN.

WEATHER, Change of : Dul; Pho-ac; Psor.

Hot Agg : *Bry;* Cam; Castr; Chin; Crot-t; Fer;Fer-p; Gamb; Kre; Nux-m; Old; *Pod.*

cold drinks, from : Nux-m.

eruptions, with : Hypr.

DIGESTION, AFFECTED : Aeth; *Ant-c;* Arg-n; Ars; *Bry; Calc;* CHIN; Fer; Lyc; Merc; NUX-V; Old; Pho; PUL.

BRAIN Exhaustion, from : Aeth; Calc-f.

Children : Calc-f.

COITION, After : Dig; Pho.

DIETETIC Errors, from : See Errors in diet.

EATING, Hurriedly, from : Anac; Cof; Old.

MASTURBATION, Emission, from: Bar-c.

OVEREATING, from : Rut; Sep.

SPRAIN, From : Rut.

WEAK : Lyc; Old.

DIGGING : See Pain, Boring.

DINNER AGG : *Alo; Bry;* Grat; Mag-m; Merc-i-r; Sul-ac; *Zin.*

AMEL : Chel; Cinb.

DIPLOPIA: See Vision, Double.

DIPSOMANIA : See Delirium, tremens.

DIPHTHERIA : AP; *Ars;* Bro; *Diph;* Kali-bi; Kali-chl; Kali-io; *Lac-c;* LACH; *Lyc;* -M E R C - C Y ; *Merc-i-f;* Merc-i-r; Mur-ac; *Pho; Phyt; Rhus-t;* Spo; Sul-ac.

CARRIER : Lach.

+ EFFECTS : Pyro.

+ FEVER, Intense : Tarn-c.

LARYNGEAL : *Bro; Iod; Kali-Bi;* Lac-c; *Lach;* Merc-cy.

NASAL : Am-c; *Kali-bi;* Manc; Nit-ac.

PAINLESS: Ap; Carb-ac; *Diph.*

RELAPSING : Diph.

DIRECTION OF SYMPTOMS

ALTERNATING : See Alternating States, Sides, etc.

APPEAR On one side, go to other, and there AGG :

Arg-n; Fer; Iris; Lac-c; LYC; Mang; Nat-m; Tub.

ASCENDING : Aco; ASAF; *Bell;* Calc; Cimi; Con; Croc; Cup; Dul; Gel; Glo; IGN; Kali-bi; Kalm; Kre; LACH; *Led; Naj;* Op; PHO; *Pul;* Saba; SANG; SEP; SIL; Strop; *Sul;* Thu; Zin.

BACKWARD : Bar-c; *Bell;Bry; Chel;* Con; Crot-t; Cup; Gel; *Kali-bi;* Kali-c; Kali-io; Lil-t; Merc; Nat-m; Par; Pho; Phyt; Pru-s; Pul; *Sep;* Spig; SUL.

CROSSWISE, **A**CROSS : *Bell;* Berb; Calc; *Chel; Chin;* Fer; Hell; Kali-bi; Kali-m; *Lac-c;* Sep; *Sil; Sul;* Val; *Ver-a;* Zin.

DIAGONAL : *Agar; Alu;* Amb; Ap; Bor; Kali-io; *Kalm;* Lach; Lyc; *Mang;* Murx; Nat-c; Nux-v; *Pho;* RHUS-T; Stic; Sul-ac; Tarx.

DOWNWARD : Alo; Arn; Aur; Bar-c; *Berb;* Bry; Caps; Cic; Cof; Hypr; KALM; Lach; Lyc; Pul; Rhod; Rhust; Sele; Zin.

FORWARD : Berb; Bry; Carb-v; *Gel;* Lac-c; *Sabi; Sang;* Sep; Sil; SPIG.

HERE And There : Aco; Agar; *Am-c;* Bar-c; Calc; Chel; Chin; Cimi; Cina; COCL; Grap; IGN; Lyc; Mag-c; Mag-p; Op; Pho; Pho-ac; Rat; Rhus-t; Sec; Stan; Stap; *Sul; Thu; Val;* Ver-v; Zin.

INCREASE **G**RADUALLY, and decrease gradually : Arg-n; Ars; Gel; *Glo;* Kali-bi; Kalm; Lach; *Nat-m;* Pho; PLAT; Pul; *Sang; Spig;* STAN; STRO; Sul; Syph.

And Decrease suddenly : *Arg-m;* Caus; *Ign; Pul; Sul-ac.*

INCREASE, Suddenly, and de crease suddenly : Arg-n; *Bell; Kali-bi; Nit-ac;* Spig; Sul.

And decrease gradually : Pul; Sabi.

INCREASE With the sun : Kalm; *Nat-m; Sang;* Sele; Spig.

OUTWARD : *Asaf;* Bell; Berb; Bry; Chin; Kali-bi; Kali-m; Kalm; Lith; Pru-sp; Sep; Sil; *Val;* Zin.

RADIATING, Spreading : Agar; Arg-n; Ars; Bap; *BERB;* Caus; Cham; Cimi; *Colo; Cup; Dios;* Kali-bi; Kali-c; Kalm; Mag-p; *Merc;* Mez; Nux-v; Phyt; Plat; Plb; Sec; Sil; Spig; Xanth.

Distant Parts to : Berb; Cup; Dios; Mag-p; Plb; Tell; Val; Xanth.

SIDE, Lain on, go to: *Ars; Bry;* Calc; Hep; Kali-c; Mar-v; Merc; Mos; Nux-m; *Pho-ac;* PUL; Sep; Sil.

Not, lain on, go to : Bry; Cup; Flu-ac; Grap; *Ign;* Kali-bi; Kali-c; Mar-v; Pul;

Rhus-t.

Right : AP; Arg-m; Ars; Aur;
Bap; BELL; Bor; *Bry;*
CALC; *Canth; Chel;* Colo;
Con; Crot-h; *Gel;* Iris;
Kalm; LYC; Lyss; Naj;
NUX-V; Psor; PUL; Ran-sc;
Rat; Rum; Sang; Sars; Sec;
Sil; Sul-ac; *Tarn.*

left, to : Aco; Amb; Am-c;
Ap; Bell; Calc-p; Caus;
Chel; Cup; Lil-t; LYC;
Merc-i-f; Pho; Rum;
Saba; Sang; *Sil;* Sul-ac;
Syph; Ver-a.

paralysed, or weak as if :
Elap.

upper, left lower : Amb;
Pho; Sul-ac.

Left : Arg-n; ASAF; Asar;
Calc-f; Caps; *Cina; Clem;*
Croc; EUPHOR; Grap; Kre;
LACH; Lil-t; MEZ; Nat-s;
Old; *Pho; Rhus-t;* Scil;
Sele; SEP; Spig; *Stan;* SUL;
Thu.

does not belong to her :
Sil.

right, to : Ars; Bro; Calc;
Cep; Fer; *Lach;* Merc-i-r;
Nux-m; Pul; *Rhus-t;*
Saba; Stan; Tarx.

upper, right lower : Agar;
Led; Rhus-t; Tarx.

weak or paralysed as if :
Lach; Pod.

Up And Down (Rising and
Falling) : Ars; Bap; Bar-c;
Bry; Calc; Cimi; Echi;
Eup-p; *Gel; Glo;* Kali-c;

Lach; Lil-t; Lyc; Osm;
Pho; Plb; Pod; Pyro;
Sul; Ver-a.

Uppermost Agg : *Bry;* Grap;
Ign; Rhus-t.

DIRTY : See Gray.

Habits : Am-c; *Caps;* Chel;
Grap; Lach; Merc;Nux-v;
Pho; Psor; Sep; Sul.

He is : *Lac-c;* Lycps; Rhus-t;
Syph.

DISAPPOINTMENT : Alu;
Cocl; Nat-m.

Loss of Ambition, from :
Nux-v.

DISBEHAVIOR Of Others
: See Misdeeds.

DISCHARGES, Loss of vital
Fluids Agg : Aco; Agar;
CALC; Calc-p; CARB-V; CHIN;
Chin-s; Cimi; Grap; Ip;
Kali-c; Lach; Pho; *Pho-ac;*
Pul; Sec; Sele; Sep; *Stap;*
Ver-a.

Amel (Suppression Agg):
Ars; Bell; Bry; *Calc;* Cam;
Cham; Chin; Colch; Cup;
Dul; Hell; *Ip;* LACH; Lyc;
Mill; Nux-v; *Op;* Petr;
Pho-ac; Psor; PUL;
Rhus-t; Sep; Sil; Stic;
Stram; SUL; Ver-a; *Zin.*

Increased in general, moist
ness increased : Ant-t;
Ars; CALC; Carb-v;
Cham; *Chin; Dul; Fer;*
Grap; *Hep;* Ip; Iris; *Jab;*
Kali-io; Lyc; *Med;* MERC;
Nat-m; *Nat-s;* Nux-v; Op;
Pho; Pho-ac; Pul; *Rhus-t;*

Samb; Scil; Sele; SEP; *Sil; Stan;* SUL; Sul-ac; *Tab;* Thu; *Ver-a.*

ACRID, Excoriating: *Am-c;* ARS; Ars-io; Aru-t; *Bro;* Carb-an; Carb-v; Caus; Cep; Cham; Cist; Colch; Eucal; Euphr; Flu-ac; *Grap;* Hep; Hydr; *Iod;* Iris; Kali-io; Kre; Lil-t; Lyc; *Med;* MERC; Merc-c; Mez; Mur-ac; *Nit-ac;* Pho; Pru-sp; Ran-sc; *Rhus-t;* Sabi; Sang; *Sep; Sil;* SUL; Sul-ac; Sul-io; Tell; Thu; Tub.

ALBUMINOUS : Alu; *Am-m;* Berb; BOR; Calc-p; Coc-c; Jat; *Nat-m;* Pall; Petr; Phyt; Seneg; Sep; Stan; Tarn.

ALMONDS, Bitter, smell like : Benz-ac.

AMMONIACAL, Odour of : Am-c; Asaf; Aur; Benz-ac; Iod; Lac-c; Lach; Mos; *Nit-ac;* Pho; Stro.

BLACK : See Black.

BLAND : Euphr; Kali-m; *Hep; Merc; Pul;* Sil;Sul.

BLOODY: See Haemorrhage.

↖ Water, like : See Meat-water like.

BLOOD Streaked : Ars; Asaf; Bry; Chin; Crot-h; *Fer;* Hep; Ip; Lach; *Merc;* Nit-ac; *Pho;* Rhus-t; Sang; Senec; Seneg; Sil; *Sul;* Tub; Zin.

BRINY, Fishy odour : Bell; Calc; Grap; Iod; Med; Olan; Sanic; Sele; TELL;

Thu.

BROWN : See Brown.

BURNING : Ars; Calc; Cep; Kali-io; Kre; *Merc;* Merc-c; Pul; Sinap; Sul.

CURDY : Bor; Helo; Merc; Til.

DESTROYING, Hair: Bels; Lyc; Merc; Nat-m; Nit-ac; Rhus-t; Sil.

EXCESSIVE : Ars; Pod; Ver-a.

FOAMY, Frothy : Ap; Arn; Ascl; Chel; Elat; Grat; *Ip; Kali-bi;* Kali-c; Kali-io; Kob; Kre; Laur; Led; *Mag-c;*Merc; Nat-s; Oenan; *Pod;* Rhe; Rhus-t; Rum; Saba; Sep; VER-A.

Bloody : Op.

+ FOUL : Eucal; *Kre;* Meph.

GELATINOUS : *Alo; Arg-n;* Berb; COLCH; Colo; Dig; HELL; *Kali-bi;* Laur; Pod; *Rhus-t;* Sabi; Sele; Sep.

GLUEY : Ars-io; Grap; Merc; Mez; Vio-t.

GREEN : See Green.

GUSHING : Ars; Bell; Berb; Bry; CROT-T; Elat; *Gamb;* Grat *Jat;* Kali-bi; Mag-m; *Nat-c;* Nat-m; *Nat-s;* Pho; Pod; Sabi; Stan; *Thu;* Tril; Ver-a.

HOT : Aco; *Am-c; Bell;* Bor; Cham; Euphr; Iod; Kre; Op; *Pul;* Sabi; Sul.

INVOLUNTARY : See Incontinence.

ITCHING, Causing : *Calc;* Flu-ac; Led; Mang; *Med;*

Par; Rhod; *Rhus-t*; Sul; Tell.

LUMPY : Aeth; Alo; *Ant-c;* Calc-s; *Cham; Chin;* Coc-c; Croc; *Grap;* KALI-BI; Kali-m; Kre; LYC; Mang; *Merc; Merc-i-f;* PLAT; Rhus-t; Sep; Sil; Stan.

MEAT-Water, Like : Ars; Calc; Fer-p; Kali-io; Kre; Mang; Merc-c; Nit-ac; Rhus-t; Stro.

Acrid : Canth.

MILKY : Calc; Kali-m; Kali-p; Nat-s; PHO-AC; *Pul;* Sep.

MOLASSES, Like : Croc; Ip; Mag-c; Pho.

MUCOUS, Altered : *Ant-t;* Arg-m; Arg-n; *Ars;* CALC; Calc-s; Caus; *Cham;* Grap; Hep; Hydr; KALI-BI; *Lyc; Merc;* NAT-M; *Nit-ac;* Nux-v; *Pho;* PUL; SEP; Sil; *Stan; Sul.*

MUSTY, Mouldy : *Bor;* Carb-v; *Colo;* Crot-h; Mar-v; *Merc;* Nux-v; *Pho; Pul; Rhus-t;* Sanic; *Stan;* Stap; Thu; Thyr.

OFFENSIVE : See Offensiveness.

PERSISTENT : Iod.

RED (See Red) : Ars-io; Kre; Merc; Rhus-t.

REDDEN Parts : Ars; Kre; Merc.

RETAINED, Ceasing : Bur-p; Cam; Hyd-ac.

SCANTY, Bringing great Amel : Ap; Arg-m; Lach; Scil.

SEXUAL Excitement, from :

Senec.

SLIMY : Bor; Calc; Chin; *Kali-bi;* Lyc; Mag-c; Merc-d; Nat-m; Par; Pho; Pho-ac; *Pul.*

STAIN Indelibly, fast : *Bur-p;* Carb-ac; Lach; *Mag-c;* Mag-p; Med; Merc; Pulex; Sil; Thu; Vib.

Yellow : Bell; Carb-an; Grap; Kre; Lach; Merc; Sele.

STICKY, Pasty, Stringy : Ant-t; Arg-n; Bov; Bry; Caus; Coc-c; Croc; *Grap;* Hydr; KALI-BI; Kali-c; Kali-m; *Lach;* Lapp; Lyc; Mez; Myr; Nat-m; Osm; *Pho;* Phyt; Plat; *Pul;* Rum; Stan; Sul-ac; Thu; Ust; Ver-a.

SUPPRESSED : Hyd-ac; Stram; Ver-a.

TARRY : Lept; Mag-c; Mag-m; Nux-m; Plat.

THICK : Arg-m; *Ars;* Ars-io; Bor; *Calc;* Calc-s; Canth; Carb-v; Con; Croc; Dul; Grap; *Hydr; Kali-bi;* Kali-io; Kali-m; Merc; Merc-cy; Nat-m; Psor; PUL; Sil; Sul.

TURN Grass, Green: Calc-f.

URINOUS Odour: Benz-ac; Canth; *Colo;* Nat-m; Nit-ac; Ol-an; Sec; Urt.

VICARIOUS : *Bry;* Con; Dig; Fer; Ham; *Lach;* Lycps; Mill; Nux-v; *Pho; Pul;* Sec; Senec; *Sep;* Sul.

WATERY, Thin : Ars; *Asaf;* Canth; *Caus;* Cham; Crot-h; Cup; Flu-ac; Gamb; *Grap;* Grat; Iod; Iris; Kali-io; Mag-m; *Merc;* Mur-ac; Nat-s; Pho; *Pod;* Rhus-t; Sabi; Sec; Sil; *Sul;* Ver-a.

WHITE : See White.

YELLOW : See Yellow.

Green : See under Yellow.

Tenacious : Sumb.

DISCOLOURED : See under Different colours, and mottled.

DISCONTENT, Displeased, Dissatisfied : Anac; Asaf; *Bism;* Calc-p; Cham; *Hep;* Kali-c; Kali-m; Kre; Led; Lil-t; Merc; Nat-m; PUL; Rut; *Sul;* Tub.

+ CAUSE, Without : Clem.

EASILY : Caul.

EVERY-THING, With : Kre; Nat-m.

HER Own Things, with : Lil-t.

HIMSELF, With : Asaf; Con; Hep; Rut.

OTHERS, With : Hep; Rut.

WEEPING Amel : Nit-ac.

DISCORDANT : See Confusion, Co-ordination disturbed.

DISCOURAGED (See Despair) : Kali-m; Myr; Stan.

DISGUST (See Aversion) : Merc; *Pul; Sul.*

+ ALL Food : Asaf.

BODY, One's own for : Lac-c.

Odour, of : Pyro.

DISLOCATED, SPRAINED, As if : Asaf; Arn; Calc; Cham; *Chel;* Grap; *Ign;* Nat-m; Petr; *Pho; Pul; Rhus-t; Sul;* Thu.

PARTS, Lain, on : Mos.

DISLOCATION Easy, Spontaneous : Ars; *Calc;* Carb-an; Chel; Grap; Lyc; Nat-c; Pho; Pru-sp; Rhus-t; Rut; Sep.

+ ILL EFFECTS : Psor.

LAMENESS, After : Rhe.

DISOBEDIENCE : Chin; Tarn.

DISORDERLY : Stram.

DISPLEASED : See Discontent.

DISPLEASURE, *RESERVED* : See Under Reserved.

DISSATISFIED : See Discontent.

DISTENSION, Feeling of (See swelled, enlarged as if) : *Glo;* Mag-c; Ran-b; Rut.

PAIN, During: Pul.

DISTORTIONS : See Contortions.

DISTRACTION, Cannot collect -ideas, concentration difficult : ACO; Aeth; Agn; Alu; Am-c; Anac; Cocl; Hell; Lach; Nat-c; Old; Pho-ac; Senec; Sul; Thu; Zin.

DISTRUSTFUL : See Suspicious.

DIVERSION AMEL : Con; Hell; Helo; Ign; Lil-t; Nat-c; Orig; Pall; Pip-m; Sep.

DOMINEERING : Lil-t; Lyc; Pall; PLAT; Sul; VER-A.

DOTAGE : Aeth; Ars.

DOUBTING PEOPLE : Alu; *Calc;* Sul-io.

DOWNWARD : See Under Di - rections.

DRAFT AGG: See Wind Agg.

DRAGGING, SENSATION : Lil-t; Sep.

+ LOAD, As from a : Alo.

WAIST Down : Visc.

DRAWING : See Pain Drawing.

UP, LIMBS AGG : Carb-v; Pul; Rhus-t; Sec.

AMEL : Calc; Merc-c; Ran-b; Sep; Sul; Thu.

DRAWN BACK : See Retraction.

TOGETHER : Carb-v; *Chin;* Merc; Naj; Nat-m; *Nux-v;* Par; Pul; *Rhus-t; Sele; Sul.*

DREAMINESS, Revery, Ec stasy: ACO; Agar; Amb; Anac; *Ant-c* Cann; *Lach; Nux-m;* Old; OP; PHO; Sep; Sul;Ver-a.

DREAMS : Am-m; Arn; Ars; Bry; Calc; *Chin; Grap;* Lach; Lyc; *Mag-c; Nat-m;* NUX-V; PHO; PUL; *Rhus-t; Sil; Sul;* Thu.

ACCIDENTS : Ars; Grap.

+ AFFAIRS, Household : Bry.

AGREEABLE, Pleasant : *Calc; Nat-c; Nux-v;* OP; *Pul;* Sep; *Stap; Vio-t.*

AMOROUS, Erotic : Am-m; Arg-n; Bism; Cact; Cam; Lach; Nat-c; Nat-p; Nux-v; Op; Pho; Pho-ac; Senec; Stap; Vio-t.

Coition, of : Bor; Sumb.

Emission, with : Stap.

Leucorrhoea, with : Petr.

Menses, before : Calc; Kali-c.

ANIMALS, Of : Arn; Merc; Nux-v; Op; Pho; Pul.

Cats, black : Daph.

ANXIOUS Frightful: Am-m; Arn; Cact; Calc; Chin; Cocl; Crot-h; Grap; Kali-c; Kali-m; Lach; Lyc; Nat-m; Nat-p; Paeon; Pul; Ran-sc; Sil; Tub.

Menses, before and after : Sul-ac.

Same over and over again : Ign.

AWAKE, On falling to sleep : Bell; Lach; Sil; Sul.

+ BLACK Forms : Op.

BLOOD, Of : See Fire.

+ BODIES, Mutilated : Arn.

+ CARE And Toil : Ap.

+ CONFUSED : Rut.

DAY'S Work, Difficulties : Am-m; Ars; *Bry;* Nux-v; Pul; RHUS-T.

DEAD, Of the : Ars; Cann; Crot-h; Elap; Mag-c; Nat-p; Pho; Thu.

Bodies : Anac; Chel; Ran-sc.

+ Funeral : Chel.

DEATH, Of : Lach.

DRINKING, Water : Med.

Emission, followed by :
Merc- i-f.

DROWNING, Of : Ver-v.

EVENTS, Previous day, of : Bry.
Long past: Sil.

FALLING : Bell; Cact; Dig;
Sumb; Thu.

+ From, high place : Nux-m.

FANTASTIC : Calc; Calc-io;
Carb-an; Lach; Nat-m; Op.

+ FIGHTING : Nat-s; Ran-b.

FIRE, Blood, Vivid : *Anac*; Aur;
Cann; Carb-v; Grap; Hep;
Hyo; Laur; Lyc; Mag-c;
Mag-m; Manc; Meny; *Pho*;
Radm; *Rhus-t*; Ruta; *Sil*;
Sul; Tub.

+ Continued, after waking :
Psor.

+ Remembered well : Mang.

FLYING : Ap; Latro; Stic.

FRIGHTFUL : See Anxious.

GLOOMY : Plant.

+ HORRIBLE : Adon.

+ HORRID : Chlo-hyd.

JOURNEY : Kali-n.

+ JUMPS, Bed, out of, in : Calc-f.

LABORIOUS, Exhausting : Arn;
Bry; Echi; Pul; Rhus-t.

LACHRYMATION, With: Plant.

LOATHSOME : Lach.

LYING, Left side, on: Sep.

MANY : Ars; Senec.

+ MENSES, During : Nux-m.

NAUSEA, In : Arg-m.

PIECING, Bodies of her children, together : Dict; Pho.

PURSUED, Being : Nux-m.

QUARRELSOME : Echi.

SHAME : Con; Tub.

SLEEP, First : Sil.

SNAKES : Arg-n; Lac-c; Lach;
Ran-sc.

THIEVES, Robbers : Alu;
Mag-c; Nat-m; Sanic.

TRUE, Seem on waking :
Arg-m; Radm.

URINATING, Of : Kre; Lac-c;
Seneg; Sep.

VIVID : See Fire.

+ VOLUPTOUS : Bor.

WATER, On, Being : Ver-v.

WEEPING : Calc-f; Glo; Kre;
Plant; Sil; Stram.

DREAMY : See Dreaminess.

DRINKING AGG : *Arg-n; Ars*;
Bell; *Canth; Chin; Cocl*;
Crot-t; Fer; *Lach*; Merc-c;
NUX-V; *Pho; Phyt*; Pod; *Pul*;
Rhus-t; Sil; Stram; Sul-ac;
VER-A.

AMEL : Bism; *Bry; Caus*; Cist;
Coc-c; Cup; Lob; Nux-v;
Pho; Sep; *Spo*.

Little Amel : Lob.

EXCITES, Urination and stool :
Caps.

HASTILY : Anac; Bry; Hep.

RAPIDLY AGG: Ars; Nit-ac;
Nux-v; Sil.

SIPS, In AGG : Merc.

AMEL : Bell; Cist; Kali-n; Scil.
Difficulty, with : Spo.

Milk Amel : Diph.

WARM AGG : Rhus-t.

WATER, Bad AGG : All-s; Zing. Seems to run outside, not going down oesophagus : Ver-a.

Too much AGG : Grat.

DRINKS COLD AGG and AMEL : See Under Food.

+ AGG, when over heated : Bels.

AS IF : Elap.

Warm, Seem : Nat-m.

DESIRE, For : See Thirst.

HOT AGG : Ap; *Bry*; Grap; Lach; *Pho*; *Pul*; Phyt.

AMEL : Ail; Ars; Lyc; Nux-v; Sul-ac.

Seems cold : Cam.

LITTLE, Eats much but seldom : Ars.

MUCH, Eats, little : Dig; Sep; Sul.

NEITHER, Or eats for weeks : Ap.

OFFENSIVE, As if : Arn.

THIRST, Without : Calad; Cam; Cocl.

URINATION, Profuse, after : Lycps.

DRIVING : See Riding.

DROPPING Like Water : See Trickling.

DROPS THINGS : See Awkward.

DROPSY OEDEMA : *Acet-ac;* Agar; Ant-c; AP; ARS; Aur; Bell; Bry; Canth; Card-m; CHIN; *Colch; Como; Dig;* Dul; Fer; *Grap;* HELL; Iod; Kali-c; Kali-io; Led; Lyc; Med; MERC; *Old; Op; Pho;* Pul; Rhus-t;

Samb; *Scil; Sep;* Sil; Stro; SUL; Terb; Til; Zin.

ALCOHOLISM, From: Ars; Flu-ac; Sul.

DIARRHOEA, With : Acet-ac; Ap; Apoc; Hell.

EXANTHEMA, After : Ars; Hell; Rhus-t; Sul.

GENERAL : See Anasarca.

GLANDS, Pressure of, from : Kali-io.

HAEMORRHAGE, After : Acet-ac; Apoc; Chin; Fer; Helo; Senec.

HEART, Affection, with : Adon; Cact; Conval; Cratae; Dig; Iod; Lac-d; Pru-s; Scop; Strop.

JAUNDICE, With: Merc-d.

KIDNEY Affections, with: Apoc; Ars; *Dig*; Helo; *Mer-c;* Terb.

Heart, and with : *Merc-d.*

LIVER Affection, with : *Apoc;* Card-m; Flu-ac; Lac-d; Lach; Lyc; Mur-ac.

MORNING Agg : Ap; Aur; Kali-chl; Pho; Sep; Sil.

Amel : Bry.

NEWBORN : Ap; Carb-v; Dig; Lach; Sec.

NUMBNESS, With : Flu-ac.

PUBERTY or MENOPAUSE, at : Pul.

QUININE, From : Apoc.

SACCULAR : Ap; Ars; Kali-c.

SERUM Exudes : Ars; Lyc; Rhus-t.

Skin, Red, with : Como.

Spleen Diseases, from : Lach.

Sprains, From : Bov.

Thirst, With: A*cet-ac; Apoc;*
Ars.

Without : Ap; Hell.

Urination or Secretion, profuse, with : Scil.

Urine Suppressed, fever, and
debility : Hell.

DROWSINESS : See Sleepiness.

DRUGS, Abuse, of, in general
: Alo; Ars; Cam; *Carb-v;*
Cham; Colo; Hep; *Hyds;*
Kali-io; Mar-v; Nat-m;
Nit-ac; NUX-V; *Pul;* Sec; *Sul.*

Anaesthetic Vapour : Acet-ac;
Amy-n; Hep; Pho.

Antityphoid Injections : Bap.

Aspirin And similar : Arn;
Carb-v; Lach; Mag-p.

Bromide : Cam; Helo;
Nux- v; Zin.

Castor Oil *: Bry; Nux-v.*

Codliver Oil : Hep.

Cosmetics : Bov.

Digitalis *:* Chin; Laur; Nit-ac.

Disease, and *A*gg: Alo; Carb-v;
Nux-v.

Heart Remedies : Lycps.

Iodides : Ars; Bell; *Hep;* Hyds;
Pho.

Iron : Chin; *Hep; Pul;* Sul;
Zin.

Lead*: Alu;* Caus; Colo;
Kali-io; Op; Plb.

Mercury *: Aur; Bry; Carb-v;*
Chin; Guail; *Hep;* Iod;
Kali-io; *Lach;* Mez; Nat-s;
NIT-AC; Phyt; Sars; *Stap;*
Sul.

Narcotics : Am-c; Bell;
Carb-v; *Cham; Cof; Lach;*
Merc; *Nux-v;* Pul.

Opium : Cham; Mur-ac;
Nat-m; *Pul;* Ver-a.

Purgatives : Hyds; Lyc;
Nux-v; Op; Sul.

Quinine : Arn; *Ars;* Carb-v;
Fer; Ip; *Nat-m;* Nux-v; *Pul;*
Sul; Ver-a.

Sulphur : Calc; Merc; *Pul.*

Tar Locally : Bov.

Terpentine : Nux-m.

Tetanus, Antitoxin : Mag-p.

DRUNKARDS : Asar; Caps;
Cocl; Sul-ac.

DRY CLEAR Or **COLD WEATHER**

Agg : See Air, Cold,
Dry Agg.

DRYNESS: Aco; Alu; *Ars; Bell;*
Bry; *Calad;* Calc; Canth;
Fer; Iod; Lach; Lyc; Mag-m;
Meli; *Nat-m;* Nat-s; NUX-M;
Pho; Plb; Pul; *Rhus-t;* Sanic;
Sang; Sec; Sep; *Sul;* Thyr;
Tub; Ust; Visc.

Internal : Aesc; *Bell;* Bry;
Grap; Op; Petr; Rum.

Partial, Local : Aco; Alu;
Bell; Bry; Grap; Kali-bi;
Lyc; Nat-m; NUX-M; Petr;
Pho; PUL; Rhus-t; Stram;
SUL; Ver-a.

PROFUSE Secretion, with :
Euphr; Lyc; Merc; Nat-m.

DUALITY,In pieces, Seperated
as if someone else : *Anac*;
Arg-n; BAP; Calc-p; Cann;
Cyc; GEL; *Lach*; Lil-t; Nux-m;
PETR; Pho; Pyro; Sil; *Stram*;
Ther; Thu; Tril; Xanth.

As IF Divided into half and
left side does not belong to
her : Sil.

DULL, BECLOUDED, Difficult
comprehension, Stupefied :
Ail; Ant-t; Ap; Arg-n; Arn;
Bap; *Bar-c*; BELL; BRY; CALC;
Carb-v; Cocl; GEL; GLO; *Hell*;
HYO; Kali-br; Kali-c; Lach;
LAUR; LYC; NAT-C; *Nux-m*;
NUX-V; Old; Op; Petr; Pho;
PHO-AC; Psor; Pul; RHUS-T;
SEP; SIL; STRAM; *Sul*; Tub;
Ver-a; Zin.

CHILDREN : Arg-n; Bar-c;
Calc-p; Sul.

EMISSION, After : Caus.

OLD PEOPLE : Amb; Bar-c.

PUBERTY, At (Girls) : Ap.

STUDYING, Reading : Aeth;
Hell; Nux-v.

WHAT He reads or hears,
about : Sele.

DUODENUM, Affection of
: Ars; Chin; Hyds; Kali-bi;
Merc-d; Nat-p; Pod; Uran.

OBSTRUCTION Of : Canc-fl.

ULCERATION : *Kali-bi*; Symp;
Uran.

DUPLICITY : See Deceitful.

DUSK : See Twilight.

DUSKY COLOUR (Pale) : Ail;
Ant-t; Ars; *Bap*; Cam;
Crot-h; *Gel*; *Hell*; Lach;
Nit-ac; *Nux-v*; Op; Sec.

DUST, FEATHER, as of a : Ars;
Bell; CALC; Chel; Chin;
DROS; Hep; Ign; *Lyc*;
Pho-ac; Pul; Rum; Sul.

AGG : Am-c; Ars; Bell; *Bro*;
CALC; Chel; Chin; DROS;
Hep; Ign; Just; *Lyc*;
Pho-ac; Pul; Rum; Sil; Sul.

FINE, Air, in AGG : Bell.

DWARFISH : Amb; BAR-C;
Bar-m; Calc; Calc-p; *Con*;
Med; Ol-j; Sil; *Sul*; Syph;
Thyr.

DYSENTERY : Aco; Alo; Ars;
Canth; *Caps*; Carb-v; Colch;
Colo; Gel; Ham; Ip; Mag-c;
Merc; MERC-C; NUX-V; *Pho*;
Rhus-t; Stap; *Sul*.

AFTER, AGG : Alo; Colch.

AUTUMNAL : Arn; Colch.

CLIMAXIS, At : Lil-t.

DIARRHOEA, After: Lept.

EMACIATED, Undersized
Chil-dren : Bar-m.

FEVER, With : Bap; Fer-p;
Nux-v.

FOOD or DRINK, least Agg :
Stap; Tromb.

HEAD HOT, Limbs cold, with
: Ip.

+ HIGH Altitude : Coca.

OLD PEOPLE, In : Bap.

PERIODIC (in summer) : Arn;

Kali-bi.

+ Potbellied Children : Calc.

Rheumatic Pain, with : Ascl.

+ Tenesmus : Calc.

DYSMENORRHOEA : See Menses Painful.

DYSPEPSIA : See Digestion Affected.

DYSPHAGIA : See Swallowing difficult.

DYSPNOEA : See Respiration Difficult and Asthma.

DYSURIA : See Urination, Dif ficult.

EARS : Aur; *Bell; Calc*; Cham; FER-P; *Grap*; Hep; Lyc; Mang; MERC; Petr; Pho; Pho-ac; Plant; *Psor*; PUL; SIL; SUL; *Tell*; Zin-chr.

Right: *Bell*; Flu-ac; Iod; Kali-c; Kali-n; Nit-ac; Nux-v; Plat; Sil; Spo.

Skin, stretched over, as if : Asar.

Left : Anac; Asaf; Bor; Grap; Guai; Ign; *Old; Vio-o.*

Right, to : Grap; Mur-ac.

Tickling over : Zin-val.

Alternating : Bell; *Bry*; Caps; Caus; Chel; Cocl; Fer-p; Glo; Kali-c; *Mag-m*; Med; Mos; *Nit-ac*; Sul.

Abdomen, with : Radm.

Teeth, with : Plant.

Behind : Aur; Bar-c; Calc; Caus; Canth; *Caps*; Caus; Glo; *Grap*; Lach; Lyc; Merc; Old; Petr; *Pho*; Psor; Sanic; Sil; Stap; Zin-chr.

Body, hard, as of : Grap.

Cracks : *Grap.*

Eczema : Tell.

Herpes : Sep.

Moisture: *Grap;* Lyc; *Petr; Psor.*

+ Screw, sensation : Ox-ac.

Throbbing : Zin-chr.

Tumour : Berb.

Below: Bell.

Between (Ear to ear) : Plant.

Everything Affects : Cann; Gel; Mang; Plant.

External : Alu; Kali-c; Kre; Merc; Pho-ac; *Sep; Spig.*

Blue : Tell.

Boils on : Merc.

Itching : Agar; Pul; Rhus- t; Sul; Tell.

Painful : Petr.

Red : *Aco*; Agar; Ap; Caus; Chin; Ip; Nat-p; *Pul*; Pyro; Sul.

left : Ant-c; Carb-v; Kre.

menses, during : Agar.

Swelling, sudden : Calc-p.

Veins, distended : Dig.

Internal : *Calc;* Caus; Grap; Kali-c; Mang; *Nux-v;Pho; Psor; Pul; Sep; Spig.*

Glands, Of : Bell; Cham; Con; Lach; *Merc*; Rhus-t; Sil.

Lobules : Bar-c; Caus; *Chin;* Kre; Pul.

Cysts : Nit-ac.

Herpes, on : Sep.

Hot and red : Cam.

Itching : Arg-m.

Red : Cham.

Ulceration of ring hole
: Kali-m; Med; Stan.

Ossicles, Sclerosis of : Thyr.

Outward In : Agar; Calc;
Canth; Chel; Merc; Psor.

Tympanum, Drum, burning :
Ang.

Calcareous deposit, on :
Calf-f; Syph.

Coated white: Grap.

Exudation, serous, on : Jab.

Injury, to : Tell.

Perforated : Caps; Hep;
Kali-bi; Sil; Tub.

Retracted : Merc-d.

Scaly : Grap.

Thickened : Ars-io;
Merc-d; Mez.

Abscess : Calc-pic; *Merc;*
Syph.

Aching : CHAM; Dul; FER-P;
Nux-v; Plant; PUL; Sul;
Tell.

Both, in : Phyt.

Faints : Hep; Merc.

Head, with : Psor; Sang.

Hiccough, with : Tarn.

Nausea, with : Dul.

Swallowing Agg : Gel.

Throat, extending, to : Cep.

Writing Agg : Phyt.

Air, As if, in : Grap; *Mez.*

Cold : Kali-c; Mill.

Hot, from : Aeth; Canth.

Rushing out, as if : Chel;
Stram.

Bleeding : Cic.

Easy, polyp : Calc.

Blood, Hot, rushing in, as if
: Cyc.

Blowing Nose Agg : See
Nose, Blowing Agg.

Body, Between, as if :
Plant.

Boil, In : Bov; Pic-ac.

Boring, Fingers, with Amel:
Chel; Colo; Lach; *Mez;*
Nat-c; Spig.

Tendency : Sil.

children, in : Cina;
Psor; Sil.

Bubble Bursting in : Nat-c.

Burning, In : Caus.

Chewing Agg : Anac; Ap;
Seneg; Sul.

Cold Agg : Caps; *Hep;* Sil.

Amel : Bell.

Heat, or Agg : Cic.

Colds Agg : Fer-p; Kali-m;
Merc-d; Pho.

Coughing Agg : Calc; Caps;
Dios.

Crawling, Out : Chel.

Crusts, On : Bar-c.

Discharge, From: Bar-m;
Calc; Calc-p; Calc-s;
Carb-v; Caus; *Con;* Grap;
Hep; Kali-bi; Kali-c;
Kali-s; LYC; MERC; Petr;
PSOR; PUL; *Sil;* Sul; Tell;
Vio-o.

Birth, from : Vio-o.

Black : Naj.

Briny : Grap; Naj; Sele; *Tell.*

Deafness, with : Asaf; Elap; Lyc.

Diarrhoea, offensive, with : Psor.

Eruptive disease, after : Cist.

Green : Lac-c.

Headache, after : Abs. with : Psor.

Itching, with : Crot-t; Elap.

Mastoid, swelling, with : Carb-an.

Polypus with : Kali-s.

Pus : CALC; Calc-s; *Con; Hep;* Kali-bi; Kali-c; Kali-s; Lyc; *Merc;* Pho; Psor; *Pul; Sil.*

bloody : Rhus-t.

Recurring : Vio-o.

Stopped, Suppressed : Aur; Carb-v; Merc; PUL.

DRYNESS : *Grap;* Lach; Petr.

ECHO, In : Caus; Colo; Nit-ac; Pho.

Peculiar noise with every : Lyc.

Sneezing, on : Bar-c.

Sounds unnatural : Terb.

Voices : Caus; Pho.

Words, one's own : Sars.

ERUCTATION Agg : Grap.

EXCORIATED, Raw : *Ars;* Cep; *Kali-bi; Merc;* PSOR; Sul; Tell.

EYES, And : Vio-o.

FLUTTERING, Sudden : Merc-d.

FOETOR, From : *Calc;* Carb-v; *Caus;* Hep; Kali-p; Nat-c; PSOR; *Sil; Sul;* Thu.

FOREIGN Bodies, as if in : Pho; Plant.

FRONT in, something : Pho.

HAEMATOMA : Bell.

HEAD Turning, Agg : Carb-v; *Mag-p.*

HEAT Emanating, from : *Aeth;* Caus.

HOLLOW, As if : Nux-v.

HOT : Caps; Chin; Nat-p.

INFLAMMED : FER-P; Merc; Merc-c; Pho; Pul; Sul; Tell.

Slap, after : Calc-s.

INSERTING Finger and drawing parts apart Amel : Aeth.

ITCHING In : Aur; Hep; Kali-c; Mang; Nux-v; Petr; Sep; Sil; Sul.

Boring with fingers Amel : Bov; Colo; Zin.

Cerumen, increased, with : Cyc.

+ Frozen, as if : Agar.

Laughing, when : Mang.

Scratch, must, until it bleeds : *Arg-m;* Nat-p.

Sneezing, with : Cyc.

Swallowing Amel : Nux-v.

Talking, when : Mang.

JERKING : Plat.

KIDNEYS, And : Thu; *Vio-o.*

LAUGHING Agg : Mang.

LEAF, Sensation of a : Sul-ac.

LYING, Face, on Amel : Radm.

MOUTH Opening Amel : Nat-c.

MUSIC Agg : Pho-ac; Tab.

NECK, Down, to : Tarx.

NODES, On : Berb.

NOISE Agg : Aco; *Bell;* Cof; Con; Nux-v; OP; Spig; Sul; *Ther.*

Least Agg : Cimi.

Amel : Calend; Grap; Jab; Nit-ac.

NOISES, In : See Hearing.

NOSE, Blowing Agg : Act-sp; Calc; Dios; Pho-ac; Sul.

NUMB : Plat; Verb.

OPEN And Close, as if : Bor.

Cool air, to, as if : Mez.

Ear to ear : Alet.

PREGNANCY Agg : Caps.

PRESSED Apart : Par.

Out, something, from : Pul.

PUFFY : Tell.

PULSATION : Lach; Mag-m; Med.

QUIVERING In : Bov; Kali-c.

Bad news, from : Kali-c; Sabi.

RED : See under External.

RIDING In Carriage Amel : Grap; *NIT-AC;* Pul.

SCABBY : Grap; Radm.

SCARLATINA, After : Mur-ac; Sul.

SINGING Agg : Pho-ac.

SIZZLING or Frying, as if, in : Calc-hyp.

SKIN, As if, stretched over : Asar.

SLAP, After : Calc-s.

SPEAKING, Loudly Agg : Mang; Terb.

Painful : Terb.

STITCHES : BELL; Caus; *Cham;* Chin; *Con;* Dul; Grap; KALI-C; Kali-io; *Merc; Nux-v;* PUL; *Sul.*

STOPPED, As if : Asar; Carb-v; *Con;* Kali-m; *Lyc; Merc;* PUL; Sil.

Blowing nose, on : Sul.

Chewing, when : Sul.

Fullmoon, at : Grap.

Plug, as from : Asar; Led.

Swallowing Amel : Sil.

Valve or membrane, with, as if : Bar-c; Iod; Nat-s.

Yawning Amel : Nat-m; *Sil.*

+ STUFFED, As if : Spig.

SURGING, In : Kali-p.

SWALLOWING Agg : Ap; Bov; Gel; Lach; Mang; Nit-ac; Nux-v; Phyt.

Moving, something, in : Nat-c.

TOOTHACHE, With : Glo; Plant; *Rhod.*

TREMBLING In, sad news, after : Kali-c; Sabi.

TWITCH, Blowing nose or sneezing : Act-sp.

URINATION, Profuse Agg : Thu.

VERTEX, To : Mur-ac.

VOICE Echoes in : Caus; Pho.

One's own sounds unnatural : Terb.

WATER Falling, height from :
Nat-p.

Cold, coming out, as if :
Merc.

Drop of, as if, in : Aco.

Hot, coming out, as if : Aco;
Cham.

Sipping Amel : Bar-m.

Swashing, as if, in :
Ant-c; Grap; Merc; *Sul.*

WAVES, In : Kali-p.

WAX, Blackish : Pul.

Chewed paper, like : Con;
Lach.

Dark, flowing : Calc-s.

Decreased : Lach.

+ Dry : Lach.

Falling, small balls, in :
Dios.

Foul : Caus.

Hardened : Lach; Pul.
black : Elap.

Increased : Caus.

Red : *Con;* Psor.

Whitish : Lach.

Yellow : Carb-v; Kali-c.

WIND Agg : *Cham;* Lach.

WORM, In, As if : Rhod.

EAT, AVERSION, or refusal to
: Anac; Kali-chl; Hell; *Hyo;*
Pho-ac; Phyt; Tarn; Ver-a;
Vio-o; Zin-chr.

CHOKES, On attempting to :
Zin-val.

EVERYTHING and anything :
Plat; Sul.

EXCRETA, His own : Ver-a.

GREEDILY : Lyc; Zin.

HUNGER, Without : Calad.

+ Drinks, thirst without :
Calad.

LITTLE, Is sufficient : Rhe.

MORE Than he drinks :
All-sat.

NEITHER Drink nor, for weeks
: Ap.

TOO Tired, to : Bar-c; Stan.

WHEN, Asked, only : Ant-c.

EATING AGG : *Alo;* Am-c;
Anac; ARS; Bell; Bry; CALC;
CARB-An; CARB-V
Caus; Chin; Colo; CON;
Fer; Hep; Ign; KALI-BI;
KALI-C; Lach; *Lyc;* Mag-m;
Merc; Nat-c; NAT-M; NIT-
AC; NUX-V; Petr; *Pho;* Pod;
Pul; Rum; *Sep; Sil; Sul;*
Ver-a; Vio-t; Zin.

AMEL : *Anac;* Bov; Cham;
Chel; Con; Flu-ac; Grap;
Hep; IGN; IOD; Kali-bi;
Kalm; Lach; NAT-C; Nat-m;
PHO; Plb; Psor; Radm;
Rhod; Sep; Spo; Val; *Zin.*

A LITTLE AGG : Bry; Carb-an;
Chin; Con; *Kali-c;* LYC;
Nat-p; *Nux-v;* Petr; *Pho;*
Pul; *Sul.*

AMEL: Lob; Spo.

BREAKFAST AGG And AMEL
: See Breakfast.

FATIGUE AGG : Ars; Bar-c;
Carb-an; Kali-c; Lyc;
Nat-m; Pho-ac; Zin.

FREQUENTLY Agg : Aeth.

Amel : Flu-ac; Sul.

+ Wants, but least food oppresses : Kali-c.

HASTILY Agg : Sil.

LONG After AGG : Aeth; Anac; Carb-v; Fer; *Kali-bi; Kre;* Nat-m; PHO; PUL; Sul; Zin.

NIGHT, At AGG : See Dinner.

SELDOM And Much : Ars.

+ SLEEPY, While : Kali-c.

TOO Much, overeating *AGG* : Aeth; *Ant-c;* Ant-t; Bry; Calc; *Carb-v; Lyc;* Nat-p; Nux-m; NUX-V; *Pul; Sul.*

UNTIL Satisfied AMEL : Ars; *Iod;* Pho.

EBULITIONS : See Waves.

ECHYMOSIS, PETECHIAE, Purpura, etc. : ARN; Ars; Bry; Crot-h; Ham; Kre; LACH; Led; Mur-ac; *Pho;* Pho-ac; Pyro; Rhus-t; Sec; Solid; *Sul-ac;* Tarn; Terb.

ADVANCING : Terb.

BLOW, Slight, from : Agar; Arn.

OLD AGE : Sars.

URTICARIA, With : Lob.

ECLAMPSIA : *Bell;* Cham; *Cic;* Cup; Hell; *Hyo;* Ign; Passif; *Stram; Stry;* Thyr; Ver-a; *Ver-v.*

DELIVERY, Immediately after : Amy-n; Ant-t.

LABOUR Pains, ceasing, from : Op.

ECSTASY (See Dreaminess) : Cof.

ECTROPION (Eyelids turned up) : Ap; Arg-m; Arg-n; Grap; Psor; Spig.

ECZEMA : Alu; *Ars;* Ars-io; Bell; BOV; Calc;Calc-s; *Carb-v;* Cic; *Clem;* Crot-t; DUL; GRAP; *Hep; Kre; Lyc; Merc; Mez; Old; Petr; Pho;* Psor; Radm; *Rhus-t;* Solid; Stap; *Sul;* Sul-io.

BEARD, Of : Ars-io.

CRUSTS, Thick, with : Stap.

DIGESTIVE Affections, with : Lyc.

DRY, Children, in : Calc-s; Dul; Frax; Tarn; Vio-t.

FINGER, Toe, of, with loss of nail : Bor.

FOUL : Lapp; Vinc.

HAIR, Margins, at : Hyds.

ITCHING Without : Cic.

LIVER, Affections, with : Lyc.

MENSTRUAL Affections, with : Mang.

MOIST : Kre; Lapp; Sul-io; Vinc.

Foul : Lapp.

NEUROTIC : Anac; Zin.

RECURRENT : Como.

SCURFY : Kre.

SUN, Exposure, from : Mur-ac.

SUPPRESSED, Head, of Agg : Mez.

URINE, Affections, with : Lyc.

Suppressed Agg : Solid.

WASHING Agg : Ars-io.

EDGE, ON, As if : Rut; Val.

EFFECTS, SINGLE : See Single Parts.

COMPENSATORY : Pru-sp.

EFFUSION, Deposit : Abro;
Ap; Bels; *Bry;* Canth; Hell;
Kali-n; Ran-b; Sul; Sul-io.

Bᴸᴏᴏᴅʏ : Carb-ac.

EGG Aᴸʙᴜᴍɪɴ Dried on, as if
: Alu; Ol-an; Sul-ac.

Rᴏᴛᴛᴇɴ Odour of : Arn; Ascl;
Cham; Psor; Stap; Sul.

EGOISM : See Pompous.

ELBOWS : Caus; Kali-c;
Rhus-t; Sep; Sul.

Aɴᴋʏʟᴏsɪs : Sil.

Axɪʟʟᴀ, To : Ars.

Bᴀɴᴅᴀɢᴇᴅ, As if : Caus.

Bᴇɴᴅ Of : Kali-c.

Eruptions yellow, scaly
: Cup.

Straightening Agg : *Caus;*
Hep; Pul.

Warts : Calc-f.

Bᴜʙʙʟɪɴɢ, In : Rhe.

Cᴀʀʀʏɪɴɢ Weight Agg : Cham.

Cʀᴀᴄᴋɪɴɢ : Kalm.

Cʀᴜsᴛs, Thick, on : Sep.

Dʀᴀᴡɪɴɢ : Ars.

Eʀᴜᴘᴛɪᴏɴs : Syph.

Hᴀɴᴅ, To : Cinb.

Hᴇʀᴘᴇs : Pho; Sep; Stap; Thu.

Iᴛᴄʜɪɴɢ : Nat-c; Syph.

Kɴɪᴛᴛɪɴɢ Agg : Mag-c.

Nᴜᴍʙ : Nat-s; Pul.

Pᴀɪɴꜰᴜʟ Heart, disease, in :
Arn.

Pᴀʀᴀʟʏsɪs : Rhus-t.

Sʜɪɴʏ : Ant-c.

Sʜᴏᴜʟᴅᴇʀ, To : Ther.

Sᴘʀᴀɪɴ : Fer-p.

Sᴛɪꜰꜰ : Bry; Lyc.

Sᴡᴇʟʟɪɴɢ : Bry; Merc.

Tᴇɴᴅᴏɴs, Inflamed : Ant-c.

Tɪᴘ, Of : *Hep.*

Touch Agg : Grap.

ELECTRIC Sʜᴏᴄᴋ ᴀɢɢ : Pho.

Sᴘᴀʀᴋs Sensation : Agar;
Arg-m; Calc; *Calc-p;* Lyc;
Nat-m; SEC; Sele.

ELECTRICITY Aᴍᴇʟ : Sil.

ELEPHANTIASIS : Ars;
Hydroc; Grap; Iod; Lyc; Sil.

ELEVATING, Lɪᴍʙs Aᴍᴇʟ (See
also Hanging down limbs
Agg) : Calc; CARB-V; Pul;
Ran-sc; *Sep; Vip.*

ELONGATED, As if : Alu; Hypr;
Kali-c; Lac-c; *Pho;* Stram;
Tab.

EMACIATION, Aᴛʀᴏᴘʜʏ : Abro;
Arg-n; ARS; Ars-io; *Bar-c;*
Bism; Bor; CALC; Calc-io;
CALC-P; Caus; *Chin; Fer;*
Grap; Hell; IOD; Led; LYC;
Med; NAT-M; NIT-AC; *Nux-v;*
Op; *Pho;* PLB; Sanic; Sars;
Sele; *Sil;* Stan; Stram;
Stro; SUL; Syph; Thu; Thyr;
Tub.

Aꜰꜰᴇᴄᴛᴇᴅ, Part : See Partial.

Aᴘᴘᴇᴛɪᴛᴇ, With : Abro; Ars;
Calc; Cina; *Iod;* Lyc;
Nat-m; Petr; Psor; Sul;
Thyr; Tub.

Asᴄᴇɴᴅɪɴɢ : Abro; Arg-n.

Cᴏᴜɢʜ, With : Amb.

Dᴇsᴄᴇɴᴅɪɴɢ : Lyc; Nat-m;
Sanic; Sars.

Fʟᴇsʜ Fell off from bones, as

115

if : Tarn.

GLANDS, Of : Con; Iod.
Enlarged, with : Iod.

GRIEF, After : Petr; Pho-ac.

INFANTILE Marasmus : *Abro;*
Ars; Ars-io; *Aur;* Bor; CALC;
Calc-hyp; Calc-p; *Chin;*
Iod; Kre; *Lyc; Mag-c;*
Nat-m; Plb; Sanic; Sil; SUL;
Syph; Ther; Tub.

INSANITY, With : Nat-m; Sil.

LOSS Of Vital fluid, from :
Chin; Lyc; *Sele.*

NEURALGIA, After : Plb.

PAINFUL : Caps; Plb.

PARTIAL, Affected parts, of, etc
: Bry; Calc; Grap; Led; *Mez;*
Pho; *Plb ; Pul;* Sec; *Sele;*
Sul.

PINING Boys: *Aur; Lyc;* Nat-m;
Pho-ac; *Tub.*

PROGRESSIVE, Acute diseases,
in : Arn; Guai; Ver-a.

RAPID : Ars; Calc-hyp; Chlor;
Fer; Thu; Thyr.

SENILE : Amb; Bar-c; Chin;
Flu-ac; Iod; Lyc; Op; Sec;
Sele.

SENSATION, Of : Naj.

UPPER Parts : Calc; Plb.

UPWARDS : Abro; Arg-n.

WELL-NOURISHED, Persons, of
suddenly : Bar-c; Grap;
Samb.

EMBARASSMENT AGG : Amb;
Gel; Ign; Kali-br; Op; *Sul.*

EMBRACES : Agar; Plat.

EVERYBODY, even objects :
Ver-a.

EMBOLISM : Kali-m.

EMISSION AL : See Seminal
Emission.

EMOTION : *Aco;* Ant-c;
ARS; *Aur;* Bell; *Cham;*
Cina; Cof; Colo; Croc; Gel;
Hyo; IGN; Lach; *Lyc; Nat-m;*
Nit-ac; NUX-V; Pall; Pho;
Pho-ac; Plat; Psor; PUL;
Stap; Stram; Sul; Sumb;
Ver-a.

EMOTIONS, MENTAL Excite-
ment AGG : ACO; Amb;
Amy-n; Anac; *Arg-n;* Aur;
Bell; *Bry;* Caus; Cham; Cof;
COLO; Con; Fer; *Gel;* Hyo;
IGN; Kali-c; Kob; *Lach;*
Nat-m; NUX-V; *Op; Pho;*
PHO-AC; Phyt; Plat; Psor;
PUL; Sep; Sil; Stan; STAP;
Stram; Tub; Ver-a.

DULL: Anac.

LIVELY AGG : Pall.

LONG-LASTING, Effects of :
Petr.

SEXUAL AGG : Plat.

SLIGHT AGG : Psor.

EMPHYSEMA : See Chest.

EMPTY, HOLLOW, Sinking
: *Chin; Cocl;* Dig; Hyds;
IGN; Kali-c; Murx; Nux-v;
Old; PHO; Podo; SEP; *Stan;*
Sul; Tell; Ver-a.

BODY, As if whole : Aur;
Kali-c.

EATING, After : Grat.

ORGANS : Tab.

EMPROSTHOTONOS : Canth;
Ip.

EMPYEMA : See under Chest.

EMPYOCELE: Kali-s; Sil; Sul.

ENAMEL Thin : Flu-ac; Sil.

ENERVATED: See Delicate.

ENLARGED, SWELLED, As if
: Aco; Alu; ARAN; ARG-N;
Bap; *Bell;* Bov; Cocl; Coll;
Gel; *Glo;* Guai; *Ign;* Lach;
Merc; Merc-i-f; Nux-v; Op;
Paeon; Par; Pul; *Ran-b;*
Rhus-t; Sanic; Spig.

ENTROPION (Eyelids turned
down) : Bor; Grap; Nat-m;
Psor; Pul; Sil; Tell.

ENURESIS : See Urnination
Involuntary, and Bed-wet-
ting.

ENVY : See Jealousy.

EPIGASTRIUM : ARS; *Calc;*
Chel; Cocl; Colo; *Ign;* Ip;
KALI-C; *Lach;* Lob; Lyc;
Nat-m; NUX-V; Pho; *Pul;*
Sep; Sul; Tab.

ABOVE : Nat-m; PHO; Pul.

ACHING : See Pain.

ANXIETY At : *Ars;* Lyc; Nux-v;
Pul.

AXILLA, To: Kali-n.

+ **B**ACK, To : Sabi.

BURNING : Ars; Med; Nux-v;
Sep; Sil; Terb; Ver-a.
Hot coal as if from : Ver-a.

CHILL, From : Arn.

COLD : Cam; Hep; Kre.

COUGH, From : Bry; Nit-ac;
Pho; Pho-ac.

EMPTY, Sinking, faint : Ant-t;
Apoc; Dig; Glo; Hyd-ac; Ign;

Kali-c; Latro; Lob; *Sep;*
Strop; *Sul;* Tab.

Eating Agg : Myr.

Meeting a friend, when :
Cimi.

Nausea, with : Lac-c.

Urination, after : Apoc.

Vertigo, with: Adon.

Walking fast, Amel : Myr.

EVERYTHING, Affects : Sul.

LUMP, Above, as if : Nat-c;
Nat-m; Pho; Pul.

In : *Agar;* Arn; Chel; Con;
Cup; *Lach; Sep.*

PAIN, Aching : Ars; Nux-v; Sil;
Ver-a; Vip.

Cramp, pinching : Lach;
Laur; Merc; Sil; *Ver-a;*
Vip.

down bowels : Arn.

taking breath away :
Cocl.

Cutting : Pul.

Heavy, suffocating : Rum.

Stitching : Arn; Bry; *Nit-ac;*
Rhus-t; *Sep;* Sul.

PRESSURE, Sense of : Cup; Lyc;
Nat-m; Nux-v; *Pho; Pul;*
Ver-a.

RADIATING From : Arg-n.

RED Spots on : Nat-m.

+ **S**CAPULA or **V**ERTEBRA, to :
Bad.

SENSITIVE, Sore : Bry; Calc;
Carb-v; Chel; Chin; Hyo;
Kali-c; *Lach;* Lyc; Nat-m;
Nux-v; Pho; *Ver-a.*

Spot : Pho.

SHOCK Felt in : Dig.

STOPPAGE In : Guai.

SWEAT : Kali-n.

SWELLED : *Calc;* Manc; Nat-m; Nux-v.

TALKING Agg: Nat-c.

TENSE : Sang.

THROAT, To, upward : *Aco;* Ars; Calc; Carb-v; Fer; Kali-bi; *Kali-c;* Lyc; Nat-m; Nux-v; Pho.

Worm, crawling : Zin.

THROBBING, PULSATION : Ars; Asaf; Bry; Chin; Kali-c; Lach; *Nat-m;* Nux-v; Old; Pul; Rhus-t; Sep.

Distension like a fist, with : Cic.

Visible, perceptible : Asaf.

TICKLING, In : Pul.

TORN Loose, as if : Berb.

TRANSFIXED Pain : Latro.

TREMOR : Sul-io.

TUMOUR : Hyds.

WRIGGLING In : Chel.

EPILEPSY (See Convulsions) : Agar; Arg-m; Arg-n; *Ars;* Art-v; Bell; *Buf; Calc;* CAUS; Cic; Cina; CUP; Glo; Hyd-ac; Hyo; *Lach;* Oenan; Op; PLB; *Sil; Sul;* Visc; Zin-p; Zin-val.

AURA, Without : Art-v.

CHRONIC, Marked aura, with : Plb.

COITION, During : Buf.

CONSCIOUSNESS, With : Hell; Nux.m; Pho.

CONTRADICTION, From : Ast-r.

DRUNKARDS : Ran-b.

+ GLOW Rise from feet to head : Visc.

HAEMOPTYSIS, Ending in : Dros.

HEART, Diseases, with : Calc-ar.

INJURY, After : Con; Cup; Nat-s; Oenan.

Blows to head, from : Art-v; Meli.

+ JEALOUSY, From : Lach.

MASTURBATION, After : Buf; Stram.

MENSES Absent, with : Pul.

During : Buf.

After : Syph.

MINOR : Art-v; Bell; Caus; Pho; Zin-cy.

Injury to head, from : Nat-s.

+ OPISTHOTONUS, with : Stan.

PREPUCE, Adherent, removed from : Raph.

PRIAPISM, with : Oenan.

PUBERTY, At : Caul; Caus.

RAGE, Then : Arg-m.

SEXUAL : Bar-m; Buf; Calc; Stan; Visc.

SHUDDERING, With : Mos.

+ SLEEP, During : Lach.

STATUS Epilepticus : Abs; Aco; Buf; Hell; Oenan.

STOOLS, During : Nux-v.

+ THUMBS, Clenching : Stan.

TOOTH Extraction, after : Buf.

TUMOUR In brain, from : Plb.

VERTIGO, Before : Hyo.

EPISTAXIS (See Haemorrhage)
: Arn; *Fer-p*; HAM; Nit-ac; *Pho;* Vip.

AFTER, Agg : Pho.

AMEL : Bro; Elap; Meli; Psor; Rhus-t; Tarn.

BED, In, morning : Alo; Caps.

BLOW Or fall, from : Acet-ac.

+ CHILDREN (fat) : Calc.

CORYZA, With : Senec; Sil.

COUGHING, From : Bell; *Dros;* Lach; Led; Merc; Nat-m; Nux-v; PHO.

Night, at : Nat-m.

Whooping Cough in : Arn; Dros; Ip; Led; Merc.

+ DRUNKARDS : Sec.

EASY : Con.

EATING, After : Am-c.

FACE, Washing Agg : Amb; Am-c; Arn; Bry; Kali-c.

FAINTING, With : Croc; Lach.

FEET, Washing Agg : Carb-v.

FEVER, During : Rhus-t.

+ FREQUENT : Meli.

GOOSESkin, with : Cam.

HABITUAL, Young persons, in : Card-m.

HANDS, Washing Agg : Am-c.

HAWKING, After : Rhus-t.

HEADACHE, During : Aco; Agar. After : Ant-c; Sep.

HEAT, With : Thu.

HEMIPLEGIA, In : Ham.

HOT WEATHER : *Croc.*

INFANTS, In : Sil.

JARRING, From : Carb-v; Sep.

LYING, Right side, on : Sul.

MENSES Absent, with: Ap; Bry; Carb-an; Cham; Dul; Fer; *Lach;* Lyc; Pho; *Pul;* Senec; Sil.

Agg : Amb; Grap; Lach; *Nat-* s; Pul; Sep.

Profuse, with : Aco; Meli.

MORNING, Rising, on : Chin. Early : Bov.

NIGHT : Carb-v; Nat-m; Nit- ac; Rhus-t; Sul.

Nostril, right, from : Kali-chl; Ver-a.

NOSE, Blowing, on : Arg-m.

NURSING Child, when : Vip.

OLD People, in : Agar; Carb-v; Ham; *Sec.*

+ ONANISM, From : Lach.

OPERATIONS, After : Bur-p.

OVERHEATED, Being Agg : Thu.

OZOENA, In : Sang.

PERSISTENT : Led.

PILES, Suppressed, from : Nux-v.

With : Sep.

PREGNANCY, During : Sep.

+ PROFUSE : Merc-cy; Meli.

+ But, ceases soon : Cact.

+ PROSTRATION, With : Sec.

PUBERTY, At : Abro; Kali-c; Pho.

SALIVATION, With : Hyo.

SINGING, After : Hep.

SLEEP, During : Bov; Merc; Nux-v; Ver-a.

SNEEZING, When : Bov; Con.

SPASMS,With : Caus; *Mos.*

STOOLS Agg : Pho; Rhus-t.

Straining at, when : Cof.

STOOPING, On : Nat-m; Rhus-t.

SWEAT, With : Bry; Caus; Con; Nux-v; Op; Pho; Tarx; Thu.

TOUCH, Slight, nose, to, on : Cic; Sep.

TYPHOID Fever, in : Arn; Bap; Crot-h; Lach.

VERTIGO, With : Bell; Carb-an; Lach; Sul; Vip.

VOMITING, With : Ox-ac; Sars. After : Ars.

WAKING On : Am-c.

WASHING Face, Feet, Hands, Agg : See Face, Feet, Hands washing.

WEEPING, When : Nit-ac.

YOUNG Girls : Croc.

Women : Abro; *Pho;* Sec.

EPITHELIOMA : See Cancer.

EPULIS: Calc; *Thu.*

ERECTION (of Penis) : *Canth;* Grap; Merc; Nat-c; Nat-m; *Nux-v; Pho;* Pic-ac; Plat; Pul; Thu.

CHILD, In a : Lach; Merc; Tub.

COITION, After : Sep.

COUGHING, When : Cann; Canth.

DYSURIA, After: Radm.

EMISSION, After : *Pho-ac.*

EXCESSIVE, Strong, Violent : Canth; FLU-AC; *Pho; Pic-ac;* Plat; Sabi.

Lascivious thoughts, during : *Pic-ac.*

+ FREQUENT, During day : Chel.

INCOMPLETE, Deficient, falling : Agn; *Arg-n; Bar-c;* Calad; Calc-s; Chin; CON; Grap; *Lyc;* Med; *Nux-v;* Pho; Sele; Sep; *Sul;* Sul-io; Tab.

Coition, during : Grap; Lyc; Sul.

+ LASTS All night : Dios.

PAIN, Abdomen, in, with : Zin.

PAINFUL (Priapism, Chordee) : *Arg-n; Cann; Canth; Caps;* Grap; Merc; Merc-c; Nux-v; Oenan; Pho; Pic-ac; *Pul;* Sabal; Štap; *Terb.*

Coition, during : Hep.

Cutting In, with : Arg-n.

+ Dreams, in : Cam.

Emission, after : Grat; Kali-c.

Epilepsy, during : Oenan.

Sleep, in : Merc-c.

Urethra, burning in with : Calc-p.

PERSISTENT : Am-c.

RIDING, In carriage, when : Bar-c; Calc-p.

SHIVERING and Sexual desire with : Bar-c.

SLEEP, During : Flu-ac; Nat-c; Op.

SLOW, Delayed : *Bar-c;* Calc; Sele.

STANDING Agg : Sul-ac.

STOOLS, During : Ign; Thu.

TOOTHACHE, with : Daph.

URINATION, Copious, after : Lith.

Urging, with : Mos.

ERETHISM False : Merc; Mur-ac; Pho.

EROTIC : See Amorous.

ABILITY, Without : Lach.

ERRATIC : See CHANGING Moods.

EFFECTS (Motion) : Ign; Lac-c; Med; Mos; Tarn; Ver-v.

ERRORS, DIET, in Agg : All-s; Calc-ar; Cep; Dios; Flu-ac; Grap; Nat-c; Sul-ac.

ERUCTATIONS : Amb; ARG-N; Arn; Asaf; *Asar;* Bell; BRY; CARB-V; Chin; *Cocl; Con;* Cup; Guai; Iod; Iris; Kali-bi; Kali-c; LYC; Mag-c; Med; *Merc; Nat-m;* NUX-V; Pho; Psor; Pul; Rhus-t; *Saba; Sep; Sul;* Tarn, *Ver-a.*

AGG : Bry; Carb-an; Carb-v; CHAM; *Chin;* Cocl; Jal; Lach; Nux-v; Pho; Rhus-t; Sul.

AMEL : Ant-t; *Arg-n;* CARB-V; *Grap; Ign; Lach; Lyc Nux-v;* Pul; Sang.

ABORTIVE, Incomplet e: Ars; Chin; Con; *Grap;* Lyc; Med; Nat-m.

ACRID, Hot : Ap; Carb-v; Con; Fag; Gym; Kali-bi; Lac-c; Lyc; Merc; Nat-m; Pod.

Eating Agg : Nat-m.

Foul air : Naj.

Smoking Agg : Lact-ac.

APPLES, Tasting like : Agar.

BALL Moving up and down during, as if : Bar-c.

BARLEY Water, tasting like : Naj.

BITTER : Arn; Chin; Nat-s; Nux-v; Pho; Pul; Sep; Tarx.

Hysteria, in : Tarx.

Milk, after : Chin.

BLOODY : Sep.

BUGS, Odour of : Phel.

COLD : Cist.

COLIC, With : Hyo.

CONTINUOUS : Chel; Con.

CONVULSION, After : Kali-c.

Before : Lach.

COUGHING, When, after : *Amb;* Arn; Carb-v; Chin; Kali-bi; Lob; Sang; Sul-ac; Ver-a.

DIFFICULT : *Arg-n;* Calc-p; Cocl; Con; Grap; Nux-v.

DRINKING, Water, after : Ap; Hypr.

EGGS Like, bad : Agar; Ant-t; *Arn;* Cham; Mag-m; Plant; Psor; Sul; Val.

EMPTY: Bry; Calc; *Carb-v; Con;* Grap; Iod; Pho; Sep; Sul.

+ EPILEPSY, Before : Lach.

FAINTNESS, Causing : Arg-n.

FECAL : Plb.

FEVER, In : Lach; Ran-b.

FOAMY, Frothy : Kre; Sep; Ver-a.

FOOD, Of : See Regurgitation.

FORCIBLE, Oesophagus would split, as if : Coca.

GALLSTONES, with : Dios; Lyc.

GARLICKY : *Asaf;* Mag-m.

Spasms, after : Mag-m.

GREASY : Alu; Asaf; Caus; Iris; *Mag-c;* Thu; Val.

HEADACHE, With : Calc; Cimi; Mag-m.

HICCOUGH, Like : Cyc.

Alternating, with : Agar.

HOT : See Acrid.

INCOMPLETE: See Abortive.

INGESTA, Tasting of : ANT-C; Ap; Bism; *Bry;* Carb-an; Caus; Chin; Fer; Nat-m; *Pul.*

Drinking water Agg : *Ap.*

LONG-CONTINUED : Glo.

LOUD, Noisy : ARG-N; ASAF; *Chin;* Kali-bi; Petr; Pho; *Plat;* Thu; Vib.

Violent and : Coca.

LYING Amel : Aeth; Rhus-t.

MEAT, From : Rum.

MENSES, At : Lach.

MUSK, Tasting of : Caus.

NAUSEOUS, Foul : Arn; *Asaf;* Bism; Carb-v; Grap; Pul;Sul.

ONIONS, Like : Mag-m.

PAINFUL : Bry; Carb-an; *Cham;* Par.

PRESSING Painful part, on : Bor.

Stomach, on : Sul.

+ PUNGENT : Petr.

PUTRID : Acet-ac; Arn; Bism; Kre; Plb; Psor; Val.

RADISH, Tasting like : Osm.

RANCID: *Asaf;* Carb-v; *Chin;* Lyc; Merc; Sep; Tell; Thu.

RELIEF, Without : Carb-v; *Chin;* Lyc.

SALTY : Carb-an; Kali-c; Nux- v; Sul-ac.

SHIVERING, With : Dul.

SLEEP Amel : Chel; Chin.

SMOKING, After : Sele.

SOUR : CALC; Carb-v; *Chin;* Grap; Gymn; Ign; Kali-bi; LYC; *Mag-c;* Nat-c; *Nat-m;* NAT-P; NUX-V; Pho; Psor; *Pul;* Rob; Sep; *Sul;* Sul-ac.

Bitter : Iris; Nux-v.

Cabbage, after: *Mag-c.*

Eating, after : *Nat-m.*

Hot : Fag; Gymn; Pod.

Intermittent fever, in : Lyc.

Milk, after : Chin; Sul.

Sugar, after : Caus.

Vertigo, during : Sars.

Vomiting, sour, after : Caus.

STALE : Flu-ac.

SUPPRESSED : Am-c; Calc; Con.

Followed by pain, in stomach : Con.

SWALLOWING, Difficulty, with : Ox-ac.

SWEETISH : Dul; Plb; Sul-ac.

Menses, before : Nat-m.

Pregnancy, during : Nat-m, Zin.

+ TASTELESS : Bry.

TEA, Tasting like : Lycps.

TOUGH, Mucus, of : Sep.

URINOUS : Agn; Ol-an.

VIOLENT : *Mos.*

VOMITING, With : Cimi.

WATER, Tasting of : Naj.

ERUPTIONS (Tendency to)
: *Aco*; ARS; Ars-io; Bar-c;
Bell; CALC; Calc-s; *Caus*;
Clem; Dul; Grap; Kali-c;
Kali-s; *Lach*; LYC; MERC;
Mez; Nat-m; Nit-ac; Petr; *Pho*;
Psor; *Pul*; RHUS-t; SEP; SIL;
SUL.

ACNE : Ast-r; Bar-c; Bell;
Carb-v; Cyc; Grap; *Hep*;
Kali-br; *Merc*; Nux-v; Sele;
Sep; Sul; Sul-io.

Black : Ars; Ast-r.

Cheese Agg : Nux-v.

+ Cosmetics, from : Bov.

Emaciation, with : Abro.

Face, disfiguring : Cop.

Hard : Ars-io.

Masturbation, from :
Crot-h; Pho-ac.

Menses, after Agg : Med.

before Agg : Grap;
Mag-m; Psor; Sep.

delayed : Crot-h.

scanty, with : Sang.

Nose, on : Ars.

Obstinate : Lapp.

Pustular : Berb; Sul-io.

body, all over : Calc-hyp.

menses, during : Kali-br.

Rosacia: Psor; Radm;
Rhus-t.

Scars, remaining, after :

Carb-an; Cop; Kali-br.

Sore : Arn.

Summer Agg : Bov.

Women, young : Cyc.

ACUMINATE, Conical : Ant-c;
Ant-t; *Ars*; Hyds; Pul; *Sil.*

ALTERNATING, other complaints,
with : Ant-c; Ars; Calad;
Grap; Hep; Stap; Sul.

Dysentery, with : Rhus-t.

Joints, with : Stap.

BLACK-TIPPED : Carb-v.

BLEEDING : Am-m; Merc; Sul.

BLUE : Ant-t; Hyd-ac.

CHALKY, white : Mez.

CIRCULAR : See Herpetic.

CLUSTERED : Agar; *Calc* :
Crot-t; Nat-m; Rhus-t.

COLD Bathing Agg : Thu.

CONFLUENT : Ant-t; Bell; Caps;
Cic; Pho-ac; Rhus-t.

COPPERY : Ars; *Carb-an*; Kre;
Merc-d; Rhus-t; Sars.

COSMETIC Agg : Bov.

COVERED, Parts, on : Led; Thu.

DELAYED : Ant-t; Ars; B*ry*;
Stram.

DRY : Ars; Ars-io; Aur;
Bar-c; Calc; Calc-s;
Carb-v; Hep; Led; MERC;
Mez; Pho; *Sep*; Sil; SUL;
Ver-a.

ECZEMA : See Eczema.

ERYTHEMATOUS : Ars; Merc;
Sul.

FAVUS : Ars; Sul.

FINE : Carb-v; Nat-m;
Rhus-t.

FISH, After : Ars; Sep.

FLAT : *Bell;* Lach; Pho-ac; Sep.

FRECKLES : *Ant-c; Calc;* Kali-c; *Lyc;* Nat-c; Nit-ac; *Pho; Pul;* Sep; *Sul.*

Sun, from : Mur-ac.

GRANULAR : Agar; Ars; Carb-v; Hep.

Honey-coloured : Ant-c.

HAIR, In apex of : Kali-bi.

HEATED, When : Bov; Carb-v; Con; *Nat-m;* Psor; Pul.

HEREPETIC (Ringworm) : Aco; ARS; Bacil; Bell; Bov; Calc; Calc-s; Clem; Con; *Dul;* Grap; Hep; Lyc; Manc; *Merc;* NAT-M; Petr; Phyt; Ran-b; RHUS-T; *Sep;* Sil; *Sul;* Tell; Vario.

Body, all over : Psor; Ran-b.

HORNY : Ant-c; Ars; Bor; Grap; Ran-b; Sil; Sul.

IMPETIGO : *Ant-t;* Ars; *Aru-t;* Calc; Grap; Rhus-t; *Sul;* Tarn; Vio-t.

INDENTED : Bov; Thu; Vario.

INTERTRIGO : Cham; Lyc; *Merc; Sul.*

Dentition, during : Caus.

ITCHING,Without : Cic; Cup-ac.

ITCH-LIKE, Scabies: Ars; *Carb-v; Caus;* Hep; Lyc; MERC; Psor; *Sele; Sep;* SUL.

LEAVE, a Blue stain : Abro; Ant-t.

a Brown stain : Berb.

a Purple stain : Abro.

a Red Stain : Aru-t.

LICHEN : Aco; Agar; Bry; *Cic;* Cocl; *Dul; Lyc;* Mur-ac; Nat-m; *Sul.*

Fiery : Cic; Lyc; Rhus-t.

MENSES, Before Agg : See Skin.

MENTAGRA : Calc; Grap; Sep.

MILIARY : Aco; Ars; Bry; Cof; *Dul; Ip;* Merc; Phyt; *Sul.*

MOIST : *Calc;* Caus; *Cic: Clem; Grap;* Kre; *Lyc;* MERC; Pho-ac; *Rhus-t; Sep; Sul.*

NEWBORN : Dul.

NODULAR : Ap; Calc; Caus; Dul; Lach; Mez; Kali-io; *Nat-s;* Rhus-t; Sil.

OBSTINATE : Mang; Sul-io.

PAINFUL : Arn; BELL; Hep; Lach; Lyc; Merc; Nux-v; Pho; *Pho-ac;* Sil; Sul.

PAINLESS : Amb; Cocl; Con; *Lyc;* Old; Sec; Sul.

PAPULES : *Aco; Bry; Dul;* Kali-io; *Merc; Sul.*

PARTS, Covered, on : Led

PATCHES, In (See Mottled) : Ail; Ap; Sec.

PEARLY : Nat-m.

PEDUNCULATED : Thu.

PEMPHIGUS : Ars; *Aru-t;* Canth; *Dul; Hep;* Lach; Manc; Ran-b; Ran-sc; *Rhus-t.*

PETECHIAE, With : Ail; Mur-ac.

PIMPLES : *Ant-c;* Ars; *Caus;* Merc; Nat-m; NIT-AC;

Pho; Pho-ac; Pul; Rhus-t;
Sep; Sul; *Zin.*

+ Liquor, excessive use of,
from : Nux-v.

Red, small, menses scanty,
with : Con.

Small, body all over :
Mag-s.

White, areola, red, with :
Bor.

PSORIASIS : *Ars-io;* Berb-aq;
Bor; *Clem,; Dul; Grap;*
Kali-m; Mang; Merc; *Pho;*
Phyt; Psor; Radm; *Ran-b;*
Sep; Sul; Thyr; Tub.

Itching, without : Cup-ac.

+ Scales, shining   : Iris.

PUSTULATING *: Ant-c; Ant-t;*
Ars; Cham; *Cic;* Clem; Dul;
Grap; Lyc; *Merc;* Nat-c;
Nit-ac; Petr; *Pul; Rhus-t;*
Sep; Sil; Stap; *Sul;* Thu;
Thyr; Vario.

Apices, black : Anthx;
Kali-bi; Lach.

brown: Ver-a.

bloody : Carb-ac.

foul : Vario.

+ sunken : Thu.

RECEDING : Ant-t; Ars; Bry;
Cam; Caus; Cup; Lyc; Op;
Sul; *Zin.*

REPELLED *:* Plb.

RINGWORM : See Herpetic.

ROSEOLA : Aco; Bry; *Kali-io;*
Pul; *Sars;*

Syphilitic : *Kali-io;* Pho.

RUBELLA : Aco; *Bell;* Bry; Pul.

RUPIA : *Ars;* Cham; Grap;
Merc; Petr; Sep; *Sul.*

SCABBY, Crusty (See Crusts) :
Calc; Con; Grap; Hep; *Lyc;*
Merc; *Rhus-t;* Sars; Sil;
Sul.

Bloody : Merc; *Sul.*

SCALY : Calc; *Clem;* Pho; Sul.

SCARLATINOUS : Ail; Am-c; *Ap;*
BELL; Lach; Lyc; Merc ;
Nit-ac; Rhus-t; Stram; *Sul.*

Maligna : *Ail;* Am-c;
Carb-ac; *Lach.*

SCARS, Unsightly, from :
Carb-an; Cop; Kali-br.

SERPIGENOUS : Ars; Sul.

+ Symmetrical : Thyr.

SKIN, Under : Hypr.

SOAP, Application of Agg : Nat-c.

SPARSE : Ail; Mur-ac.

SPRING Agg : Nat-s; Psor;
Sang; *Sars;* Sep.

STAB Wound, after : Sep.

STICKY : Lapp.

SUMMER Agg : Kali-bi.

SUPPRESSED, Undeveloped :
Ail; Ap; Ars; Asaf; BRY; *Cup;*
Dul; Ip; Petr; Pho-ac; Psor;
Stram; SUL; *Zin.*

Childhood, in : Kali-c.

SYPHILITIC : Ars-io; Kali-io;
Merc; Merc-c; Merc-i-f;
Merc-i-r; Nit-ac; Syph.

TETTERY: Alu; *Ars;* Bov; Calc;
Cham; Con; *Dul; Grap;*
Lyc; *Merc;* Mez; *Nat-m;*
Petr; Pho; *Rhus-t;* Sep; Sil;
Sul; Vib.

Touch Agg : Ap; Chin; Coc-c; Cof; Hep; Lach; Mang; Plb; Thu.

Trade : Bor.

Urticarious : See Urticaria.

Vesicles, Blisters : ARS; ARU-T; CANTH; *Caus;* Clem; CROT-T; *Dul;* Euphr; *Grap; Lach;* Manc; Med; *Merc;* NAT-M; Nat-s; Nit-ac; *Pho;* RAN-B; RHUS-T; *Sep; Sul;* Urt.

Abscess over : Rhus-t.

Air, in : Asaf.

Bloody : Carb-ac; Sec.

Blue : Anthx; Ran-b.

Dark : Ail; Anthx.

Discharges, from : Tell.

Large : Buf; Manc.

Yellow : Anac; Euphor; Nat-s; Ran-sc.

Winter Agg : Alu; Ars; *Petr; Psor;* Saba; Tub.

Amel : Kali-bi; Sars.

Yellow : Cup.

Zoster : Ars; Crot-t; Grap; Lach; Merc; Mez; Pru-sp; *Ran-b; Rhus-t; Vario.*

After : Kali-m.

Gastric disturbances, with : Iris.

Pain, after : Zin.

before : Stap.

ERYSIPELAS : Aco; AP; Arn; *Bell;* Canth; Crot-h; Euphor; *Grap; Lach; Merc;* Pul; *Rhus-t;* Sec; Sul.

Brain Affections, with : Ver-v.

Bullosum : Euphor.

Gangrenous : Ars; Carb-v; Lach; Sec.

Menses, During : Grap.

Navel about, injury, after : Ap.

Newborn Babies : Bell; Cam.

Receding : Lyc.

Recurring : Ap; Fer-p; *Grap;* Hyds; Nat-m; *Rhus-t;* Sul.

Senile : Am-c; Carb-an.

Swelling, Great : Ap; *Bell;* Merc; Rhus-t.

Traumatic : Calend; Psor.

Urticaria, With : Canc-fl.

Vesicular : Canth; Euphor; Rhus-t.

Turning, dark : Canth; Ran-b.

Wandering, Creeping : *Grap;* Hyds; Rhus-t; Sul; Syph.

ERYTHEMA : See Under Eruptions.

ESCAPE, Impluse, to : *Bell;* Bry; Cup; *Hyo;* Mez; Nux-v; Op; Stram.

Hide, and : Meli.

EUSTACHIAN TUBES : Bar-m; Fag; *Fer-p; Kali-m;* Merc-d; Nux-v; Petr; Sil.

Right : Hyds.

Left : Sang.

Catarrh : Asar; Calc; Kali-s; Merc-d; Petr; Pul.

· Hypertrophy : Ars-io.

Inflammation : Calc;

Kali-s; Pul; Sil.

ITCHING : Nux-v; Petr; Senec; Sil.

OBSTRUCTED : Kali-m; Merc-d; Petr.

OPEN, With a pop : Merc-i-r.

STRICTURE : Lach.

EXACTING : See Critical.

EXAGGERATES, Her Symptoms : Asaf; Cham; Plb.

EXALTATION : See Cheerful.

EXANTHEMATA, In general : *Aco;* Ap; *Bell; Bry;* Cof; Euphr; *Merc;* Pho; *Pul;* Rhus-t; Sul.

BLUE : Hyd-ac.

+ CHECKED : Hell.

DIARRHOEA, During : Ant-t.

+ NON-*APPEARANCE* : Stram.

UNDEVELOPED : Saba.

EXCESSIVE USE : See Overuse.

EXCITABLE : See Anger.

EXCITEMENT Mental, Nervous : ACO; *Bell;* COF; Gel; Hyo; Lach; Mar-v; NUX-V; Op; Pyro; *Stram;* Val; *Ver-a;* Zin; *Zin-val.*

EASY : Ign.

PLEASURABLE AMEL : Kali-p; Pall.

EXCORIATION : See Discharges Acrid.

EXCRESCENCES : See Fungus Growth.

EXCRETIONS : See Discharges.

EXERTION MENTAL AGG : Agar; Anac; Arg-m; *Arg-n;*

Aur; CALC; Calc-p; *Ign;* Kali-p; *Lach; Lyc; Nat-c; Nat-m;* Nat-p; NUX-V; Pho; Pho-ac; Pic-ac; Pul; Rhus-t; Sele; *Sep; Sil;* Stap; Sul.

AMEL : Fer; Gel; Helo; Nat-c.

PHYSICAL AGG : Alu; ARN; ARS; Ars-io; *Berb;* BRY; CALC; Calc-s; Carb-an; COCL; *Con; Dig; Fer;* Gel; Iod; Laur; *Lycps;* Nat-c; *Nat-m; Nat-s; Nit-ac;* Pic-ac; RHUS-T; Sele; Sep; Spig; Spo; Stan; *Stap;* Strop; *Sul;* Tub; *Ver-a.*

AMEL: Adon; Aesc; Bur-p; Flu-ac; Hep; *Ign;* Kali-br; *Lil-t;* RHUS-T; SEP. Mental Symptoms AMEL : Calc; *Iod.*

Slight AGG : Sul-io; Thyr.

Violent AGG : Lapp; Mill; Symph.

WILL, Of Amel : Phyt.

EXHALATION AGG : Ant-t; Arg-m; Ars; Caus; CHLOR; Colch; Dros; Med; Meph; *Pul; Samb;* Vio-o.

AMEL : ACO; Agar; Bry; Rhus-t; Sabi.

FORCIBLE : Chin; Gel; Ox-ac.

HOT (See Breath Hot) : Kali-bi.

EXHAUSTION : See Weakness.

EXHILARATION : See Cheerful.

EXOSTOSIS : See Bones.

EXOPHTHALMIC GOITRE :

See Goitre.

CHOKING : Meph.

TREMBLING, with : Meph.

EXPECTORATION (See Discharges) AGG : Coc-c; Dig; *Led; Nux-v.*

AMEL : *Ant-t; Ap;* Aral; Coc-c; Grind; Hypr; Kali-bi; Kali-n; Sep; *Stan;* Sul-io; Zin.

ASTRINGENT : Chio.

BALLS, Of : Agar; Arg-n; Coc-c; Sang; Sil; *Stan.*

Bitter, green : Med.

Feels like a round, and rushes into mouth : Syph.

Round, flying from mouth : Kali-c.

BITTER : Cham; Pul.

BLEEDING From mouth, with: Dros.

+ BLOOD, Pure,Cough after : Am-c.

BLOODY (See Haemorrhage) : Bry; Chel; Laur; Mag-c; Stan; Sul-ac.

Chest, burning, in with : Psor.

Chronic : Sul-ac.

Erection, violent, after : Nat-m.

Fall, after : Fer-p; Mill.

Lactation, during : Fer.

Lumpy : Sele.

Menses Agg : Pho; *Zin.*

before : Zin.

suppressed or instead of : Carb-v; Dig; Led; Lyc;

Nux-v; Pho.

Plugs : Sang.

Water : Gel.

BLUISH : Amb; Kali-bi; Pho.

CASTS : See Membranous.

COLD (Cool) : Cor-r; Pho.

CORROSIVE : Iod; Kali-c; Sil; Thu.

CREAMY : Amb.

CURDY, Cheesy : Kali-c; Thu.

DIFFICULT : *Ant-t; Caus;* Ip; Just; Kali-bi; Mag-c; Pul; Sang; Scil; Seneg.

Cough, loose, with : Hep.

DRINKING Amel : Am-c.

EASY : Agar; *Arg-m;* Dul; Nat-s; Pho; Scil; *Stan;* Tub.

By day : Euphr; Mang; Pho.

EPISTAXIS, with : Dros.

FLIES From mouth : Arg-n; *Bad; Chel:* Kali-c; *Kali-m;* Mang; Mez.

FOAMY, Frothy : *Ars; Ip;* Kali-io; Kali-p; Pho; Rum.

FOUL Taste : Asaf; Lach; Pul.

GRANULAR : Bad; Calc; Chin; Kali-bi; Pho; Sil.

Offensive : Sil.

Sneezing, when : Mez.

GRAYISH (See Grayish) : Amb; Arg-m; Lyc; Stan.

GREASY : Caus.

GREENISH (See Green) : Benz- ac; Par; Psor; Sul-io.

HARD : Nat-c.

Calcareous : Sars.

HEAVY : Scil.

HOT : Aral.

LOOSE : See Cough, expectoration, with.

LUMPY : Calc-s; Kob; Lyc; Sil.

LYING Amel: Cist; Thu.

MEMBRANOUS, Casts : Brom; Iod; Kali-bi; Merc-c; *Spo.*

MILKY : Ars; Kali-chl; Sul.
Odour, of : Spo.

MORNING and EVENING : Scil.

MOUTHFUL : *Euphr;* Pho; Rum.

MUSTY : Bor.

OFFENSIVE : Ars; Ars-io; Bor; Calc; Guai; Lyc; Meph; Nat-c; Phel; Sang; Sil; Stan.
Bedbug, like : Phel.

ORANGE-COLOURED : *Kali-c;* Pul.

PROFUSE, Copious : Am-c; Ars; Cact; Calc; Calc-s; Coc-c; Euphr; Hep; Lyc; Mag-c; Pho; Pul; Rum; Sep; Sil; Stan; Tub.
Glairy : Cist.
Nasal discharge, with : Sabal.
Old Age : Alum; Bar-c.

PURULENT : Bro; Bry; Carb-v; *Chin; Con;* Dros; Fer; *Kali-c;* Led; *Lyc;* Nat-c; Nit-ac; Pho-ac; Plb; Pul; RHUS-T; Samb; Sang; *Sep; Stan;* Sul.

RETCHING, With : Carb-v.

RUSTY : *Bry; Lyc;* Sang; Scil.

SAGO, Like : Sil; Stan.
Yellow : Calc-f.

SALTY : Aral; Ars; Lyc; Mag-c; Nat-c; Pho; Pul; Sep.

SLIPS, Back again: CAUS; CON; *Kali-s;* Sang; Seneg; Zin-chr.

SMEARY : Nit-ac; Phel; Thu.

SOUR : Kali-c; Kali-n.

SPITTING, With : Zin-chr.

STICKY, Tough, viscid : Coc-c; *Hep;* KALI-BI; Sang; *Stan;* Sul-io; Zin-chr.

SWALLOW, must (See Slips back) : Caus; Con; Kali-s; *Lach.*

SWEET : Ap; Calc; Lycps; Scil; Zin-chr.
Frothy : Kob.

SYRUP, Like : Carb-an.

THICK : Arg-n; Bro; Hep; Hydr; Kali-bi; Kali-s; Sil;Tub.

VOMITING, With : Dig.

WARM : See Hot.

WEAK, Too, to cough out : Caps.

YELLOW : Hep; Sil; Stan; Sul-io; Tub.
Green : Ars-io; Lyc.

EXPIRATION : See Exhalation.

EXPLOSIONS : See Blows and Shattered.

EXPRESS HERSELF, cannot : Pul.

EXPRESSION : See Face.

EXTENSION : See Stretching.

EXTREME GOES, to : Bell; Caus; Con; Val.

EXTREMITIES : See Arms, Legs.

EXUDATION : See Effusion.

CONTINUOUS : Merc.

FIBRINOUS : Iod; Kali-chl; Kali-m; Merc-d.

HARD : Kali-m; Nit-ac.

EYEBROWS : See Brows.

GUM, Sticky : Euphr; Kali-bi.

LASHES Falling : Ars; Med; Petr; Rhus-t.

Dandruff : Sanic.

Ingrown : See Entropion.

Long ,curved : Pho.

Stiff, points towards nose : Nit-ac.

EYELIDS : Aco; Agar; Ap; Bell; Calc; *Caus*; Hep; Merc; Rhus-t; *Sep*; Spig; *Sul.*

EDGES : See Tarsi.

INNER Surface : *Arg-n*; Ars; Rhus-t.

UPPER : *Caus*; GEL; Kalm; *Sep*; Spig.

Foreign body between eyeball and : Berb; Coc-c; Fer-p.

Hard : Med.

Swelled : *Kali-c*; Sep.

between brows, and *Kali-c.*

LOWER : *Calc*; Pho-ac; Rut; Seneg.

Contraction : Colch.

Swelled : Ap; Arn; Ars;

Merc-i-f; Pho.

AGGLUTINATED, Suppuration : Arg-n; Asaf; Calc; *Caus*; Cham; Euphr; Glo; Grap; Guai; Kre; *Lyc*; NUX-V; Pho; PUL; RHUS-T; *Sep*; Sul.

Menses, during : Calc.

Sneezing, with : Gamb.

BLEEDING : *Hep*; Nat-m; Nux-v; *Sul.*

BLUE : Dig; Kali-c.

BURNING : Colo; Ran-b; Stic.

Closing, on : Manc.

Fiery : Phyt.

CHEMOSIS : Ap; Arg-n; Kali-io; Lyc; Rhus-t.

CLOSED, Shut : *Colo;* Mur-ac; Nux-m; Rhus-t.

Headache, with : Nat-m.

Sleepiness, without : Vio-o.

Tightly, Spasms : *Ars;* Bell; Cham; Colo; Croc; Cup; Euphr; HYO; Ip; Kali-c; *Merc; Nat-m;* Sil; Stram.

COLD : Kali-c.

CRUSTY : Bor.

CYST, on: Fer-p.

DRY : Rhus-t; Ver-a.

ECZEMA : Kre.

EPITHELIOMA : Sep.

EVERTED : See Ectropion.

EYEBALL, Stick to : Asaf; Sanic.

Sneezing, when : Gamb.

GRANULAR : Ap; Arg-n;Ars; Bor; Grap; Kali-bi; Lyc; Merc-i-r; Nat-s.

GUMMY : Bor; Psor.

HEAVY, Falling, drooping, pa
ralysis : Alu; *Caus;* Cham;
Chlo-hyd; Cocl; Con; GEL;
KALI-P; Manc; Naj; Nit-ac;
Nux-v; *Rhus-t; Sep;* Spig;
Syph; Thu; Ver-a.

Right : Caus.

Left : Bar-c; Buf; Colo;
Kali- p; Thu.

Bending head backward
Amel : Seneg.

Coal gas from : Sec.

Leucorrhoea, with : Caul.

Lying Agg : Nat-m.

Sore, and : Manc.

Weekly : Stan.

HALF OPEN, As if: Bell.

INFLAMMED : Aco; Ars; Bell;
Lyc; Pul; Stap; Sul.

Gonorrhoeal : Aco; Pul;
Sul; Thu.

INVERTED : See Entropion.

ITCHING : Arg-n; Gamb; Tell.

+ JERKING : Cocl.

MOTION OF, AGG : Colo.

NARROWING, Space between
: Agar.

NODES : Grap; Stap.

OEDEMA : Ap; Ars.

PRICKING : Spig.

PUFFY : Fer.

+ QUIVERING, Constant :
Caus; Kre.

RED : Aco; Lyc; Myr.

RETRACTED : Iod.

RUBS : Gamb; Ign.

SPASMS, Of : Ars.

+ Lower : Rut.

STICKS, In, as if : Med.

Eye balls, to : Asaf; Sanic.

STIFF : *Ap; Kalm;* Nat-m;
Onos; Rat; RHUS-T.

STYES : Calc-f; Con; *Grap;*
Kre; Lyc; PUL; Sep; Sil;
Stap; Sul; Zin.

Crop of : Lapp.

Recurrent : Ap.

TENSE : Phys.

THICK : Alu; Arg-m; Arg-n;
Bar-c; Merc; Tell.

TWITCH : AGAR; Bell; Calc;
Cic; Colo; Ol-an; *Phys;* Plat;
Rhe;   *Sul.*

Asthma, during : Cup.

Closed, when : Polyg.

Cold, air, in : Dul.

Constant : Kre.

Convulsions, during :
Kali-bi.

Lower : Iod; Kali-io; Rut.

Lying, when : Polyg.

Opening, on : Kali-bi.

Painful : Colo.

Rapid succession, in : Myg;
Rat.

Reading, when : Berb.

Vertigo, with : Chin-s.

ULCER On : Ars; Lyc.

WARTS On : Caus; Thu.

EYES : Aco; *Agar;* Ap; *Arg-n;*
Ars; BELL; CALC; Caus;
Euphr; *Gel;* Grap; *Lyc;*
MERC; NAT-M; Nux-v; Pho;

PUL; *Rhus-t;* *Rut;* Sep; *Spig;* SUL; Ver-a; Zin.

RIGHT : Am-c; *Bell;* Calc; Cann; *Colo;* Euphr; *Lyc;* Nat-m; Nit-ac; Petr; Pho; Plat; Rhus-t; Seneg; Sil.

Closed, Hemiplegia, in : Ap.

Protruding, looks larger than left : Arn.

LEFT : Ap; Ars; Asar; Bry; Chel; Chin; Hep; Laur; Mez; Nux-v; Plb; Scil; *Spig; Spo;* Stan; Sul; Tarx; Thu.

Drawn, inwards : Cyc.

Pain, periodical, overb : Mur- ac.

Smaller, than right : Arn; Flu-ac; Scil.

Vertex, to : Vio-o.

ABDOMEN, With : Arg-n.

ABOVE, Something, as if cannot look up : Carb-an.

AIR, Cold, blowing on, as if : See Wind.

streaming out, as if : Thu.

Hot, streaming out, as if : Dios.

ALTERNATING Between : Aco; Agar; *Ars;* Bell; *Chin;* Cup; *Lyc;* Pul; *Ran-b;* Seneg; Sil.

Abdomen, with : Euphr.

Limbs, with : Kre.

AROUND : Asaf; *Cinb;* Hep; Ign; Kali-bi; Merc.

Bluish : Ant-t; Ars; Bism; *Chin;* Ip; Merc-i-f; Old; , Rhus-t; Sec; Stap; Thu; Ver-a.

Crawling : Cist.

Dark circles under : Fer; Sep; Thu.

Eruptions : Ant-c; Ap; Ars; Bar-c; Caus; Hep; Merc; Sil; Sul.

pimples, hard : Guai.

Numb : Asaf.

Red : Ap; Bor; Chin-ar; *Elap;* Lapp; MALAN; Pul; Rum; Sil.

Swelling : Ap; Kali-c; Kali-io; Rhus-t.

Yellow : Coll; Mag-c; Nit-ac; Nux-v; Spig.

ASCENDING, into Right : Sang.

Left : Spig.

BACKWARDS (drawing etc) : Ast-r; Bry; *Crot-t;* Grap; Grind; Hep; *Lach;* Old; *Par;* Pho; Pru-sp; Pul; Radm; *Rhus-t;* Seneg; Sil; Spig.

+ BALL, round, in, or stick, as if : Dios.

BEHIND : Bad; Bry; Chel; *Cimi;* Gel; *Lach;* Lith; Manc; Merc; Pod; Pul; *Rhus-t;* Sep; Ther.

BENDING Head backwards Amel : Seneg.

BIG, As if : Arg-n; Chel; Chlo-hyd; Cimi; Como; Glo; *Guai;* Lyc; Meli; Mez; Par; Pho; Pho-ac; Seneg; Spig.

BLEEDING : Both; Crot-h; Lach; Nux-v; Pho.

Blowing nose, on : Nit-ac.

Bᴌɪɴᴋɪɴɢ Amel : See Winking.

Bʟᴏᴏᴅsʜᴏᴛ : Aco; *Arn;* Cact; Chlo-hyd; Ham; Led; *Nux-v* Phys; Thu.

Water, from, in newborn : Cham.

Bʟᴏᴡɪɴɢ Nose Amel : Aur.

Bᴏɪʟs, Over, left : Nat-m.

+ Bʀɪʟʟɪᴀɴᴛ : Ap.

Bᴜʀɴɪɴɢ, Heat : ARS; BELL; Bro; Bry; *Cham; Chin;* Cimi; Grap; *Kali-c;* Kali-p; Lil-t; *Lyc;* Mag-p; Merc-c; Pho; Rum; *Rut; Sul;* Zin.

Closing, on : Echi; Manc.

Cold iron, thrust, as if from : Til.

Dry : Aru-t; Croc.

Fever, in : Sep.

Fiery : Ced; Clem.

Hot, Painful : Naj.

vapour coming out, as if : *Cham;* Clem; Dios.

Indoors : Rum.

Moving, eyes, on : Stic.

+ Red : Stro.

Sand, as if, from : *Caus;* Nat-m.

Sneezing, with : Como.

Weeping, as from : Croc.

Bᴜʀsᴛɪɴɢ : Pho; Pru-sp; Sul.

Cʟᴏsɪɴɢ ᴀɢɢ : Arn; Bry; Carb-an; Chel; Con; LACH; *Sep;* Stro; THER.

Aᴍᴇʟ : Con; Gel; Kali-c; Sil; Tab; Zin.

Difficult : Caus; *Nux-v; Par;* Pho; Sil.

Frivolously on being questioned : Sep.

Heart affection, in : Spo.

+ Light, penetrating the brain : Kali-c.

Must : Croc.

Sees vision, on : Bell.

Sitting, on : Mur-ac.

+ Tightly, for relief : Meli.

Walking in open air, when : Calad.

Cᴏɪᴛɪᴏɴ Agg : Kali-c; Nat-m; Pho; Sep.

Cᴏʟᴅ Application Agg : Ars; Clem; *Merc;* Thu.

Amel : Ap; *Arg-n;* Asar; Bry; Nux-v; Pho; *Pul;* Syph.

Iron pressed through, as if

: Til.

Water, as if, in : Scil.

Cᴏʟᴅɴᴇssn : Alu; Berb; *Calc;* Croc; Fu-ac; Mez; Plat.

Icy : Seneg.

Pain, with : Mez.

Cᴏʟᴅ-ᴛᴀᴋɪɴɢ Agg : Dul; Merc; Pul; Rhus-t.

Cᴏᴍʙɪɴɢ, Hair Agg : Nux-v.

Cᴏᴛᴛᴏɴ, Piece, as if, in : Radm.

Cᴏᴜɢʜɪɴɢ Agg : Seneg.

Cᴏᴠᴇʀᴇᴅ, As if : Pul.

Cʀᴀᴍᴘ : Vio-o.

Cʀᴀᴡʟɪɴɢ, In : Nat-s.

Cʀᴏssᴇᴅ, As if : Bell; Calc; *Con;* Kali-bi; Nat-m; Op; Pod; *Pul;* Zin.

CRUSHING : *Bry; Pru-sp.*

DARK Amel : Con; Lil-t.

DERMOID : Nit-ac.

DISTORTED : Hyd-ac.

Spasms, during : Sil.

DRAWN, Back : See Backward.

+ Downwards : Aeth.

Together, as if : Lach; Lyc; MERC; *Nat-m;* Op; Sul; Zin.

DRY : *Aco;* Alu; Ars; *Bell;* Glo; Ign; Lith; *Lyc;* Mez; NUX-M; Op; *Pul;* Stap; SUL; Ver-a; Zin.

+ Lachrymation, with : Stap.

Using, them, as if from : Lith.

DULL : Ant-t; Cep; Nux-v; Op; Stan.

EARS, And : Vio-o.

EXERTION, Physical Amel : Aur.

FALLING Out, as if : Bro; Carb-an; Colo; Guai; *Ign;* Hell; Lyc; *Pul; Sep;* Tril.

+ FINGERS, Before: Psor.

+ FIXED : Hyd-cy; Merc-cy.

+ Staring : Cup.

FORCED Out, as if : Ham.

Pressing throat; on,as if : Lach.

FOREIGN Body, as of a : Ap; Calc-p; Dios; Flu-ac.

Between, lids and : Berb.

FORMICATION : Nat-s.

FOUNDRY, Work Agg : Merc.

+ GLASSY : Pho-ac.

GLAUCOMA : Aco; Aur; Bell; Berb; Bry; *Colo;* Gel; Osm;

Pho; Plb; Phys; Spig.

Injury, after : Phys.

Iridescent vision: Osm.

GREEN : Canth; Cup-ac.

HAEMORRHAGE, Intraocular : Ham; Sul-ac.

+ HAIR, Before : Euphr; Plant.

HAND Covering with Amel: Aur; Thu.

HEAT Agg : Ap; Arg-n; Cof; *Merc;* Pul; Zin.

Fire, of Agg : *Ant-c;* Arg-n; Merc; Pho.

Amel : Flu-ac.

Steaming out : Dios.

HEAVY, As 'if : Ars-io.

HICCOUGH, Vomiting Agg: Ap; Arn; Asar; Bry; Chin; Lyc; Nux-v; Pul; Sep; Sil; Ver-a.

INJECTED : Aco; *Ap;* Arg-n; Arn; *Bell;* Cep; Glo;Led; *Merc;* Nat-m; *Nux-v.*

INJURIES : Arn; Erig; Euphr; Ham; Led; Stap; *Symp.*

INTO, Pains : Stap.

ITCHING : Calc; *Pul; Sul;*

JERK, Stare, and : Cic.

KIDNEYS, And : Vio-o.

LACHRYMATION Amel : Pru-sp.

LARGE, As if : See Big, as if.

LIGHT Agg : Bar-c; *Bell;* Calc; Chin; Con; Nat-s; Rhus-t.

Amel : Am-m.

Artificial Agg : Ars; Pic-ac.

LIVER Symptoms, with : *Corn.*

LOOKING, Fire, at Agg : Ap;
Merc; Nat-s.

Down Agg : Nat-m.

Amel : Bar-c.

Intently Amel : Petr.

Pieces of paper, at Agg :
Calc-s.

Red objects, at Agg : See
Sun.

Sun, At or anything white
or red Agg : *Ap; Lyc.*

Up Agg : Ars; Carb-v; Chel.

White object at, Agg : See
Sun.

LOOKS Down before him :
Stan; Ver-a.

LOOSE, As if : Carb-an.

MENSES, At Agg : Croc; Naj;
Nit-ac.

MOONLIGHT Amel : Aur.

MOTION Of : Agar; Caus; Bell;
Cham; Cup; Hyo; Mag-p;
Stram.

Constant : Kali-io.

Directions, in all : Kali-br.

Of one, other motionless :
Apoc; Phyt.

Oscillations : Agar; Benz-n;
Cocl; *Cup;* Elap; Gel; *Zin.*

eyes, closed with : Cocl;
Stic.

closing quickly on : Aeth;
Cup.

Sleep, in : Aeth; Ap.

NEEDLES, as if in : Cimi; Rhod;
Spig.

Red hot : Rhod.

NEURALGIA, operations, after

: Mez.

NUMB around : *Asaf.*

NYSTAGMUS : See Motion.

OPENING, Amel : See Closing
Agg.

OPEN, Half open, etc : Bap;
Bell; Colch; *Cup;* Hell;
Hyd-ac; LYC; *Op; Pho;* POD;
Samb; Stram; Thu.

One: *Ant-t;* Chin; Ign;
Ver- a.

Rapid succession, in : Myg.

OPENING DIFFICULT (See
Eyelids closed tightly) : Ars;
Caus; Gel; *Nux-m;* Rhus-t.

Faceache, with : Chel.

Headache during : Nat-m;
Tarn.

Melancholy, in : *Arg-n.*

Menses, during : Cimi.

Sneezing, after : *Grap.*

Swallowing Amel : Terb.

OPERATIONS, After : Alum;
Asaf; Mez; Stap; Zin.

OVARIES, With : Onos.

OVER : Am, *Ars; Bell;*
Bism; Bry; Calc; *Carb-v;*
Ced; Chel; *Chin-s; Gel;*
Iris; Kali-bi; *Lach; Lil-t;*
Lyc; Naj; *Nat-m; Nux-v;*
Pho; Pul; Sang; Sil; *Spig;*
Thyr; *Zin.*

Right : Bell; Ced; Chel; Lyc;
Nat-m; Pul; *Sang;* Senec;
Sep; Syph.

Left : Ars; Bry; Fer; Kali-c;
Nux-m; Sele; Sep; *Spig.*

pain periodically : Mur-ac.

veins distended : Dig.

warm flowing : Nit-ac.

PARALYSIS, Post-diphtheritic : Phys.

PINK : Euphr.

PRESSED Apart : Asar; Pru-sp.

Forward : *Bry*; Kali-m; Merc-c; Nux.v; Pru-sp; Sang; *Spig*.

throat, pressing, on : Lach.

Outward : Ced; Glo;

Gy m; Lach; Nat-m.

PRESSING Amel : Asaf; Caus; Chel; Pic-ac.

PROTRUDING : Aco; Ars; BELL; Bro; Chlor; Cocl; Fer-io; Glo; *Guai*; HYO; IOD; Jab; Laur; Lycps; Nat-m; Stram.

As if : Med; *Par*; Spo.

Brilliant, and : Aeth.

Convulsions, during : Dros.

Cough, during : Caps; Dros.

Injury, from : Led.

Mania, during : Cam.

Measles, during : Dros.

Right more than left : *Como*.

Trembling, with : Meph.

Tumour behind eyeball, from : Thu.

PUCKERED, As if : Ars.

PUFFY : Kali-io.

PULSATING, Throbbing : Bell.

Night : Asaf; Merc.

QUIVERING : Sul.

RADIATING Pain : Mez; Spig.

RAW : Arg-n; Kali-io; Lyc.

READING and Writing Agg :

Chin; Phyt.

RED : Asar; Bell; Merc; Merc-i-r; Radm; Rhus-t; Spig; Thu.

Bluish : Plb.

+ Bulging : Ap.

Lower : Glo.

Prostate, enlargement, with : Sabal; Solid.

Reading, sewing Agg : *Arg-n; Nat-m*; Radm; Rut.

Sexual excess, after : Stap.

Styes, with : Sep.

Vision, yellow, with : Alo.

Vomiting Agg : See Hiccough.

REFLEX Symptoms : Kali-p.

RESTLESS : Chin-s; Stram; Ver-a.

RUBBING Amel : Caus; Cina; Croc; *Pul*; Ran-b.

RUBS : Cep; Gamb; Gym; Ign; Sanic; Scil; Seneg.

Brain affections, in : Scil.

Measles, in : Scil.

SAND, As if, in : Ars; Calc; Caus; Chin; Flu-ac; Nat-m; Sul.

Headache, during : Lac-d.

Right : *Sep*.

Night : *Zin*.

SEEING, Sight, cinema, etc. Agg : Arn.

SEWING Agg : Mang.

SKIN Overhanging, as if : Ol-an.

SLEEP, Afternoon, Amel : Am-c.

Sᴍᴀʟʟ, As if : Lach.

Left than right : Arn;
Flu-ac; Scil.

Sᴍᴀʀᴛ : Manc; Radm; Ran-b.

Lids, closing, on : Manc.

+ Sᴍᴏᴋᴇ In, as if : Croc.

Sɴᴇᴇᴢɪɴɢ Amel : Lil-t.

Sɴᴏᴡ, Exposure, to Agg : Aco;
Cic.

Sᴏʀᴇ, Bruised, aching : Arn;
Bap; *Bry;* Chio; *Cimi;*
Como; EUP-P; *Gel;* Mag-p;
Merc; Onos; Pho; Pul; *Phyt;*
Rhus-t; Sang; Spig; Tub.

Sᴘᴀʀᴋʟɪɴɢ : *Bell; Cam;*
Stram; Strop.

Sᴘʀᴀɪɴᴇᴅ, As if : Lil-t.

Sǫᴜɪɴᴛ : *Alu;* BELL; Calc;
Cic; Con; Cup; *Cyc;* HYO;
Nat-m; Spig; Stram; Zin.

Brain diseases, after :
Kali-p.

during : Stram.

onvergent : *Cic; Cyc.*

Convulsions, after : Cyc.

during : Stram.

Day, alternate, on : Chin-s.

Dentition, during : Alu.

Diarrhoea, with : Stram.

Divergent : Agar; Colo;
Con; Hyo; Jab; *Nat-m.*

Double : Alu.

Meningitis, with : Tub.

Menstrual irregularities,
with : Cyc.

Night terrors, after :
Kali-br.

Operations, after : Jab.

Sensation of : Calc.

Terror, fear, from: Stram.

Sᴛᴀʀɪɴɢ : Ant-t; *Bell; Cic;*
Cup; Glo; *Hell;* HYO; *Ign;*
Iod; Laur; Lyc; Merc; Naj;
Op; Sec; *Stram;* Ver-v.

Everything, at, as if : Med.

+ Eyes wide open : Scil.

Headache, during : *Bell;
Glo; Stram.*

Person, at, but does not
understand what he
speaks : Merc-c.

Unconscious, when : Caus.

Vacantly, in space : Bov.

Sᴛɪꜰꜰ: *Kalm;* Nat-m; Onos.

Sᴛɪᴛᴄʜɪɴɢ : Pru-sp; Spig.

Coughing Agg : Seneg.

+ Sᴛᴏɴᴇs, little, full of, during headache : Lac-d.

Sᴛᴏᴏʟs Agg : Nat-c.

Sᴛʀᴀɪɴ Agg : See Reading
Agg.

Sᴜɴᴋᴇɴ : *Abro;* Ant-c; Ant-t;
Ars; Cam; *Chin;* Cina; Cup;
Fer; Glo; Iris; Merc-cy;
Pho-ac; Sec; Spig; Stan;
Stap; Sul; Ver-a.

Menses, during : Ced.

+ Sᴜɴʟɪɢʜᴛ, Bright, com-
plaints from : Clem.

Sᴜɴʀɪsᴇ to Sunset Agg :
Kalm; Nat-m.

Sᴡᴀʟʟᴏᴡɪɴɢ Agg : Arg-n;
Tarn.

Sᴡᴇᴀᴛ On : Mag-c.

Under : Con.

Sᴡᴇʟʟᴇᴅ, As if : Como; *Guai;*
Mez; *Nat-m;* Par; Pru-sp;

Rhus-t; Rum; Seneg; SPIG; Spo.

SWELLING Between, and brows : *Kali-c.*

Morning : Rum.

One, of, coma in : Terb.

Under : Ap; Arn; Ars; Med; Merc; Merc-i-f; Pho.

right : Merc-i-f; Polyg.

SWIMMING, Cold water, as if in : Scil.

TENSION : Rut.

Decreased : Nat-m.

THINKING of it Agg : Lach; Spig.

TINGLING : Clem; Pic-ac; *Phyt.*

TONGUE, Protruding Agg : Syph.

TOUCH Agg : Aur; Bry; Hep; Pho.

TURNED Down : Aeth; *Hyo.*

Left, to : Dig; Pho.

+ Outwards : Pho.

Up : Buf; Cam; Cup; Glo; Hell; Mos; Op.

fever, in : Hell.

TURNING Agg : Sang; Sil; Spig; Tub.

TWISTING, Revolving as if : Pho; Phys; Pop-c.

UPWARD, From : Berb; Grap; Lach.

URINATION Amel : Gel; Ign; Kalm.

VEIL Falling over, as if : Con.

VEINS, Distended, on: Dig.

VERTEX, To : Bur-p; Lach; Vio-o.

VOMITING Agg : See Hiccough Agg.

WATER, Warm, flowing over : Nit-ac.

WATERY : Tell; Thu.

+ **W**EIGHT, On, as if : Carb-v.

WILD LOOK : Bell; Lil-t; Lyss; Nux-v; Sec; Ver-v.

WIND Blowing on, as if : Cham; Flu-ac; Lach; Mez; Pul; Sep; Syph; Thu.

Cold : Croc; Syph.

WINE Agg : Gel; Zin.

WINKING : Bell; Croc; Euphr; Flu-ac; Merc-d; Mez; Spig.

Amel : Bell; Croc; Euphr; Old.

Absent : Caus.

Convulsions during : Kali-bi.

Inclination to : Mez; Spig.

+ Must : Flu-ac.

Painful : Kali-io.

Rapidly : *Ast-r*; Merc-d.

Reading, while : Calc; Croc.

Writing, after : Hep.

WIPE, Must : Calc; Croc; Euphr; Nat-c; Nat-m; Pul; Seneg.

WIPING, Amel : *Calc*; Cina; Cyc; Euphr; *Nat-c.*

WRITING Agg : Calc-f; Nat-m; Phyt.

YAWNING Agg : Agar; Saba.

YELLOW : Chin; Crot-h; Lach; *Nux-v*; Plb; Sep; Spig.

Lower part : Nux-v.

Spots : Agar; Pho-ac.

FACE : Aco; Ant-c; Ap; Ars; *Bell;* Bry; Caus; Cham; Chin; Fer; Hyo; Lyc; Mag-p; *Merc; Nux-v; Rhus-t;* Stram; *Sul;* Ver-a.

RIGHT : Ap; *Bell;* Cact; Calc; Canth; Chel; *Kalm;* Lyc; Nat-c; Nux-v; *Sang;* Zin.

Left, to : Grap.

LEFT : Aco; *Colo;* Con; *Lach;* Rhus-t; Sep; *Spig;* Stap.

ALBUMIN, Covered with, as if : Alu; Petr; Pho-ac.

Dried on, as if : Mag-c; Sul- ac.

ALTERNATING Sides : Chin; Lyc; Pho.

ANGIOMA : Abro.

BESOTTED, Stupefied : Arn; *Bap;* Bry; Crot-h; Gel; Hyo; Op; Stram.

+ BLACK Pores, in : Sabi.

BLEMISHES, Clearing for: Berb-aq; Cimi; Sars.

BLUISH : Aco; Ant-t; ARS; Asaf; Bap; *Bell;* Cam; Carb-v; Con; CUP; Dig; Hyo; *Ip;* Kali-m; LACH; *Op;* Samb; VER-A; VER-V; Zin.

Chill during : Nux-v; Stram.

Cough, whooping cough, with : Dros; Ip; Samb.

Laughing, when : Cann.

Menses, before : Pul.

Pregnancy, during : Pho.

Red, evening, in : Phel.

BLUSHING : See Red.

BOILS : Bro.

Small, menses, at : Med.

BROWN : See Earthy.

CHANGING Colour : Aco; Bell; Fer; IGN; *Pho; Plat;* Sep; Stram.

CHEWING Agg : Pul; Stap.

Amel : Cup.

+ CHILDISH : *Anac.*

CHLOASME : Caul; Kali-p; Sep.

COBWEB, On : Alu; Bar-c; Bor; Bro; Calad; *Grap;* Ran-sc; Sumb.

COLD : Abro; Ant-t; *Ars;* Cam; *Caps;* CARB-V; *Cina;* Cocl; Colch; Hell; Lyc; Plat; VER-A.

Children, fleshy, in : Iod.

Drops of water, were

spurting out, as if : Berb.

One side, with severe pain, in other : Dros; Polyg.

Water, holding, in mouth Amel : Clem.

running about, which Amel : Bism.

Wind, Amel : Arg-n.

CONGESTED : Aco; Amy-n; Aur; *Bell;* Glo; Hyo; Nux-v; Op; Pul; *Stram.*

COUGHING Agg : Kali-bi; Samb.

CRAMP : Colo; Mez; *Plat; Verb.*

CRAWLING : See Flies or Spider.

DESIRES To wash with cold water : Ap; Asar; Flu-ac.

Thereby Amel : Asar; Calc-s; Pho.

DEATH-LIKE, Pinched,

collapsed : See Hippocratic.

DIRTY : See Earthy.

DISTORTED : Ars; BELL; Cam; Cocl; *Colo*; Hyd-ac; *Hyo*; Ign; Ip; Lyc; Nux-v; *Op*; Sec; STRAM; Tell; Ver-a.

+ Pain, by : Cham.

Speaking, when : Ign.

Waking, on : Crot-h.

DOWN, On, hysteria, in : Nat-m; Psor.

DRAWN : Aeth; Ant-c; Ars; Bell; Lyc; Op; Sec; Stram; Tab; Ver-a.

To, a point : Bism; Bro; Kali-n.

root of nose : Bro; Par.

DUSKY, Dark, sooty : Alu; Ant-t; *Bap*; Colch; Crot-h; Gel; Hell; Iod; Mur-ac; Op; *Pho*; Psor; Stram; Tub.

EARTHY, Dirty brown : Anthx; Ars; Calc-p; *Chin*; *Fer*; Iod; Lyc; Merc; Nat-m; Nux-v; Op; Psor; Sul; Terb; Thu.

Yellow : Lycps.

EATING Agg : Mez; Pho.

Amel : Kalm; Rhod.

EGG, White of, on : See albumin.

ELONGATED, As if : Stram.

EMACIATED, Thin : Acet-ac; Alu; Ars; Calc; Carb-v; Fer; Iod; Nat-m; Sele; Stap; Tab; Tarn.

Neuralgia, after : Plb.

+ EMBARASSMENT : Amb.

+ EPITHELIOMA : Kali-s.

ERUPTIONS : *Ant-c*; Calc; Caus; Dul; Kali-br; Kali-c; *Kre*;

Led; Merc; Mez; Nat-m; Petr; Psor; Pul; *Rhus-t*; *Sep*; Sul.

Burning : Am-m.

Coryza, with : Mez.

Eczematous : Ars; Bor; Calc; Cic; Grap; Hypr; Kre; Merc; Mez; *Rhus-t*; Sars; Vio-t.

Fine : Aur.

Menses, at : Am-c; Grap; Sars.

Nodular : Chel.

Pimples : Carb-an; *Carb-v*; Nat-c.

red : Led.

EXPRESSION Changed : Aco; Ap; Arg-n; *Ars*; Bell; Cam; *Gel*; Hyo; Lyc; Mang; *Op*; Pho; Pho-ac; Sec; STRAM; Ver-a.

Expression Less : Anac; Gel; Kali-br; Lycps.

FLIES or Spiders, crawling on, as if : Calad; Coc-c; Gym; Laur.

+ FOOLISH Look : Abs.

FORMICATION: Crot-t; Gym; Nux-v; *Plat*; *Sec*.

Prickling, and : Ap.

FRECKLES : See under Eruptions

FRIGHTENED Look : *Aco*; Cup; Spo; Stram; Ver-a.

FROWNING : Cham; Hell; Hyo; *Lyc*; Sep; Sul; *Stram*; Ver-a.

FUZZY : Caus; Psor.

GLISTENS, Shining, waxy :

Ap; Ars; Med; Sele; Thu.

GREEN : Carb-v; Chel.

GRIMACES : See Grimaces.

+ HAGGARD Look : Ant-c; Ars; Cam.

HAIR, On, as if : Sumb.

HAND Passes constantly over : Nux-v.

HECTIC Spots : Aco; *Ars;* Calc; *Chin;* Fer; Iod; Kali-c; Kre; *Lyc; Pho;* Pho-ac; Pul; *Sang;* Sil Stan; *Sul;* Tub.

HEAT : BELL; Bry; CALC; *Cham;* Cina; Fer; Grap; Hep; *Nux-v;* Pul; Stram; Tub.

Affected side : Tub.

Eating, after : Petr.

Feet, cold, with : Samb.

Hands, cold, with : Arn; Dros; Stram.

Headache, with : Chin-s.

One side, other cold : Cham; Dros; Ip.

Palpitation, with : Mag-m.

Rises, into : Kali-bi; Sang.

Sitting, while : Val.

HIPPOCRATIC, Death-like, pinched : Aeth; Ant-t; ARS; Carb-v; Chin; Sec; Tab; VER-A.

+ IDIOTIC : Agar.

INJURIES : Symp.

ITCHING : Calc; Caus; Rhus-t.

JERKS, Talking, while : Sep.

MASK-LIKE, immobile : Lycps; Mang.

MISERABLE : Zin.

MOUTH, Opening, Agg : Cocl.

NOISE Agg : Spig.

NUMB : Aco; Asaf; Caus; Cham; Gel; Kalm; Mez; PLAT; Sep; *Verb.*

Affected side : Caus; Nux-v; Plat.

Right : Chel; Gel; PLAT.

OLD LOOK : *Alu; Arg-n-;* Bar-c; *Calc; Con;* Guai; Lyc; OP; Sanic; Sars; Sep; Sul; Syph; Tub.

Few weeks old infant : Op.

+ Wrinkled : Pulex.

PAIN, Neuralgia, prosopalgia, aching : Aco; *Ars;* Aur; Bell; *Bry;* Calc; Cam; *Caus;* Ced; *Chin;* COLO; Gel; Kalm; MAG-P; *Mez;* Nat-m; *Nux-v; Pho;* Plat; Pru-sp; *Rhus-t; Sep;* SPIG; *Stan; Stap;* Stram; *Verb.*

Alternating with pain in coeliac region : Colo.

pain in stomach, with : Bism.

Boring : Aur; Hep; Mag-c; Mez; Plat.

Chewing Agg : Alo; Hell; Kali-chl; Pul; Stap.

Chilliness, with : Colo; Rhus-t.

Cold washing Agg : Fer; Mag-c.

Ame l: Caus.

body becoming Agg : Mag-p.

water, holding in mouth, Amel : Clem.

+ Coming and going : Spig.

Cramp : Colo; Mez; *Plat; Verb.*

Eating Amel : Kalm.

Eye symptoms, with : Colo.

open, cannot : Chel.

Heated, when Agg : Fer.

Kneeling and pressing the head firmly against ground Amel : Sang.

+ Lachrymation, with : Plant; Pul.

Linear : Caps; Cep.

+ Lips, from : Stap.

Lying Agg : Fer.

Menses, scanty, with : Caus; Lob; Mez.

Mouth, opening Agg : Mag-p.

Nasal discharge, with : Spig.

Noise Agg : *Spig.*

Paralysis, with : Caus; Cur; Gel; *Nat-m.*

Pregnancy, in : Ign; Mag- c; Sep.

Radiating : Sang; Spig.

fingers, to : Cocl.

Tea Agg : Spig.

Teeth, carious, or extraction, after : Hekla.

chattering, with : Sul-ac.

+ Temples, to : Plant.

Urination, frequent, with : Calc.

+ Yawning : Alo.

PALE and Hot : Cimi; Cina; Croc; Hyo; Op.

+ Cachectic : Sil.

Cough, during : Cina.

Deathly : Crot-h; Sul-ac.

Exertion, from : Spo.

Red, alternately : *Aco;* Cam; Caps; *Fer;* Fer-p; Glo; *Lac-c;* Op; Stram; Stro; Zin.

Linea nasalis : *Aeth;* Ant- t; Carb-ac; *Cina;* Ip; Merc-cy; *Pho; Stram;* Tarn.

Menses absent, with : Lob.

during : Ign.

Migraine, with : Amy-n; Ars.

Rising, on : Aco; Ver-v.

+ Sickly : Pho-ac.

+ waxy : Mag-c.

udden : Nat-c.

Wilted : Nat-c.

Yellow : Kali-bi.

PARALYSIS : *Cad,M; Caus;* Grap; Kali-io; Merc; Seneg; Syph.

Distortion of muscle, with : Grap.

Eyes, Close, cannot : Cadm.

closed, with : Ap.

Chewing, difficult, with : Syph.

Goitre, suppression, from : Iod.

Mouth, opening Agg : Caus.

Neuralgia, after : Kali-m.

Swallowing, difficult : Cadm.

Talking difficult : Cadm; Syph.

Twitching of muscle, with : Kali-m.

eyelids of, with : Syph.

PEAKED : Stap.

PINCHED : Cam; Carb-v; Sec.

PUFFY, Bloated : Acet-ac; *Aco;* AP; Apoc; *Ars; Bry; Calc;* Crot-h; *Lach;* Laur; Lyc; Manc; Merc; Merc-d; Pho; Psor; Samb; Stram; Tarn; Ver-v.

Lying Agg : Apoc.

Pale : *Ap; Ars; Calc;* Grap; Hell; Lyc.

coughing, when : Samb.

Red : *Aco;* Arn; Chin; Fer; Lach; Op; Stram.

RED (See Cheeks, Eyes around) : Aco; *Bell; Caps;* Hyo; Nux-v; Op; Stram; Stro; Tarn.

One side : *Aco; Arn;* Bar-c; Bell; CHAM; Chel; *Ign;* Lac-c; Merc; Mos; Nux-v; *Pho;* Pul; Ran-b; Spig; Sul.

other pale : Cham; Ip.

right : *Ars; Calc;* Lachn; Merc; Mos; Nat-c; Sang; Sul-ac; Tab.

left : Acet-ac; Agar; Am-c; Ap; Bor; Cham; *Lyc; Nat-m;* PHO; *Rhus-t;* Stram; *Sul;* Thu; Ver-a.

Alternating : Chel; Lach; Nat-p; *Pho.*

Asthma, in : Caps.

Blotches : Iod; Kre; Oenan.

Circumscribed : Chin; Fer; Lyc; Pho; Sul; Tub.

Cold, but : Asaf; Caps; Fer; Mos.

Coma, in : Chin.

Convulsions, during : Glo; Op.

Cough Agg : Bell; Sang; Tub.

Eating, after : Caps; Lyc; Nux-v; Sul.

Fiery : Amy-n; *Meli;* Saba; Tarn.

Flushes, blushing : Amy-n; Coca; Strop; Tell.

Glowing : Mur-ac.

Headache, during : Bell; Glo; Meli.

Hot, and : Bell; Chin; Hell; Stram.

Loss of vital fluids, from : Chin.

+ Old men : Fer.

Spots : Am-c; Bell; Elap; Pho; Saba; Strop; Sul.

Stool, during : Caus.

Toothache with : Bell; Cham.

Unconsciousness, during : Glo; *Mur-ac.*

Vertigo, during : Kalm.

+ Walking, when : Pho.

Yellow spots : Kre.

REDDISH YELLOW : *Chel;* Gel; Lach; NUX-V.

RUBS, Fist, with, coughing, while (children) : Caus; Pul; *Scil.*

Hand with : Nux-v.

RUDDY, Florid : Arn; Fer.

+ SALLOW : Ant-t; Arg-m.

+ Sunken : Chel.

SHAVING Agg : Aur-m; Carb-an.

SICKLY : Ant-t; Arg-n; Ars; *Chin;* Cina; Lach; Lyc; *Nit-ac; Nux-v;* Stap; Sul-ac.

Cough, during : Cina.

SKIN Tight, as if : Cann.

+ SPIDERLETS, Red : Med.

SPOTTED, Blotched : Aco; Aeth; Ars; Carb-an; *Kali-bi;* Lach; Manc; *Rhus-t;* Sil; Sul.

STUPID Look : Bar-c; Cann; Hell; Kre.

SUFFERING : Ars; Cact; Kali-c; Lyss; Mang; Sil; Sul.

SUNKEN : Ant-t; Arg-n; ARS; Berb; *Cam;* Carb-v; CHIN; Dig; Hyds; Ign; Kali-m; Mang; Op; Par; *Rhus-t;* Sec; *Ver-a.*

SUNRISE to Sunset Agg : Kalm; Spig; Stan; Verb.

SWALLOWING Agg : Kali-n; Pho; Stap.

SWEAT On (See Sweat partial) : Bell; Cam; Cina; Ign; Merc; Lyc; Op;Spo; Val.

Cold : Ant-t; ARS; Cam; *Carb-v; Cina; Merc*-c; Spo; Tab; VER-A.

diarrhoea, in : Apoc.

Convulsions, during : Buf; Cocl.

Drinking Agg : Cham.

Eating Agg : *Cham;* Ign; *Nat-m;* Sul.

Hot : Cham.

One side, on : Nux-v; Pul.

Spots on, while eating : Ign.

SWOLLEN, Turgid : Ail; Am-m; *Ap;* ARS; BELL; *Bry;* Cham; Kali-c; Lac-d; *Lyc;* Lycps; *Manc; Merc; Nux-v;* Oenan; Op; Pho; Rhus-t; Stram; Tarn; *Ver-v.*

+ Dark, and : Ail.

Morning : Kali-chl.

One side : *Arn; Bell; Bry; Cham; Merc; Merc-c;* Sep; Spig.

right : Arn; Merc-i-f; Polyg; Sang.

Stiff : Rhus-t.

TALKING Agg : Bry; Kali-chl; Mez; Pul; Sep; Tell.

Amel : Kali-p.

TENSION : Pul; Verb; Vio-o.

TERRIFIED Look : ACO; Ap; Spo; Tarn; Ver-a.

THINKING of it Agg : Aur.

TIRED : Hell.

TONGUE, Protruding Agg : Hyo; Syph.

TOUCH Agg : Lapp.

TWITCHING, Trembling : *Agar;* Ars; BELL; Cham; Gel; Ign; Laur; LYC; Myg; Oenan; *Op;* Plb; Rhe; Sele; Senec; STRAM; Tell; Thu.

Asthma, before : Bov.

Coughing, while : *Ant-t;* Kali-m.

Eating, when : Kali-m.

Sleep, in : Rhe.

Speaking, when : Kali-m.

+ Spreads, all over body : Sec.

Tongue, protruding, when : Hyo.

Vision, misty, with : Mill.

ULCER, Cancerous : *Con.*

VEINS, Distended : Chin; Dig.

Spider-like : Thu.

WALKING Amel : Mag-c; Rhus-t.

WARTS On : Dul; Sep.

WASH, Desire to, in cold water : See Desire to wash.

+ WAXY : Acet-ac; Sil.

+ WILD Look : Anac; Sec; Val.

WIND, Cold, blowing on, as if : Colo; Mez.

WRINKLED (See Forehead) : Abro; Alu; Calc; *Lyc;* Syph.

YELLOW : *Ars;* Bry; Card-m; *Chel; Chin;* Fer; Kre; Lach; *Lyc; Merc;* Nat-s; *Nit-ac;* NUX-V; *Plb;* Pod; SEP.

Hair, at the edge of : Caul; Kali-p; Med.

Spots : Nat-c.

Red : See Reddish yellow.

spots : Kre.

FAG, ENERVATION : See Delicate.

FAILURE, Feels himself a : Naj; Sul.

FAINT, FAINTING (See also

Unconscious) : ACO; ARS; *Asaf;* BRY; Cam; *Carb-v;* CHAM; Caus; CHIN; Cof; Croc; *Crot-h; Dig;* Glo; Hep; IGN; Iod; LACH; *Mos;* NUX-M; NUX-V; Op; Plb; Pod; *Pul;* SEP; Stram; Strop; SUL; Sumb; Tab; Thyr; Val; VER-A.

ACCOMPANIMENT, As a : Lach.

AFTERPAINS, after every : Nux-v.

ARMS Extending, head, above,on : Lac-d; Spo.

ASCENDING Stairs : Anac.

BATH, Hot Agg : Lach.

BLINDNESS, After : Nux-m.

BLOOD, At the sight of : Nux-m.

CAUSE, Without : Asaf.

CHILL, During : *Sep.*

CLOSE, Crowded room, in : Asaf; Plb; *Pul.*

COITION, After : *Agar;* Dig; Nat-p; Sep.

During, women, in : Murx; Orig; *Plat.*

DIE, As if would : Vinc.

DINNER, During, after : Mag-m; Nux-v.

DISTURBED, When : Asaf.

+ EASY : Ign; Mos.

+ EATING, While : Mos.

EMISSION, After : *Asaf;* Pho-ac.

EMOTIONS, On : *Ver-a.*

EXERTION, On : *Sep.*

Slight : Ver-a.

FEVER, During : Arn; Nat-m;

145

Pho; *Sep.*

FREQUENT : *Ars*; Pho; *Sul.*

Sweat, profuse, with : Hyds.

GASTRIC Origin : Ol-an.

HAEMORRHAGE, With : Ver-a.

HEAT, Then coldness, with : *Sep.*

HEATED, When : Ip; Tab.

HOUR, At a certain : Lyc.

INJURIES, Slight : Ver-a.

LOOKING Up : Tab.

Steadily at, any object : Sumb.

MEDICINE, Taking, on : Asaf.

MENSES, During : Lach; Laur; Mag-c; Mos; *Nux-m*: Nux-v; Sep; Tril.

Coldness, with : Laur.

Pain,from : Kali-s; *Lap-lab.*

Start, at : Merc.

Suppressed from : Nux-m.

MUSIC, From : Sumb.

NURSING, Child, when : Vip.

ODOURS, From : Colch.

PAIN, From : Asaf; *Cham*; Cocl; *Hep*; Mos; *Nux-m*; Nux-v; st Ran-sc; Stro; Val.

PALPITATION, During : Lach; Nux-m.

PROLONGED : Hyd-ac; Laur.

+ READING, when : Merc-i-f.

RISING, on : *Bry; Cadm;* Merc-i-f; Phyt; *Ver-v*; Vib.

ROOM, Entering : Plb.

Hot : Ip; Lil-t; Pul; Sep.

SITTING, Up, on : Vib.

STANDING, On : *Alu;* Lil-t; Nux-m.

STOOL, At : Con; *Nux-m;* Nux-v; Ox-ac; Pod; Spig; Sul; Ver-a.

STOOPING, On : Elap; Sumb.

SUDDEN : Ip; Pho; Ran-b; Sep.

SUMMER : Ip.

SWEAT, with: Dig; Hyds.

Cold : Lach.

THINKING After : Calad.

TRIFLES, From : Sep; Sumb.

VERTIGO, With : Berb.

VOMITING, From : Cocl; Nux-v; Ver-a.

WAKING, On: *Carb-v.*

WALKING, Open air, in : Seneg.

WASHING Clothes on : Ther.

WOUND, From slight : Ver-a.

WRITING, After : Calad.

FALLING : Bro; Caus; Coll; Con; Kre; Laur; Nat-c; Pho-ac; Rat.

AS if : BELL; Thu.

BACKWARD, As if : Bry; Chin; Led; Rhus-t.

DOWN, As if : Laur.

EASILY : Calc.

FORWARD, As if : Alu; Dig; Elap; Mang; Nat-m; *Nux-v;* Rhus-t.

GROUND To, when walking or standing, suddenly : Mag-c.

+ suddenly, cries, and : Hyo.

Rolls about and : Cic.

Through, as if : Benz.

Unconscious : Cocl.

screams,and : Buf.

HEIGHT, From as if : Caus;
Gel; Mos.

+ Sleep in, as if : Caps.

INWARD, Wall as if, epilepsy
before : Carb-v.

OUT, As if : *Bell;* Cocl; Laur;
Lil-t; Nux-v; Pod; Sep.

RISING and Falling : See
Directions Up and Down.
As if : Bar-c; Lach.

SIDEWAYS, As if : Calc; Cocl;
Nux-v.

STREET, in: Chin-s.

WITHOUT Any cause or from
least obstacle : Nat-c.

FALTERING : See Hesitates.

FALLOPIAN TUBES, Inflam
mation of (Salpingitis) : Ars;
Coll; Lach; Merc; *Pul; Sep;*
Stap.

CUTTING Along : Polyg.

SERUM Or Pus, escapes from
uterus : Sil.

FANATICISM : Thu.

FANCIES : See Perceptions
Changed.

FANNED, As if : See Air,
Blowing, on part.

FANNING AGG : Mez.

AMEL : Ant-t; Ap; Arg-n; Bap;
Carb-v; Chin; Chlo-hyd;
Crot-h; Fer; Kali-n; Lach;
Med; Sec; Xanth.

FANTASY : See Imaginations.

FAR OFF FEELING : Med; Syph.

FASTIDIOUS : *Ars;* Grap;

Nux-v.

FASTING AGG : *Calc; Croc;*
Dios; *Flu-ac;* IOD; Kre; Lach;
Laur; Nat-c; Pho; Plat; Plb;
Ran-b; Sep; Stap; Sul; Tab;
Val.

AMEL *: Cham; Con;* Kali- s;
Nat-m;

AS If : Ars; Bry; Chin; Cocl;
Ign; Pul; Ver-a.

meals, after : Lyc.

FATIGUE AGG : Actea; Berb;
Cof; Epip; Helo; Nux-v; Pho-ac.

SCIENTIFIC Labour, from AGG
: Grap.

FATS : See Food.

FATTY : See Greasy.

DEGENERATION *: Ars;* Aur; Cup;
Kali-c; *Lyc;* Mang; Merc;
Pho; Vanad.

FAUCES, ITCHING : Phyt; Rhus-t.

NUMB : Arg-m.

SENSITIVE : Coc-c.

FAULT FINDING : Ars; Helo;
Sul; Ver-a.

FAVUS: See under Eruptions.

FEAR, ANXIETY, **F**RIGHT : Abro;
ACO; *Arg-n;* ARS; *Bell;* Bor;
Calc; Calc-p; *Carb-v;* Cist;
Cocl; Cof; *Dig;* Gel; Grap; Hyo;
IGN; *Lyc;* Lyss; Med; Merc-c;
Mos; Murx; Nat-c; Nat-m;
Nit-ac; *Nux-v; Op;* PHO; Psor;
Pul; Rat; Rhus-t; Samb; *Sec;*
Spo; Stram; Sul; Ther; Tub;
Ver-a.

ALONE, Of being : Ant-t; Con;
Naj.

Lest, he injures himself :

Ars; Merc; Nat-s.

Darkness, in : Kali-br; Radm; Val.

ANIMALS, Dogs etc : *Bell;* Buf; *Chin;* Tub.

APPEARING In public, (Stage fright etc) : Anac; Arg-n; *Gel.*

APPROACH, Of : *Arn;* Bar-c; Caus; Cup; Ign; *Lyc;* Petr; Pho; Plb; Sep; Tarn; Ther.

ARREST, Of : Ars; Meli; Plb; Tab; Zin.

ASCENDINGING, Steps on : Nit-ac.

ASSASSINS : Plb.

BAD NEWS : Ast-r.

BED or Coach, of : Alum Cann; Cedr.

Wetting: Alu.

BITTEN, By beast, being : Hyo.

BRILLIANT Shining objects mirrors,etc. : Canth; Lach; Lyss; Stram.

CAUSE, Without : Plb; Zin-val.

CHILDREN, About one's : Rhus-t.

COITION, At the thought of in women : Kre.

CORNERS, to walk past, certain : Arg-n; Kali-br.

Something, creeping out of : Pho.

CROSSING Streets : Aco; Hyd-ac; Plat.

CLOSED Carriage, Riding in : Cimi; Succi.

CROWD : Aco; Arg-n; Aur; Fer-p; Gel; Nat-m; Pul.

CRUELTIES, Hearing : Calc.

DARK : Arg-n; Cam; *Cann;* Carb-an; Kali-br; Sanic; STRAM; *Val.*

Eyes, Closing on : Carb-an.

DEATH, Of : ACO; Arn; ARS; Cact; *Calc;* Cimi; *Gel;* Hyd-ac; Kali-c; Kali-n; Lac-c; Mos; Nit-ac; *Pho;* Plat.

Starvation, from : Ars.

DESIRE, To escape, from : Merc.

DISEASE, Of : Arn; Calad; *Calc; Kali-c; Lac-c; Lil-t;* Nux-v; *Pho;* Sele.

Cholera : Lach; *Nit-ac.*

Contagious : Bor.

Incurable, being : Cact; Lil-t.

Lungs, of : Aral.

Pneumonia : Chel.

Small-pox : Vario.

Syphilis : Hyo.

Tuberculosis : Calc.

DOOR, Bell, ringing : Lyc.

Opening, on: Cic; Con; Lyc.

DOWNWARD, Motion : See Falling.

EMISSION, After : Carb-an; Petr.

ENDURE, Can not : Lyss.

EVERY Thing, of : Calc; Hyd-ac; Lyc.

+ EVIL, Of : Kali-m.

EXAMINATION, Of : Aeth; Anac; Gel; Pic-ac.

EYES, Closing on : *Carb-v;* Mag-m.

FALL Upon him, High walls and buildings : Arg-n; Arn.

FALLING, Downward motion of : *Bor; Gel;* Hypr; Lac-c; Sanic; Sil; Zin.

Forwards : Alu.

Height, from : Hyo.

Houses, of : Hyd-ac.

Stairs, down : Lac-c.

up, and : Onos.

FEVER, During : Aco; Amb; Ars; Bar-c; Ip; Sep.

FINANCIAL, Loss of: Ars; Calc-f; Stap.

FRIENDS, Of : Cedr.

FRIGHT, Of, remains : Op.

FUTURE, Misfortune, evilforebodings : ACO; ARS; Ast-r; CALC; Caus; Cham; Chin-s; Cimi; Dig; Grap; Grat; Kali-c;Kali-m; Lil-t; Merc; Nat-m; *Nux-v;* Pho; Plat; PSOR; PUL; Thu; *Ver-a.*

Imaginary : Kali-c; Laur.

Sense, of : Merc.

Twilight Agg : Caus.

GHOSTS : Carb-v; Kali-c; Pho; Pul; Ran-b; *Stram.*

GLISTENING Objects : See Brilliant.

GREEN Stripes, seeing on : Thu.

HEALTH, Of others, about : Cocl.

. One's own : Arg-m; Kali-p.

+ HEART, will stop : Lach.

HURT, Being : *Arn;* Chin;

Hep; Kali-c; Rut; Spig.

HUSBAND Will never return, something will happen to him : Plat.

IMAGINARY Things: *Bell;* Hyd-ac; Laur; Pho.

IMPULSE Of his own : Alu.

INSANITY, Of : Alu; *CALC; Cann;* Chlor; *Cimi;* Kali-br; Lil-t; Lyss; Manc; Med; *Pul;* Sumb.

KNIVES, Of : Alu; Ars; Chin; Hyo; Lyss; Nux-v.

LIGHTNING *:* Sil.

LONG LASTING *: Aco;* Hyo; Op; Petr.

LYING Down of, lest one die : Mos.

Heart will stop : Lach.

MANIACAL : Sec.

MIRRORS, Of : See Brilliant.

MURDERED Of being : Cimi; Op; Pho; Pl; Stram; Tab.

Somebody : Ars.

NARROW or shut places : *Arg-n;* Cimi; Lac-d; Stram; Succi; Val.

NEVER, Get well : All-s.

NIGHT, At, can not lie in bed : Rhus-t; Syph.

NOISE : Bor; Cocl; Mos; Ther.

Door, at : Aur; Lyc.

Least : Aur.

Street, in: Bar-c; *Caus.*

OBSERVED, Her condition being : Calc; Chel.

OPEN Air, of : Cyc.

Space : See Agoraphobia.

ORDEALS : Arn; *Arg-n; Gel;*
Kali-br; Lyss; Strop.

PAIN, Becomes unbearable :
Cep.

From : Sars.

PARALYSIS, Of : *Anac;* Arn; Bap;
Syph.

PEOPLE, of : See
Anthropophobia.

Yet if alone Agg : Ars; Clem;
Con; Kali-br; Lyc; Sep;
Stram; Tarn.

menses during : Con.

PHYSICIAN : Iod; Thu; Ver-v.

PLACES, Buildings : Arg-n;
Calc; Kali-p; Visc.

POINTED, Things, needles, pins
: Ap; Ars; Bov; Merc; Plat;
Sil; Spig.

POISON : *All*-s; Anac; Ap; Bell;
Glo; *Hyo;* Lach;Kali-br;
Rhus-t; Ver-v.

POVERTY : Bry; Calc; Calc-f;
Nux-v; Psor; Sep.

PURSUIT : Hyo.

RAIN : Elap; Naj.

RATS : Cimi.

RIDING Carriage, in : Bor; Lach;
Psor; Sep.

ROBBERS : Ars; Ign; Nat-m.

SAY Something wrong, lest
he should : Lil-t; Med.

SELF Control, losing: Arg-n;
Gel; Stap.

SHADOWS : Calc.

His own : Calad; Lyc; Stap.

SHARP Things (See pointed
things) : Alu; Ars; Merc;
Plat.

SHUT Places : See Narrow.

SLEEP, Loss of, from : Cocl;
Nit-ac.

Falling to : Calad; Lach;
Sabal.

SOCIETY : Cup; Cup-ac;
Sele; Til.

Position, his own in :
Ver-a.

STOOL, After: Calc; Caus;
Kali-c; Nit-ac.

STRANGERS : *Bar-c;* Buf;
Carb-v; Caus; Cup; Thu.

SUDDEN, Wakes from sleep:
Arn.

TALKING, Loudly : Meli.

TELEPHONE : Visc.

THUNDER Storm, Lightning
: Bor; Lyc; Nat-c; Nit-ac;
Pho; Rhod.

TOUCH, Of (See Approach) :
ANT-C; *Arn;* CHAM; Cina;
Con; Cup; Ign; Kali-c; Lyc;
Tarn.

Others passing, by : Aco.

Sore parts : Tell.

TREMBLING And Chattering
of teeth, with : Elap.

TREMULOUS : Mag-c.

TRIFLES, Over : Aco; Ign;
Sep; Thu.

TUNNEL : Stram.

TWILIGHT Agg : Caus.

UNDERTAKING Any new thing
: Arg-n; Ars; Lyc; Sil.

VEHICLES, Approaching of :
Hyd-ac.

150

WAKING, On: Ant-t; Arn; Ars; Cina; Lach; Psor; Spo; Tub.

Slowly must, otherwise something will happen : Cup.

WATER (See Water) : Hyo; Lyss; Stram.

WOMEN : Pul.

FEARLESSNESS (See Boldness) : Agar.

FEATHER : See Dust.

FEATHER BED *AGG* : Cocl; Colo; *Mang*; Merc; Psor; Sul.

FEEBLE : See Weak.

FEELS TOO HOT : See Heat Agg.

GOOD and **B**AD by turns : Alu; Psor.

NOT **N**ORMAL, but can not tell why : Bro.

FEET : Arn; Ars; Bell; Bry; Caus; Kali-c; Lyc; *Pul;* Sep; Sil; Zin-ch.

ARCHES : Rut; Sil.

BED, Out of: Ars; Cham; Sang; Sec; *Sul.*

BLOTCHY : Led.

BONES : Chin; Cup; Hypr; *Led*; Mez; *Rut*; Stap.

Broken, as if : Zin.

BORDER, Of: Grap; Kali-bi; Led; Lith; Zin.

BRACES, **S**TRETCHING, Amel : Ign; Med; Pul.

BROKEN, As if : Hep; Zin.

BUNIONS : Grap; Lyc; Paeon; *Sil.*

BURNING : Cham; Med; Pho-ac; *Pul;* Sec; *Sul.*

Hands cold, with : Sep.

Menses during, night at : Nat-p.

CLUBBY : Nux-v.

COLD Agg : Bar-c; Con; Lach; *Nux-v; Pul;* Sil.

As if, though warm : Sul.

Water, as if, in : Gel; Sanic; *Sep.*

Wet Agg : See Wetting Agg.

COLDNESS (See Coldness partial) : Kali-chl; Raph.

Bed in : Am-c; Calc; Grap; Psor; Rhod; Senec; *Sep;* Sil.

right : Lyc; Raph.

left : Ars; Tub.

icy : Bell.

Chorea, in : Laur.

Colic, with : Colo.

+ Constant : Old.

Day time, burn at night : Nat-p.

Fever, during : Arn; Lach; Stram; Sul.

Headache, during : Gel; Meli; Sep; Vario.

Hot days, summer in : Asar.

Icy : Cam; Carb-v; Elap; Lach; Pho; Samb; Sep; Sil; Ver-a.

menses during : Nat-p.

Menses, with : Nux-m.

One of : Chel; Con.

right : Bar-c; *Lyc*; Pul; Sabi.

left : Carb-v; Psor; *Sul;* Tub.

other, hot : *Lyc*; Pul.

Pregnancy, during : *Lyc*; *Ver-a.*

Smokers : Sec.

Soles burning : Cup.

Urnination, during : Dig.

Walking only, while : Anac; Chin; Plb.

CRAMP : Bell; Caus; Cup; Frax; Lac-c; Rum; Sanic; Sec; Val; Ver-v.

Pregnancy during : *Calc*; Frax.

CRAWLING : See Formication.

CRIPPLED : Ant-c.

DAMP : CALC.

DESQUAMATION : Manc.

DORSUM, of : Calc; *Caus*; Hep; Led; *Pul*; Spig; Tarx.

Cramp: Anac; Lach; Ver-v.

Itching : Caus; Led.

Stitches, in : Berb.

Sweat : Iod.

Swelled : Bry; Pul; Thu.

DRY : *Sul.*

EMACIATION : Caus.

ENLARGED, As if : *Ap*; Colo.

FANNED, Wants : *Med.*

FIDGETY : Kali-p; Tarn; Zin.

FLAT : Calc-p.

FLOATING, As if : Spig.

FORMICATION : Agar; Hypr; Sec.

FROST Bitten, as if : Kali-p.

FURRY : Hypr.

GALLED : Cep.

GLUED To floor, as if : Pho.

HANGING Down Agg : See

Hanging down limbs Agg.

HARD Floor Agg : Rut.

HEAD To, Glowing sensation : Visc.

HEAVY : *Alu; Ars*; Cyc; Ign; Mag-c; NAT-M; Pho; Pic-ac; *Pul; Rhod; Rut;* Sep; SUL.

Walking Amel : *Mag-c;* Nat- m; Sul.

Weight, hanging, as if : Rhus-t; Rut.

HELD To The EARTH, by magnet, as if : Led; Pho.

HIGHER Than head, as if : *Spig.*

HOT : See Burning.

Cold and, alternately : Gel; Polyg.

Water in AMEL : Buf.

INSTEP : Sang.

INVERSION : Cic; Nux-v; Sec.

ITCHING : Led; Pic-ac; Sep; Strop; Sul.

KNEE, To : Cedr.

MOTION Amel: Ars; *Rhus-t;* Zin.

Spasmodic of left foot : Cina.

NUMB : Ap; Arg-n; ARS; *Cocl;* Con; Form; Grap; Lyc; NUX-V; Pho; Pio-ac; Pic-ac; *Plat*; Sep.

Right : Alu; Am-c; Ant-c; Ars; Cam; Kali-bi; Mang; Rhus-t; Sep.

Left : Grap; Kali-c; Med; Nat-m; Pho; Psor; Thu.

Legs crossing, on : Laur.

Sitting, when : Ant-t; Helo.

OFFENSIVE, Sweat without : Grap; Sil.

PAINFUL, Menses during : Am-m; Ars; Mag-c.

Sciatica, with : Mag-p.

Standing, from : Scil.

PARALYSIS : Caus; Plb; Vip; Zin.

As if : Cham.

PRESSES To floor AMEL : Cup-ar; Ign; Med; Zin-io.

PRICKING : Kali-p.

RESTLESS : Ars; Rhus-t; ZIN.

SHOP Girls, of : Scil.

SPASMS : Bism; Ver-a.

STAMPS : Ant-c; Stram; Ver-a.

STIFF In A.M. : Led.

STRETCHING AMEL : See Braces.

Spasmodic : Cina.

SWEAT : *Bar-c; Calc;* Calc-s; *Carb-v;* Cocl; Colo; Grap; *Iod; Lyc;* Mag-m; Merc; Psor; *Pul;* SEP; *Sil; Sul; Thu;* Zin.

Acrid : Flu-ac; *Grap;* Manc; Sep; Sil; Thu.

Burning, with : Calc; Lyc; Sul.

Cold : Aur; *Bar-c; Calc;* Calc-s; Carb-v; Kali-m; Lach; Lyc; Mur-ac; Pul; Sec; Stap; Tarn; Ver-a. bed in, morning : Merc.

Destroys shoes : Grap; Hep; Naj; Sanic; Sec; Sil.

Foul, offensive : Aur; *Bar-c;* Calc-s; Grap;

Kali-c; Lach; Lyc; *Nit-ac;* Ol- an; Psor; *Pul;* Sec; Sep; SIL; Tell; *Thu.*

menses, after : Sep; Sil.

Injuries of spine, after : *Nit-ac.*

Sour, toes between : Kob.

Sticky, hose stiff : Am-c; Calc; Kali-c; Lyc; Manc; Sanic.

Stubborn: Psor.

Suppressed: *Bar-c;* Ol- an; Pho; Sep; *Sil; Zin.*

Swelling, with: Lyc.

Toes, sore with : Grap; Zin.

Walking Agg : Carb-v.

Warm : Led.

Wilting the skin: Ant-c.

SWELLING, Oedema etc.: *Ap; Ars;* Caus; Chel; Grap; Led; *Lyc; Med;* Merc-c; Pul; Pru-sp; Samb; Sil.

Right : Bov; Lac-c; Lach; Lyc; Sars; Sec; Spig; Spo; Stro; Sul.

Left: *Ap;* Colo; Como; Kali-c; Kre; Lyc; Sang; Sil; Tell.

Cold : Ap; Calc.

Diarrhoea, after or Amel by : Med.

with : Acet-ac.

Hands of, with : Fer.

Hot : Ars; *Bry;* Lyc.

Menses, during : Ap; Grap; Lyc; Pul.

One foot, only : Kali-c.

Paralysis, with : Cocl.

Sensation of : *Ap.*

Soles, painful, with : Saba.

Sprain, after : *Bov.*

SWING, Half circle in, walking while : Cic.

TINGLING : Cocl.

TOUCH Agg : Ars; Calc; Chin; Kali-c; Sep; Sul.

+ TOUCH, Do not, ground, as if : Calc-ar.

TREMBLING : Aur; Bar-c; Merc; Ox-ac; Pul.

Menses, during : Hyo.

TURN INWARD : Cic.

Under : See Ankles Weak.

ULCER, On : Sil.

UNCOVER, Must : Cham; Flu-ac; Med; Pul; *Sul.*

VEINS, Distended : Sul-ac.

VESICLES : Nat-c.

WEAKNESS : Ars; Mag-c; Ox-ac; Sil .

Sitting Agg : Card-m.

WEIGHT, Hanging : See Heavy.

WETTING Of AGG : Cep; Cham; Cup; *Dul;* Merc; Nat-c; Nat-m; *Pho;* PUL; Rhus-t; *Sep;* SIL.

WINTER Agg : Caus.

WOOD, As if were: Plb.

FEIGNING SICK : See Malingering.

FELON : See Fingers.

FEMALES AFFECTIONS In
General : Aco; Ap; *Bell;* Calc; Caps; Cham; Chin; Cimi; Cocl; Con; Croc; Helo; *Lach;* Mag-m; Mos; PUL; Sabal;

SABI; SEP; Val; Vib.

AFTER PAINS : See After Pains.

COITION Agg : Ap; *Arg-n;* Fer; Fer-p; Hep; Kre; Lyc; Lyss; Nat-m; Pul; Sep; Sul; Tarn; Thu.

After Agg : Ap; Plat; Stap.

Aversion to : Agn; Bor; Caus; Grap; *Nat-m; Sep.*

menses after : Caus; Pho.

orgasms painful, from : Nat-m.

Enjoyment absent : Berb; Caus; Kali-br; Sep.

First Agg : Stap.

Haemorrhage, after : *Arg-n;* Arn; Hyds; *Kre;* Nit-ac; Sep; Tarn.

CONCEPTION , Easy : Bor; Merc; Nat-m.

Promotes : Canth; Nat-c.

DESIRE, Sexual, diminished: Agn; *Caus; Grap;* Helo; Ign; *Nat-m;* Onos; Sabal; Sep.

Increased : AGN; *Calc;* Calc-p; Cam; *Canth;* Con; Flu-ac; Grat; HYO; Lach; *Murx; Nux-v; Orig; Pho;* PLAT; *Pul;* Stram; Tarn; *Ver-a.*

contact, least, from : Lac-c; Murx.

dysmenorrhoea, with : Cann.

menses, before: Ars; Calc-p; Pho; Stan; Stram; Ver-a.

during : Ars; Canth; Hyo; Lach; *Lyc*; Plat; *Pul.*

after : Ars; Kali-p.

suppressed, from : Ant-c.

must keep busy to repress it : Lil-t.

nursing, while : Calc-p; Pho.

old women in : Mos.

parturition, after : Chin; Ver- a; Zin.

pregnancy, during : Pho.

scratching, distant parts from : Stan.

women, sterile, in : Cann.

worms, from : Saba.

Perverted : Sabal.

Suppressed, ill effects from (See Sexual desire male) : *Con;* Sabal.

Violent, insatiable, nymphomania : AGN; Ast-r; Calc; Grat; *Hyo;* Lach; Murx; Orig; *Plat;* Stan; Stram; Sumb; *Ver–a;* Zin.

love, disappointment from : Ver-a.

lying in women : Ver-a; Zin.

masturbation, driving her to : Orig ; Plat; Zin.

unsatisfied sexual desire from : Ver-a.

virgins, in: Con; *Plat.*

widows, in : *Ap; Orig.*

+ FRIGIDITY : Ign.

ORGASM, Delayed, wanting : Berb; Brom.

Easy : Stan.

SEXUAL, Excitement easy: Bur-p; Lac-c; Manc; Orig; Sumb; Zin.

STERILITY: Agn; Aur; *Bor;* Merc; Nat-c; *Nat–m;* Pho; Sep.

Acid vaginal secretion from : Nat-p.

Atrophy of mammae and ovary, from : Iod.

Excessive sexual desire from : Kali-br; Orig; Pho; Plat.

Menses, copious, from : Calc; Merc; Mill; Nat-m; Sul.

Non retention of semen, from : Nat-c.

Ovarian atony, from: Eup-pur.

Sycotic : Med.

+ Uterine torpor, from :*Goss.*

Weakness, from : Merc; Sil.

TO COMPLETE, Full Term, in delicate and sheer nervous women : Rat.

WOMEN Who deliver, still born children : Cimi.

For pregnancy, late in life : Bell.

FEMALE ORGANS in General : Amb; Ap; BELL; *Calc;* Cham; *Cimi;* Con; Grap; Kali-c; Kre; *Lach; Lil-t;* Lyc; Nat-m; *Nux-m;* Nux-v; Onos; Pho; *Plat;* PUL; *Sabi;* Sec; Senec; SEP; *Sul; Thu;* Til; Tril; Ust; *Vib;* Visc.

BACKWARD, Pains : Bell; Lil-t; Sep.

BURNING : Ars; Berb; *Canth;* Carb-an; *Kre;* Nit-ac; Sec; Sul.

COLD : Plat.

CONSCIOUSNESS, Of internal : Vib.

CROSSING Legs, Amel : Lil-t; Sep.

DRYNESS : Berb; Lyc; *Nat-m;* SEP.

GANGRENE : Sec.

HARD : Con; *Kre;* Merc.

HEART, To : Naj; Xanth.

HEAVY : Lob; Plat.

Menses, during : Plat; Sep.

ITCHING : Amb; Am-c; CALAD; *Calc; Carb-v; Con;* Kre; Merc; NAT-M; Nit-ac; Petr; Plat; Rhus-t; SEP; Sil; *Sul;* TARN.

Burning : Am-c; Calc.

Coition Agg : Nit-ac.

+ desire for: Sabi.

Cold water Amel : Calad.

+ Desire Strong, to embrace : Alu.

Intolerable : Agar; *Amb;* Calc.

Lying Amel : Berb.

Menses, after Agg : Nit-ac; Tarn.

from : Sul; Tarn.

Pregnancy during : Calad; Flu-ac; Helo; Merc; Sabi; *Sep.*

Urine, contact of Agg : *Merc.*

Voluptuous : *Orig; Plat.*

Walking Agg : *Nit-ac;* Thu.

LABOUR LIKE, Bearing down pains : Agar; Alo; BELL; *Caul;* CHAM; GEL; *Lil-t;* Murx; Nat-m; NUX-V; Plat; PUL; *Sabi; Sec;* SEP; Stan; Vib.

Colds Agg : Hyo.

Fear of death with : Cof.

Menopause, after : Agar.

Noise Agg : Cimi.

Riding in carriage Agg : Asaf.

Rubbing Amel : Pall.

Standing Agg : Dict.

Amel : Bell.

LYING Agg : Amb; Fer; Kre; Murx; *Pul.*

Back, on Amel : Onos.

Doubled up, Amel : Cact; Cimi; Nux-v.

MOIST, As if : Petr.

PRESSURE, Back, on Amel : Mag-m.

Vulva on, Amel : Lil-t; Murx; Sanic; Sep.

SITTING Agg : Sul.

SORE, Sensitive, painful : Ap; Bell; Canth; Cof; *Con; Kre; Lach;* Lil-t; Mur-ac; *Plat;* Stap; Sul; Thu.

+ Redness of : Til.

STOOLING Agg : Amb; Pod; Stan.

SWELLED : Ap; Ars; Bell; Canth; *Kre; Nit-ac;* Nux-v; *Pul;* Rhus-t.

THIGHS, To : Cham; Stap; Xanth.

TINGLING, Voluptuous: *Orig; Plat.*

UPWARD, Going: Alu; Cact; Calc-p; Coc-c; Elap; Lach; Lil-t; Nit-ac; Pul; Sabi; *Sep.*

Right : Alu; *Ap;* Croc; Lach; Lyc; Murx.

Left. : *Bro;* Caul; Cimi; Kali- c; Lac-c; LACH; LIL-T; NAJ; Sul.

mammae, to : Murx.

FEROCIOUS : See Delirium, Maniacal.

FESTERING, As if : Buf.

FESTINATION : Alu; Mang; Syph; Tarn.

FEVER : ACO; Ant-t; *Ap;* Arn; ARS; BELL; BRY; *Canth;* Caps; *Carb-v; Caus;* Cham; Chin; Chin-s; Con; Fer-p; *Gel;* Ign; Ip; Kali-s; Lach; LYC; Med; *Merc;* Merc-c; Mez; *Nat-m;* NUX-V; Op; PHO; Pic-ac; PUL; RHUS-T; Sang; *Sul;* Tarx; Ver-a.

+ ADYAMIC : Ail; Bap; Mur-ac.

AFTER AGG : *Ars;* Bell; *Chin;* Hep; Nux-v.

ALTERNATING, Chill, with : See Chill alternating with fever.

BEFORE AGG : Arn; *Ars;* Calc; *Carb-v; Chin;* Cina; Ip; *Pul;* Rhus-t; Spig; Sul.

BLACK WATER : *Ars;* Crot-h; Lyc.

CATARRHAL : See Coryza.

CHILL Absent : Ap; Ars; Bell; Bry; Cham; Gel; Rhus-t.

COITION, After : Grap; Nux-v.

CONTINUED : See Blood Sepsis, Typhoid etc.

CONVERSATION, From : Sep.

COUGHING Agg : Arn; Ars; Chin; Ign; Mur-ac; Nat-m; Thu.

Whooping, with : Dros.

COVERS, Warmth, Agg : Ap; Chin; *Ign;* Mur-ac; Nat-m; Op; *Pul.*

Amel : Bell; Nux-v; Pul; Pyro; Rhus-t; Stram; Stro; Tub.

DENTITION, During : Aco; Calc; *Cham;* Nux-v; Sil; Sul.

DRINKS, Warm Agg : Sumb.

DRY, Burning : ACO; *Ap;* Ars; *Carb-v;* Dul; Gel; *Mur-ac; Nux-v;* Op; Pho; *Pul;* Sec; Tub.

Night, at : Samb.

DURING AGG : *Ars;* Bry; Calc; Cham; *Chin;* Ip; Kali-c; Lyc; Nat-m; *Nux-v;* Op; *Pul;* Rhus-t; *Sep;* Sul.

DYSENTERIC : Bap; Fer-p; Nux-v.

EATING Agg : Pho; Tub.

Amel : Anac; Chin.

EMOTIONS, From : Caps.

EXTERNAL : *Aco;* Ars; *Bell;* Bry; *Canth;* Cham; *Ign;* Pul; Rhus-t; Sil; Stram.

FANNED Desire to be, in place of thirst : *Carb-v.*

FEET, Cold with : Tarn.

FRIGHT, From : Cheno.

GASTRIC : Ant-c; Ant-t; Ars; *Bap;* Bry; Fer-p; Ip; Pul.

HANDS, Cold, with : Thu.

HECTIC : Ars; Ars-io; Bap; Caps; Chin-ar; Fer-p; Iod; Pho; Sang; Sep; Sil; Tub.

HIGH, Hyperpyrexia : ACO; Bap; Chin-ar; Iod; Mur-ac; Pho; *Pyro;* Sul; Ver-v.

Erratic, rise of: Pul.

Evening in, below normal in morning : Ver-v.

HOME SICKNESS, From : Caps.

INSIDIOUS : Ars; Chin; Sec; Sul; Tub.

INTERMITTANT Ague : Aran; ARS; Calc; Calc-ars; Caps; Ced; *Eup-p;* Fer; Ign; *Ip;* Kali-s; Lyc; *Nat-m;* Nat-s; Nit-ac; *Nux-v;* Pho-ac; Psor; Pul; Pyro; Sul; Tarn; Tub; *Ver-a.*

INTERNAL : *Aco;* Am; *Ars; Bell;* Bry; Laur; Mag-c; Merc; *Nux-v;* Pho; Pho-ac; Rhus-t; Sul; *Ver-a*

External coldness with : *Aco;* Ars; Cam; Mos; Sul-io; Ver-a.

cold parts, with : *Aco;* Ant-t; Ap; Am; *Ars;* Bell; Calc; *Cam;* Carb-v; Cham; Cina; Cof; Dig; Dros; Hyo; Ign; Ip; Kali-c; Mez; *Mos;* Nit-ac; Nux-v; Pho-ac; Plat; Rhus-t; Sul; *Ver-a.*

INTOLERANCE Of both, cold and warmth : Cocl; Cor-r.

+ MALIGNANT : Crot-h.

MENSES, With: Calc; Grap; Pho; *Pyro;* Rhod; *Sep.*

MENTAL Exertion Agg : Old; Spo.

MILK (Fever) : *Aco; Bry; Calc;* Cham.

Delirium with : Aco.

MOTION Agg : Cam; *Chin;* Sep.

Amel : Caps; Lyc; Pho; Pul.

NIGHT Agg : *Ars;* Bap; Bell; Bry; Calc; Cham; Grap; *Hep;* Iod; Lach; Merc; Petr; Pho; *Pul; Sil;* Sul; Urt.

Periodically: Flu-ac.

NOISE, From : Bry.

ONE SIDED : Alu; Bry; Cham; Dig; Lyc; Mos; Nux- v; Pul.

Right : Alu; Bry; Cham; Pho.

Left : Lyc; Rhus-t; Stan.

Lain on : Mag-m.

OSCILLATING : Chel; Chin-ar; Echi; *Pyro;* Sul-ac; Ver-v; Zin.

PAIN, From : Carb-v; Cham.

Abdomen, in : Sec.

PAINFUL : Bry; Canth; Rhus-t.

PAINLESS : Pho; Pho-ac.

PAROXYSMS, Irregular : Ars; Nux-v; Psor; Pul; Sep.

PUERPERAL : See Puerperal Sepsis.

PULSATIONS, With : Urt.

RELAPSING : *Calc; Fer; Psor; Sul;* Tub.

REMITTENT : Aco; Ars; Bell;

Bry; Cham; *Gel*; Merc.

Bilious : Merc-d.

Infantile : Ip.

SEPTIC : See Blood Sepsis.

SHIVERING, With : Arn; Caus; Gel; Kali-io; Nux.v; Sul.

SLEEP Agg : *Calad*; Mez;Op; *Samb*.

Amel : *Calad*; Pho; Sep.

STUPID Form : Bap; Carb-v; Hell; Hyo; Mur-ac; Op; Pho-ac.

SUBNORMAL, Persistent : Cact; Chin-s; Kali-p; Nat-sal.

SUPPRESSION, From : Cham; Merc.

SWEAT Absent : Ars; Bell; Bry; Cact; Gel; Nux-m; Scil.

Amel : Ars; Lyc; Rhus-t.

Thighs on, with : Spo.

cold : Caps.

With, continues, after : Calc; Chin; Hell; Merc; Op; Pho; Pho-ac; Pul; Pyro; Stram; Sul; Tub; Ver-v.

THEN Sweat, then chilliness : Calad; Kali-bi.

THIRST, Without : Cham; Cina; Ign; *Pul*.

TRAUMATIC : Cof.

VERTIGO, With : Urt.

+ WEAKNESS, Disproportion-ate : Sul-ac.

YELLOW: Ars; Cadm; Canth; Carb-v; Crot-h; *Nux-v*.

FIBROIDS (See New Growths)

: CALC; Calc-f; Calc-s; Con; Grap; Kali-br; *Pho; Sil*; Thyr; Tril; Ust.

BLEEDING : Bur-p; Calc; Hyds; Led; Nit-ac; Pho; Sul-ac; Tril; Vinc.

BURNING : Lap-alb.

+ CRAMPS, With : Bur-p.

HARD, Stony : Merc-i-r.

FIBROID TISSUE, Ligaments : *Bry; Calc*; Calc-f; Colch; FLU-AC; *Grap;* GUAI; *Kali-m; Lyc*; Phyt; Rhod; RHUS-T; Rut; Sabi; *Sec; Sil*; Stap.

FICKLE : See Persevere can not.

FIDGETY : Ap; Bor; Cimi; *Grap*; Kali-br; Meny; Pod; Sep; Sil; Sumb; Tarn; Vib.

WOMEN, Urinary troubles, with : Meny.

FIGWARTS : See Fungus growths.

FILM : See Valve.

FINANCIAL LOSS AGG : Arn; Ars; Aur.

FINE PAIN : See Pain Stitch-ing, Needles, Hair, Hair sensation, Thread sensation.

FINGERS : Am-m; Lyc; Ran-b; Rhus-t; Sil; Sul; Thu.

ALONG : Fago.

ALTERNATING, With gastric symptoms : Kali-br.

AROUND : Calc-p; Kali-bi; Lith.

Ulceration: Grap; Pul; Sil.

ATROPHY : Sil.

BACKWARD, Bent : Sec.

BETWEEN :Grap; Nit-ac;

BITES : Med; Plb.

BLUE *:* Agar; *Carb-v;* Sec.

BONES, Developed,
imperfectly : Stap.

Pain, pressing, in : Vio-o.

BURNING : Kali-c; Mag-c;
Mur-ac.

Between, touching water on
: Laur.

CHILDREN, Put in mouth : Calc;
Cham; *Ip.*

CLENCHED : Aeth; Arg-n; Sec.

CLOSED *:* Cup; Merc; Plb.

Motion, constant, with :
Colch.

CLUBBING : Laur.

COLD : Abro; Agar; Chel; Grap;
Kali-c; Tarx; Thu.

CONTRACTED, Hysterical : Zin.

Sprain, from : Cann.

CONVULSIONS, Spasms : Agar;
Chel; Cup; Sec.

CRACKS : Calc; Nat-m; Petr;
Sanic; Sars.

Nails, around : Nat-m.

CRAMPS : Arn; Chel; Merc; Sec;
Ver-a.

Contraction, with : Cyc.

Cutting with shears : Con.

Dysmenorrhea, alternating
with : Dros.

Periodical : Pho.

Picking small objects : Stan.

Single, in: Tab.

Washing Agg : Tab.

Writing, while : See Working

with; Writing Agg.

CROOKED *:* See Deformed.

CROSSED : Carb-v; Grap.

DEFORMED : Kali-c; Lyc.

Sprain, from : Cann.

DESQUAMMATION : Am-m;
Elap.

DRAWN Together : Pho.

ECZEMA, loss of nails, with
: Bor.

ELECTRIC current flowing
through, on touching any
thing, as if : Alu.

EMACIATED *:* Sil.

EXTEND, Can not : See
Straighten Can not.

FELON, Runround, panaritium
: Am-c; Anthx; *Ap;* Ars;
Dios; *Flu-ac;* Hep; *Lach;*
Merc; NAT-S; Nit-ac; Psor;
Sil; Sul; Syph; TARN-C;
THU.

Chronic tendency : Dios;
Hep; Sil.

Cold water Amel : Ap;
Flu- ac; Led; *Nat-s; Pul.*

Deep : Calc; Merc-c; *Sil;*
Sul.

Injury, from : Led.

Parturition, after : Cep.

FLEXED, constant motion,
but : Colch.

Spasmodically : Rhod.

FORMICATION : Lyc; Sec; Thu.

Extending to lower limbs
: Thal.

FUZZY, Smokers, of : Sec.

GRASPING Amel : Lith.

GROWTH Stunted : Stap.

HAIR, Back on, as if : Flu-ac.

HEAVY : Plb; Strop.

HYPERTROPHY : Am-m.

ITCHING : Anac; Psor; Sul; Urt.

JERKING : Caus; *Cic; Cina;* Cyc; Rhe; Stan; Sul.

Sleep during: Sul-ac.

Writing, when : Sul-ac.

JOINTS : Ant-c; Calc; Calc-f; *Caul ;* Caus; Lyc; Nat-m; Sep; Spig; Sul.

Closing Agg : Caul; Nat-m.

Dark, dirty : Pic-ac.

Dislocation, easy : Hep.

Distorted : Colch.

Nodes, on : Stap.

Swollen : Nit-ac.

Ulcers, on : Bor; Mez; Sep.

KNITTING Amel : Lyc.

LAME : Calc; Kali-m; Sep.

LIFT, Can not : Cur.

MASHED : Hypr.

MIDDLE :Calc; Nat-m; Syp.

MOBILITY, Affected : Calc.

MOTIONS, Of : Kali-br; Mos.

Flexed, with : Colch.

NAILS : See Nails.

NODES : Abro; Benz-ac; Berb; Calc; Caul; Kali-m; Led.

NUMB : Abro; Aran; Bar-c; *Calc;* Dig; Grap; LYC; Merc; Nat-m; PHO; Plat; *Rhus-t;* Sec; Sil; Sul; Thu; Thyr.

Extending to other parts : Thal.

Left, then right leg : Thyr.

Night, at waking on : Nat-m; Thu.

Ring and little : Arg-n.

PALE : Kre.

PARALYSIS, Of : Mez.

PEELING Of : See Desquammation.

PICKS, Plays with : Aru-t; Calc; Con; Hyo; Kali-n; Lach; Tarn; Ther.

PRICKLING : Abro.

RED : Mur-ac.

ROUGH, Everything feels: Par.

SENSITIVE : Berb; Lac-c; Led; Sec.

SIDES : Sars.

SINGLE : Tab.

SKIN, Tight : Mag-p.

SPREAD Apart : Glo; Lac-c; Lyc; Med; *Sec.*

STIFF: Kali-c; Led; Lyc; Rhus-t.

Book holding while : Lyc.

Grasping anything when : Carb-an; Dros.

Paralytic : Lil-t.

Scissors, Cutting with, while : Con.

STRAIGHTEN, Can not : Ars; Cam; Colo; Cup-ar.

SWEAT, On : Lyc.

SWELLED : Mur-ac.

As if : Kali-n.

TENSE : Crot-h; Mag-p; Pho; Pul.

THUMBS, As if were : *Pho.*

TINGLING : Aco; Ars; Cact;

Nat-m; Ran-b; Sil.

TIPS : Am-m; *Calc-p;* Kali-c;
Lach; Mar-v; Pho; Sec; Thu.

Brown : Tub.

Burn : Canth; Mar-v; Med;
Nat-m.

Bursting : Caus.

Cold : Chel; Lac-c; *TARX.*

dry : Ant-t.

icy : Ant-t; Lac-d.

Cracked : Am-m; Bar-c;
Bell; Grap; Med; Merc;
Nat-m; *Petr;* Ran-b; *Sars;*
Sil.

Dead : Mag-m.

Dry, as if made of paper :
Ant-t; Sil.

Formication : Am-m; Mag-s;
Nat-m; Sec.

Fuzzy : Tab.

Heavy : Plb; Strop.

Knobby : Laur.

Numb : Arg-m; Arg-n;
Kali- p; Lach; Nat-m; *Pho;*
Spo; Stap; Sul.

chill, with : Stan.

Painful : Calc; Cist; Kali-c;
Lac-c; Sil; Sul.

Peeling : See Desquammation
under Fingers.

Pricking, grasping when :
Rhus-t.

Red : Aco.

Sensitive: Berb; Calc-p;
Cist; Lac-c; Nat-c; Sars;
Sul; Tarn.

Sweat, on : Carb-an; Carb-v;
Pho; Sep; Sul.

Tearing, fine : Stap.

Tingling : Am-m; Kali-c.

Ulcers : Ars; Pho; Psor;
Sars.

Vesicles: Nat-c.

Warts, on : Caus.

TOUCHING One another un-
bearable : Lac-c; *Lach;* Sec.

TWITCHING : Cic; Lyc.

Cough, with : Osm.

Sleep, during : Lyc; Rhe.

USING Agg : See Working
with, Grasping Agg.

WATER Soaked : Sec.

WEAK : Calc; Carb-v; Kali-m;
Sep.

WORKING With, Grasping,
Sewing, playing
instrument etc., AGG :
Agar; Bov; *Calc;* CAUS;
Cham; Cimi; Cocl; *Cyc;*
Dros; Gel; KALI-C;Mag-p;
NAT-M;Pho; Pic-ac; Plat;
Sep; *Sil; Stan; Val;* ZIN.

WRITING Agg : Anac; Arg-m;
Arn; Caus; Cyc; Dros;
Kali-c; Mag-p; Pic-ac;
Stan; Sul-ac.

Amel : Fer; Nat-c; Zin-ar.

YELLOW Spots, on : Saba.

FIRELIKE : See Burning,
fiery.

FISHY ODOUR, Taste etc. :
Calc; Grap; Med; Ol-an;
Sanic; Sep; Tell; Thu.

FISSURE : See Cracks.

FISTULA : *Berb*; Bry; CALC;
Calc-f; Calc-p; Carb-v;
CAUS; Con; *Flu-ac;* Hep;

Kali-c; LYC; Nat-c; Nit-ac; Petr; *Pho*; *Pul*; SIL; Stram; SUL.

CHEST, Symptoms and : Berb; Calc-p; Sil.

CLOSING, After : Kali-c.

RECTO VAGINAL : Thu.

+ **FITFUL** : See Changing Moods.

+ **FIT OF PASSION** : Mag-c.

ILL EFFECTS : Nat-m; Plat.

FIXED IDEAS : See Ideas.

FLABBY FEELING : See Relaxation.

FLATULENCE : Alo; *Amb*; ARG-N; Arn; Ars; *Asaf*; Calc; Carb-an; CARB-V; CHAM; CHIN; *Cocl*; Colch; GRAP; Hyds; *Ign*; *Kali-c*; LYC; Mag-c; Nat-s; *Nit-ac*; Nux-m; NUX-V; Old; Op; *Pho*; Pic-ac; *Pul*; *Sil*; SUL; Tarn; Terb; Val; Ver-a; Vib.

ABDOMEN, Upper in : Carb-v; Pul.

Lower, in : Aco; Lyc; Nat-m; Nux-m; Sil; Sul; Zin; Zin- val.

Right side : Bism; CALC; Grap; Lil-t; *Nat-s;* Ox-ac; *Pho*; Thu.

Left side : Am-m; *Aur; Carb-v;* CON; Crot-t; Dios; Euphor; Lyc; Nat-m; Pho-ac; Seneg; Stap; SUL.

+ AIR HUNGER, with : Kali-io.

BACK, Felt in : Rhod.

BATH, After : Calc-s.

CROAKING : Arg-m; Colo; Lyc; Saba.

DISCHARGE, Of : *Carb-v*; Chin; Grap; Kali-c; *Old.*

DYSMENORRHOEA With : Vib.

FERMENTING, As if: Chin; Lyc; Rhus-t.

FOOD, All turns to gas : Carb-v; Kali-c; Nux-m; Nux-v.

GENERATION, Of : Carb-v; Kali-c; Mar-v.

HERE AND THERE : See Wandering.

HYSTERICAL : Asaf; Ign; Pul; Raph; Val.

+ INCARCERATED : Calc; Mos; Nat-s.

MENSES, With : Kali-p; Nux-m; Vib.

NOISY, Rumbling, growling, Borborygmy : Agar; Anac; Ant-c; CARB-V; *Caus; Chin; Hell;* Hep; *Lyc;* Nat-m; NAT-S; NUX-V; *Pho; Pho-ac; Pul;* Sep; SIL; *Sul;* Ver-a.

Annoying, women, in : Rum.

Empty, feeling with : Sars.

Lying, left side on : Colo.

Sleep, during : Agn; Cup.

Stools, before : Mag-c.

after : Petr.

NUMBNESS, With : Med.

OBSTRUCTED, Retained : Ant-t; Arg-n; Carb-v; Cham; CHIN; COCL; Colch; Grap; IGN; LYC; Nat-c; *Nit-ac;* Nux-v; Plb; *Pul*; RAPH; Sil; STAP; Tarn Ver-a.

Left Side : *Aur.*

Stools, after: Lyc; Pic-ac.
 before : Lyc.

PAINFUL, Wind, colic : Carb-v;
 Cham; Chin; Coll; Lyc;
 Mag-p; Nat-s; *Nux-v;* Ox-ac;
 Pul; Rhod; Stap;Ver-a;
 Zin-val.

Hot drinks Amel : Pho.

POST OPERATIVE : Chin; Raph.

PRESSING, Bladder, on : *Carb-v;*
 Ign; Kali-c.

+ Out : Lyc.

 Rectum, on : Calc; Ign; Nat-s.

 Upward : Arg-n; Asaf;
 Carb-v; Grap; Thu.

PUSHING : Nat-s.
 Upward : Asaf.

RECTUM, In : Hep; Nux-v; Sep.

ROLLING : Thyr.

SOUR Food, from: Pho-ac.

SQUEAKING : Kali-io.

VEGETABLES, From : Caps.

WANDERING : *Carb-v;* Chin;
 LYC; Nat-m; Pul; Sil.

FLATUS Back, felt, in : Rhod.

COLD : Con.

COUGHING, On: Sang.

HOT : Agar; *Alo;* Carb-v; Mar-v;
 Stap; Zin.

INVOLUNTARY : Pho.

MOIST : Ant-c; Carb-v.

OFFENSIVE, Foul: Alo; Arn;
 Ars; Asaf; Bry; CARB-V;
 Caus; *Cocl;* Lach; Nat-m;
 Nat-s; Nit-ac; *Pul; Sil;* Spig;
 Sul; Zin.

 Eggs like, spoiled : Arn;
 Stap; Sul.

Garlicky : Agar; Pho-ac.

Urine, like: Agn.

Writing, after: Ant-c.

PASSING AGG: Chin; Cocl;
 Flu-ac.

 AMEL : CARB-V; Colo; *Lyc;*
 Nat-s; *Nux-v;* Pul; Sang;
 Scop; Stap; Sul.

 Difficult : Op; Ox-ac.

 Up and Dowm AMEL :
 Arg-n; Grap; Kali-c;
 SANG; Ver-a.

 walking when : Myr.

+ PROFUSE, Inodorous : Agar.

SOUR : Calc; Mag-c; Nat-c;
 Rhe.

+ UPWARDS, Not down: Asaf.

FLEETING *PAINS* : See
under Pain.

FLESHY : See New
Growths, Fungus Growths.

FLEXURES : See Skin, Folds.

FLOATING, *FLYING* As if : Aco;
Arg-n; Asar; Calc-ar; Cann;
Cocl;Cof; Hyo; Hypr;
LAC-C; Lach; Nat-m;
Nux-m; Op; *Pho-ac;* Phys;
Spig; Stic; Stram; Thu; Val;
Zin-io.

 LYING, Left side, on Agg :
 Zin-io.

FLOWING : See Trickling as
of water.

FLUCTUATION : See Waves.

FLUIDITY : See Discharges,
Increased.

FLUSHES : See Waves.

FLUTTERING : See Vibrations.

FLYING To Pieces : See Shattered.

FOAMY, *FROTHY* : See Discharges, Foamy.

FOETID : See Offensive.

FOETUS, + *EXPELS*, Dead: Canth.

LYING Crosswise, as if : Arn.

MALDISPOSITION : Pul.

MOVEMENT, As if : Nat-c; Tarn.

Causes nausea and vomiting : Arn.

Disturb sleep : Con.

Intolerable : Sep.

Lively : Lyc; Op.

Painful : Con; Croc; *Sil*.

Somersault, like : Lyc.

Violent : Lyc; Op; Psor; Sil; Thu.

vomiting, with : Psor.

FOGS : See Cloudy Weather.

FOLDS : See Skin.

FONTANALLES : See Under Children.

FOOD & DRINKS AGG & AMEL *Acid*; See Sour.

ALCOHOLIC Agg : *Ars*; Asar; Bar-c; Calc; *Carb-v*; Chin; Cimi; Hyo; *Kali-bi*; *Lach*; NUX-V; *Op*; *Pho*; Pul; *Ran-b*; Sele; *Stram*; *Sil*; *Sul-ac*; Terb; Zin.

Amel : Aco; Agar; Canth; *Con*; *Gel*; Lach; Op; Sele; Sul-ac.

ALL Disagree : Arg-n; Carb-an; *Carb-v*; Fer; Lach; Mos; Nat-c; Syph.

APPLES Agg : Ars-io; Bell; Bor.

Amel : Guai.

Sour Agg : Merc-c.

ARTIFICIAL AGG : Alu; Calc; Mag-c; Sul.

BACON Amel : Ran-b; Ran-sc.

BAKED Agg : Carb-v; Pul.

BEANS Agg : See Legumes.

BEER Agg : Bap; Card-m; *Kali-bi*; Led; Nux-v; Rhus-t.

Amel : Nat-p; Ver-a.

BERRIES Agg: Ip.

BITTER Agg: Nat-p.

BRANDY Agg : Nux-v; Op; Sul.

Amel : Old.

BREAD Agg : *Bry*; Hyds; Lyc; Nat-m; *Nux-v*; *Pul*; Sul.

Amel : Caus; Nat-c.

Butter, and Agg : Acet-ac; Chin; Nit-ac; *Pul*; Sep.

BUCK WHEAT Agg : Ip; *Pul*; Ver-a.

BUTTER Agg: Carb-an; *Carb-v*; Nat-m; *Pul*.

Milk Agg : Bry; Pul.

Tastes too sweet : Ran-b.

CABBAGE Agg : *Bry*; Carb-v; Kali-c; *Lyc*; Mag-c; *Petr*; Rob.

CAKES Agg : Ant-c; Ip; Pul.

Hot Agg : Kali-c; Pul.

CARROT Agg : Calc; Lyc.

CEREAL Agg : See Farinaceous.

CHEESE, Old Agg : Ars; Bry; Ptel; Rhus-t.

CHERRIES Agg : Merc-c.

CHILLI (Green or Red) Agg : Pho.

CHOCOLATE Agg : Bry; Calad; *Kali-bi;* Lyc; *Ox-ac*; Pul.

COFFEE Agg : Ars; Canth; Caus; *Cham;* Colo; IGN; Merc; NUX-V; Ox-ac; Pul.

Amel : Arg-m; Cham; Colo; Fago; *Ign.*

Odour of, Agg : Flu-ac; Lach; *Nat-m;* Osm; *Sul-ac;* Tub.

COLD Agg : ARS; Bell; Calc; *Canth;* Caps; Cham; Chel; Chin; Dul; Fer; *Hep;* Kali-io; Kali-m; Kre; Lach; LYC; Manc; Merc-i-r; NUX-V; *Rhus-t;* Saba; Samb; Sep; *Sil;* Stap; Ver-a.

Amel : *Ap;* Arg-n; *Bell; Bism; Bry;* Cann; CAUS; Cup; Ign; Kali-m; LACH; Merc-i-f; *Pho;* Phyt; *Pul;* Radm; Sang; Sele; Sep.

Drinks, in hot weather Agg : Bry; Kali-c; Nat-c; Ver-a.

CONDIMENTS, Spices Agg: *Nux-v;* Pho; Sele.

Amel : Hep; Nux-m.

CUCUMBER Agg: Ars; Cep; Pul; Ver-a.

DAINTY Agg : Pul.

DRY Agg: *Calc;* Lyc; Nat-c; Pul.
Too, seems, while eating : Calad; Chin; Fer; Ign; Kali-io; Ox-ac; Raph.

EGGS Agg : Calc; Colch; Fer; Led; *Pul;* Sul.

FARINACEOUS Agg : Bry; Caus; *Lyc;* Nat-c; NAT-M; NAT-S; Pul.

Children in Amel : Nat-c.

FAT Oils Agg : Ant-c; Ars; Calc; CARB-V; *Chin;* CYC; *Fer; Grap;* Kali-m; Lyc; Nat-p; PUL; Rob; Sep; Tarx.

Amel : Nux-v.

FISH Agg: Ars; Carb-an; Carb-v; Kali-c; Nat-s; *Plb; Pul;* Urt.

Amel : Lac-c.

Fried Agg : Kali-c.

Herring Agg : Fer-p.

Pickled Agg : Calad.

Salmon Agg : Flu-ac.

Shell Agg : Carb-v; *Lyc;* Urt.

Spoiled Agg : Ars; Carb-an; Carb-v; Pul.

FLATULENT Agg : *Bry;* Chin; *Lyc; Petr.*

FROZEN : See Ice.

FRUITS Agg : *Ars; Bry;* Caus; Chin; Colo; Elap; Glo; Ip; Nat-c; Nat-s; *Pul;* Rum; Sep; VER-A.

Amel : Lach.

Banana Agg : Rum.

Canned Agg : Pod.

Grapes Agg : Ox-ac.

Guava Agg : Sep.

Juicy Agg : Ant-c; Calc; Iod; Pul; Sul.

Oranges Agg : Pho-ac.

Peach Agg : Cep; Flu-ac; Glo; Psor.

Pears Agg : Bor; Bry; *Ver-a.*

Plantains Agg : Rum.

Plums and prunes Agg : Rhe.

Sour Agg : Ant-c; Ip; Lach; Ox-ac; Pho-ac; Pod; Psor.

Amel : Lach; Naj.

Unripe Agg : Ip; Rhe; Rob; Sul-ac.

GARLIC, Odour of Agg : Saba.

HONEY : Nat-c; Pho.

HOT Agg : Bry; Chlo-hyd; Nat-s; *Pul; Sep.*

+ Amel : Chel.

Drinks Amel : Ail; Ars; Lyc; Nux-v; Sul-ac.

ICE, Frozen things Agg : Arg-n; *Ars;* Calc-p; Carb-v; Dul; Ip; Kali-bi; *Pul;* Rob.

Amel : Xanth.

Water Agg : Dig.

INDIGESTIBLE Agg : *Iod;* Ip; Rut.

Amel : Ign.

LEGUMES Beans, peas Agg (See Flatulent) : *Bry;* Calc; *Lyc;* Petr.

LEMONADE Agg : Phyt; *Sele.*

Amel : Bell; Cyc; Phyt.

LEMONS Amel : Bell; Stram.

Peel Agg : Ip.

LIQUIDS Agg : ARS; *Chin; Cocl;* Colo; Crot-t; *Fer;* Ign; *Lach; Nat-m;* PHO; *Rhus-t; Sil; Ver-a.*

+ MALT Liquor: Kali-bi.

MAPLE Sugar Agg : Calc-s.

MEAT, Mutton Agg : Arg-n; *Ars;* Caus; Carb-v; Chin; *Colch; Fer;* Kali-bi; Lept; Lyss; Merc; Ptel; *Pul.*

Amel : Ver-a.

Fresh Agg : *Caus;* Chin.

Spoiled, Agg : See Ptomaine Poisoning.

MELONS Agg: Ars; *Flu-ac;* Zing.

MILK Agg : Aco; AETH; Amb; Bry; CALC; Calc-s; *Chin;* Con; Lac-d; Lyc; Mag-c; *Mag-m;* Merc; Nat-c; *Nit-ac;* Nux-m; Ol-j; Pho; *Pul;* Sep; Sul.

Amel : Aco; Ars; Chel; Cina; Fer; Iod; Merc; Mez; *Nux-v;* Pho-ac; Scil; Stap; Ver-a.

Boiled Agg : Nux-m; Sep.

Cold Agg : Kali-io; Spo.

Amel : Iod.

Sour Agg : Pod.

Sweet Amel : Ars.

Warm Agg : Amb.

Amel : Chel; Crot-t; Grap.

MIXED Agg : Ant-c; Ip; *Pul.*

NUTS Agg : See Fats.

ODOUR Of cooking Agg : Ars; *Cocl; Colch;* Dig; Ip; Merc-i-f; Sep; Stan.

ONIONS Agg : Bro; *Lyc;* Nux-v; *Pul;* Thu.

Amel : Cep.

OYSTERS Agg : Alo; Bro; Carb-v; *Lyc;* Pul; Sul-ac;

Amel : Lach

PASTRY : Ant-c; Ip; Kali-chl; Lyc; Pho; *Pul.*

PEPPER Agg : Ars; *Cina;* Nat-c; Sep; Sil.

Cayenne Agg : Pho.

PORK Agg : *Ant-c;* CARB-V; *Cyc; Grap;* Ham; Ip; PUL;

Sep.

POTATOES Agg : *Alu;* Colo; Mag-c; Nat-s; Pul; Sep; Ver-a.

Amel : Acet-ac.

Sweet Agg : Calc-ar.

POULTRY Agg : Carb-v.

PUDDING Agg : Ptel.

RAISINS Agg : Ip.

RAW Agg : Pul; *Rut;* Ver-a.

RICH Agg : Ars; Bry; *Carb-v;* Ip; Kali-m; Nat-s; Nit-ac; PUL; Sep.

SALADS Agg : Ars; Bry; *Calc;* Carb-v; Ip; Lach; Lyc.

SALT Agg: Alu; Ars; Carb-v; Dros; Mag-m; NAT-M; *Pho;* Sele.

Amel : Mag-c; Nat-m.

SAUSAGE Agg : Acet-ac; *Ars;* Bell; Bry; Pul.

SEASONED, Highly Amel : Nux-m.

SIGHT or Smell Agg : Ars; Colch; Nux-v; Pho; Sul.

SOUP Agg : Alu; Kali-c.

SOUR Agg : *Ant-c;* Ant-t; Arg-n; Ars; Carb-v; Dros; Flu-ac; Merc-c; Nat-m; Nat-p; Pho-ac; Pod; *Pul;* Sep; Sul.

Amel : Arg-n; Ign; Lach; Ptel; Pul; Sang.

Becomes : Lapp.

Odour Agg : Dros.

SOURKRAUT Agg : Bry; Lyc; Petr; Pul.

SPICES : See Condiments.

SPOILED Agg : See Ptomaine Poisoning.

STARCHY Agg : Colo; Mag-c;

Nat-c.

STAWBERRIES Agg : Ant-c; Bur-p; Ox-ac; Sep.

SUGARCANE Juice Agg : Ars.

SWEETS Agg : Ant-c; *Arg-n;* Ars; Cham; Cina; Grap; *Ign;* Ip; Lyc; Med; Merc; Nat-p; Ox-ac; Sang; Sele; Sul; Zin.

Amel : Bell.

TAMARIND Water Agg : Sele.

TEA Agg : Ars; Calad; Chin; Cocl; Dios; *Fer;* Pul; *Sele;* Strop; THU.

Amel : Alo; Dig; Fer; Glo; Kali-bi.

THOUGHT Of Agg : Carb-v; Grap; Nat-m; *Pul; Sep.*

TOBACCO Agg : See Tobacco.

TOMATO Agg : Lith; Pho.

TURNIPS Agg: Calc-ar; Bry; Lyc; Pul; Rob.

UNCOOKED : See Raw.

UNRIPE Agg : Rhe.

VEAL Agg : Calc; Caus; *Ip; Kali-n;* Sep; Zin.

VEGETABLES (Green) Agg : Alu; Ars; Bry; Caps; Hell; Hyds; Lept; Lyc; Nat-c; *Nat-s;* Ver-a.

Decayed : Carb-an.

+ Potatoes except : Acet-ac.

VINEGAR Agg : *Ant-c; Ars;* Sul.

Amel : Asar; Hell; Pul.

WARM Agg : *Bry; Lach; Pho;* Phyt; *Pul.*

Amel : *Ars;* Lyc; *Nux-v;* Rhus-t.

WATER Agg : Ars; Chin-ars.

Drinking too much Agg : Grat.

WINE Agg : LED; Nux-v; Ox-ac; Rhod; Zin.

FOOLISH : See Childish, Silly.

HAPPINESS And PRIDE : Sul.

FORCED APART : See Separated as if.

OUT As if : See Pain Pressing.

THROUGH NARROW OPENING, As If : BAR-C; Bell; Buf; Carb-ac; Coc-c; Cocl; Dig; Glo; *Lach*; Op; *Plb*; Pul; Sul; *Tab;* Thu; Val.

Fluids, as if : Coc-c.

FORCEPS DELIVERY After : Bur-p; Hypr.

FORE ARM : See Under Arms.

FOREBODINGS : See Fear of future.

FOREHEAD : *Aco; Am-c;* Arn; Ars; BELL; *Bry;* Chin; Ign; Lach; Lyc; *Merc; Nat-m;* NUX-V; *Pho;* Phyt; Pru-sp; *Pul;* Sep; Sil; *Spig; Sul;* Thu.

ACHING : Merc-i-f.

ADHESIONS Of Skin : Sabi.

ALTERNATING Sides : *Iris;* Lil-t; Pho; Saba.

ASCENDING, Into : Lach; Zin.

BALL, Lump, Knot : Ant-t; Carb-ac; Caus; Kali-c; Stap.

Hot : Carb-ac.

BAND, Constriction : *Cact;* Gel; Merc; *Sul.*

BLOCK, Solid, as of a : Kali-bi; Kre.

BLOOD Boils : Led.

+ BOARD, Pressed against : Dul; Rhus-t.

BROWN Yellow : Kali-p; Sep.

At the edge of hair : Caul; Kali-p; Med; Nat-m.

BUBBLES : Form.

CENTRE : Crot-h.

COLD : Cimi.

+ Perspiration, in all complaints : Ver-a.

Spot, on : Arn.

CRACKLING : Aco.

CRAWLING, As of a worm : Alu.

+ DEEP, Pigmented patches, in liver complaints : Van.

+ EYES, Close must : Pod.

FLATTENED, or Pressed flat, as if : Cor-r; Ver-a.

FORMICATION : Colch; Zin.

FROWNING : Lyc; Ver-a.

+ Brain, diseases, in : Stram.

FULLNESS : Carb-s; Cinb.

+ FURROWS, Deep : Lyc.

HEAT, Burning : Ap; Bell; Kali-io; Nux-v; Pho.

HEAVY : Ant-c; Rut; Stap.

HOLLOW : Caus.

LOOSE : Sul-ac.

MENSES Amel : Cep.

NASAL Discharges Amel : Cep;· Kali-bi; *Lach;* Zin.

NAVEL, With : Lept.

NODES : Caus.

NOSE, To : Lach; Phys.

NUMB : Mur-ac; *Plat.*

OCCIPUT, To : Caus; Tub.

Right : Pru-sp.

Left : Senec.

OILY, Greasy: Hyds; Psor.

PIMPLES, Disappear in open air : Hep.

PRESSES, Against something : Nux-v.

PRICKING : Mur-ac; Vio-o.

PROJECTING : Apoc.

PULSATION : Bell; Glo; Iris; Lac-d; Pul.

Right : Ant-t; Bell; Ign.

Left : Aco.

RUB, Inclination,to : Glo;Ver-a.

SKIN, Drawn in folds, as if : Grap.

SWEAT, Cold : Ant-t; *Carb-v*; Chio; Cina; Dros; Ip; Op; Stap; *Ver-a*.

Drinking Agg : Cup; Ip.

Amel : Ver-a.

Epistaxis, with : Croc.

Sudden: Val.

Vomiting, with : Chio.

SWELLED : Ap; Hell; *Nux-v*; Rhus-t.

TONGUE, Protruding Agg: Syph.

UPPER : Colo.

VEINS : Abro; Calad; Cam; Chin; Cub; Sul.

VERTIGO Felt in : See Vertigo.

WARTS, On : Cast-eq.

WATER, As of : Plat.

WAVING, Shaking, as if : Bell; Merc; Sep.

WEIGHT In, as if: Rut.

WRINKLED : Hell; Hyo; LYC;

Rhe; Sep; *Stram*; Ver-a.

Brain symptoms, with : Grat; Hell; *Stram*.

Chest symptoms, with : Lyc.

Headache, during : Caus; Grat; Stram; Ver-a.

FOREIGN BODIES : Aco; Anac; Calc-f; Hep; Lob; Sil.

FORGETFUL : See Memory Bad.

EVERYTHING, For, busy when : Ant-c.

+ EXTREME : Stro-carb.

FORGETS ERRAND : Bar-c; Manc; Med.

EVENTS, Recent : Abs; Ail; Grap; Rhus-t.

+ EVERYTHING : Gymn; Merc.

NAME, His own : Med.

Objects, of : Lith.

Persons, of : Chlor; Guai.

SENTENCE, Finish can not : Med.

+ SUDDENLY : Anac.

TIME And PLACE : Merc.

WHAT, He wishes to do next : Manc; Mill.

She wanted to say : Hypr; Iod.

WORDS, In mouth: Anac; Arn; Bar-c; Cann; Med; Pho-ac; Rhod.

Hunts, for : Thu.

+ WORDS, Whole, while writing : Rhod.

FORGOTTEN Something, constantly as if, he had :

Caus; *Iod*; Mill.

THINGS come to mind in sleep : Calad; Sele.

FORMICATION Crawling (See also Skin) : *Aco; Agar;* Arn; Bar-c; Bor; Calc; Carb-an; Colch; Lyc; Merc; *Nux-v;* Oenan; Op; Osm; *Pho;* Pic-ac; *Plat; Rhus-t;* Saba; Sang; SEC; Sep; Spig; Stram; Stro; *Sul;* Tell; Vario; *Zin.*

AFFECTED Part : Colo.

ANGINA, During : Dig.

ANXIETY, With : Cist.

BAD News, After : Calc-p.

BODY, ALL OVER : Ail; Aran; Cist; Dig; Mag-m; Med; Zin-p.

COLD : Frax; Lac-c.

Body around : Helod.

Menses, before : Ant-t.

DYSPNOEA, With : Cist.

HERE And THERE : Op.

INTERNAL : Med.

KNOCKING Against Anything Agg : Spig.

PAIN, After : Sec.

With : Hypr.

PARALYSED Part : Cadm; Pho.

ROOT Of Hairs, at : Pho-ac.

RUBBING Amel : Sec.

SKIN, Under: Cadm; SEC; Zin.

SWEAT, With : Rhod.

FORSAKEN, LONELY : Arg-n; *Aur;* Bar-c; Calc; MENY; Plat; *Psor; Pul.*

FRACTURES : See Bones broken, brittle.

FRAGILE : See Broken Feeling and Bones brittle.

FRAIL As if body were : Sars; Thu.

FRANTIC : See Besides himself.

FRECKLES: See Under Eruptions.

FRETFUL : See Anger.

FRICTION AGG : Con; Sep; Tell.

FRIGHT (See Fear, Emotions Agg) Complaints, from : Aco; Acte; Anac; Ap; Caus; Cup; Hyo; Hypr; Ign; Lyc; Nat-m; *Op;* Pho; Pho-ac; Pul; Sil; Stram; Ver-a; Vib; Zin.

ANIMALS, From : Stram.

CAUSE, Without: Plb.

+ SUDDEN, Pleasant surprise : Cof.

TENDENCY to take : Sul-ac.

FRIGHTENED EASILY : Aco; Arg-n; *Arn;* Ars; Bar-c; Bor; Cact; Carb-an; Carb-v; *Cocl;* Grap; IGN; Kali-c; Kali-p; *Lyc;* Nat-c; *Nat-m;* Petr; *Pho;* Saba; *Stram;* Ther; Zin.

EMISSIONS, After: Alo.

NOISE, Every : Bor.

+ SUFFOCATIVE Attack, follow : Samb.

TRIFLES, At: Ant-t; Kali-c; Kali-s; Lach; Lyc; Nit-ac; Pho.

FROST AIR AGG : *Agar; Calc;* Caus; CON; Lyc; Nux-v; *Pho-ac; Pul;* Rhus-t; SEP; *Sil; Sul;* Syph.

BITE : See Chilblains.

FROTHY : See Discharges Foamy.

FULLNESS : See Congestion.

FUMES : See Vapour.

FUNGUS GROWTH, Excrescences, warts, condylomata, proud flesh, Haematodes Etc. : Ant-c; Ars; Aur; Bar-c; *Calc; Carb-an; Caus;* Clem; *Dul;* Lach; *Lyc; Merc;* Merc-c; Med; Nat-c; *Nat-s;* NIT-AC; Petr; *Pho; Pho-ac;* Phyt; Ran-b; Rhus-t; *Sabi;* Sang; *Sil; Stap;* Sul; *Thu.*

BLEEDING : Nit-ac; Pho.

BURNING : Sabi.

FLESHY : Calc; Stap; Thu.

FOUL : Sabi.

GRANULAR : Calc; Nit-ac; Stap; Thu.

ITCHING : Sabi.

PEDUNCULATED : Lyc; *Nit-ac; Sabi;* Stap; Thu.

RAGGED : Nat-c; Pho-ac; Rhus-t; Thu.

SPONGY : Calc; Lyc; Nit-ac; Stap; Thu.

SUMMER Disappear, winter reappear : Psor.

FURIBUND : See Delirium Maniacal.

FURRY : See Coated.

FURY : See Rage

FUSSY : Ap; Calc-p; Samb; Sele; Zin.

GAGGING : See Retching.

GAIT, BODY Trembles while walking : Lact-ac.

BENT : See Stooped.

DRAGGING : Lach; Lathy; *Myg;* Naj; Nux-v; Pho; Rhus- t; Tab.

FEET, Swing at each step : Cic.

FESTINATION : See Festination.

HEELS, Do not touch ground when walking : Lathy.

KNEES, Knock against each other : Arg-n; Caus; Colch; Con; Glo; Lathy; Zin.

LEGS, Apart : Pho.

Involuntarily thrown forward, when walking : Merc.

LIMPING : Caus; Colo; Dul; Kali-c; Rhus-t; Tab.

Involuntary : Bell.

MISSING Steps when going down stairs : Stram.

REELING : Agar; Alu; Cocl; Lol-t; Pho.

SHUFFLING : Ol-an; Op; Sec; Stap; Tab; Vip.

SLAPPING : Mang.

SLOVENLY : Sil.

SLOW, Sluggish : Gel; Pho; Pho-ac; Tab.

SPASTIĆ : Lathy; Zin. Nat-c; Onos; Pic-ac; Pul; Ver-v.

STAGGERING : Alu; Buf; Calc; Helod; Lil-t; Mur-ac; Nat-c; Onos; Pic-ac; Pul; Ver-v.

Coition, after : Bov.

Places one foot over the

other : Mar-v.

Unobserved, when : Arg-n.

Walking in dark or closed eyes when : Alu; Ap; Arg-n; Gel; Iodof; Stram; Zin.

STAIRS Ascending Agg : Tab.

STEPPING, Backwards : Mang; Oxytr; Stram.

Down from high step Agg : Phyt.

High: Agar; Bell; Carb-v; Merc; Nat-m; Onos; Rhus-t.

Left, towards : Lach.

Puts down heel hard : Helod.

STOOPED, Bent : Am-m; *Arg-n; Carb-v;* Cocl; Colo; Con; Gel; Lathy; Mang; Nat-m; *Pho; Sul;* Terb; Ver-a.

STUMBLING : Agar; Arg-n; Bar-c; Caus; Con; Hyo; Ip; Nat-c; Nux-v; Pho; Pho-ac; Rut; Zin.

+ Against everything : Ip.

Ascending and descending when : Phys.

Easily : Agar; Pho;Pho-ac; Rut.

TOTTERING : Op; Pho; Rhod; Ver-a; Zin.

Drunkards : Ran-b.

UNSTEADY: *Agar;* Arg-n; Ast-r; Bar-c; Caus; Cocl; Con; Kali-br; Lol-t; Nat-c; Ol-an; Sec; Stan; *Sul;* Tab; Tarn-c.

Sciatica, in : Kali-cy.

WADDLING : See Legs apart.

GALL BLADDER BURNING : *Lept;* Myr.

Anger, After Agg : Stap.

BURSTING : Bap; Lept; Myr.

CLAWING : Lyc; Med; Nat-s.

DUCT : Hyds.

Obstruction, duodenum at : Canc-fl.

EATING Amel: Mag-m.

FULLNESS : Myr.

GRIPPING : Sep.

INFLAMMATION : Lach; Pho.

Septic : Bry; Buf; *Lach; Pho.*

SORE : *Bap;* Lept; Myr.

+ STOMACH, To : Berb.

STONES: Bell; Berb; *Bry; Calc; Card-m; Chel;* Chio; Euon; *Lach; Lept;* Lyc; Mag-p; MERC; Merc-d; Myr; Nat-s; Nux-v; *Pho;* Pod; Sang; Sul; Tarx; Ver-a.

STOOPING Agg : Sep.

GANGLIA (Bursae) : Am-c; Ap; *Arn;* Benz-ac; Carb-v; *Nat-m;* Pho; RUT; Sil; *Stic;* Sul.

GANGRENE : Anthx; ARS; Bell; Canth; CARB-V; Chin; Cist; Crot-h; Kre; LACH; Mur-ac; Plb; *Sec; Sil;* Solid; Sul-ac, Tarn-c; Sec. Vip.

BURNS or Scalds from: DRY

COLD HOT Sic

DIABETIC original

LEECHES, Application from : Sec.

MOIST : Carb-v; *Chin;* Hell; Pho.

MUSTARD, Application from :

Calc-p; Sec.

SENILE : Carb-v; Cep; Euphor; Pho-ac; SEC; Sul-ac.

THREATENED, With blue parts : Ars; Asaf; Aur; Con; Hep; *Lach;* Merc; Sil; Ver-a.

TRAUMATIC : Arn; Lach; Sec; Sul-ac.

GARGLING AGG : Carb-v.

GARLICKY, ODOUR of discharges, taste, etc : Art-v; Asaf; Cup-ar; Kali-p; Lach; Osm; Petr; *Tell.*

GASTRIC *FEVER* : See Fever.

GASTRITIS : Aco; Ars; Bry; Merc-c; Nux-v; Pho; Ver-v.

ALCOHOLIC : Arg-n.

ENTERITIS : See Vomiting, Purging with.

GATHERED Together : See Constriction.

GAY : See Cheerful.

GELATINOUS : See Discharges.

GENITALS (In general, both sexes) : Agn; Am; Berb; Calad; Cof; Erig; Gel; Hyo; Merc; Nat-p; Nit-ac; *Pul;* Rhus-t; Sabal; Sele; *Sep;* Sul.

RIGHT : Ap; Calc; Caus; *Clem;* Hep; *Lyc;* Merc; Nux-v; Pall; Spo; Sul-ac; Ver-a.

LEFT : *Lach;* Naj; *Pul;* Rhod; *Thu.*

ALTERNATING Between : Cimi; Colo; Lac-c; Lycps; Ol-an; Onos; Rhod.

BURNING, Heat : Cof; Tarn; Tub.

Eating Agg : Tub.

COLD : Berb; Calad; Sabal.

CRAWLING : Calc-p; Plat.

DRY : Tarn.

ERUPTIONS : Petr; Radm; *Rhus-t..*

+ FLABBY : Bar-c.

FLOWING, Everything towards (male) : Colo.

FUMBLES, Grasps : Aco; Bell; Buf; Canth; *Hyo;* Merc; Sep; *Stram;* Zin.

Constantly : Stram.

Coughing when : Zin.

INFLAMMED : *Merc.*

ITCHING : Cof; Plat; Radm; Sabi; Tarx.

Burning : Nat-m; Urt.

MOTION Agg : Sabi.

NUMBNESS : Bar-c.

Ascending : Form.

OFFENSIVE : Psor; Sars; Sul; *Thu.*

Briny, coition, after : Sanic.

PULSATING, Coition, after : Nat-c.

RAW : Merc; Tarn.

SENSITIVE : Cof; Plat; *Stap;* Tarn; Zin.

SITTING Agg : Sul.

SWEAT, Moisture, on : Dios; Sars; Sele; *Sep;* Thu.

Coughing Agg : Thu.

SWELLED : *Rhus-t;* Tarn.

THIGHS, Down : Cham; Chel;

Cimi; Kali-c; Ox-ac; Rhus-t; Sep; Ust.

TICKLING : Alu; Plat.

UPWARD : Murx.

VARICOSE : Zin.

WEAKNESS, Stool, after : Calc-p.

GENTLE : See Timid.

GESTURES, MAKES : Bell; Cocl; Hyo; Mos; Nux-m; Stram; Tarn.

RIDICULOUS : Cic; Hyo; Nux-m.

GHOSTS : See Fear.

GIDDY : See Vertigo.

GIRDLE *PAINS* : See under Pain.

SENSATION : Stan.

Yawning, with : Stan.

GIRLS : See Puberty

+ DRIED UP and WRINKLED : Alu.

+ PAMPERED : Mos.

GLABELLA, ACHING, Fulness, and : Kali-bi.

NODES : Caus.

PUFFY : Flu-ac; Kali-c; Sele; Sil.

GLANDS (In General) : Ap; Ars; Aru-t; Aur; BAR-C; *Bell;* Bro; *Bry;* CALC; Carb-an; Chin; *Clem;* Cist; Con; Hep; Iod; Kali-m; *Lach; Lyc;* MERC; Nit-ac; *Pho; Phyt;* PUL; Rhod; Rhus-t; SIL; Spo; Stap; Sul; Tab; Tub.

BEAD LIKE, Knotted : Aeth; Aur; Bar-io; Bar-m; Berb;

Calc-io; Nit-ac; Sul-io; Tub.

BURNING : Ars; Pul.

CERVICAL : Am-m; Bar-c; *Calc;* Canc-fl; Cist; Grap; Kali-c; Lap-alb; Lyc; *Merc;* Merc-i-f; Rhus-t; *Sil; Sul;* Vio-t.

Malignant : Cist.

Milk crusts, with : Canc-fl; Vio-t.

Neck, moving Agg : Ign.

CONSTRICTION : Calc; Ign; Iod; Plat; Pul.

DUCTLESS : Spo.

EMACIATED : Con; Iod.

ENLARGED, Swelled : Bell; Calc; Carb-an; Cist; Dul; Iod; Kali-m; *Merc;* Phyt; *Rhus-t;* Sil; Sul; *Sul-io;* Syph; Tub.

Atrophy, or : Kali-io.

Body, all over: Med.

Emaciation, with : Ther.

Fever, during, over body : Bell; Kali-c; Sep.

Many : Tub.

Menses, during : Kali-c; Lac-c.

Painful : Merc-i-r; Stap.

FLACCID : Cham; Con; Iod.

FORMICATION : Con; Spo.

HARD : Alum; Bad; Bar-m; Bro; Calc; Calc-f; Carb-an; Clem; Con; Iod; *Phyt;* Sele; Sil; Spo; Sul.

+ HOT And Throb, all over : Asaf.

INFLAMMED : Aco; Bell; Bry;

Calc; Merc; Pho; Sul.

INGUINAL : See Groins.

ITCHING : Anac; Caus; *Con;* Kali-c; Pho; Sil; Spo.

MESENTERIC : Calc; Iod.

PULSATION : Con; Merc.

SORE, Bruised : Con.

STITCHES : Bell; Ign; *Merc;* Nit-ac; Pul;; Thu.

SUBMENTAL : Led; Sil; Stap.

Hard : Anthx.

Head, moving Agg : Calend.

Swallowing Agg : Chin.

TEARING : *Chin;* Merc; Pul; Thu.

TENSION, In : Pho.

ULCERATIVE Pain : Pho; Sil.

UTERINE Haemorrhage, with : Carb-an.

GLANS (Penis) : Merc; Nit-ac; Rhus-t; Thu.

ACHING, Steady : Chel; Osm.

BURNING, Urinating, when : Anac.

COLD : Berb.

CRACKS : Ars.

CRUSHED : Rhod.

DRY : Calad.

FLACCID : Mag-m; Nat-c.

INFLAMMATION: Cinb; Kali-chl.

INTO : Par-b.

ITCHING : Chel; Mez; Sul.

NUMB : Berb.

PIMPLES, Small, red : Cinb.

PULSATION : Coc-c; Pru-sp.

RAG Like : Calad.

SORE, Slight rubbing, on : Cyc.

Nat-c.

SWELLED : Merc.

TUMOUR, Yellow behind : Lyc.

Soft : Bell.

URINATING Agg : Ox-ac; Pru-sp.

URINE, Reaches and then returns : Pru-sp.

WARTS, On : Ant-t.

GLAUCOMA : See Under Eye.

GLEET : See Urethra, discharge gleety.

GLISTENING, Shining : Aco; AP; *Aur; Bell; Bry;* Calc-f; Carb-ac; Caus; Cist; Euphr; Glo; *Kali-bi;* LAC-C; Lach; Mang; Nat-m; *Pho;* Rhus-t; Sabi; Sil; Syph; *Terb.*

OBJECTS AGG : Bell; Canth; Hyo; Lyss; Mur-ac; Stram.

GLOBUS : See Ball, Hysteria.

GLOOMY : See Sad.

GLOSSITIS : See Inflamm-ation, Tongue.

GLOTTIS Spasms of (Laryngismus Stridulus) : *Bell;* Calc; Calc-p; *Gel;* IGN; *Mos.*

ALTERNATING, With constriction of fingers and legs : Asaf.

GLUEY : See Discharges, Gluey.

GLUTTONY : Ab-c; All-s; Ant-c; Bry; Chin.

GNAWING : See Pain Gnawing.

GODLESS, Want of religious feeling : See Irreligious.

GOITRE : Ars-io; Bro; Calc;
Flu-ac; Hep*; Ign; Iod;* Iris;
Nat-m*; Spo;* Strop; Thyr; Vip;
Zin-io.

RIGHT Side : Hep.

LEFT Side : Chel.

AIR, Passing through, as if on
breathing : Spo.

CARDIAC Pain, with : Spo.

Symptoms, with : Cact.

CHOKING, From : Grap; Merc-i-f;
Spo.

DIARRHOEA, with : Cist.

EXOPHTHALMIC *: Bell;* Buf;
Fer-p*; Iod;* Jab; Lycps;
Nat-m; Strop.

Grief, from : Amy-n; Chlo-
hyd.

Trembling, with : Meph.

HARD : Buf; Iod; Nat-c; Spo.

HEART, Action, rapid with :
Buf.

LUMPY *:* Grap.

MENSES Agg : Calc-io; Cimi;
Iod.

Suppressed, from:Fer;
Fer-io.

NODULATED : Grap; Phyt.

PAIN, Into head, with : Hep.

PALPITATION, With : Pho.

PINCHED, As if : Nat-ar.

PREGNANCY, During : Calc-io;
Hyds.

PRESSING, Inward : Zin-io.

PUBERTY, During :,Calc-io;
Hyds.

SMALL Causing Agg : Bar-c;
Bro; Caus; Crot-h; Grap;

Lach; Pho.

SUFFOCATION, With : See Choking.

TOUCH, Pressure Agg : Kali-io.

TOXIC : Bell; Cact; Crot-h;
Lycps.

VASCULAR : Ap.

GONORRHOEA : *Arg-n;*
Calc; CANN; Canth; Dig;
Fer-p; Kali-chl; *Med; Merc;*
Nat-s; Nit-ac; Petros; *Pul;*
Sep; Sul; THU.

+ **C**HRONIC *:* Kali-io.

+ Thick, green discharge :
Kali-io.

HAEMATURIA, With : Mez.

ILL Effects : See Sycosis.

SUPPRESSED : Agn; Clem;
Nat-m; Med; PUL; *Sars;*
Thu.

GOOSE SKIN: Buf; Hell;
Nux-v; Par; Ver-a.

DRINKING, After : Cadm.

HANDS, Hot with : Cadm.

HEARTBURN, With: Cadm.

NOSE Bleed, With: Cam.

GOSSIPING: Hyo.

GOUT : *Colch;* Colo; Kali-io;
Led; Lyc; Nux-m; Radm;
Ran-sc; Sul; *Urt.*

ACUTE *:* Colch; Sabi; Urt.

+ **A**STHMA, And : Benz-ac.

DIARRHOEA, After : Ant-c;
Benz-ac; Colch; Merc-d;
Nat-s.

JOINTS, Small of : Ran-sc.

METASTASIS, From : Abro; Ant-c.

RHEUMATIC : Rhod.

GRACILE : Pho.

GRANULAR A<small>PPEARANCE</small> :
Carb-v; Grap; Hep; Nat-m;
Pho-ac.

GRANULATION P<small>OOR</small> :
Carb-v; Hep; Kre; Nit-ac; Sil.

W<small>ARTY</small> : Arg-n.

GRAPES Like : See Growth.

GRASPED And **RELAXED**
: See Opening and Shutting.

GRASPING *AGG* : Caus. (See
Fingers, working with).

A<small>MEL</small> : Anac; Cimi; Lith; Spig.

C<small>OLD</small>, Objects A<small>GG</small> : *Hep;* Merc;
Nat-m; Pho; Sil; Thu; *Zin.*

I<small>NVOLUNTARILY</small> : Sul.

S<small>MOOTH</small> Objects A<small>GG</small> : Plb.

T<small>IGHTLY</small> A<small>GG</small> : Rhus-t.

A<small>MEL</small> : Mez; Nux-v.

GRAY, Dirty (Discharges,
discolouration etc) : Arg-m;
Ars; Berb; Calc; Caus; *Chel;*
Cup; Dig; Diph; Fer-p;
KALI-C; Kali-m; Lach; *Lyc;*
Merc; Merc-cy; Ox-ac; PHO;
Pho-ac; Sil; Sul.

GREASY, Oily, Fatty (Skin
discharges etc) : *Bry;* CAUS;
Flu-ac; *Iod;* Iris; Kali-p;
MAG-C; Malan; *Merc;*
Nat-m; Ol-an; Pho; Psor; Pul;
Sele; *Thu;* Val.

GREEDY : See Avaricious.

E<small>ATING</small> In : Nat-c; Zin.

GREEN, *GREENISH* (Skin
discharges etc.) : *Aco;* Ap;
ARS; *Carb-v;* Cham; Con;
Ip; Kali-bi; Kali-io; Lyc;
Mag-c; Med; MERC; *Nat-s;*

Par; Pho; PUL; Rhus-t; Sec;
Sep; Stan; *Sul;* Sul-ac;
Ver-a.

S<small>POTS</small> : Arn; Buf; *Con;* Lach.

T<small>URNS</small> : Arg-n; Bor; Calc-f;
Nat-s; Psor; Rhe; Sanic.

Y<small>ELLOW</small> : *Merc;* Pul.

GRIEF Sorrow : Am-m; Ars;
Aur; *Caus;* Cocl; Colch; Colo;
Con; Cyc; Grap; IGN; Lach; Lyc;
Naj; Nat-m; Petr; *Pho-ac; Pul;*
Samb; *Stap;* Zin.

B<small>OISTEROUS</small> : Nat-m.

B<small>ROODING</small> : Ign.

C<small>AN NOT CRY</small> : Am-m; Gel;
Nat-m.

F<small>INANCIAL</small>, Loss, from : Arn;
Aur.

I<small>MAGINARY</small>, Broods over :
Cyc; Ign.

P<small>ARALYTIC</small> State of Body and
Mind, from : Phys.

P<small>ROLONGED</small> : Nat-m; Pho-ac.

S<small>ILENT</small> : *Ign; Nat-m*; Pho-ac;
Pul.

T<small>RIFLES</small>, Over : Bar-c.

GRIMACES : Agar; Cup; *Hyo;*
Plat; Stram.

GRINDING : See Pain
Cramping.

GRISTLY : Nit-ac; Sil.

+ **GRIT W**<small>ANT</small> Of : *Sil.*

GRITTY F<small>EELING</small> : Con.

GROANING : See Moaning.

E<small>VERY</small> Little thing from :
Bar-c.

GROINS : Alo; Am-m; Cocl;
Gran; Guai.

R<small>IGHT</small> : Calc; Cham; Kali- c;

Lach; *Lyc*; Nux-v; Pul;
Rhod; Rhus-t; Sul-ac; Thu.
Swelling painful, leg
extending, on : Ars-io.

LEFT : Euphor; Mag-c; Naj;
Zin.

AFTER Pains, felt in : Caul;
Cimi.

ALTERNATING Between : Colo;
Phys.

BODY, As of a : Carb-an; Plant.

CLOTHES, Feel uncomfortable
: Hyds.

COITION Agg : Ther.

CORD Like swelling, to knee
: Buf.

COUGHING Agg : Bor.

CREEPING Cold, menses
before : Ant-t.

CUTTING : Thu.

DRAGGING : Calend.

ERUPTION, Moist, menses
before : Sars.

EXTERNAL Ring : Ars; Merc.

INTERNAL Ring : Am-m; Aur;
Lyc; *Nux-v*; Sul-ac.

Coughing Agg : Nat-m.

GLANDS : Calc; *Hep; Merc*;
Nit-ac; Oci-c; *Thu*.

+ Indurated: Tub.

Swollen : Calc; Clem; *Hep*;
Lach; *Merc*; Nit-ac; *Sul*.

Colds Agg : Merc.

Pain, jerking, with : Clem.

legs in, with : Calc-ar.

Visible : Tub.

HOLLOW : Con; Nux-v; Pall.

JERKING, Penis, to : Zin.

KNEES, To : Pod.

LUMPS, Hard, painful : Pul.

OPERATIONS, After : Naj.

+ PRESSING In, both, to sexual
organs : Alu.

RASH, Menses, before : *Ap*;
Ars.

SORE, Menses, before :
Ant-t; Bry.

SPRAINED, As if : Hyds.

STITCHES, Menses, during:
Bor.

SWELLING, As if : Am-m.

Fall, after : Aur.

Painful, extending to legs :
Ars-io.

TENSE, Sprained : Am-m;
Nat-m.

GROPING In dark, as if : Croc;
Hyo; Op; Plb.

GROUND Gives way : Arg-n;
Con; Kali-br; Sul; Visc.

OR STAIRS, Came up to meet
him : Bell; Calc; Cann;
Pic-ac; Sil.

GROWING PAINS : Calc;
Calc-p; Guai; Mang; Pho-ac.

GROWLING : See Howling.

GROWTH, AFFECTED, Disorders
of : Bar-c; Calc; Calc-p; Pho;
Pho-ac; Sil; *Thyr*.

RAPID : Guai; Pho.

GROWTHS NEW, TUMOURS,
etc. (See Cancer, Cysts) :
Ant-c; Ars; Bell; Bels; Calc;
Carb-an; Carb-v; Caus;
Clem; Con; Grap; *Lyc*; Med;
Nit-ac; Ran-b; Sil; *Stap*; Sul;
Thu.

ANGIOMA : Abro; Lyc; Sul.

BURNS After : Calc.

DISPERSING, For : Croc.

ENCEPHALOMA : Croc

ERECTILE : *Lyc*; Nit.ac; Pho.
Menses, before Agg : Lyc.

FLESHY : Merc; Nit-ac; *Stap*; Thu.

FUNGUS : See Fungus Growth.

GRAPES Like: Alo; Calc; Dios.

HORNY : Ant-c; Ran-b; Sil; *Sul.*

LIPOMA (See Cysts): Aur; Croc; Lap-alb; Pho; Phyt.

LYMPHANGIOMA : Vip.

LYMPHOID : Radm; Sec.

NEUROMA : Calend; Cep.

PAIN severe : Stram.

RAPID : Iod; Pho.

SENSITIVE, Convulsions from least touch : Stap.

GRUMBLING : Alu; Aur; Sang; Thyr; Val.

HIS VALUE is not understood by others : Calc-s.

GUILT, SENSE Of : Alu; Arn; *Ars;* Aur; Chel; *Cocl*; Con; Croc; Cyc; Dig; Hyo; Kali-br; Kalm; Kob; *Med*; Psor; VER-A.

TRIFLES, About : Sil.

GULLET : See Oesophagus.

GUMMATA : Carb-an.

GUMMY : See Discharges, Gluey.

GUMS : Bor; Carb-v; Kali-c; Kre; Merc; Nux-v; Stap.

LOWER : Sars.

UPPER : Calc; Rut.

INNER : Pho; *Stap.*

ALTERNATING Sides : Aeth.

ABSCESS : Bell; Calc-f; Echi; Hep; Merc; *Sil.*

Recurrent: Caus.

BLACK, Wedges, on: Bism.

BLEEDING : Amb; Am-c; Bar-c; Bov; Cist; Kre; *Merc;* Nat-m; Nit-ac; Pho-ac; Psor; Stap.

Easily : Ant-c; Caus; Lach; Sul-ac.

Pressing with finger large quantity oozes : Bap; Grap.

Sour : Grap.

Sucking them : Bov; Carb-v.

Touch, on: Lyc; Merc; Pho.

BLUE : *Kre.*

Line along margin : Plb.

BORING : Calc; Merc.

CLENCHES : Lyc; *Phyt;* Pod.

EDGE, At : Am-c; Calc; Flu-ac; Mez; Syph; Thu.

EPULIS : Nat-m; Thu.

EXCORIATED : Carb-v; Sep.

EXCRESCENCES : Nat-m; Stap.

Hard : Plb.

GRASPS, At : Sil.

INCISORS, Behind : Merc-cy; *Pho.*

ITCHING : Kali-c.

NODES, Painful : Pho-ac.

White, small, on : Berb.

PAINFUL : Ars; Kre; Merc; Stap.

RAGGED : Merc.

RECEDING, Detached,

Scorbutic : Ars; *Carb-v;*
Caus; Kali-chl; *Kali-p;* Kre;
Merc; Mur-ac; Psor.

SORE, Sensitive : Am-c; Ars;
Carb-v; Merc.

Chewing, while : *Carb-v;*
Nit-ac.

Cold and Warmth Agg :
Nat-m.

Eating, while: Clem; Pho.

SPONGY : Kali-p; Kre; Lach;
Merc; Merc-c; Mez; Psor;
Sep; Thu.

SUCKING AGG : Bov; Nit- ac;
Nux-m; Sil.

SUPPURATION, Pyorrhoea :
Calc; Carb-v; Cist; Hep;
Kali-c; *Merc;* Merc-i-f;
Pho; PUL;*Sil;* Stap.

SWELLED : Merc; Nux-v; Sep;
Stap; Sul.

White : Nux-v.

TUBERCLES, on: Plb.

VESICLES : Sil.

GURGLING : Agar; ALO; Berb;
Cic; Cina; *Crot-t;*Cup; *Gamb;*
Hyd-ac; Jatr; Kali-c; Kre;
Laur; Lil-t; *Lyc; Pod; Pul;*
Scil; Sul; Thu.

GUSHING : Ars; Bell; Berb;
Bry; CROT-T; Elat; *Gamb;*
Grat; Ip; *Jatr;* Kali-bi;
Mag-m; *Nat-c;* Nat-m; *Nat-s;*
Pho; *Pod;* Sabi; Stan; *Thu;*
Tril; *Ver-a.*

HABITS, INTEMPERATE AGG :
Arg-n.

DIRTY : See Dirty.

HACKING, Like a Hatchet : Am-c;

Ars; Aur; Clem; Kali-n; Lyc
Pho-ac; Rut; Stap; Thu.

HAEMATEMESIS : See
Vomiting, Blood, and
Haemorrhage.

HAEMATOCELE : Arn; Con;
Ham; Rut.

HAEMATODES : See Fungus
Growth.

HAEMATOMA: Calc-f; Merc;
Sil.

EAR, On: Bell.

HAEMATURIA : See Urine
Bloody and Haemorrhage.

GONORRHOEA With : Mez.

MENSES, Suppressed, from :
Nux-v.

HAEMOPHILIA: Arn; Ars;
Carb-an; Crot-h; Ham; Kre;
Lach; Nat-s; *Pho;* Sil; Visc.

SUPPURATION, With: Hyds.

HAEMOPTYSIS (See
Haemorrhage) : Aco; Am-c;
Ars; Bell; Bry; Chin; Fer;
Hyo; Ip; Mill; Nit-ac; Pho;
Plb; Pul; Rhus-t; Sabi;
Sec; Sul; Sul-ac; Terb.

BLOOD, Black, watery : Elap.

CHEST, Heat in, with: Psor.

CONVULSIONS, After : Dros.
With: Hyo.

DRUNKARDS : Ars; *Nux-v.*

DYSPNOEA, With : Arn.

EXERTION, Violent, after : Urt.

INTERMITTENT : Kre.

MASTURBATION, From : Fer.

MENSES, Before : Dig.
Suppressed, with : Ars;

Senec.

PALPITATION, With : Mill.

+ **P**ERIODICAL : Kre.

+ **R**EPEATED : *Pho.*

RHEUMATISM, Alternating with : Led;

VALVULAR Heart Disease,in: Cact; Cratae; Lycps.

HAEMORRHAGE (Bloody discharges) : Acet-ac; *Aco;* ARN; Ars; BELL; Bur-p; *Cact;* CALC; Canth;*Carb-v;* CHIN; Croc; *Crot-h;* FER; Ham; Hyds; Ip; *Kre;* Lach; Led; Lept; Lyc; Lycps; Mang; MERC; Merc-c; *Mill;* NIT-AC; *Nux-v;* PHO; PUL; Rhus-t; Sabi; *Sec; Sep;* Solid; Sul; *Sul-ac;* Terb; Tril; Urt; Ust; Vib; Vip.

ACRID : Kali-c; Sil.

ACUTE : *Aco; Bell;* Croc; Fer; Hyo; Mill; Pul.

AGG & AMEL, from : See Bleeding.

ALTERED Blood of : Crot-h; Pul; Sec.

BRIGHT : *Aco;* Arn; *Bell;* Carb-v; *Dul; Erig; Fer; Hyo; Ip;* Led; Meli; Mill; Nit-ac; Pho; Plb; *Sabi;* Sul; Tril.

Clots, dark with : Fer; Sabi; Sang; Ust.

gelatinous, with : Laur. Frothy : Led.

CLOTTED (See Discharges lumpy) : Arn; Bell; Bur-p; Canth; Chin; Fer; Hyo; Ip; Nux-v; Pul; Sabi; Sul.

Rapidly : Ip.

CLOTS, Mixed with : Sabi; Ust.

DARK : Aco; Bur-p; Canth; Carb-v; Cham; Chin; Croc; Crot-h; Elap; Ham; Helo; Kre; Lach; Nux-m; Nux-v; Pul; Sec; Sep; Sul-ac; Ust.

Thin : Am-c; Sul-ac; Ust.

EASY : Kali-chl.

EFFECTS, Chronic : Stic; Stro.

FACE, Flushed with : Amy-n.

+ **F**AVOURS, Absorption : Ham.

FROTHY : Led.

GUSHING : Aco; *Bell;* Cham; Erig; Ham; Ip; Lac-c; Pul; Sabi; Sec; Tril.

Intermittently : Psor; Sul.

HEART Symptoms, with : Cratae; Lycps.

HOT : *Bell;* Sabi.

+ **L**EECH Bite, from : Alum.

LIFTING Agg : Petr.

+ **M**IND Tranquil, with : Ham.

OFFENSIVE : Bell; Bry; Carb-v; Helo; Sabi.

ORIFICES Of the body, from : Bothr; Crot-h; Ip; Pho.

PASSIVE, Oozing : Bov; Buf; Carb-v; *Chin;* Crot-h; Fer-p; Ham; Kre; Pho-ac; Sec; Terb; *Ust.*

Mucous mixed, with : Caps.

Wounds, closed, edges from : Mill.

+ **P**OST-PARTUM : Mill.

RIDING Carriage in Agg : Petr.

SCRATCHING Agg : Psor.

SLIGHT, Causing great Agg :

See under Bleeding.

STICKY, Stringy : Croc; Merc; Naj; Ust.

THICK : Agar; Bov; Croc; Cup; *Nux-m*; Plat.

THIN, Watery : Carb-v; Crot-h; Grap; Laur; Nit-ac; Rhus-t; Sabi; Sec; Sul-ac.

Clot, won't : Lach; Pho.

   mixed, with : Arn; Bell; Caus; Pul; Sabi.

VIOLENT : Mur-ac.

WEAKNESS, Undue : Alu; Bry; Carb-an; Ham; Hyds.

HAEMORRHOIDS : See Piles.

HAIR AFFECTIONS Of : Bell; Bor; Calc; Carb-an; Carb-v; Con; *Grap; Hep; Kali-c; Lyc*; Merc; *Nat-m*; Nit-ac; *Sul*; Ust.

BLOND : Bro; *Calc;* Caps; Cocl; Hyo; *Pul*; Sele; Seneg; Sil.

BODY, All over : Med; Thu; Thyr.

BRISTLING, Erect : Aco; *Bar-c;* Cham; Canth; Chel; Glo; *Laur*; Meny; Mur-ac; Sul-io; *Ver-a; Zin*.

+ BRITTLE : Grap; Zin.

CHIN and UPPER Lip, on (women) : Ol-j.

COLD : Sul.

DARK : Aco; Cina; Iod; Nit- ac; *Nux-v*; Pho; Pho-ac; Plat; Sep.

DRY : Alu; Kali-c; Psor; Sul; *Thu*.

Oily, becomes : Lyss.

FALLING : Alu; *Ars*; Ars-s-fl; Aur; *Calc*; Carb-v;Flu-ac; GRAP; Hell; *Hep; Kali-c;* Kali-s; Lach; *Lyc*; Nat-m; Nit-ac; PHO; Sep; Sil; Stap; SUL; Thal; Thu; Thyr; *Ust*.

Beard, of : Grap; Kali-c; Plb; Sele.

Bregma, from : Ars; Nat-m; Pho.

Children, in : Nat-m.

Climaxis, at : Sep.

Colour changes, after : Kali- io.

Combing, when: Canth.

Fevers, after : Flu-ac.

Genitals, from : Sele.

Gray, hair replaced by : Vinc.

Grief, from : Pho-ac.

Handfuls, bunches, in : Carb-v; Mez; *Pho*; Syph; Thal.

Headache, after : Ant-c; Hep; Nit-ac; Sep; Sil.

Illness, severe after : Carb- v; Manc; Thal.

Itching of Head, with : Ant-c.

Lactation, during : Nat-m.

Nails, with : Hell; *Ust*.

Occiput, from : Carb-v; Chel; Merc; Petr; Stap.

Parturition, after : Carb-v; Lyc; Sul.

Pregnancy during : Lach.

Pubis, from : Nat-m; Nit-ac; Zin.

Rapidly : Thal.

Sides, from : Grap; Pho; Stap.

Spots, in : Alu; Flu-ac; Grap; Hep; Lyc; *Nat-m; Pho.*

Sweat, offensive from : *Sul.*

Temples, from : Kali-c; *Nat-m.*

Vertex, from : See Bald under Head.

GRAY, Early : *Ars; Lyc; Nar-m; Pho-ac;* Sil.

LETTING Down, **A**MEL : Bell; Cina; Fer; Kali-m; Kali-n; Kali-p; Pho.

MARGINS, Edge at : Hyds; Kali-p; Med; Nat-m; Old; Petr; Sep; *Sul;* Tell.

Brown, stripe : Kali-p.

Moisture : Diph.

Yellow : Med.

MATTED : Ant-c; Grap; Lyc; Ust; Vinc; Vio-t.

Secretion, sticky, from : Ust.

OFFENSIVE, Foul : Vinc.

OILY, Greasy: Bry; Merc; Pho-ac.

PAINFUL, Touch to, etc : Ap; *Ars;* Bry; *Chin;* Hep; *Nux-v;* Sele; *Ver-a;* Zin.

Root, at : Colo.

Vertex, on : Zin.

PULLED, As if : ACO; Aeth; *Arg-n;* Kali-n; Lach; Mag-c; *Pho;* Sele.

PULLS Her : See Desire to pull her hair.

SENSATION, Of : Arg-n; Ars; Kali-bi; Pul; Sil; Sul.

SOPPY, Wet : *Rhe.*

SPLIT : Thu; ZIN.

STANDING, As if : Mur-ac; Rhod; Spo; Sul-io.

*S*TIFF : Sele.

TANGLED, Tousy : Bor; Flu-ac; *Lyc;* Med; Mez; Nat-m; *Pho-ac;* Psor; Sul.

THICK : Ant-c; Grap; Lyc; Ust; Vio-t.

HAIR COMBING or Brushing **A**GG : Bry; *Chin;* Carb-ac; Form; Glo; Ign; Mez; Sele; Sil.

AMEL : Form; Tarn.

Back Agg : Pul; Rhus-t.

Electric crackling, when : Sanic.

CUTTING AGG *: Bell;* Glo; Led; Pho; Sep.

TOUCHING AGG : Ap; *Ars;* Bell; *Chin;* Fer; Lach; Nux-v; Pul; SELE; Sep; Ver-a; Zin.

HALLUCINATIONS : See Perceptions Changed and Imaginations.

HAMMERING : See Pain, Hammering, Head.

HAMSTRINGS, SHORT, Tense : Am-m; Bry; Dios; Guai; Nat-m.

LEFT : Sul.

HAND LAYING On part **A**MEL : Carb-an; Croc; *Cup;* Meny; Pho.

MOVING, Body on, as if : Carb-v.

HANDS : *Calc;* Caul; Lyc; Nux-v; Pho; *Sul.*

BACK Of : Kre; Nat-c; Rhus-t;
Sep.

Brown : Iod.

Cramp: Mag-c; Ver-a.

Eruptions : Kre; Mez;
Mur-ac; Nat-c; Petr; Pul.

Spiders, were crawling :
Visc.

Sweat, cold : Bothr; *Chio*;
Zin-s.

Swollen, as if : Iod.

Warts : Nit-ac.

Wrinkled : Pho-ac.

BEHIND HIM AGG : Ign; Sanic.

BITES, Sleep, during: Elap.

BURNING Heat: Agar; Asar;
Carb-v; *Lach*; Med; Mur-ac;
Petr; Pho; Sang; Sep; Spig;
Stan; Sul.

Body, spreads to, from
: Chel.

Chill, with : Kali-c.

Cold, feet, with : Sep.

Agg : Caps.

weather in : Rhod.

Fanning, desires : *Med.*

Feet, and : Flu-ac.

One : Mez.

Then, cold : Cocl.

CALLOSITIES : Grap; Sul.

Cracked : Cist.

CLAMMY : Sanic; Tarn; Sul.

Feet, and : Sanic.

CLAPPS : Bell; Stram.

Head over : Sec.

COBWEB Sensation : Bor.

COLD (See Coldness of Single

parts) : Bro.

One : Chin; Dig; Ip; Lyc;
Pul; Rhus-t; Sul.

other warm : Chin; Ip.

Right : Gel.

then, left : Med.

Left : Thyr.

Coughing, when : Rum.

+ Dead, as if : Ox-ac.

Diarrhoea, during : *Pho.*

Face, dark red, with : Mur-ac.

Feet, and : Kali-m; Sanic.

Headache, during : Amb;
Vario.

Hot, feet, with: Calc; Sep.

weather, in : Asar.

Icy : Cact; Hyd-ac; Nux-m;
Thyr; Ver-a.

emissions, after : Merc.

fever, in : Thu.

headache, with : Vario.

Room, warm, in : Sep.

Smoker's : Sec.

Sweat, during : Thu.

Uncovering on : Mag-c.

Water, in AGG : Con;Lac-d;
Mag-c; Mag-p; Pho; Tarn.

AMEL : Flu-ac; Gel; Jat.

CONTRACTION, Involuntary, as
if grasping : Sul.

COVER , Cannot : Mag-c.

CRACKS (See also fingers) :
Alu; *Calc; Grap*; Hep;
Nit-ac; *Petr;* Rhus-t; Sanic;
Sars; Sep; Sil; Sul; Zin.

CRAMPS : Anthx; *Bell; Calc*;
Lyc; Pyro; Sec; Val.

Broom, can not let go : Dros; Stan.

Closing, on : Chin.

Feet, and : Lyc; Lyss.

Grasping Agg : Amb.

cold things Agg : Nat-m.

+ Sleep prevents : Val.

Writing, while : Nat-p.

CRAWLING : Hypr.

+ DEAD, While sewing : Crot-h.

DRY : Anac; Bar-c; *Lyc; Sul.*

ECZEMA : Berb; Cor-r; Grap; Nat-c; Sep; Zin.

Dorsum : Mur-ac.

Trade : Bor.

+ EMACIATION : Sele.

+ FORMICATION : Hypr.

HEAVY : Bell; Pho.

HOT : See Burning.

Constant : Lyc.

ITCHING : Agar; Anac; Sul.

JERKING : Nat-c.

LAME : *Caus;* Cup; Kali-bi; Mez; Sil; Zin.

Exertion or writing while : Mez; Sil.

LARGE TOO, As if : Cact; Hyo.

LAYING, Affected part on : See Hand laying on.

MOTION, Automatic, towards mouth : Nux-v.

NUMB : Ap; Calad; Carb-an; Cocl; Form; Kali-n; Lyc; Stro.

Alternating : Echi.

Chest affections, with : Carb-an.

Cold, and : Lach; Ox-ac.

Electric shock, as from, as if : Flu-ac.

Grasping anything : Calc; Cham; Cocl.

Heat, insensitive to : Plb.

Left, formication, with extending up : Grap.

Putting in pocket : Nat-m.

Sewing when : Crot-h.

Ulnar nerve, along : Cup-ac.

OFFENSIVE : Phys.

OPEN And Shut: Stram.

PARALYSIS : Plb.

PINS And Needles : Colch.

PRICKING : Kali-p.

PUFFY, Feet and : Naj.

A.M. in : Just.

PURPLE : Sep.

RESTLESS, Busy :Kali-br; Sul; Tarn; Ther; Thyr; Ver-v.

Delirium, during : Ver-v.

Feet, and : Stic.

RUBS : Bap.

+ SOFT : Cact.

STIFF, Knitting when : Kali-m.

Writing, when : Kali-m.

SWEAT, On : Agn; Ars; CALC; Naj; Nit-ac; Pho; Sep; Sil; *Sul*; Thu; Thyr; *Tub.*

Cold : Canth; Nit-ac; Sep.

feet on, with : Cimi; Ip; Kali- bi; Tarn.

heat, during : Am-c; Fer-p; Nit-ac.

stools, during : Chin.

vomiting, with : Chio.

Cough, with : Naj.

Feet, and: Flu-ac; Naj;
Nit- ac.

Injuries to spine, from :
Nit-ac.

Opthalmia, during : Flu-ac;
Sul.

Palms, put together, when
: Sanic.

Profuse   : Stic; Sul.

SWELLED, As if : Coll; Kali-n;
Stro; Terb.

Ankles, and   : Stan.

Feet, and : Fer; Just.

Hanging down, arms when
: Am-c.

Left, heart disease, in : Cact.

Opening and closing on :
Mang.

TREMBLE : Glo; Lach Lol-t;
Mag-p; Ox-ac; Tarn; Zin.

Carrying something to
mouth : Merc; Plb; Sil.

Concomitant, as a : Calc-p.

Grasping, objects : Led;
Merc; Plb.

Menses, during : Hyo; Zin.

Moving, when : Led.

Palpitation, with : Bov.

Vomiting, with : Calc-p.

Waking : Nat-s.

Writing, when Agg : Cimi;
Merc; Nat-m; Nat-s; Plb;
Sul; Zin.

fast Amel : Fer.

presence of others
Agg : Ign.

ULNAR Nerve, along: Cup-ac.

USING : See Fingers, Working
Agg.

VEINS, Swelled : Am-c; Arn;
Chin; Ham; Laur; Nux-v; Op;
Pho; PUL; Thyr; Vip.

Chill. during : Chel.

VESICLES : Kre; Ver-v.

WANTS, Covered : Ign.

Fanning : Med.

WARTS, On : Dul; Nat-m.

+ Horny : Ant-c.

WASH, Tendency to: Coca;
Lac-c; Psor; Syph.

Dry, when : Pho.

WATER, In AGG (See Cold of
single parts) : Ign; Nat-m;
Pho.

Cold : See Under Cold.

WEAK : Bov; Caus; Kali-bi;
Med; Ox-ac; *Zin.*

Drops things : Bov; Stan.

Menses, during: Alum.

Writing, while : Mez; Sil.

+ WENS : Pho-ac.

WITHERED, Skin: Lyc.

WOODEN Sensation: Kali-n.

WRINGS : Ars; Kali-br;
Stram; Sul; Ther.

Walks the floor, and: Buf.

YELLOW, Colic with : Sil.

HANGING AFFECTED PARTS AGG
And AMEL : See Hanging Limbs
Agg and Amel.

DOWN, LOOSE, suspended as
if : Alu; Aur; Bar-c; *Ign;*
Ip; Kali-c; LACH; Lil-t;
Med; Merc; PHO; Saba;

Sep; Sul; Val.

LIMBS AGG : Alu; Am-c; Bar-c;
BELL; *Calc;* CARB- V; Con;
Pul; Ran-sc; Sabi; Thu; Vip.

AMEL : Aco; *Arn;* Asar; Berb;
CON; *Lyc;* Mag-c; Mag-m;
Mang; Mar-v; Merc; Pho; Rat;
Rhus-t.

HAPPY SEEING OTHERS AGG :
Hell; Helo.

HARD BED Sensation: See Bed.
Pain : See Pain Aching.

PARTS, Feel soft : Merc; Nit-ac;
Nux-m.

HARDNESS, INDURATION : Alu;
Ant-c; Ars; Bad; Bar-c; Bell;
Bro; *Bry;* Calc; CALC-F;
CARB-AN; Carb-v; Chin; Cist;
Clem; CON; Flu-ac; Grap; Iod;
KALI-M; Lach; *Lyc;* Mag-m;
Merc; Merc-i-r; *Pho; Phyt;*
Plb; *Rhus-t;* Sele; *Sep; Sil;*
Spo; Stap; *Sul;* Tarn-c.

INJURY After : Calc-f.

PRESSURE Constant, from : Sep.

STONY : Calc-f; Carb-v; Kali-bi;
Kali-m; Merc-i-r; Sul;
Tarn-c.

HARSH : Kali-io.

HASTE : See Hurry.

HATEFUL : Led; Lyc; Nat-m;
Nit-ac; Tarn.

HATRED : See Malice.

MALE, FEMALE, each other for
: Sep.

OTHERS, By as if : Lach.

HAUGHTY : See Insolent.

HAUTEUR : See Pride.

HAWKING (Mucus) : Arg-n;

Caus; Con; Cor-r; Hep;
KALI-BI; *Kali-c;* LACH; LYC;
Mang; Merc; *Nat-c; Nat-m;*
Nux-v; PHO; Pul; Rhus-t;
Rum; Sele; *Sep.*

AGG : Am-m; Arg-n; Coc-c;
Nux-v; Sil.

AMEL : Kob; Lach.

BITTER : Arn; Ars; Cist;
Menis; Nat-m.

BLOOD, Bright red : Saba.

BROWN, Gluey: Ol-an.

Effort, with : Bry.

CLEAR, Morning, in : Sele.

COLD : Sinap.

CONSTANTLY : Mang; Spo.

COPPERY : Cimi.

DRAWN From posterior nares
: Cinb; Cor-r; *Hep;* Hyds;
Kali-bi; Mag-c; Nat-c;
Nat-m; Nit-ac; Nux-v;
Sele; Sep; Spig; Sul; Tell.

Brown : Bry.

Vomits, from : Sep.

EATING Agg : Sil; Tub.

GLAIRY : Pall.

GREEN : Colch; Par; Syph.

Comes involuntarily in
mouth : Colch.

LUMPS, CHEESY, of : *Agar;*
Hep; *Kali-bi;* KALI-M;
Kali-p; *Mag-c;* Merc;
Merc-i-f; PSOR; Sanic;
Sep; *Sil.*

Foul : Kali-m; Lach; Med;
Petr; Sil.

Solid : Calc; Lith; Mar-v;
Merc; Merc-i-f; Sep.

Nausea, From : Stan.

With : Lil-t.

Salty : Calc; Nat-m; Tell.

Singing, Before : Calc-p.

Sleep, During : Calc-p.

Sour : Tarx.

Sticky : Arg-n; Cinb; Coc-c; Hyds; KALI-BI; *Lach;* Mag-m; Phyt; Rum.

Sweetish : Aesc; Mag-p.

Talking, While : Arg-m; Calc-p.

Tough : Aesc; Kali-c; Ol-an; Par; Rum.

Vomiting, With : Calc-p.

HAY *FEVER* : See Coryza, Annual.

Asthma : See Asthma.

HEAD Affections In General : BELL; *Bry;* Calc; *Carb-v;* Chin; Gel; *Glo; Lach; Lyc; Nat-m; Nux-v;* Par; *Pho; Pul;* Sang; Sep; *Sil;* Spig; Sul; Tub.

One Sided : Alu; Anac; Arg-n; *Ars;* Asaf; Calc; *Chin; Chin-s;* Con; IRIS; Kali-c; Kali-io; Nux-v; *Pho-ac;* Plat; PSOR; *Pul;* Saba; SANG; Sars; *Sep;* Spig; Sul-ac; Verb; Zin.

Begins on one, goes to and Agg on other : Arg-n; Fer; Iris; Lac-c; LYC; Mang; Nat-m; Tub.

Right : *Bell;* Cact; *Calc;* Carb-v; Chel; IGN; *Iris;* Kalm; Lyc; Nat-c; Plat; Plb; Pru-sp; Pul; Rhus-t; *Saba;* SANG; Sars; *Sil.*

cut off, as if : Lach.

Left: Arn; Ars; Asaf; Bro; Chin-s; *Colo;* Ip; Kali-c; *Lach;* Lil-t; *Merc;* Mur-ac; Naj; Nit-ac; Nux-m; *Nux-v;* Onos; *Rhod;* Sele; *Sep;* SPIG; Sul.

growth retarded : Flu-ac.

Absent, As if : Asar; Calc-io; Nit-ac.

Aching : See Pain.

Active, When Amel : Merc-i-f.

Alternating, With : Alo; Alu; Ars; Cina; Gel; Glo; Ign; Psor; Strop.

Back, with : Ign; Meli.

Lumbago, with : Alo.

Pelvis, with : Gel.

Stomach, with : Ars; Bism; Ox-ac; Plb; Ver-a.

Air, Wind, through : Aur; Cor-r; Ver-a.

Blowing on, as if : Petr.

Cold Amel : Seneg.

Streaming through eyes : Thu.

Anger Agg: Mez.

Arms Over : Ars; Lac-c; *Pul.*

Ascending Agg : Bell; Bry; Calc; Sil; Spig.

Into : Aco; BELL; Bry; *Calc;* Canth; Chel; Chin; Cimi; Gamb; *Gel; Glo;* Kalm; Mang; *Meny;* Merc; Nat-m; Pho; SANG; Sep; SIL; SPIG.

Right : Alo; *Bell;* Gel; Ign; Meny; Nat-m; Nux-v; Pho; SANG.

Left : Arg-n; Chel; Cimi; Colch; Lac-c; Lil-t; Par; Petr; Sabi; Sil; SPIG.

Stairs Agg : Ant-c.

BACKWARD, Extending : Arn; BELL; BISM; BRY; *Cimi; Glo;* Kali-bi; Lac-d; Lach; Lyc; Med; Mur-ac; Nat-m; *Nit-ac;* Par; Pru-sp; Rut; Sep; Syph; *Thu;* Tub; Ver-v; Verb; Zin.

Pulled, as if : Syph.

BALD : Alum; Aur; Bar-c; Flu-ac; Grap; Lyc; Syph; Zin.

+ Gonorrhoea, from : Kali-s.

Premature : Bar-c; Sil.

Soreness of Scalp, with : Zin.

Spots, covered with wooly hair : Vinc.

   lock of white hair : Psor.

BALL, Lumps, knot : Con.

Striking in, talking while : Sars.

Throat, rising from, to : Plb.

BAND, constriction : Anac; Ant-t; Carb-ac; Carb-v; Caus;Coca; Cocl; Gel; Glo; Grap; *Merc;* Nit-ac; Ox-ac; Sars; Sul.

+ Amel, green tea and smoking : Carb-ac.

Hot : Aco; Chlo-hyd.

+ Tight, around : Xanth.

Tight, painful, removes the hat involuntarily, without Amel : Sars.

BANDAGING, Binding Amel : Ap; *Arg-n;* Glo; Lac-d; Mag-m; Pic-ac; *Pul;* Pyro; *Sil.*

BASE, Of : Cimi; Gel; Syph; Ver-v.

BATHING, Washing Agg : Canth.

Feet Amel : Ascl.

BEATS, The : Aco; Ap; Hyo; Mill; Syph; Tub.

BED, Early, in Agg : Hell; Rhod.

BELONGS To another, as if : Ther.

BEND, Backwards, must : Ant-t; Arn; *Cham;* Kali-n; Nat-c; Stram;

Amel : Seneg; Thu.

Sneezing, when : Lyss.

BIG, With big belly : Calc.

Body, wasted with : Sil.

Jaws, small with : Kali-io.

BLOW, Shock, Thrusts etc. as of : *Ap;* Cann; Croc; *Glo;* Ign; Naj; *Nat-m;* Nux-v; *Spig;* Sul-ac; Tarn.

Biting, chewing, while : Am-c.

Talking, when : Sars.

BLOWING Nose Agg : Amb.

Amel : Chel.

BOILING Water, side lain on as if : Mag-m.

BORES Into pillow : See Drawn Backwards.

BREATHING, Deep Agg : Anac; Cact; Rat.

BURNING, Heat : *Aco;* Ap; *Bell;* Bor; Bry; Cact; Calc; *Frax; Grap;* Lach; Merc; *Merc-i-r;* Nat-c; Oenan; Pho; *Pic-ac;* SUL.

Mental exertion, from :
Calc.

Amel : Cham.

Spot, in : Con.

CAP, Hat, aversion to : Iod;
Led; Lyc.

On, as if : Berb; Eup-p;
Phys; Pyro.

CARRIAGE, Riding in Amel :
Kali-n.

CATARRHAL : Kali-bi; *Merc;*
NUX-V.

CHILDREN, Thin Agg : Lyc.

CHRONIC : Arg-n; Ars; Calc;
Nat-c; Nat-m; Psor; Sep;
Sil; Zin.

+ CLOTHES, Warm Agg : Aru-t.

+ COFFEE, Hot Agg : Aru-t.

COITION Agg : Bov; Pho-ac;
Sil.

COLD Application Amel : Alo;
Ars; Bry; Cyc; *Glo;* Pho; Sul.

Water Agg : Ant-c.

poured over, as if : Cup;
Tarn.

COLDNESS : Agar; *Bell; Calc;*
Calc-p; Cann; Chel; Cup;
Dul; Hypr; *Laur;* Lyc;
Merc-c; Nat-m; Pho;
Rhus-t; Sep; Sil; Stan;
Stro; Tarn; VER-A; *Ver-v.*

Hand, cold as from, as if :
Hypr.

+ Hands and feet : Vario.

Heated, from being : *Carb-v.*

Upper part : Val.

Warm room, in : Laur.

COMMOTION, Painless, in :
Caus.

COMPRESSION, Cap, Squeezing
: Agn; Arg-n; *Berb;* Bry;
Cact; Glo; Ign; Lach; *Meny;*
Merc; Onos; Pho-ac; Plat;
Pul; Stap.

Vise like : Arg-n; Nit-ac;
Pul.

CONGESTION : *Aco;* Amy-n;
Ap; Ars; BELL; *Bry;* Calc;
FER; *Gel;* GLO; Hyo; *Lach;*
Meli; NUX-V; *Op;* Pho; *Pul;*
Psor; Rhus-t; *Sang;* STRAM;
Sul; VER-V.

Palpitation, with : Scop.

CONSTIPATION Agg : *Bry;* Colch;
Nux-v; Op.

CONVERSATION Amel : Dul;
Eup-p; Lac-d.

COUGH Agg : Bell; *Bry; Caps;*
Carb-v; Con; Fer; Iris;
Kali-c; Lac-d; NAT-M;
Nux-v; Pho; Psor; Scil; *Sul;*
Vio-o.

Amel : Chel.

COVER, Must : Bro; *Rum.*

CRASH, Explosion, in : Alo;
Dig; Glo; Pho; Zin.

Sleep, falling to, on: Dig;
Zin.

CRAWLING, FORMICATION : Aco;
Arg-m; *Arg-n;* Colch; Cup;
Hyo; Pho; *Plat; Pul; Rhus-t;*
Sul.

CROWDED Room in, company
etc. Agg : Lyc; Mag-c; *Plat;*
Plb; Stap.

CRUSHED, Down, as if : Dios.

CRUSHING, In : Bry; Nat-s;
Nit-ac; Syph.

CUT OFF, As if : Lach.

DAMP, Day Agg : Glo.

DANCING, From Agg : *Arg-n*

+ DARK Room Amel : Nat-s.

Working in Agg : Ced.

DEEP, In : Aco; Arg-n; Bov; Calc; Dul; Lach; Nux-v; Pho; Sul; Tub.

+ DELICATE Literary Persons : Arg-n.

DESCENDING Agg : *Bell;* Fer; Rhus-t.

DIARRHOEA, Alternating with : Alo; Pod.

Amel : Pod.

With : Iris.

DIURESIS, Polyuria, with : Aco; *Gel;* Glo; *Lac-d;* Ol-an; Phys; Sele; Sil; Vib.

DOWNWARD To nose, face, neck etc. : *Agar;* Ant-t; Bism; Calc; Calc-p; Cham; *Chin;* Dul; Guai; Hypr; Ign; IP; *Lach; Led;* Mang; *Med;* Meny; *Mez;* NUX-V; *Pho;* Pic-ac; Plat; *PUL;* Rhus-t; Sep; *Stap;* Stro; VERB; *Zin.*

DRAFT Agg : *Bor;* Chin; Hep; *Mag-m; Naj;* Nux-v; *Psor;* SIL.

DRAWN, To a point, as if : Grap; Hypr; Lachn; Stro; Ther.

Backward, Bores into pillow, etc. : Ap; Aru-t; Bell; Cic; *Cimi;* Cup; Hell; Med; Op; Pod; Syph; Tub; Ver-v; *Zin.*

Shoulder, to : Agar.

Side to, glands enlarged from : Cist.

DRINKING, Hot tea Amel : Fer-p; Glo.

Iced drinks Agg : Con; Dig.

Amel : Alum.

+ EAR to EAR : Pall; Plant.

EAR, With : Fer-p; Merc; Pul; Sang.

Jarring Agg : Med.

EATING Amel : Cist; Elap; Lith; Lyc; Mag-c; Pho; Phyt; Psor; Rhod; Sang; Sil; Thu.

Frequently Amel : Sul.

ELECTRIC, Shocks, spasms before : Cep; Hell; Mag-p.

All parts of body : Mag-p.

EMISSION Agg : Ham.

EMPTY, Hollow : Arg-m; *Cocl;* Cor-r; Manc; Naj; Pho; Pul.

Menses, during : Fer-p.

Vertigo, with : Manc.

Walking Agg : Manc.

ENLARGED, As if : Agar; *Arg-n;* Arn; *Bell;* Bov; Cor-r; Gel; *Glo;* Lith; Nat-c; Nux-m; *Nux-v;* Ran-b.

Pain during : Cup.

Pregnancy, during : *Arg-n.*

Stools Agg : Kob.

EPILEPSY, After : Caus; Cup; Kali-br.

Before, and : Cina.

EXPANDING And CONTRACTING : Calc; Glo; Lac-c.

EXPLOSIONS : See Crash.

EYES, Extending into : Carb-v; *Chin;* Cimi; Ign;

LACH; Lith; Mang; Nat-c; NIT-AC; PHO; Pho-ac; Pul; *Sil*; SPIG; *Sul;* Val; *Zin.*

Closing Agg : Cep; Chin; Sil; Ther.

half Amel : Alo.

Motion of Agg : Bell; Bry; Nux-v.

lids of Agg : Colo.

Out through, as if : Nat-c; Sil.

Over head, to nape : Bur-p.

Pressure, on Amel : Nat-m.

Straining of, exertion Agg : Gel; Nat-m; *Onos;* Pho-ac; Rut.

Symptoms, with : See Visual Symptoms, with.

FEAR, Fright Agg : Aco; Chin-ar; Cimi; Glo.

FEET, And : Mag-m.

Bathing Amel : Ascl.

FINGERS, Tip to : Cam.

FIXING Attention, on, Amel : Pall.

FLATUS Passing Amel : Aeth; Cic; Sang.

FORWARD, Extending : Aco; Alu; Arg-n; *Bell;* Canth; *Carb-v; Chin;* Cimi; *Con; Gel;* Laur; Lyc; Mur-ac; Pho-ac; *Rhus-t;* Saba; Verb.

Right : Kali-c; SANG; *Sil.*
Left : Chel; Sabi; SPIG; Thu.

FROWNING Agg : Ars; Mang; Nat-m.

Amel : Caus; Pho; Sul.

FULNESS : *Aco*; Bry; *Glo*; Merc; Sul.

FUNGUS : Ap; Calc-p; Pho.

+ GASTRIC Symptoms : Tarx.

GOING, Food without Agg : Ars; Cact; Cist; Lach; Lyc; Sang; Sil.

HAIR, CUT Agg : *Bell*; Glo; Pho; Sep.

Binding Amel : Sul-io.

Down Amel : Bell; Cina; Fer; Kali-m; Kali-p; Pho.

+ Dragged by, as if : Alu.

Washing Amel : Bell.

HAMMERING : See Pain.

HANDS, Holding near Amel : Carb-an; Glo; Petr; Sul-ac.

HAT, Head on Agg : Nit-ac.

HEART symptoms, with : Cact; Crot-h; Dig; Glo; Kalm; Merc-i-f; Naj; Spig.

Pain after : Merc-i-r.

HEATED If Agg : *Aco*; Ant-c; Bell; *Bry*; Carb-v; *Glo*; Lyc; Nit-ac; *Ver-v;* Zin.

HEAT Of SUN Agg : See Sunlight, Shine.

- HEAVY : Ap; Carb-v; Chin; Gel; Lach; Lol-t; Mang; Mur- ac; Nat-m; Nux-v; Petr; Pic-ac; Sul.

Pillow, on : Buf; Glo; Sang.

HOLD, Unable to (See Wobbling about) : Ap; Cocl; Cup; *Gel*; Sanic; Ver-a.

HOLDS, While coughing : Bry; Nic; Nux-v.

Groans, and : Cimi.

HOT, AIR, about : Ast-r; Flu-ac; Plant; Pul; Ver-a.

Application Amel : Arg-n;

Aur; Bry; Gel; Kali-c; *Mag-p*; Pho; *Sil.*

Cold limbs, with: Aco; *Arn;* BELL; Bry; Calc; Carb-v; *Chin;* Fer; Gel; Lach; Mur- ac; *Sul.*

Spots, on : Con.

Vapour, rising to top : Buf; Ol-an.

Vertigo, after : Aeth.

Weather Agg : Nat-c.

HYSTERICAL, Young women : Arg-n.

INJURIES, To : *Arn;* Calc; *Cic;* Con; Glo; Hep; Hypr; Lach; *Nat-s*; Pul; Rhus-t; Sil; Sul-ac; Symp.

Delirium, after : Bell; Hyo; Op; Stram; Ver-a.

Distress in, after : Lac-d.

Stupefaction, after : Arn; Cic; Con; Pul; Rhus-t.

Tender, after : Nat-m.

INWARD Extending : Agar; Anac; Arn; Ars; Calc; Canth; Hep; *Ign;* Nit-ac; *Stan;* Thu.

IRONING Clothes, Agg : *Bry;* Pho; Sep.

JARRING : Ther.

Cars, in Agg : Med.

JAW, Into : Lach; Pho; Stro.

JERKS : *Bell;* Bry; Caus; Cic; PUL; Sep.

Sexual excitement, with : Ver-v.

Up, and drops it again : Stram.

KNEELING And pressing the to floor, Amel : Sang.

KNOTTED, Up, as if : Cam.

LARGER Than body, as if : Bap; Hypr; Lith; Mang; Nux-v; Ran-b.

LAUGHING Agg : Nat-m; Zin.

LEAN On something, desires to or AMEL : Bell; Fer; Kali-c; *Merc;* Nux-v; Saba; Spig.

Hand, on : Iod.

Side to, one : Cina.

Table, on, AMEL : Ign; Saba.

LEFT To, face and neck : Tarn.

LIFT It up, desire to : Ther.

+ LOOSE, In, as if : Kali-c.

LYING Agg : Ther.

Amel : Con; *Nat-m;* Nux-v; Sang; Sele.

Dark in Agg : Onos.

Occiput, on Agg : Bry; Cact; *Cocl;* Kali-p; Onos; PETR; Pho; *Sep;* Spig.

Amel : Kali-p; Pho-ac.

Right side, on Agg : Pho.

With head low Agg : Pul; Sang.

Amel : *Bry;* Phys; Ver-v.

+ LYING, Something, in : Plant.

MALE VOICE, Hearing Agg : Bar-c.

MEALS, Missing Agg : See Going food without Agg.

MENSES, Before and After Agg : Glo; Kali-p; Lil-t.

During Agg : Croc;Glo; Kali-p; Lac-d.

Instead, of : Croc; Glo; Lith.

Profuse, after Agg : Glo.

Suppressed Agg : Lith; Naj; Psor.

MENTAL Exertion Agg : *Anac;* Cimi; Glo; *Iris; Kali-br;* NAT-C; Nat-p; Pho-ac; *Pic-ac;* Pul; *Sep; Sil;* Zin.

MILK Agg : Bro; Lac-d.

Amel : Bry; Ver-a.

MOTIONS, Of : Alu; *Bell* ; Cam; Cic; Cina; *Cup;* Hyo; Ign; Sep; Spo; Stram; Ver-v.

Agg : Tub.

Convulsive, can not talk or swallow : Nux-m.

Eyes, of Agg : Nat-m.

Nodding to and fro : *Agar;* Chin; Hyo; Hypr; Ign; Nat-m; Sep; Stram; Ver-v.

bending, forwards, when : Hyo.

Rolling : See Rolling.

Swinging backwards and forwards, as if : Pall.

Writing, while : Caus.

MUSIC Agg : Cof; Pho; Pho-ac.

NARCOTICS Agg : Acet-ac; Cof.

NECK, To : Bry; Cimi; Cocl; Kali-c; Lach; Nux-m; Nux-v.

NOISES, Clang, Reverberations etc. in : Ars; *Aur;* Calc-f; Chin; Cop; Iod; Kali-c; Kalm; Kre; Lyc; *Phel;* Pho; Plat; PUL; Sars; Sil; *Stap; Sul;* Zin.

Seminal emission, after : Carb-v.

Sleep, falling to, on : Zin.

Talking, when: Sars.

NOSE, Bleeding Amel : Bry; Buf; Fer-p; Meli; Pic-ac; Psor;

Boring, in Amel : Tarn.

Discharge, from Amel: Cep; Kali-bi; *Lach;* Zin.

Into : Cimi; *Lach;* Mez.

NUMB : Grap; *Kali-br;* Nit-ac; Petr; Plat.

Side, one : Mez.

ODOURS, Strong Agg : Anac.

OPENING And SHUTTING, As if: Calc; Cann; Cimi; *Cocl;* Glo; Lac-c; Sep; Sul; Vib.

OPENS, And Cold air enters in. as if : Cimi.

+ OPERA, Seeing after : Cact.

OUTWARD Extending : Aco; Arn; *Asaf;* BELL; Bism; *Bry;* Canth; Cham; Chin; Con; Dul; Ign; Lach; Lyc; *Mez;* Nat-c; Rhus-t; Sep; Sil; Spig; Sul; Val.

OVER LIFTING Agg : Calc.

+ OVER TAXED, School child : Zin.

+ OVER WORK : Pul.

PAIN, Aching, dull heavy : Aco; Agar; Alo; Am-c; Ars; Bell; Bism; Bry; Cact; Calc; *Carb-v; Chel;* Chin; *Gel;* Glo; Meny; NAT-M; *Nux-v;* Petr; Pho; Pho-ac; *Pul;* Rhus-t; Sep; Sil; *Sul;* Thu; Zin.

Boring, digging : ARG-N; *Caus;* Colo; Hep; IGN;

Sep; Spig.

Bruised, Crushed : Bry; Chin; *Ign;* Ip; Nit-ac; *Nux-v;* Syph.

Bursting, distended : Aco; Arn; *Bell;* BRY; Chin; Fer; *GlO;* Lach; Meli; Merc; Nat- m; *Nux-v;* Spig.

Coition, desire for, with : Sep.

Coldness with : Mos.

hands and feet : Vario.

Crampy : Aco; Ign; Plat.

Cutting Sharp, shooting : Arn; *Bell;* Calc; Lach; Tub.

right : Spig.

left : Sep.

Drawing : Carb-v; Cham; Chin.

Eructation, with : Calc.

Eye, inflammation, with : Bad.

over, one : Pho.

Hair, being pulled as if : *Chin;* Mag-m; Sul.

Hammering : Calc; *Fer;* Lach; Manc; Nat-m; Psor; Sul.

Heart pain, after : Merc-i-f.

Hunger, with : Kali-p.

Lachrymation, with : Mez.

+ scalding : Pul.

Linear : Tell.

Maddening, Shrieks, with: Aco; Ap; Ars; *Bell; Cham;* Colo; Cup; Gel; *Meli;* Sep; *Stram.*

Nail. Clavus, Plug : Cof; *Ign;* Nux-v; Thu.

coryza, with : Form.

Persistent : FER; Lac-d; Terb.

for years : Lac-d.

Pressing, Pressure: *Bry;* Chin; Ign; *Nux-v;* Saba; Stan; Sul.

+ Screwed as if : Kali-io.

Shattered, as if : Aeth; *Arg-m;* Bar-c; *Bell; Bry;* Calc; *Chin;* Cimi; *Ign; Iris;* Merc; *Nux-v;* Pho; Rhus-t; Sil; Sul.

Shooting : Kali-c; Tub.

Sleep, felt during : Ther.

Sore : *Chin;* Gel; Ip; Nux-v; Phyt.

Spot, in a : Cann; Colch; *Ign;* Kali-bi; Kali-io.

Squeezing : See Compression.

Stitching, Stinging : *Arn; Bry;* Caus; *Kali-c;* Nat-m; *Pul* Sul.

sun, standing, in: Bar-c.

Stools pressing at : Lyc; Rat.

Stuperfying, Stunning : *Bell;* Calc; Cocl; Flu-ac; Gel; Hell; Hyo; *Nux-v;* Pho- ac; Spig; Stan; Stap; Verb.

Sutures, along : *Calc-p; Flu-ac.*

Tearing, Rending : *Chin; Lyc; Merc;* Nux-v; Pul; Sul.

Throbbing, Pulsating : *Aco; Bell;* Bry; Cact; Calc;

Chin; GLO; Jab; LACH; Laur;
Led; Lyc; Meli; Nat-m; Pyro;
Sep; *Sil;* Stap; Sul; Ver-v.

cough, after : Lyc.

+ painless : Pyro.

Twinging : Bell; *Bry;* Chin;
Pul; Sul.

vertigo, with : Rhus-t.

Waked, by : Aco; Ars; Chin;
Kali-c; Lach; Nux-v; Sil;
Sul.

OPERA, Seeing, after : Cact.

PRESSURE Amel : Am-c; Ap;
ARG-N; Bell; *Bry;* Cact; Fer;
Lach; Mag-m; Mag-p;
Meny; *Nat-m;* Nux-m; *Pul;*
Stan; *Ver-a.*

Back, on Amel : Sang.

Eyes, on Amel : Nat-m.

Hand, of cold Amel : Calc.

Hat, of Agg : Carb-v; Nit-ac.

Nose, root at Amel : Kali-bi.

Vertex, on, Agg : *Chin;*
Lach; Phys; Ther.

PULLED, Back, as if : Syph.

PUSHED, Forward, as if : Fer-p.

RAIN Agg : Phyt.

Amel: Cham.

READING Amel : Ham; Ign.

RECLINES : Carb-v.

REMOVE, Desire to : Ther.

RETCHING Amel : Asar.

REVERBERATION : See Noise.

ROLLING, Of : Agar; Ap; *Bell;*
Cina; *Hell;* Hyo; *Lyc;* Merc;
Nux-m; POD; Pyro; Tarn;
Ver-v; *Zin.*

Bending, forward, when :
Hyo.

Brain, Concussion of from
: Hyo.

Business worry, from : Pod.

Moaning, and : Merc; Pod.

Side to Side, from Amel :
Agar; Kali-io; Med;
Pho-ac.

Teeth, grinding with : Zin.

ROOM, Crowded Agg : See
Crowded Room Agg.

RUBBING Amel: Ars; Chin;
Tarn; Thu.

Soles, Amel : Chel.

RUBS, Against something :
Tarn.

Hands, with : Ver-a.

RUNNING Agg : *Pul.*

SCHOOL GIRLS Agg : Calc;
Calc-p; Cimi; Mag-p;
Nat-m; Pho-ac; Pul; Saba;
Zin.

Diarrhoea, with : Calc-p.

SCRATCHING Amel : Mang.

SEMINAL Emission Agg : Ham.

SEPERATED From body, as if :
Alo; Alu; Ant-t; Cann; *Daph;*
Nat-c; Nat-m; *Nux-m; Psor;*
Ther.

SEWING Agg : *Lac-c;* Petr.

SEXUAL Desire, suppression
from Agg : Con; Pul.

SHAKING Agg : Bell; Glo;
Nux-m.

Amel : Cina; Gel; Lach; Pho.

Up and down Amel Chin.

+ SHAKES, Without cause :
Lyc.

197

+ Involuntarily : Lyc.

+ Slow, then rapid : Lyc.

SHOPPING, Exertion Agg : Epip; Sep.

SINKING, Downwards, from : Arg-n.

SITTING Erect Amel : Cic; Gel.
Still Amel : Nat-m.

SKULL CAP, Sensation of : Carb-v; Cycl; Grap; Lach.

+ SKULL, Small for brain : Glo.

+ SKULL, Small, too : Cof.

SLEEP During Agg : Ther.
Amel : Nat-m; Sang.

SMOKING Amel : Calc-p; Carb-ac; Lycps.

SNEEZING Agg : Carb-v; Kali-c; Nat-m; Nit-ac; *Pho;* Spig; *Sul.*
Amel : Calc; Calc-p; Lil-t; Lyc; Mur-ac.

SOUP, Warm, Amel : Kali-bi.

SOUR THINGS Agg : Bell; Sele.

SPEECH, Hearing Agg : Bar-c; Lyss; Mag-m.

+ Incoherent : Stram.

STANDING, (Head) on, as if : Ars; Dios; Elap; Glo; Lach; Pho; Pho-ac; Thu.

STIFF : Caus.

STOOL Agg : Manc; Ther.
Amel: Aeth; Agar.
Pressing at Agg : Lyc; Mang.

STOOPING Agg : Fer; Kali-c.
Amel : Cina; Con; Hyo; Ign; Meny; Mez; Nat-s.

STUDENT'S : Ars-io; Aur; Cimi; Iris; Kali-p; Pic-ac.

SUN DOWN Amel : Gel; Lac-d; Sul-io.

Light, Shine Agg : Ant-c; *Bell; Bry;* GLO; *Lach;* *Nat-c;* Nux-v; Pul; Val.
Amel : Grap; Stro.

Shade in Amel : Bro.

SUPPORTS, Hand, with, when Rising or Stopping : Stram

SUPPRESSION, From : Ant-t.

Sexual excitement : Pul.

+ SWASHING of Water, as if : Hell.

SWEAT, On : Am-m; Anac; CALC; CHAM; *Chin;* Guai; Kali-m; Mag-m; MERC; Mur-ac; Pho; *Pul;* Rhe; Sanic; SIL.

Air open, in, walking when : Chin.

Cold : Hep.

Musty : Ap.

Palpitation, with : Calc.

SWEET Things Agg : Ant-c.

+ SWIMMING, In, as if : Ab-c.

TALKING AGG : *Aco;* Cact; *Chin;* Cof; Ign; Mez; NAT- M; *Sil;* SUL.
Amel : Dul; Eup-p; Ham; Lac-d; Sil.

Hearing, distant Agg : Cact; Mur-ac.

TEA Green Amel : Carb-ac.

TEETH, Pressing together Agg : Am-c.
Amel : Sul.
With : Merc; Plant.

THICK, As if : Ther.

TIGHTNESS : Nit-ac; *Nux-v.*

TIP, Fingers of, to : Cam.

TIRED, Weary, as if : Pho; Psor.

+ TOBACCO Smoke Amel : Calc-p; Lycps.

TONGUE, Protruding Agg : Syph.

TOUCH Agg : Aur; *Chin;* Hep; Lyc; Mez; Nit-ac; *Nux-v.*

TURNING AGG : *Calc; Cic;* Kali-c; Pul; Spig; *Spo.*

Quickly Agg : Sang.

Side to side Agg : Cina.

TWISTING, In : Kali-c; Mur-ac; Til.

Side, one, to : Cic; Cup.

UNCOVERING AGG : Ars; Aur; *Bell;* Calc-p; Colch; Con; *Hep;* Hyo; Kali-bi; Lach; Mag-c;Mag-p; Nux-m; Nux-v; *Psor; Rhus-t;* Samb; SIL; Stro.

UNSTEADY, As if : Sul.

URAEMIC : See Urination, suppresion, from.

URINATION, Before, if call is not attended to Agg : Flu-ac; Sep.

During Agg : Colo; Nux-v; *Tab.*

After Amel : Agar; Flu-ac; Gel; Ign; Meli; Sang; Sil.

Frequent, and profuse Amel : Kalm.

Frequent, and scanty then Agg : Iod; Ol-an.

Profuse Agg : Mos.

Amel : *Gel; Ign.*

with : Aco; *Gel; Ign;* Lac-d; Mos; Ol-an; Sele; Sil.

Suppression, from : Arn; *Glo;* Hypr; Sang.

UTERUS, With : Cimi; Helo; Plat; Pul; Sep.

VARIABLE Intensity : Zin.

VERTIGO, After Agg : Calc; Rhus-t.

+ VISE, In as if : Arg-n.

VISUAL Or Eye symptoms with : Bar-c; Bell; Bry; Cocl; Cyc; *Gel;* Hyo; Kali-c; Lach; Lil-t; Nat-c; Pul; Sang; Sep; Sil; Stram; Zin.

VOMITING Agg : Phyt.

Amel : Eup-p; Nat-s; Sang; Stan.

With : Dig; Eup-p; Ip; Sang.

WAKED, By pain : See Under Pain.

WALKING, Motion Agg : Bell; Bry; Carb-v; Led; Mez; Nit-ac; Tub.

Amel : Guai; Rhus-t.

Jarring, of Agg : Stan.

WALKS, With head thrown backward : Arn.

Tip toe on : Crot-h.

WASHER Women's of Agg : Bry; Pho.

WASHING Agg : Canth; Tarn; Zin-chr.

Cold water, with Amel : Ant-t.

Feet, with cold water Amel : Nat-s.

WATER Were poured over : Cup.

WAVING In, as if Glo; Sep.

  Occiput to sinciput : Senec.

WEAK, Persons : Sabal.

WEEKLY Agg : Calc; Epip.

+ WILD Feeling : Lil-t.

  + Sleep, prevents : Lil-t.

WIND Through : See Air.

WINTER Agg : Bism.

WOBBLING About : Abro; Aeth;
Bell; *Calc-p;* Cham; Dig;
Hyo.

  Falls backwards : Dig.

  forwards, or : Colch.

Whooping cough, in : Ver-a.

WRAPPING Agg : Iod; Led; *Lyc;*
Pho; Pul.

  Amel : Cor-r; HEP; Led;
Nux-v; Pho; *Rhus-t.*

WRINKLING Forehead Agg and
Amel : See Frowning.

WRITING Amel : Fer.

YAWNING Agg : Kali-c.

  Amel : Mur-ac; Nat-m; Stap.

HEAD EXTERNAL (SCALP and
SKULL) : *Aco;* Ap; *Ars; Arn; Aur;*
Bar-c; Bell; CALC; CALC-P;
Caps; Chin; Clem; Hep; *Lyc;*
Merc; Mez; *Nit-ac; Nux-v; Old;*
Pho;Pho-ac; Rhod; RHUS-T;
Ru; Sil; Stap; Sul; *Vio-t.*

RIGHT : *Calc;* Canth; Con; Mez;
Sil.

LEFT : Clem; Rut; Thu.

FRONT : Hep; Led; Pho-ac; Sul.

  Bregma : Ars; Merc.

OCCIPUT : Carb-a; *Carb-v; Petr;*
Sil.

SCALP, Contracted, as if : Carb-v.

  Boils, on : Aur; Sanic.

+ Crawling : Arg-m.

  Creeping : Ran-b.

  Damp Agg : Led.

  Drawn back and forth, as
if : Nat-m.

  Eruptions, on : ARS; Bar-c;
Calc; Grap; HEP; *Lyc;*
Merc; Mez; OLD; *Petr;*
RHUS-T; *Sul;* Vio-t.

  ringworm : Dul.

  Fissure : Kali-io.

  Gathered, as if : Chin; Sele.

  Hard : Fer-p.

  Ice cold : Calc. :

  Itching : Anac;

Bar-c; Calc; Calc-s;
GRAP; *Lyc;* Mez; NAT-M;
Old; Pho; Saba; *Sep;* SUL.

+ damp weather : Mag-c.

  day and night : Old.

  Lice : Carb-ac; Merc; *Psor;*
Stap.

+ as if : Led.

  Lumps, Nodes : Caus;
Daph; Grap; Sil.

  headache, with : Sil.

  sore : Hep; Kali-io.

  under : Aur.

  Milk crusts : *Calc; GRAP;*
Lyc; Old; Ol-j; Psor; Sep;
Sul; Tub; Ust; Vio-t.

  cervical glands swelling
of, with : Canc-fl; Vio-t.

  eroding : Stap.

  foul : Calc; Stap; Sul.

  suppressed Agg : Vio-t.

Numb : Plat.

one side : Mez.

Oedema : Ap; Ars.

Sensitive, Painful : Ars;
Bell; Bry; Chin; Hep;
Kali- io; Merc; Merc-d;
Nit-ac; Nux-v; Par; Sil;
Spig; Tub.

  hair, combing, on : Kre;
Nat-s.

Shivering : Mos.

Stiff : Rhus-t.

Sweats : *Calc*; Cham; *Pul*;
Rhe.

+ gushing : Stry.

Swelling, puffy, on : Nit-ac.

  beneath : Sil.

Tension: Alo; Asar; Merc;
Plat; Vio-o.

+ Tight : Adon; Caus.

Under : Rhod.

Wounds, bleeding, from :
Calend.

SIDES : Zin.

SKULL, Lifted, as if : Lac-d.

+ Must press : Carb-an.

Painful : Mez.

Small, too, as if : Chel; Cof;
Glo; Grat.

Tumours, painful : Kali-c.

  perforating : Lach.

TEMPLES : Nat-m.

+ **T**UBERCLES, All over : Syph.

VERTEX : Carb-v; Grap.

Itching : Ver-a.

HEADSTRONG : See Stubborn.

HEALING DIFFICULT (Wounds,
ulcers, etc.) : *Arn; Ars*; Bor;

Calc; *Cham*; Con; Grap; *Hep;*
Kali-bi; *Lach; Lyc;* Merc;
Petr; Sil; *Sul*; Visc.

+ **H**ELPS : Manc.

HEARING ACUTE, Sensitive to
noise : ACO; Aur; BELL;
Caus; Cham; *Chin;* COF;
Con; *Lach; Lyc;* Mur-ac;
Nat-c; Nit-ac; *Nux-v; Op;*
Sabal; Sep; *Sil;* Spig; Tab;
THER; Zin.

  Distant sound : Calend;
Nux-m.

  Dull, and alternately : Cic.

  Heat, during : Caps; Con.

  Menses, during : Hypr.

  Nausea, causing : Cocl; Ther.

  Rumpling of paper, to : Bor;
Nat-c; Nat-s.

  Scratching on linen and
silk, to : ASAR.

  Voices and talking, to : Zin.

  her own (autophoney) :
Bell.

  seem too loud : Caus.

BAD, Deafness, impaired :
Aur; Bar-c; BELL; CALC;
Carb-an; Carb-v; *Caus*;
Chin; Chin-s; CIC; CON;
Cup; Grap; *Hyo*; Kali-m;
Led; LYC; Med; MERC-D;
Nat-m; NIT-AC; *Op; Petr;
Pho*; PHO-AC; PUL; *Sec*;
Sep; SIL; SUL; Ver-v; Verb.

  Abdomen, coldness, in with
: Amb.

  Adenoids, from : Stap.

  Adhesions, in middle ear,
from : Iod.

Bending head backwards
Amel : Flu-ac.

Blowing nose Agg : Sul.
Amel : Mang; Merc; Sil.

Cause, without : Syph.

Cholera, after : Sec.

Colds Agg : Fer-p; Gel;
Kali-m;Mag-c; Merc-d;
Pho.

menses, during Agg : Fer-p.

Concussions, blows, after
: *Arn*; Chin-s; Croc.

Confusion of sounds : *Carb-an.*

Convulsions, after : Sec.

Cotton, stuffed with, as if,
from : Led.

Coughing Agg: Chel.
Amel : Sil.

Direction of sound, can not
tell : Arg-n; Carb- an;
Kali-bi.

Discharges, suppressed
from : Lob.

+ Earache, recurring, from
: Nat-c.

+ Eating Agg : Sul.

Enlarged tonsils from : Hep;
Kali-bi; Merc; Nit-ac; Stap.

Eruptions, suppressed after
: Lob; Mez.

Eustachian tubes, hyper-
trophy, from : Ars-io.

+ occlusion, from : Kali-m.

Exanthemata, after : Carb-v.

Hear, can distant sound :
Calend.

Human voice, to : Ars;
Cheno; Pho; Sul.

except for : Ign.

Indistinct : Bov.

Infectious diseases, after
: See Typhoid fever, after.

Leaf or membrane before
the ear, as if from :
Ant-c; Verb.

shaking and boring in
ear Amel : Sele.

Measles, after : Nit-ac; Pul.

Menses, at : Fer-p; Kre.

absent with : Nat-c.

Misunderstanding, of :
Bov; Pho.

Morning Amel : Rhod.

Moving quickly, on : Ver-v.

Nervous : Aur; Jab; Syph.

Night, at : Elap.

Noise Amel : Calend;
Grap; Jab; Nit-ac.

Old people, in : Bar-c; *Cic*;
Petr.

One, in, noises in other :
Amb.

Otalgia, after : Caps; Nat-c.

Paralysis of auditory
nerve from : Caus; Glo;
Hyo; Kali-n; Kali-p; Sil.

+ Periodically : Spig.

Pressure, ear on, Amel :
Pho.

+ Quinine : Calc.

Riding in carriage Amel :
Calend; Grap; *Nit-ac*; Pul.

Room, warm in Amel : Pul.

Rubbing Amel : Pho.

Scarlet fever, after : Carb-v;
Lyc; Sul.

Sexual excess, after : *Petr.*

Snap, report Amel   : Sil.

Sound seem far off : Lac-c.

Speech, embarassed,
with : Aur.

Spinal fever, after : Sil; Sul.

Stooping Amel : Croc.

Sudden : Elap; Gel; *Mag-c;*
Plb; Sep; Sil.

plugs as from : Sep.

Swallowing Amel : Merc.

Syphilis hereditary, from :
Lac-c.

Tympanum, injury, from :
Tell.

Typhoid fever, after : Ap;
Arg-n; Ars; Nit-ac; Pho-ac.

Walking, motion (quick)
Agg   : Chin-s; Ver-v.
Amel : Merc-i-r.

Water getting in ear, from
: Verb.

+ working, in : Calc.

Wax, hardened from : Sele.

Weather, damp Agg : Mang.

+ Wisdom tooth, cutting from
: Mag-c.

Yawning Amel : Sil.

EAR, Not his own, with: Psor

FALSE, Misunderstanding :
Bov; Pho.

FOOT STEPS, In next room : Nat-p.

FOREHEAD, Through, as if : Sul.

ILLUSORY SOUNDS, Noises : *Bell;*
Cact; *Calc;* Cann; *Caus;*
CHIN; *Chin-s;* Cimi; Grap;
Kali-io; Lyc; Mang; Petr;
Pho-ac; Psor; *Pul;* Radm;
Sang; Spig; Spo; *Sul;* Thyr;

Tub. Val.

Blowing nose on : Bar-c;
Carb-an; Mang; Pho-ac;
Stan.

Chewing, while : Bar-m;
Calc; Grap; Iod; *Kali-s;*
Meny; Nat-m; *Nit-ac;* Petr.

Climaxis, at : Sang.

Coition Agg : Carb-v; Dig;
Grap.

Confused, voices : Benz-ac.

Convulsions, after : Ars;
Caus.

Coughing, on : Kali-m.

Crackling : Ars; Cof; Dig;
Glo; *Phel.*

Crashings, Explosions :
Alo; Ars; Bar-c; *Dig;* Glo;
Grap; Kali-c; Mos; Nit-ac;
Petr; *Phel;* Pho; *Rhus-t;*
Saba; Sil; Zin.

Deafness, with : Cimi.

Door, beating at : Ant-c.

Ear, passing hand, over
Agg : Mar-v;

Echoes, reverberating :
Caus; Colo; Lyc; *Pho;* Sep.

loud   : Pho-ac.

+ music : Pho.

words : Bell; Sars.

Fever, during : *Ars;* Lach;
Nux-v; Tub.

Fluttering : Plat; Spig.

Gurgling, bubbling : Lyc;
Nat-c.

Headache, during : *Chin;*
Form; Naj; Pul; Sil.

Hissing   : Dig; Mar-v.

+ boiling water, as if : Dig; Thu.

Horn blowing : Kalm.

Humming, Buzzing : Arg-n; Calc; Cann; *Chin*; Chin-s; Kali-c; Lyc; Nux-v; Plat; PUL; Sep; *Sul.*

+ vertigo, with : Arg-n.

Inspiring, forcibly, when : Mar-v.

Lying Agg : Fer-p.

Amel : Bar-c; *Pho-ac.*

Morning Amel : Rhod.

Music, as if : Cann; Merc.

Nauseous taste, with : Naj.

Pain, with : *Ars*; Lach.

Pulsating : Bell; *Calc;* Cann; *Fer-p*; Nit-ac; *Pho;* Pul.

Ringing : Bell; Cact; Calc; Calc-s; Cann; Carb-v; CHIN; Kali-c; Kali-io; Kali s; Lyc; *Nux-v;* Petr; Plat; Psor; *Pul;* Sep; Sul.

bell : Pyro.

+ deafness with : Arg-n.

haemorrhage, during : Chin.

headache, during : Chin.

menses, before : Fer.

Roaring, rumbling : *Aur;* Bar-c; *Bell;* Bor; Carb-v; *Caus;* Chin; Chin-s; *Grap;* Lyc; *Nux-v;* Pho-ac; *Pul;* Sil; Spig; *Stap; Sul.*

music Amel : Ign.

+ pulse, synchronises with : Kali-br.

Rushing : Kali-c; Lyc; Nat- m; Nit-ac; *Pho; Petr.*

water, as of : *Cham;* Cocl; Pul; Radm; Ther.

Singing : Chin; Kali-c.

Sneezing Agg : Bar-c; Bar-m.

Stools, after : Calc-p.

during : Lyc.

Stooping on : Croc.

Swallowing, on : Bar-c; Benz-ac; Calc; Cic.

empty : Thu.

Swashing : Sul.

Talking Agg : Mar-v; Nat-c; Op; Spig.

Tickling:Chin; Grap; Zin-val.

Vetigo, during : Bell; *Chin-s;* Dig; Op; Pho; Psor.

+ Voices of absent persons : Cham.

Water boiling, as if in : Cann; Dig; Thu.

+ falling from height : Nat-p.

Yawning Agg : Mang.

+ Noise, Every, in sleep : Alum, (See Sleep light).

Perversion Of : Calc.

Sound, Seem distant, while : Lac-c; Sabal.

Variable : Cheno.

HEARING Talk Agg : See Talk Hearing Agg.

HEART : ACO; Ars; *Aur; Bell;* Bry; Buf; CACT; *Calc; Carb-v;* Chin; DIG; *Fer-p;* Glo; Iod; *Kali-c; Kalm; Lach;*

Lith; *Lil-t;* Lob; LYCPS; *Naj;*
Nat-m; PHO; Pru-sp; PUL;
Scil; Sep; SPIG; Spo; Strop;
SUL; Tab; Tarn; Thyr; Ver-a;
Ver-v; Zin-io.

ACHING : Lith; Spo; Strop; Tab;
Ver-v.

Dysmenorrhoea, with:
Crot-h.

Headache, with : Crot-h.

ALTERNATING, With : Benz-ac;
Glo; Kalm; Nat-m; Nat-p;
Strop;Visc.

Abdomen, with : Merc-i-f.

+ Aphonia, with : Ox-ac.

Piles, with : Coll.

ANGER Agg   : Cup.

ANGINA : See Angina Pectoris.

ANUS, Wiping Agg : Ap.

ANXIETY, Anguish, with :
ACO; Arn; Ars; *Aur;* Calc;
Carb-v; Dig; Ign; Ip; *Pho;*
Plat; *Pul;* Spig; Strop; Sul;
Ther; Ver-a.

Evil, something going to
happen, as if   : Meny.

APEX Region : Ap; Lil-t; Sul.

Base to : Med.

Cutting : Zinch-chr.

Painful : Lil-t.

ARMS, To : Alu; Bar-c; *Cact;*
Carb-v; Dios; Glo;Kali-n;
Kalm; Latro; Lyc; Pho; Spig;
Stic.

Right : Bor; Kre; Ox-ac;
Pho; Plb; Phyt.

Left : *Aco;* Ars; Cact; Cimi;
Dig; Kalm; Lach; *Latro;*
Lil-t; Pho; Pul; RHUS-T;

SPIG; Strop; Tab; TARN; Thyr.

shoulder, and : Fago;
Scop; Thu.

mammae, from : Lith.

ASCENDING Agg: Ars; Aur;
Calc; Nit-ac.

Descending, and : Lac-d.

AXILLAE, To : Kali-n; Latro; Thyr.

BACKWARD (To Left Scapula) :
Agar; Alo; Cimi; *Kali-c;*
Kalm; Lach; Laur; *Lil-t;* Mez;
Naj; Rhus-t; Rum; SPIG; Sul;
Tab; Ther; Thu.

From : Cimi; Kali-c; Spig;
Ther.

BALL, As of a : Lil-t.

BASE To apex : Syph.

Painful : Lob.

BEATS, Audible : Ars; Ars-io;
Bism; *Pul;* Saba; *Spig;* Sul.

Back, heard in : Abs.

Body over whole : Bell; Fer;
Glo; Kali-c; Lach; Nat-m.

Ceasing, as if : *Aur;*
Chin-ar; Cic; Cimi; *Conv;*
DIG; Gel; Lob; Rum; Vib.

and start suddenly : *Aur;*
Conv.

then heavy throbbing :
Rum.

trembles and throbs
inspiration, Amel :
Arg-m; Arg-n.

Ear, felt, in : Glo; Pyro; Thyr.

Face, felt, in: Mur-ac.

Hard : Spo; Zin.

occasional : Sep.

Head, felt, in : Phys.

Heavy: Lycps.

Neck, upto : Bad.

One hard : Sep; Zin.

Shaking the body : Ap; Arn; Mur-ac; Nat-m; Rhus-t.

Strong : Rhod.

occasional : Hyd-ac.

Throat, felt, in : Phys.

Thumping : Aur; Iod; Rhod; Spo; Zin.

Unsteady : Tab.

Violent : Gel; Ver-v.

Visible : Ars; Iber; Kalm; Lach; *Spig*; Sul; Ver-a.

Water, in as if : Sumb.

BENDING Double Agg : Lith; Spig.

BIG, Seems, too : Lach; Sul.

BLADDER (Urinary), with: Lith.

BLOCK, As of a: Stro.

BOILING, In region : Glo; Lach.

BREATH, Holding Agg : Cact.

BUBBLE Starts from, and passes into arteries : Nat-p.

BUBBLING, In region : Bell; Lach; Lachn; Lyc.

BURNING : *Aco*; Ars; Aur; Bry; Calc; Cup; Hyo; Kalm; Op; *Pho*; Pul; Rhus-t; Sul; Syph; Ver-v.

Ascends, impeding breathing : Croc.

Fire, on, as if : Kali-c; Op; Tarn.

BURSTING, Distended : Glo; Pho; Zin.

+ CAVITY, In place of : Med.

CHOCOLATE Agg : Raph.

CHURCH Bell ringing Agg : Lyss.

CLUTCHED And released alternately : *Cact* ; Iod; Lil-t.

CLUTCHING : Thyr.

Short breath, from : Thyr.

COITION After Agg : Dig.

COLD : ACO; Ars; Bov; Carb-an; Grap; *Helod*; Kali-bi; Kali-chl; Kali-m; Lil-t; Nat-m; Petr; Rhus-t; Sul-io; *Ver-a*.

Drops were falling, on, as if : Cann.

Horripilation, with : Carb-an.

Icy, chill, during : Nat-m.

COMPRESSION, Constriction Squeezed, Grasped : Am-c; Arn; *Ars*; Ars-io; CACT; Colch; IOD; Lach; LIL-T; Radm; Spig.

Cap like : Zin.

Drinking water Amel : Pho.

Walk erect, can not : Lil-t.

CONGESTION : Aco; Glo;Pho.

COUGHING Agg : Aur; Pho.

CRACKLING : Spig; Spo.

CUTTING : Ars; Colch; Sul; Ver-a.

+ DEBILITY, Influenza, after : Iber.

DILATATION :Adon; *Cact;* Chlo-hyd; Cratae; Dig; Grind; Naj; Spig; Tab.

Shock, from : Tab.

DRAWN Down, as if : Thu.

DRINKING Agg : Con; Cup.

DROP, Down, as if: Hypr.

DROPSY (Hydro-pericardium) : Ars; Ascl; Colch; Dig; Lyc.

EARS, To : Thyr.

EMPTY, Hollow, as if: Cocl; Grap; Med; Sul.

ENDOCARDITIS : Ars; Aur; Kalm; *Lach;* Naj; Spig; *Zin-io.*

Septic : Naj.

EXERTION Agg : Cact; Dig; Lil-t; Nit-ac; Strop; Tab.

EYES, With : Lith; Spig; Spo.

FALLING Down, as if : Laur.

FATTY Degeneration : Adon; Arn; Ars; Ars-io; Aur; Aur-m; Cact; Kali-c; Pho; Phyt.

FLOATS : Bov; *Buf;* Kali-io; Sumb.

FLUTTERING, Trembling : Ars; *Calc;* Chin; Cic; Cimi; Crot-h; DIG; Kalm; *Lil-t;* Naj; Nat-m; Nux-m; Nux-v; Rhus-t; SPIG; Strop; Tarn.

Air, in, as if : Buf.

Body, all over : Phys.

+ Excitement, least: Amyl-n.

Head, felt in : Phys.

Menses, after : Nat-p.

Then blood rushes to head : Cinb.

Throat, felt in : Phys.

Vexation, after : Lith.

FOOT, Sweat suppressed Agg : Aur; Bar-c.

FORAMEN OVALE, Non-closure of : Calc-p.

FORCEPS, Delivery, after : Cact.

FORMICATION, Crawling : Canth; Kalm; Nux-v.

FULNESS : Aur; Lach; Sul; Ver-v.

GOITRE, During : Ars; Buf; *Crot-h;* Lach; Latro; Lycps; Pho; *Spo;* Thyr.

GURGLING : Psor.

HANDS, Over : Buf; Cup; Hyd-ac; Laur; Lil-t; Naj; Nat-m; Pul; Tarn.

Wetting in cold water Agg : Tarn.

HANGING By the thread as if : Aur; *Kali-c;* Lach; Lil-t; Nux-m.

Rib, left, floating from : Kali-c.

HARD, As if : Nat-c.

HEAD, Alternating, with : Amy-n; Glo; Nux-m; Strop; Tab.

Congestion, with : Scop.

Extending, to : Glo; Lachn; Lith; Med; Nux-m; Pho; Sep; Spig; Spo; Strop.

Then : Merc-i-f.

With : Lach; Naj.

HEAT, Ascending to : Croc.

+ Yawning Amel : Croc.

HEAVY : Aur; Lil-t; Pul; Spig; Tub.

HOLLOW : See Empty.

HYPERTROPHY : Aco; Aur; Bro;Cact; Iber; Kali-c; Kalm; Lith; Lyc; Naj; Pru-s; Spo;

Thyr.

Compensatory : Adon.

Gymnastics, from : Bro; Rhus-t; Thyr.

Palpitation, with : Bro.

IMPEDED : Rum.

INFECTIOUS, Diseases after : Naj; Scop.

INFLUENZA, After : Adon.

JOINTS, Alternating, with : Nat-p.

JUMPING : Aur; Merc-i-f; Tarn; Thyr.

KNOCKING At : Pru-s.

+ LARGE, Feels : Buf.

LEANING, Backwards Agg : Glo.

LIFTED Up or rising up, as if : Colo; Pod; Spo; Val.

Throat, to : Caus; Glo; Phyt; Pod.

LIVELY : Strop.

LIVER Symptoms, with : Agar; Aur; Cact; Calc; Dig; Mag-m; Myr.

LOOSE, As if : Aur; Crot-h.

Walking on : Aur.

LOVE Sickness, from: Cact.

LUNG Affections, with: Pho.

LYING Agg : Aur; Spo; Thyr.

Amel : Laur; Naj; Psor; *Spig.*

Back on Amel : Cact; Fago; Psor; Tell.

Right side on Agg : Alu; Arg-n; Bad; Cimi; Kali-n; Lach; Lil-t.

Left side on Agg : Crot-h.

MASTURBATION Agg : Bar-c.

MENSES, At Agg : Lith.

METASTASIS To : Aur; Kalm; Lach; Lyc.

MOTION Agg : Con; Dig; Mag-m; Spig.

Amel :Aur; Caus; Colch; Gel; Glo; Mag-m; Rhus-t.

MUSCLE Exhaustion : Arn; Chin-ar; Zin-io.

+ MYOCARDITIS : Ars-io.

NARROW Space,as if, in : Eup-p.

NECK And Throat, to: Ars; Bad; Bell; Glo; Naj; Pho; Phys; Scop; Spig; Spo.

Electric shock : Grap.

NEEDLES, At : Cimi; Lyss; Manc.

+ NEPHRITIS, After : Adon.

NUMB : Kalm.

OCCIPUT To : Ars.

OPPRESSED: Ars; Aur; Cact; Ip; Lycps; Pul; Scop; Spig.

Walking Amel : Colch.

PALPITATION : ACO; Agar; Amy-n; Arg-n; *Ars;* Ars-io; *Aur; Cact;* CALC; *Cham; Chin;* Colch; Con; CRATAE; *Dig; Glo;* IOD; Kali-bi; *Kali-c; Kalm;* Lach; *Lil-t;* LYC; MERC; Naj; NAT-M; Nat-p; *Nit-ac;* NUX-V; *Pho;* Pho-ac; PUL; *Rhus-t;* SEP; SPIG; *Spo;* Strop; SUL; Tab; *Thu;* Thyr; VER-A; Zin-io.

Head, beating in, with : Nat-m.

congestion : Scop.

Anxious, Nervous : ACO;

ARS; *Aur*; Bro; Calc; Carb-v; Chin; *Cof*; CRATAE; *Dig*; Grap; Lach; MOS; Naj; *Nat-m*; Ol-an; *Pho*; *Pho-ac*; PUL; SPIG; Strop; Sul; Sumb; Thu; *Val*; *Ver-a*.

+ thunderstorm, after : Nat-p.

Aphonia, alternating, with : Ox-ac.

Arm, left holds, during : Aur.

Attacks of : Bar-c; Cann; Mang; Old; Pho.

Attention is directed to anything, when : Nat-c.

Audible, extending, limbs to : Aesc.

Back pain, with : Tub.

+ Bathing Agg : Bov.

Bathing, Cold Amel : Iod.

+ Body, through out : Arg-n.

Breathing deep Agg : Spig; Tub.

Amel : Arg-m; Carb-v.

holding Agg : Cact.

Breathlessness, with : Strop.

Chest expanding on : Lach.

tightness, with : Chel.

Chill, before : Chin.

during : Merc; Nat-m.

Chronic : Strop.

Climaxis, at : Sumb.+

Coition, during : Agar; Calc; Lyc; *Pho*; Pho-ac; Visc.

after : Dig; Sec; Sep.

Continuous : Calc; Carb-v; Cratae; Sul.

Convulsions, before : Cup; Glo.

Coryza, with : Anac.

Coughing Agg : Calc; Iber; Nat-m; Ol-j; Pul; Sul.

Dinner, after : Pul.

Disappointed love, from : Cact; Ign; *Nat-m*; Pho-ac.

Drinking, after : *Con*.

cold water : Thu.

Dyspnoea, with : Merc-i-f; Spo.

Emissions, after : Asaf.

+ Emotions, pleasurable : Bad.

slight Agg : Calc-ar; Lith.

Epigastrium, in : Med.

Epistaxis, with : Grap.

Eructation Amel : Aur; Bar-c; Carb-v; Mos.

Excitement, after : Arg-n; Pho.

Exertion, Slight Agg : Ars; Calc; Calc-ar; Chin-s; Con; Dig; Lil-t; Rhus-t; Spig; Sumb; Thyr.

Amel : Mag-m.

Eyes, closing Amel : Carb-an.

Face, felt, in : Mur-ac.

pale, with : Amb.

+ red : Agar.

Faintness, with : Cocl; *Crot-h*; Hyd-ac; Lach; Laur; Lil-t; *Nux-m*; Pul; Ver-a.

Fear, with : Nit-ac.

Fever, in : Ars; Calc; Nit-ac; Pul.

Fistula in ano, with : Cact.

Foetus, first movement from : Sul.

Fright, after : Dig.

  as from : Nux-m.

Goitre, with : Pho.

Grief, from : Dig; Op.

+ Growth fast, with : Pho-ac.

Haemoptysis, with : Mill.

Hammering : Thyr.

Hands, tremors, with : Bov.

+ Hands, washing in cold water from : Tarn.

Headache with: Bro; Calc-ar.

  beating in, with : Nat-m.

  congestion, with : Scop.

Hot, drinks Amel : Nux-m.

  feeling, with : Ant-c.

Hunger, from: Kali-c.

Hymn tune in church, from : Carb-an.

Hysterical : Sumb.

  nose bleeding with : Agn.

Lachrymation, with : Am-c.

Laughing, on : Iber.

Limbs, trembling, with : Cof.

Lying Agg : Kali-n; Merc; Nux- v; Ox-ac; PUL; *Sul;* Thyr.

  back on Agg : Ars; Merc-i-f.

    Amel : Kalm; Lil-t.

  left side on Agg : Bar-c; Bro; Cact; Nat-c; Nat-m; *Pho; Psor;* Pul; Sep; Zin-io.

    Amel : Ign; Mag-m.

  right side, on, Agg : Alu; Arg-n; Bad; Kali-n; Kalm;

Lil-t; Plat.

  Amel : Lach; Nat-c; *Pho; Psor;* Tab.

Maids, old, in : Bov.

Masturbation Agg : Fer.

Menses before : Cact; Cup; *Spo.*

  Amel : Eupi.

  suppressed from : Cyc.

  with : Buf; Crot-h; Ign; Phys.

Mental exertion Agg : Calc-ar; Cocl.

Metastasis, from : Abro; Aur; Cact; Colch; Dig; Iod; Kalm; Lach; Naj; *Pho;* Spig; Spo; Sul.

Morning, waking, on: Kali-c; Nux-v.

Motion, walking Agg : Aur-m; Cact; Chin; Dig; Naj; Pho; Psor; Spig.

  Amel : Arg-n; *Fer;* Gel; Lob; Mag-m; Nux-m; Rhus-t.

  every Agg : Chin.

  quick Agg : Cocl.

Mouth foul odour, from, with : Spig.

Music, when listening to : Amb; Kre; Stap.

Nausea, with : Arg-n; Bro.

Nervous : See Anxious.

Noise from every strange: Nat-c; *Nat-m.*

Occiput, to : Cimi; Sep.

Pain changing locality when : Lach.

Painful : Mag-m; Spo.

Periodical : Chel.

Pleasurable emotions, from : Bad; Cof.

Preaching Agg : Naj.

Pregnancy during : Arg-m; Lil-t.

Pressure with hand Amel : Arg-n.

Puberty Agg : Aur.

Pulsations, through the body with : Saba.

Sadness, as from : Nux-m.

Sexual excess, from : Sec.

Sighing Amel *: Arg-m.*

Sitting, when Agg : Asaf; Mag-m; Pho; Rhus-t; *Spig.* Amel : Cact; Lach.

Sleep, in : Merc-c. unable to : Cimi; *Ign;* Spig.

Stiff, as if : Aur-m.

Stool, after Agg : Agar; *Ars; Con;* Cratae; Grat. during   : Ant-t. loose, with : Ant-t.

Stooping Agg : Nat-c; Spig; Thyr.

Stop, must : Aur.

Sudden : Mos.

Suffocative feeling, with : Calc-ar.

Sun heat Agg : Cof.

Sweat, with : Jab; Spo; Tab; *Ver-a.* cold, with : Am-c.

Takes the breath, away : Chin.

Talking Agg : *Naj;* Pul. impossible : Naj.

Thinking of it Agg : Alum; Sumb. wrong of, on Agg : Iod.

Throat, to : Nat-m; Spo.

+ Thunderstorm, after : Nat-p.

+ Tobacco Amel : Agar.

+ Tumultous : Agar; Amy-n.

Urination, profuse with : Cof. affections, of, with : Laur. scanty, with : Ap.

Uterus, soreness of, with : Conv.

Vertigo, with : Adon; Aeth; Cact; Cocl; *Iber;* Spig. throat choking, with : Iber.

Violent: Arg-n; Calc; *Cratae;* Dig; Glo; Iod; Kali-c; *Lycps;* Mur-ac; Nat-m; *Pul;* Sep.

Visible: Bov; *Carb-v;* Glo; Kalm; Naj; Sep; *Spig;* Ver-a. apex beat, through, clothing : Mag-p.

Waking, on : Lach; Naj; Pho. suddenly, on : Chin-s.

Washing hands in cold water : See Hands Washing.

Water in, as if : Bov; Sumb.

Weakness with : Hyds.

Women, looking at : Pul.

Writing,when: Fer-p; Nat-c.

Wrongs, real or imaginary, from : Iod.

PLUG At : Ran-sc.

PRESSURE Of Hands Amel : See Hands over.

PURRING : Glo; Iod; Pyro; *Spig.*

RADIATING, From : Aco; Glo; *Kalm; Spig.*

REFLEX From : Asaf; Naj.

RESTLESS : Ars.

REVOLVING As if : Ant-t.

RHEUMATISM, After : Adon; Aur; Benz-ac; Gel; Kalm; *Lach;* Spig.

RIDING, Carriage, in Agg : Naj.

RIGHT Side, as if, on : Bor; Ox-ac;*Phyt.*

RISING, As if : See Lifted.

Seat from Agg : Gel.

RUBBING Amel : Lil-t.

SCAPULA, To, left : Agar; Kalm; Naj.

+ Arm, and : Kalm.

+ SENILE : Ars-io.

SHOCKS, At : Calc; Con; Lith; Nux-v.

Coughing Agg : Agar.

Electric : Sep.

Eructation Agg : Agar.

Noise, sudden Agg : Agar.

SHORT Breath : Strop; Thyr.

SHOULDER And Neck, to : Naj; Scop.

Left, arm and : Fago.

SITTING Agg : Mag-m.

Erect Agg : Aco.

SMOTHERED, As if : Stro; Thyr.

SNEEZING Agg : Agar; Bor; Dros; Merc.

SORE, Bruised : AP; ARN; Bap; BAR-C; Cact; *Cimi;* Flu-ac; Lach; *Lith; Lycps; Nat-m;* Spig.

Foot sweat suppressed Agg : Aur; Bar-c.

SPACE,Too small, as if, in: Eup-p.

SPINE, Touching Agg : Tarn.

SQUEEZED, As if : Iod.

STAGNATED Sensation: Lyc; Saba; Zin.

STAIRS, Going up and down Agg : Lac-c.

STOOLING Agg : Con.

STOOPING Agg : *Lith;* Lil-t; Old.

STOPS, As if : See Beats, ceasing as if.

SURGING Upward : See Lifted up.

SWELLED, Full, as if : Asaf; Cimi; Glo; *Lach;* Pyro; Sep; Sul.

SWAYING By the thread, as if : Tub.

SYMPTOMS, Few, with : Naj.

Vary, with : Lycps.

TENSION : Radm.

THROB, One : Zin.

TIRED, Feeling: Crot-h; Kali-bi; Lil-t; Naj; Nux-v; Op; Pho; Pyro; Rhus-t; Strop; Ver-a; Zin-io.

Lung troubles, chronic after : Ars-io.

TOBACCO Agg : Cact; Kalm; Scop.

Toe, Big, alternating, with : Nat-p.

Torn loose And swinging by thread, as if : Dig.

Tremors : See Fluttering.

Tumultous : Aco; Amy-n; Lycps.

Turns Over, twists : Ap; Arn; Cact; Caus; Crot-h; *Lach*; Rhus-t; *Sep*; Tab; Tarn.

Twitching : Aesc; Arg-m;Cam

Undulating, As if: Benz-ac; Spig.

Warm : Rhod.

Unsteady : Tab.

Urinating Amel : Lith; Nat-m.

Valves : *Bar-c*; Calc; Calc-f; *Kali-c*; Lach; Laur; Naj; Pho; *Pul*; Spo; *Strop; Tarn*; Thyr; Zin-io.

+ Aortic obstruction : Kalm.

Incompetent : Cact; Cratae; Kali-c; Spo.

Mitral and Tricuspid regurgitation : Apoc; Cact; Laur; Psor; Strop.

Walking Amel : Colch.

Water, As if in : See Floats.

Weak : See Tired feeling.

Entering cool room from a walk in hot sun : *Rhus-t*.

Whirling About, as if : Cact; Iod.

Wine Agg : Glo.

HEARTBURN : Aesc; Amb; Am-c; *Calc; Carb-v;* Cic; *Con; Croc*; Fer-p; Lyc; Mag-c; NUX-V; PUL; Sumb.

Dinner, After : Merc-i-r.

Fats Agg : Nat-c.

Horripilation, With : Calend.

Milk, After : Amb.

Palpitation, With : Nat-m.

Sweets Agg : Zin.

Water, Burning : Ars.

HEAT *AG*G (Feels Too Hot) : Aco; Alu; *Ant-t;* AP; *Arg-n; Bell; Bry; Carb-v;* Cham; Coc-c; Cyc; Dros; Euphor; *Flu-ac;* GEL; *Glo;* Guai; IOD; Kali-io; Kali-m; LACH; Led; LIL-T; Lyc; Med; Merc; Nat-c; NAT-M; *Nat-s;* Op; *Pul;* Rat; Sabi; *Sang; Sec; Sul.*

Amel (Warmth of bed, external heat Amel*)* : Ars; *Bell; Bry;* Caus; *Cham;* Chin; Clem; Cocl; Dros; GRAP; HEP; Hyo; *Kali-bi;* KALI-C; Led; *Lyc;* Mag-c; *Mag-p;* MERC; Nat-c; *Nux-m;* NUX-V; Pho; RHUS-T; Rum; *Samb; Scil;* Sep; SIL; STRO; SUL; Zin.

Cold, And Agg : Ant-c; Calc; *Caus;* Cimi; Fer; *Flu-ac;* Grap; Hell; Kali-c; Lach; MERC; *Nat-m; Pho-ac;* Phys; Sep; Sil; Sul; Sul-ac; Syph.

Amel : Syph.

Extreme Agg : Ant-c; Caus; Ip; Lach; Sul-ac; Syph.

Fire Of Amel : See Stove of Amel.

RADIATING AGG : Ant-c.
    AMEL : Mez.
STEAM, Of AGG : Kali-bi.
STOVE, Of AMEL : Ars; Bov;
    Hep; Ign; Lach; Rum; Tub.
HEAT See Burning, Fever
    EXHAUSTION : Aco; Helo;
    Nat-c; *Sele;* Ver-v; Zin-io.
    FEVER Without : Cham; Grap;
    Ign; Lach.

FLUSHES, IN : *Amy-n;* Buf; *Calc;*
    Carb-an; Caus; Cocl; Coll;
    Flu-ac; Glo; LACH; Lyc;
    Mang; Nat-s; Nit-ac; *Pho;*
    Psor; *Sang; Sep;* Stro; *Sul;*
    Sul-ac; Sumb; Thu; Thyr; TUB.
    Bone pains, with : Flu-ac.
    Cardiac pain, with : Spo.
    Chill, then : Thyr.
    Eating, after : Tub.
    Face, in : Caus; Sang; Stro.
    Fixed, ideas, with : Pho.
    Head, to : Sang.
      ache, with : Sang.
    Hot water, immersed in, as
      if : Pho.
    Menses, during : Nat-m.
    Motion Amel : Sul-ac.
    Pain, with : Cam.
    Palpitation, with : *Kali-c.*
    Piles, with: Coll.
    Sleep, falling to, on : *Con;*
      Lach.
    Steam, being over, as if :
      Pulex.
    Stooping Agg : Merc-c.

Sudden : Mang; Sep.
Sweat, with : Sep; *Tub.*
  cold, then : Amy-n;
    Sul-ac; Hyr.
  sticky : Kali-bi.
Thinking of it Agg : Spo.
Throbbing, general, with:
  Sul.
Tired, when : Helo.
Trembling, then : Sep;
  Sul-ac.
Upper parts, in : Sul-ac.
Upwards : Glo; Sep.
Waking, on : Lach.
Warm, water dashed over
  one, as if : Pul; Rhus-t.
  ingesta Agg : Sul-ac.
  were poured over one,
    as if : *Ars; Psor;* Pul;
    Rhus-t; *Sep.*
INTOLERABLE : Sabi.
ITCHING, With : Alu.
LIVELY Impression, from :
  Pho.
MENTAL, Exertion Agg : Old.
ONLY, disagreeable : Val.
PARTIAL : *Aco; Ap;* ARS; *Bell;*
  Bor; Bry; Calc; *Canth;*
  Caps; Carb-v; Caus;
  Cham; Lyc; *Merc;* Mos;
  Nux-v; PHO; Pho-ac; *Pul;*
  Rhus-t; Sep; SUL; Ver-v.
  Affected part : Guai.
  External : Ars; Bell; Merc;
    Pho; Pho-ac; Sul.
  Internal : Aco; Bell; Bry;
    Canth; Laur; Merc-c;
    Pho; Sul.
PUNGENT, Glowing : Cep;
  Rut; Tarn-c.

Head to, feet from : Visc.

SHIVERS, With : Ars; Sec.

SIDE ONE of, other cold : Ap; Par.

Lain on : Mag-m.

SPOTS, In : Tub.

STOOPING, On : Merc-c.

SWEAT, Hot, with : Glo.

WEAKNESS, With : Spo.

HEATED BY FIRE, SUN,
Becoming Heated AGG : *Aco; Ant-c;* BELL; Bor; *Bry;* Carb-v; *Gel;* GLO; Iod; Ip; Kali-c; Kali-s; Lach; Lyss; Merc; *Nat-c;* Nat-m; Op; Pul; Samb; Sele; Sil; Ther;Ver-v; Zin.

AMEL : ARS; IGN.

EASILY Bro; Kali-n; Nit-ac.

HEAVINESS, LOAD : Aesc; Alet; Alo; Alu; Ap; Arg-n; Ars-io; Bell; Bism; *Bry; Calc; Chel; Con;* GEL; Helo; Ip; Lach; Lapp; Lil-t; Lith; Lyc; Meny; *Nat-m;* NUX-V; Par; Petr; PHO; Pho-ac; Pic-ac; PUL; Ran-b; *Rhus-t;* SEP; Scop; Sil; Spig; *Spo; Stan;* Stic; SUL.

+ AFFECTED PART : Elap.

LIGHTNESS, Alternating, with : Nux-v.

PARALYTIC : Stan.

+ WHOLE BODY : Am-c;Cast-eq.

HECTIC FEVER : See Fever.

SPOTS : See Face.

+ **HEEDLESS** : Am-c.

HEELS : Am-m; Calc; Caus;

Con; Fer; Grap; Ign; Led; Mang; Nat-c; Pul; Sabi; Sep.

BONE Would push through, as if : Con.

BURNING : Cyc; Grap; Ign.

Coal red hot applied to, as if : Visc.

Near each other, when : Ign.

CALF, To : Anac.

COLD : Merc; Sang; Sep.

Touching each other when : Ign.

CONTRACTION : Colch.

CORNS : Pho.

CUTTING : Mag-m.

ELEVATING Amel : Phyt.

FORMICATION : Grap; Sul.

ITCHING : Caus; Med; Pho; Pho-ac.

KICKS : Stic.

NUMB : Alu; Ign; Lyc; Stram.

Sitting, while : Con.

Stepping on : Alu.

OS CALCIS Painful : Aran; Cinb.

PAINFUL : Am-m; *Mang;* Med; *Pul; Rhod;* Val.

Intermittent : Sabi.

Lying back, on Agg : Fer.

Standing long, after : Zing.

Walking Amel : Cyc; *Val.*

PIERCING : Nat-s.

PINCHED, By narrow shoes, as if : Chel; Ran-b.

PURPLE : Pul.

Red : Petr.

+ RED Hot Coal : See Under

215

Burning.

SHOOTING : Con; Sabi.

SITTING Agg: Cyc; *Val.*

SORE, Bruised : *Cep;* Cimi; Kali-bi; Lac-c; *Led*; Polyg.

Burning : Cyc.

STAND, Can not, on : Caus.

STICKING : Petr; *Val.*

STONE UNDER : Aur; Berb; Bro; *Cann*; Hep; *Lyc; Rhus-t.*

SWEAT, Fishy on : Ol-an.

TEARING : Am-m.

TENSION : Caus.

THROBBING : Nat-s.

TINGLING : Nux-m.

ULCER : Am-m; Aran; Ars; Cep.

WALKING Agg : Zin.

Amel : Cyc; *Val.*

VESICLES, On : Petr.

HELD BEING AMEL : See Holding Amel.

HEMICRANIA : See Head, One sided symptoms.

CLIMACTERIC : Croc.

MENSES, Instead of : Croc.

HEMIOPIA : See Vision Half.

HEMIPLEGIA (See also Paralysis) : *Arn; Aur-m; Caus;* Cheno; COCL; Elap; LACH; *Nux-v; Old; Pho; Rhus-t,* Xanth.

RIGHT Side : *Caus; Chel;* Elap; Merc-i-r; Nat-m; Plb.

Aphasia with : Canth; Cheno.

LEFT Side : Ap; Gel; *Lach;* Nux-v; Op; *Rhus-t;* Stro; Vip.

ANGER After : Stap.

APOPLEXY, After : *Arn; Bar-c; Bell; Cocl;* Lach; Nux-v; Op; PHO; Stan; Zin.

CONTRACTION Of limbs, with : Cheno.

CONVULSIONS Of other side : Hell; Stram.

DIPHTHERIA, After : Nux-v.

HYPERESTHESIA of other side with : Plb.

MASTURBATION, After : Stan.

MENTAL SHOCK, After : Ap.

NUMBNESS Of other : Cocl.

SLOWLY Advancing : Caus; Syph.

SPASMS, After : Stan.

SWEAT, With : Stan.

TWITCHING, With : Stram.

HERE AND THERE : See Directions.

HERNIA : Am-m; Aur; Cham; Lyc; *Nux-v;* Sul; Sul-ac; Ver-a.

FEMORAL: Cub; Lyc; Nux-v.

INFANTILE : *Aur;* Calc; Cham; Lyc; Mag-m; Nit-ac; *Nux-v;* Sul-ac.

Congenital : Thu.

STRANGULATED : Aco; Alu; Aur;Bell; Calc; Caps; Cham; Colo; Lach; Lyc; Nit- ac; Nux-v; Op; Plb; Sil; Sul; Sul-ac; Tab; *Ver-a.*

TENDER : Sil.

UMBILICAL : Calc; Lach; Nux-m; Nux-v; Op; Plb.

HERPES : See Eruptions.

HESITATES: Anac; Arg-n; Grap; Kali-br.

TRIFLES, At : Grap.

HICCOUGH : *Am-m*; Ars; Ars-io; Carb-an; *Cic; Cyc; Hyo;* IGN; Iod; Lyc; Mag-p; *Mar-v* ; Merc;Nat-c; Nat-m; Nux-m; NUX-V; *Pul*; Ran-b; Sec; Tab; Ver-v; Zin-val.

AGG : *Am-m*; Bry; Cyc; Hyo; Ign; Nux-v; Stro; Zin-val.

ALCOHOLIC Drinks, after or drunkards, in : *Ran-b*; Sul-ac.

ALTERNATING, Spasms of chest, with : Cic.

ASTHMA, Before : Cup.

BACK, Pain, with : Mar-v.

BRAIN, Affections, in : Arn; Cina.

Concussion, from : Hyo.

BREATH, Short, with : Phys.

CHEST, Pain, with : Stro.

COLIC, With : Hyo.

CONSUMPTION, In : Lyc.

CONVULSIONS, With : *Cic; Hyo*; Ran-b.

Before : Cup.

COUGH, After : *Tab;* Trifo.

CRAMPS, With : Cup-ar.

+ DAY and NIGHT : Mag-p.

DINNER, After and during : Mag-m.

DRINKING, After : Ign.

EAR ACHE, with : Tarn.

EATING or Nursing after : Hyo; Ign; Mar-v.

Amel : Carb-an.

ERUCTATIONS, With : Cyc; Dios; Ign; Nux-v.

Amel : Carb-an.

Bitter : Ign.

Empty : Ign.

EVENING : Gel.

FEVER, After : Ars; Lach.

During : Mag-p.

Same hour when fever ought to come : *Ars.*

Typhoid, in : Pho.

HAWKING Agg : Calc-f.

+ INCESSANT : Merc-cy.

INJURY To head, from : Hyo.

LAUGHTER Agg : Calc.

NERVOUS (Hysterical) : Gel; *Ign*; Mos; Nux-m; Zin-val.

+ OBSTINATE : Stram.

PERITONITIS,In : Hyo; Lyc.

PERSISTENT : Kali-br; Laur; Merc-cy; Sul-ac; Zin-val.

PREGNANCY, During : Cyc; Op.

RETCHING, Vomiting with : Mag-p; Merc; Nux-v.

+ SLEEP Amel : Phys.

During : Ign; Merc-c.

SMOKING Agg : Arg-m; Calend; Ign; Pul; Sele.

THIRST, With : Nicc.

UNCONSCIOUS When : Cup.

VIOLENT : Nat-m; Nicc; Stram; Ver-v.

Painful : Rat; Ver-v.

Sleep, in : Merc-c.

Thirst, with : Nicc.

VOMITING, Before : Cup; Jatr.

After : Jatr; Ver-v.

With : Bell; Bry; Lach; Rut.

YAWNING, With : Cocl; Cyc.

Stretching and with: Amy- n; Mag-c.

HIDE DESIRE To: *Bell* Hell; Pul; Stram.

CHILDREN, Behind furniture : Bar-c.

RUN Away, and : Meli.

HIGH LIVING : Dig.

PLACES (See Ascending) Agg : *Arg-n; Aur;* Coca; Gel; Pul; Stap; *Sul.*

HILLS AMEL : Syph.

HIP JOINT : Bry; *Caus;* Led; Merc; Pho-ac; Rhus-t; Stram; Thu.

BUTTOCKS, With : Card-m.

CRACKING, In : Cam; Cocl; Croc.

CRAMPS : Led.

DISLOCATION Spontaneous: Colo; Rhus-t; Thu.

LEG, Too long, as if, with: Kre.

MOTION Agg : Ant-t.

Amel : Am-m; Calc-f; Iris.

RISING Agg : Nat-s.

STOOPING Agg : Card-m.

TUBERCULOSIS (Morbus coxarious) : Calc; Calc-p; Card-m; Chin; Colo; Hep; Kali-c; Kali-s; Led; Pho-ac; Pul; Rhus-t; Sil; Stram; Tub.

Right : *Led.*

Left : Stram.

HIPS (Region) : Arn; Caus; Euphor; Lyc; Phyt; Rhus-t; Rut; Sep; sul.

ALTERNATING, Between : Euony.

ABOVE : *Caus.*

ACHING, Loss of power of legs

with : Stap.

BRUISED : Mag-m; Rut.

BUBBLING : Led.

BURNING : Mag-m.

CHANGE Of Weather Agg : Phyt.

COITION, After Agg : Mag-m.

CONTRACTED (Drawn together) : Colo; Polyg.

COUGHING Agg: *Caus;* Val.

CRAMP : Colo; Led.

DRAGGED, Down, from : Visc.

DRAWN Together : See Contracted.

FORCED Apart, disjointed as if : Agar; Calc-p; Con; Sep; Sul; Tril.

HOLLOW : Pall.

MOTION Agg : Ant-t.

Amel : Am-m; Calc-f; Iris.

PAIN, Violent : Stram.

PREGNANCY, In : Calc-p.

After : *Hypr.*

RISING Agg : Nat-s; Sep.

SITTING Down Agg :Nat-s.

SORE : Visc.

TO HIP : Arn; Cimi; Colo; Lac-c; Lil-t; Onos; Thu; Ust.

Up, Back : Pho.

URINATION Agg : Berb.

WEAK : Calc-p; Rut; Sep; Thu; Tril.

Coition preventing : Cep.

Sudden : Kob.

Walking Agg : Kob.

WRENCHED : Iris.

HIVES : See Urticaria.

HOARSENESS : See Voice.

HODGKIN'S DISEASE :
Ars; Ars-io; Bar-io; Iod;
Pho; Syph.

HOLDING Or BEING HELD
AMEL : Ars; *Bry*; Carb-an;
Diph; Dros; Eup-p; *Gel*; Glo;
Lach; Lil-t; Murx; Nat-s;
Nux-m; Nux-v; Rhus-t; Sang;
Sep; Sil; Stram; Sul; Sul-ac.

ANYTHING Agg : Caus.

ATTENDANT, To : Ant-t.

HOLE, BLOWING Through
: See Air; blowing through.

HOLLOW : See Empty.

HOMESICK : *Bry;* CAPS; Carb-
an; Eup-pur; Hyo; IGN; Merc;
Op; *Pho-ac*; Sil.

AILMENTS, From : Clem.

+ **HONOUR WOUNDED** : *Nux-v.*

HOOK WORM DISEASE :Carb-
tetra; Cheno; Thymol.

HOPEFUL : Sul; Tub.

DESPAIR, Alternating with :
Aco; Kali-c.

LUNG Disease, in : Aur.

HOPELESS : See Despair.

HORNY : See Growth, Eruptions.

HORRIPILATION : See Goose
Skin.

HORROR : *Calc;* Cic; Plat; Zin.

+ COLD WATER, Of : *Phys.*

+ SOLITUDE And Work : Cadm.

HORSE BACK : See Riding
on horse back.

HOT APPLICATION AMEL : Anac;
Ars; Calc-f; *Hep*; Kali-c;
Mag-p; Nux-v; Radm;

Rhus-t; Sil; Syph.

BALL : See, Ball, Knot.

BATH AMEL : See Bathing Hot.

AGG : Ap; Bels; Op.

DAYS, Weather Agg : See
Summer Agg.

And cold nights Agg : See
Cold Nights with hot days
Agg.

DRINKS AMEL : See Drinks hot,
under Food.

IRON, Wires, needles etc. as
if : Agar; Alu; Ap; *Ars*;
Bar-c; Lith; Mag-c; Naj;
Nit-ac; Ol-an; Rhus-t; Spig;
Vesp.

WATER, As if, in : Pho.

Breast to abdomen: Sang.

Flowing through part, as
if : Sumb.

Pain during: Terb.

Poured on part, as i f : Ver-v.

HOUR EXACT Agg : See
Periodicity.

HOUSE IN AGG : Bry; Lyc;
Mag-m; *Pul;* Rhus-t; Til.

Amel : Agar; Cyc; Ign.

HOWLING : Aco; Arn; *Bell;*
Cham; Cic; Ver-a.

ANGER, With: Arn.

HUMERUS ACHING, right :
Bry; Gel; Phyt.

BROKEN, As if : Bov; *Cocl;* Pul.

Middle : Merc-i-r.

CRAMP, Left : Val.

CRUSHING : Stan.

ELECTRIC Shock : Val.

NIGHT, Only : Dros.

WRITING Agg: Ars-io.

HUMID Damp weather **A**GG : Alo; Ars; Bap; *Bro*; Bry; Carb-s; *Carb-v; Gel*; Iod; *Ip*; Kali-bi; LACH; Lyss; Nat-m; *Nat-s;* Old; Op; Pul; Rhus-t; Sil; *Ver-a.*

AMEL : Sil.

HUMMING, Buzzing, Whizzing, Purring : Caus; Kali-m; Kre; Mos; Nux-m; Old; Op; Pul; Spig; Sul.

HUNGER : See Appetite.

AGG *: Grap;* Iod; *Kali-c; Sil;* Spig; *Sul.*

HURRY, **I**MPATIENCE : Aco; Alu; Ap; *Arg-n;* ARS; BELL; Calc-p; Cham; HEP; Hyo; IGN; Ip; Kali-s; Lach; *Lil-t;* Lycps; Med; *Merc;* Mos; Nat-m; Nit-ac; NUX-V; Rhe; Sep; *Stram* Sul; *Sul-ac;* Tarn; Thu; Val; Ver-a.

CANNOT Do things fast enough : *Sul-ac.*

COMPLAINTS, From : Arn.

DRINKING, In : Anac; Bry; Hep. Unconsciousness, during : Hell.

EATING, While : Caus; Hep; Lyc; Plat; Sul-ac.

Can not eat fast enough : Zin.

EVERY **BODY** Must: Tarn.

EXECUTION, Slow, with : Alu.

MENSES, During : Ign.

MOVEMENTS, In: Arg-n; Stram; Sul-ac; Tarn.

TIME, For the appointed, to arrive : *Arg-n.*

TO DO, several things, at once : *Lil-t.*

TRIFLE Things, in: Med; Sul; Sul-ac.

WALKING, While : Arg-n; Sul-ac; Tarn.

WRITING, When: Sul-ac.

HURT, **F**EARS **B**EING : *Arn*; Chin; Hep; Kali-c; Rut; Spig.

FEELING, Others, of: Chin.

LITTLE, Pains terribly : Colch.

HYDRARTHROSIS : See Water in Joints.

HYDROCELE : Ap; Calc; Grap; Iod; Pul; *Rhod;* Sele; SIL; Sul.

LEFT Side : Dig; *Rhod.*

BOYS, Of : Abro; Pul; Rhod; Sil; Sul-io.

Birth, from : Rhod.

+ **C**HILDREN : Aur; Calc.

GONORRHOEAL Orchitis, after : Pho.

INJURY, From : Samb.

MULTILOCULAR : Ap.

OVERLIFTING, From : Rhus-t.

SUPPRESSED, Eruptions, from : Hell.

HYDROCEPHALUS : *Ap*; Apoc; *Calc*; Calc-p; Iodof; Hell; Lyc; Merc; *Sil*; Sul; Tub; *Zin.*

+ **C**ONVULSIONS, With : Sul.

DIARRHOEA, After (infants) : Zin.

VISION. Loss of, with : Apoc.

HYDROGENOID : Dul; Nat-m; Nat-s; Thu.

HYDRO-PERICARDIUM
: See Dropsy, under Heart.

HYDROPHOBIA : *Bell;* Canth;
Cup; *Hyo;* Lyss; Pho; Saba;
Stram.

PROPHYLACTIC *: Bell;* Hyo;
Lyss; Stram.

+ **HYDRO-THORAX** : Adon;
Flu-ac; Lyc.

HYGROMA : See Ganglion.

HYPERCHLORHYDRIA : See
Sour, under Stomach.

HYPOCHLORHYDRIA. Alternating,
with : Chin-ar.

HYPERMETROPIA : See Far
Sight, under Vision.

HYPERPYREXIA : See Fever,
High.

HYPERTENSION : See Blood
Pressure, High.

HYPERTROPHY : *Ant-c;* Ars;
Calc; *Clem; Dul; Grap;*
Ran-b; Rhus-t; Sep; *Sil;* Sul.

EXERTION, Excessive, from :
Thyr.

ONE SIDED : Lyc.

HYPOCHONDRIAE : Aco; Chin;
Lyc; Merc; Nat-s; Ran-b; Stap.

LEFT : See Spleen.

RIGHT : See Liver.

ACHE : Scil; Sil.

Leucorrhoea Amel : Phyt.

ANXIETY, Felt in : Arn; Nux-v.

AROUND : Ran-b.

BALL : Bro; Cup.

BAND, About: Aco; Card-m;
Dros; Ign; Nux-v.

BRUISED, Sore : Bry; C*hin;*
Eup-p; Ran-b; Visc.

CONSTRICTION : Cact; Lyc.

COUGHING Agg : Dros; *Eup-p;*
Kali-c; Nat-s.

FULL : Sep.

HARD : Iod.

HEAVY : *Coc-c;* Zin.

HOLDS : Dros

STICKING : Sil.

TENSION : Aco; Lyc.

HYPOCHONDRIASIS : Ars;
Asaf; AUR; Card-m; Con;
Grat; Ign; *Nat-c;* Nat-m;
NUX-V; Plat; PUL; *Sep;* Stan;
Stap; *Sul;* Val.

SEXUAL : Mos.

HYPOCRISY : Pho.

HYPOGASTRIUM : *Bell;* Bry;
Carb-v; Lyc; *Merc;* Ran-b;
Scil; *Sep.*

ACHING, Painful : Ars; Plat;
Pul; *Sep;* Sul; Ver-a.

Coition, after Agg : Cep.

Heavy : Vib.

Menses, during : Calc; Sec.

BACKWARDS, Right : Caus;
Pho; *Sep;* Ust.

Left : Aco; Carb-v.

BEARING Down : Bell; Dict;
Lil-t; Lyc; Nux-v; Plat; Pul;
Sep; Sul.

BOARD, Across : Nux-m.

CLAWING : Bell.

COLDNESS : Plb.

CONSTRICTION : Bell; Chel;
Hyo.

CRAMPS : Vib.

CUTTING : Bell; Hyo; Pul; Thu.

Menses, during : *Kali-c;* Lil-t.

DISTENSION *: Kali-c;* Phys.

EMPTY : Kali-s; Sec.

　Flatus passing Amel : Kali-s.

FLATULENCE : Zin; Zin-val.

FULNESS : Aesc; Bell;

HEAVY : Med; Pho-ac; Sec;
　Sep; Sul; Tarn.

　Menses. Amel : Vib.

LEGS, Down : Con.

SORE : Calc; Lach; Phys; Terb;
　Ver-a.

　Standing Agg : Phys.

TENSION : Sep.

TREMBLING : Calc-p; *Lil-t.*

WEAK : Am-c; Apoc; Calc;
　Chio; Pho; Plb; Sul; Ver-a.

　Stools, before : Merc-i-f.

HYPOSTASIS : Am-c; Rhus-t; Sep.

HYSTERIA: ASAF; AUR; Caus;
Cham; *Cocl;* CON; Gel; Grat;
IGN; Kali-p; Lach; *Mag-m;*
Mos; Nat-m; Nit-ac; NUX-M;
NUX-V; *Plat; Pul;* Sep; *Sul;* Sumb;
TARN; Ther; VAL; Ver-a.

CLIMAXIS, At : Pho-ac; Ther.

COITION, Agg : Lac-c.

FAINTS : Cocl; Ign.

FRIGHT, After: Saba.

GLOBUS : Aco; Con; *Mag-m;*
　Mos; Plb; Senec; Val; Zin.

　Eructation Amel : Mag-m.

　Warm : Val.

HAEMORRHAGE, After: Stic.

LASCIVIOUS : Plat; Tarn.

LOOKED, At, when: Plb.

MENSES, Before : Hyo; Mos;
　Plat.

　First day, of: Raph.

MORNING Agg, Sighing Amel :

Tarn.

MUSIC Amel : *Tarn.*

PUBERTY, At : Ther.

SEXUAL, Excess, after :
　Pho-ac.

　Orgasm, at the height of :
　Lac-c.

SUPPRESSION of discharges,
　after : *Asaf;* Lach.

TWITCHINGS, Menses before :
　Cup; Kali-c; Nat-m; Pho;
　Pho-ac; Plat; Pul; Sep; Sul.

　Menses during : Aco; Bry;
　Calc; Caus; Cham; Chin;
　Cocl; Cof; Cup; Form;
　Hyo; Ign; Ip; Lyc; Mag-
　m; Merc; Nat-m; Nux-v;
　Pul; Sul.

　Menses, after : Chin; Cup;
　Pul.

+ VIOLENT : Aur.

WATCHED, When, only : Plb.

ICHTHYOSIS : *Ars-io;* Pho;
Syph; Thyr.

+ ICE FACTORY COMPLAINTS
: Dul.

ICY COLD : See Coldness, Icy.

IDEAS : See Imaginations.

COMPELLING : *Lach;* Nit-ac.

ERRONEOUS : Saba; Val.

FIXED : Anac; Ars; Chin; Hell;
　Nat-m; Saba; Stan; Sul;
　Thu.

MANY : Med.

　But uncertain in execution
　: Med.

MURDERING, Her Family, of :
　Jab; Kali-br.

PERSISTENT : Med.

222

STRANGE : Arg-n.

VANISH : Anac; *Nux-m*; Ol-an; Ver-a.

WANDER : Dul; Pho; Thu.

IDIOCY : See Childish.

IDLENESS AGG : See Busy when Amel.

ILEOCOECAL REGION : See Appendicitis.

ILEUS : See Abdomen, Paralysis of Intestines.

ILIAC DOWN Thigh : Berb.

URINATING Agg : Berb.

ILL OR SICK FEELING : Aco; Ant-t; Bap; Chel; Cimi; Lach; Lob; Nux-v; Petr; *Pod*; Psor; Pul; Sang; Stro; Tab; Tarx.

+ ALL OVER, Pelvic complaints, in : Vib.

DOES NOT KNOW, Why : Bro.

PAIN, From : Stro.

QUEER, Menses, before: Bro.

ILLUSIONS : See Imaginations.

IMAGINARY DISEASE : Arg-n; Mos; Saba; Ver-a.

BROODS Over: Cyc; Lil-t; Naj.

IMAGINATIONS, ILLUSIONS, FANCIES, Delusions : Aco; Amb; Anac; *Arg-n*; Ars; *Bar-c*; BELL; Calc; *Cann*; COCL; HYO; *Ign*; Kali-br; Lac-c; Lach; Merc; Mos; Nux-m; *Op*; Petr; Pyro; SABA; STRAM; SUL; Thu; Val;Ver-a.

ANIMALS, Objects are : Hyo.

BEHIND HIM, Somebody : See Behind.

Walking : Calc.

DEAD, He is : Lach.

DECEIVED, Being : Dros; Rut.

DEPRESSIVE : Amb; Kali-br.

DONE Something, wrong : Cina.

EAT, He can not : Myr.

FRONT Of him, someone : Con.

FURNITURE, To be persons : Nat-p.

+ HE Is not himself: Syph.

+ HEAVY Being : Alu.

HORRID : Lac-c.

+ HOUSE, Full of thieves : Ars.

HUSBAND, Neglecting her : Stram.

INSULTS, Of : Stap.

+ LARGER, Of being : Alu.

LIMBS, Talking together: Bap.

NOSE, Wears, somebody else's : Lac-c.

NUMB, Being : Alu.

ODOUR, Smell of : See under Smell.

PASS, Can not a certain point: Kali-br.

RICH, As if, he is : Pho; *Plat*; Pyro; *Sul*; Ver-a.

SMOOTH, Being : Alu.

SNAKES, Around : Hyo; Lac-c; Tub.

STARVE, He must : Kali-m.

STRANGE Surroundings : *Cic*; Hyo; Plat; Tub.

STEPPING Hard somebody, as if : Alo.

SUPER HUMAN Control, under : *Anac*; *Lach*; Op; Plat; Thu.

TOUCH, Sensory : Anac; Canth; Op; *Rhus-t*; Stram; *Thu.*

VOICES, Of : Aco; Anac; Ast-r; Cham; Chlor-hyd; Coca; *Elap;* Med; Nit-ac; Stram.

Unpleasant, about, himself : Coca.

WALKS On Knees, as if: Bar-c.

WIFE is faithless : Stram.

WORLD Is on fire : Ver-a.

IMBECILITY : See Childish.

IMITATES: Cup; Lach; Nux-m.

IMMOBILE : Lycps; Mang; Stro.

SIDE, One : Stro.

IMMORAL : See Moral Perversions.

IMPATIENCE : See Hurry.

IMPETIGO CONTAGIOSA : See under Eruptions.

IMPOTENCY (See Erections falling incomplete) : Calad; Iod; Kob.

DIABETES, With: Coca; Mos; Pho-ac.

FRIGHT, During coition, from : Sinap.

GONORRHOEA, After: Calad.

IMAGINARY : Stry-p.

+ MELANCHOLY, With : Kali-br.

+ NIGHTLY Emissions, with : Uran-n.

ONANISM, After : Arg-n; Grap.

PSYCHICAL : Onos.

SEXUAL Excess, after: Arn; Grap.

+ **IMPUDENT** CHILD : Grap.

IMPULSES CONTRADICTORY : *Anac.*

FEARS, His Own : Alu.

HORRID : Alu; Ars; Caus; Hep; Iod; Lach; Merc.

Busy when Amel : Iod.

TO DO Strange things : Cact.

TO TOUCH, Things : See under Touch.

IMPULSIVE : Arg-n; Croc; Cup; IGN; Med; PUL; Tarn.

INACTIVE, LETHARGIC, Apathetic Lies down : Ail; Alu; Ant-t; Ap; *Arn*; Ars; Bels; Bism; Calad; *Calc*; Carb-v; Caus; Chel; *Chin*; Con; Cup; Fer; *Gel;* Grap; *Hell*; Kali-c; Lach; Mar-v; *Mur-ac;* NUX-V; Old; OP; PHO; PHO-AC; Pic-ac; Psor; Radm; Rut; Sang; Sele; SEP; Sil; *Stram; Sul;* Sul-ac; Tarn; Thyr; *Zin.*

ACTIVITY, Alternating, with: Alo; Aur.

COITION, After : *Calc.*

CONVERSATION, From : Sil.

EATING, After: Lach; Lyc; *Pho-ac*; Sele.

STOOL, After, every: Arn.

STORMY Weather, in: Sang; Tub.

INATTENTION AGG : Gel; *Hell.*

INCITING OTHERS : Hyo.

INCOHERENCE : See Confusion.

INCONSTANCY : IGN.

INCONTINENCE Stool, Urine, Sexual, etc. : *Alo;* Arg-n; *Arn;* Ars; BELL; CAUS; Chin; Con; Dios;

Gel; Hyo; Mur-ac; Nat-m; *Pho;* PHO-AC; *Pod; Pul; Sele; Sep;* Stap; *Sul;* Uran-n.
FRIGHT, From : Op.

INCOORDINATION : See Co-ordination disturbed.

INCREASES AND DECREASES : See Directions.

INDIFFERENCE : Ap; Arn; Ars; *Bap;* Berb; CALC; *Carb-v; Chin;* Clem; CON; Gel; HELL; *Ign;* Lil-t; Mez; *Nat-c; Nat-m;* Nat-p; Onos; *Op;* PHO; PHO-AC; PLAT; PUL; SEP; Stap; Sul; Tab.

COMPLAIN Does not : Hyo; *Op; Stram.*

EVERYTHING, To : Carb-v; Merc; Mez; Nat-p; Pho-ac.

Done for her : Lil-t.

HOUSEHOLD Matters, to: Cimi.

LOVED Ones, to relations : Flu-ac; *Hell;* Nat-p; *Pho; Sep.*

Her own children : Lyc; *Pho; Sep.*

OPPOSITE Sex : Thu.

PAIN, To : Op.

PLEASURE, To: Fer-p; Hell; Nat-m; Op; Sul.

SOCIETY, When in : *Arg-n;* Kali-c.

STOIC : Ail; Op.

+ SULLEN : Ver-a.

SURROUNDINGS, About : Pic-ac; Rum.

WELFARE Of others, to : SUL.

INDIGESTION (See Digestion affected) : Aeth; *Ant-c.*

COITION, After : Dig; Pho.

HURRIEDLY Eating and drinking from : Cof; *Old.*

SPRAIN, From : Rut.

INDIGNATION : Ars; Calc-p; Colo; *Stap.*

PREGNANT, While : Nat-m.

INDOLENT, SLUGGISH : Alu; Bor; *Caps;* Carb-v; Chel; Chin; *Grap;* Kali-bi; Lach; *Merc;* Nat-m, Nit-ac; Nux-v; Pho; Psor; Sabi; Sep; Sil; SUL.

SUDDENLY : Calc.

INDURATION : See Hardness.

INDUSTRIOUS : Aur; Tarn.

INFANTS : See Children.

INFERIORITY : See Cowardly, Anthropophobia, Company Agg.

INFILTRATION : Calc; Carb-an; Grap; Iod; Kali-io; Kali-m; Rhus-t; Sul; Sul-io.

+ STUBBORN : Kali-m.

INFLAMMATION : *Aco;* Ap; *Ars;* BELL; BRY; Calc; Cann; *Canth;* Cham; Echi; Fer-p; GEL; Hep; HYO; *Iod;* Kali-c; *Lach; Merc;* NUX-V; *Pho;* Plb; PUL; RHUS-T; Sec; Sep; SIL; *Stap;* Sul; Terb; *Ver-v.*

INFLUENZA : Ars-io; Bap; Bry; Cam; Caus; *Eup-p;* Fer-p; *Gel;* Merc; *Nux-v; Rhus-t;* Saba.

GASTRIC : Bap.

PAIN Remaining, after: Lycps.

WEAKNESS, Remaining after : Abro; Con; Kali-p; Nat-sal.

INGUINAL GLANDS : See under

Groins.

INHALATION : See Inspiration.

INJURIES, SHOCKS, Wounds, Bruises etc. : ARN; Bels; *Calen*; Cic; *Con*; Echi; Glo; Ham; Hep; Hypr; Kali-io; *Lach*; Led; Lith; Nat-s; Nit-ac; *Pul; Rhus-t; Rut;* Stap; Stro; *Sul-ac;* Symp.

BITES Of Poisonous animals, from (Rats, Snakes, Cats, Dogs etc.) : Anthx*; Ap;* Arn; *Ars;* Ced; Cist; *Echi;* Hypr; *Lach;* LED; Mos; Pyro; Seneg; Sul-ac.

+ Bees : Tab.

Boots, tight from : Paeno.

Bruised, Sore spot, from: Lith.

+ Insects : Ced.

Mosquitoes : Calad; Tab.

Leeches : Alum.

+ Snakes : Ced; Plant.

BONES, To : Arn; Calc; Iod; *Petr;* Pho; Pho-ac; Pul; RUT; Stap; Symp.

BRUISES, Contusions : Arn; Con; Ham; Hypr; Rhus-t; Rut; Symp.

Trifles, from every : Terb.

COLD Become : Led.

CONSTITUTIONAL Effects : ARN; Carb-v; Con; Glo; Iod; Lach; *Led; Nat-s*; Nit-ac; Pho; Stap; *Stro.*

CRUSHED : Arn; Con; Hypr; Rut; Stap.

DEEP *:* Bels.

DISSECTING : Ap; *Ars; Lach.*

FALLS : Stap; Stic; Sul; Tell.

FESTER : *Anthx; Ap; Ars;* Echi; Led; Pyro.

GAPING (Wounds) : Hypr.

GLANDS, To : Bels; *Con.*

HEAD, To : See Head.

HEIGHT, Falling from: Mill.

INCISIONS, Cuts, Stabs : Arn; Lach; *Pho;* Pul; *Stap;* Sul-ac.

LACERATED : Calen; Ham; Hypr; Stap.

LITTLE, Pains terribly : Colch.

MENTAL Effects : Cic; *Glo;* Hypr; Mag-c; *Nat-s.*

MUSCLES, To : Rhus-t.

NERVES, To : Bels; Cep; *Hypr;* Pho; Pho-ac; Xanth.

OLD : Cep; Symp.

Pains, in : Cep; Kali-io; Sil; Symp.

PAINS, Returning : Glo; Kali-io; Nat-m; *Nat-s; Nit-ac;* Nux-v.

PELVIC Organs, of : Bels.

PUNCTURED, Shot gun etc. : Ap; Arn; *Hypr;* Lach; *Led; Nit-ac;* Plant; Sul-ac.

Perineum, to : Symp.

Soles and Palms to : *Hypr; Led.*

REOPENING Of **O**LD : Carb-v; Crot-h; Flu-ac; Lach; Nat-m; *Op; Pho; Sil.*

SALT, Sprinkled, on as if : Sars.

SLIGHT **A**GG : Val; Ver-a.

SLOW to Heal (See healing difficult): Carb-v; *Hep;*

Kre; Lach; Nit-ac; Petr; *Sil*; Sul.

SPLINTERS, From: Cic; Hypr.

TENDONS, To: Anac.

TWITCHING : Led.

INQUISITIVE : Agar; Aur; Lach; Laur.

INSANITY, MANIA, Craziness : Amb; Ars; BELL; CUP; *Hyo*; Kali-br; Kali-chl; Lyc; Med; *Merc; Nux-v; Op*; STRAM; Syph; *Tarn;* VER-A; Vip.

APOPLEXY, After: Hell.

BRUTAL : Abs.

BUSY *: Ap*; Kali-br.

CRAZY THINGS, Does all sorts of : Gel; Stram.

DEPRESSIVE Narcosis, alternating with : Ap; *Hyo*.

EROTIC *: Ap; Bar-m*; Buf; Canth; HYO; *Orig*; Pho;*Plat*; Stram; *Tarn*; Ver-a; Zin.

Menses, before : Dul; Stan.

FEMALES, Of : *Aco*; Ap; *Bell;* Cimi; *Orig;* Plat; *Pul;* Stram; Ver-a.

Self accusation, from : Hell.

Stupor, alternating with : Ap.

HAEMORRAGE, After : Chin; Cup; Sep.

HEAD, Washing in cold water Amel : Saba.

LOQUACIOUS : Par.

MALIGNANT : Cup.

MASTURBATION, After : Buf; *Cocl; Hyo*; Op.

MENSES, Before : Cimi.

Profuse, with: Sep.

Suppressed, with : Ap; Ign; *Pul.*

NEURALGIA, Disappearance of, after: Cimi; *Nat-m.*

OVERSTUDY, Mental labour, from : Kali-p; Lach; Pho.

PERIODICAL : Con; Nat-s; Plat.

PUERPERAL : Aur; Bell; Cam; Cimi; Cup; Hyo; Lyc; Plat; Pul; Sec; Stram; Thu; Ver-a; Ver-v.

Modesty, lost : Sec.

QUARRELSOME : Hyo.

RELIGIOUS : Cam; Lach; Nat-c; Stram; Ver-a.

SEXUAL Excess, from : *Ap.*

STRENGTH Increased : Agar; Bell; Stram; *Tarn.*

SUICIDAL : Ars; Naj.

SUPPRESSED, Eruptions, after : Caus; Sul; Zin.

SWEAT, Cold, with : Stram.

SYPHILITIC : Syph.

+ TACITURN, Alternating with: Ver-a.

URINE, Passes on the floor : Plb.

WEDDING Preparations of : Hyo.

INSECT BITES : See under Injuries, Bites, Stings.

CRAWLING : See Crawling, Formication.

INSECURITY, SENSE Of : Ail; Alo.

INSENSIBLE : See Unconsciousness and Numbness.

227

INSOLENT, *Rude*, Haughty : Lil-t; Lyc; Lyss; Med; Pall; Par; PLAT; Sul; VER-A.

INSOMNIA : See Sleeplessness.

INSPIRATION AGG : Crot-h; Ip; Kali-n; Lob; Mez; Nux-m; Spo; Sumb.

AMEL : *Colch;* Cup; *Ign;* Lach; *Spig;* Stan; Verb.

COLD Air, Amel : Sele.

Expiration, hot : Sul.

DID NOT REACH, the pit of stomach : Pru-sp.

NOSE, Through, expiration through mouth, while lying on back : Chlor-hyd.

+ SHORT, Jerking : Ox-ac.

SLOW, Expiration quick: Stram.

INSTEP ULCER : Lyc.

+ **INSULTS** On the LOOK OUT, for : Caps.

INSUSCEPTIBILITY : See Numbness.

INTELLECT : ACO; Anac; Aur; Bap; BAR-C; BELL; Cann; Cocl; HELL; HYO; Ign; LACH; Laur; LYC; Merc; Nat-c; Nux-v; OP; PHO; PHO-AC; *Plat; Pul; Rhus-t;* SEP; STRAM; *Sul;* VER-A.

INTEMPERANCE AGG : Stram.

INTERCOSTAL REGION : Aesc; Amy-n; Bry; Cimi; Mez; Ran-b; Sil; Verb.

NEURALGIA : See Pleurodynia.

PLUG Sensation : Caus; Cocl; Lyc; Ran-sc; Ver-a.

INTERMITTENCY : ARS; Calc; Chin; Ip; Lach; Nat-m; Nit-ac; *Nux-v;* Pho-ac; *Pul;* Sec; Sul.

INTERMITTENT FEVER : See under Fever.

INTERNAL AFFECTIONS : Calc; Canth; Nux-v; Pho.

INTERTRIGO : See under Eruptions.

INTESTINES BREAKING, As if, bending on : Adon.

+ BITTEN Off, as if : Pall.

BURNING : Manc.

CANCER : Rut.

COLD, As if : Plant.

Balls running through, as if : Buf.

Water flowing through, to anus : Mill.

menses, during : Kali-c.

COLDS Agg : Dul.

CONTENTS, Fluid as if were : Polyg.

CORD, Bound and loosened, as if : Chio.

+ EATING, Something, in as if : Kali-bi.

+ FALLING Out, as if : Kali-br.

FALLS To side lain on : Merc.

HANGING Down, as if: Agn; Ign; Psor; *Stap.*

Bed turning in, when : Bar-c; Merc; Merc-c.

INACTIVE : Aeth; Phys.

INFLAMMATION, High fever with: Ver-v.

INTUSSUSCEPTION : Ars; Cup; Op; Plb; Ver-a.

KNOTTED : Asaf; Elap; Saba;

Sul; Ust; Ver-a.

LIQUID, Flows from Stomach, to : Mill.

LOOSE, Shaking, and : Mang.
Walking, while : Mang.

MARBLE, Dropped down at stool as if : Nat-p.

NEURALGIA : Cup-ar.

OBSTRUCTED, As if : *Op.*

PARAYSIS Of : See under Abdomen.

RUNNING, Alive, in : Cyc.

SHIVERING, In : Arg-n.

SORE : Manc.

STRICTURE : Con.

WEAK : Merc.

WORM, Writhing along in, as if: Calad.

INTOXICATION : *Caps; Gel;* Lach; NUX-V; Op; Ran-b.

EASY : Bov; Con; Zin.

+ FEELING Of : Naj.

INTROSPECTION, Introverted : *Cocl; Ign;* Mur-ac; Ol-an; *Pul.*

INTUSSUSCEPTION : See under Intestines.

IRIS : Bell; Merc; *Merc-c;* Nit- ac; Sul.

HAEMORRHAGE, Iridectomy, after : Led.

INFLAMMATION : Arn; Merc-c; Rhus-t.

Adhesions, with : Calc; Clem; Merc-c; Nit-ac; Sul; Terb.

Hypopion, with : Hep; Merc; Sil.

Prostate gland, with : Sabal.

+ Syphilitic : Stap.

JAGGED : Sil; Stap; Thu.

PARALYSIS, Of : *Ars;* Par.

PROLAPSE, Cataract operation after : Alum; Stap.

IRREGULAR : See Coordination, disturbed.

IRRELIGIOU : Anac; Colo; Croc; Laur; Kali-br.

IRRESOLUTE, Vacillating, *Wavering : Anac; Ars;* Asaf; Bar-c; Cocl; *Grap;* Hell; *Ign;* Lach; Lyc; *Nux-m; Onos;* Op; Petr; Pho; *Pul;* Sul-ac.

IRRITABLE : See Anger, Vexation.

CHILDREN : Abro; Cham; Cina; Kali-p; Lac-c; Mag-c; Rhe.

Towards : Kali-io.

COITION Agg : Petr.

Amel : Tarn.

DAY Time, only : Lyc; Med.

DAY and NIGHT : Cham; Lac-c; Op; Psor; Stram.

HEADACHE, During : Syph.

NIGHT, Only: Ant-t; *Jal;* Lac-c; Nux-v; Psor; Rhe.

QUESTIONED, When: Arn; Cham; *Nux-v;* Pho-ac.

SENDS The doctor home, says he is not sick : ARN; CHAM.

SEXUAL Appetite, loss of, from : Sabal.

STOOLS, Before : Bor.

+ SUDDENLY, Beats anything in his way : Stro.

TAKES, Everything amiss :

See Bad Parts, takes everything.

TOUCHED When : Ant-c; Tarn.

ISOLATED EFFECTS : Agar; Gel; Ver-a; Zin.

ITCH : See Eruptions, Itch like.

BAKER'S, BARBER'S : Ant-t; Cic; Grap; Lith; Mag-p; Phyt; Rhus-t; Scop; Sul-io; Tell.

ITCHING : Aco; *Agar; Amb; Ant-c; Ap;* Ars; Bov; Bry; *Calc;* Carb-v; CAUS; Chel; Cist;Con; Fago; Grap; *Lyc;* Mag-c; *Merc;* Mez;Nat-m; *Nit-ac;* Nux-v; Ol-an; Op; Pho; Psor; *Pul;* Radm; *Rhus-t;* Sabi; Sep; *Sil;* Spo; *Stap; Sul;* Sul-io; Tarn; Thu; Urt.

AFFECTED Part, over: Agar.

AIR Agg : Ars; Hep; Old; Petr; *Rum.*

Amel : Stro.

BATHING, After : Bov; Calc; Clem; Mag-c.

Amel: Clem.

BED, In Agg: Kali-ar; Led; Pic-ac; *Psor;* Sil; *Sul.*

BITING : Agar; Led; Ol-an; *Old;* Pul; *Stap;* Urt.

+ **BODY** All over : Pall.

BURNING : AGAR; AP; Ars; Bry; *Caus;* Grap; *Lach;* Lyc; *Petr; Pul; Rhus-t; Sil;* SUL; Thu.

Hairy parts, of : Rhus-t.

+ Mosquito bites, after : Calad.

Painful part, in : Alu.

COLD Agg : Clem; Thu; Tub.

Amel : Berb; Calad; Fago; Grap; Mez.

+ **CORROSIVE** : Vinc.

CRAWLING : Agar; Colch; Lyc; Plat; Plb; Pul; Rhus-t;Sep; Spig; Stap; Sul; Tarn; Tell.

DESQUAMMATION, With : Clem.

DIABETES, In : Mang.

EATING Amel : Chel.

EROSIVE : Rut.

ERUPTIONS, Without : Alu; Ars;Cist; Cup; Dol; Mez; Thyr.

Night Agg: Thyr.

HAIRY Parts, on : Rhus-t.

HEAT Of Stove Amel : Clem; Rum; Tub.

+ **HERE AND THERE** : Am-c.

HOT Bath Amel: Syph.

INTERNAL (Tickling): Amb; Ap; Caus; Coc-c; *Cham;* Cist; *Con;* Fer; Hyo; IOD; Ip; Kali-bi; Kali-c; *Lach;* Nat-m; NUX-V; PHO; Rhus-t; *Rum;* Sang; Sep; Stan; Sumb; Sul.

Intolerable : Coc-c.

+ **INTOLERABLE** : Kali-ar.

JAUNDICE, In : Dol; Hep; Myr; Pic-ac; Ran-b; Thyr.

MEAT Agg : Rum; Rut.

MENSES Amel : Cyc.

During : Kali-c.

MOSQUITO Bite, after : Calad.

NAUSEA, With : Lob.

NERVOUS : Arg-m.

OLD PEOPLE, In (Pruriti Senilis) : Alu; Ars; Dul; Fago; Merc; Mez; Old; Sul; Urt.

PAIN, Alternating with : Stro.

PAINFUL : Bar-c; Sil; Sul.

PLEASURABLE : Sul.

PREGNANCY, In : Sabi; Tab.

PRICKLING, With: Lob.

RUBBING Slowly, Amel: Crot-t; Dios; Med.

Changes place : Tub.

SCRATCHING Agg : Ars; Crot-t; Mez.

Bumps form, after : *Dul;* Lach; *Mez; Rhus-t;* Ver-a.

Changes, places : Mez; Stap.

Eruptions, follow : Am-c; Old.

Moisture, follows : Grap; Old; Radm; Rhus-t; Sele.

SCRATCH Must : Agar; Arg-m; Cof; Psor; Stap.

Until it bleeds : Alu; Arg-m; *Ars;* Cof; Psor.

Until it is raw : Grap; Petr.

SORENESS, With : Med.

SPOTS, In : Con; *Led; Sep;* Sil; Sul-ac; Zin.

SWEAT Agg :MANG; *Merc;* Rhod.

THINKING Of it Agg: Med.

UNCOVERING, Undressing Agg : Dros; Kali-ar; Nat-s; Nit-ac; Nux-v; Old; Pall; Rhus-t; *Rum;* Stap; Tell; Tub.

VOMITS, Not relieved, until he : Ip.

WARM On becoming : Aeth; ALu; Lyc; Merc; Psor; Sul; Urt.

Bed, in Kob.

WIPING, Hand with Amel :

Dros.

JADED RAKES : *Agn.*

JARRING, Shaking, stepping hard, riding (See sensitive)

AGG : Alo; Anac; ARN; BELL; Berb; Bry; *Chin;* Cic; *Cocl;* Cof; Con; *Glo;* Hep; Kali-io; Lac-c; Lach; Led; *Nit-ac;* Nux-v; RHUS-T; Sang; SEP; SIL; Spig; Ther.

AMEL: Ars; Caps; Gel; *Nit-ac.*

SUDDEN Agg : Vib.

JAUNDICE (See Yellowness) : Aesc; Canc-fl; Card-m; Chio; Iod; Lept; Mag-m; Myr; Nat-p; Pic-ac; Tarx.

ABDOMEN, Itching, with : Cham.

ANGER, After: Nat-s; Nux-v.

BRAIN, Affection, in : Pho.

CHRONIC : Aur; Chel; *Con;* Iod; *Pho.*

Relapsing : Sul.

CIDER, From: Chio.

CONCOMITANT, As a : Pho.

DIARRHOEA, After : Chin.

During : Dig.

FEVER, With: Card-m; Vip.

FRIGHT, From : Aco.

FRUITS, Unripe, from: Rhe.

GALL STONES, With : Pod.

HAEMATOGENOUS : Pho.

HEAD Ache, with : Sep.

LOSS Of Vital fluids, from : Chin.

LUNG Symptoms, with : Card-m; Chel; Hyds.

MASTURBATION, After : Chin.

MENSES, Arrested, with : Chio.

NERVOUS Excitement, from : Pho.

NEW BORN, Infants : Aco; Bov; Chin; Elat; Myr; Nat-s.

Stool, bilious, with: Elat.

+ OBSTINATE : Choles.

OVER EATING, Or Rich food from : Carb-v.

PREGNANCY, In : Aur; Pho.

SEXUAL Excess, after: Chin.

SUMMER, Every: Chio.

URINARY Symptoms, with: Carb-v; Cham; Chin; Ign; Lyc; Nux-v; Plb.

JAWS UPPER : Am-c; Carb-v; Chin; Kre; *Pho;* Zin.

Projects : Hep.

Swelling : Nit-ac.

Throbbing : *Pho.*

LOWER : *Bell;* Caus; Cham; Cocl; Lach; Laur; Nat-c; Plb; Stap; Zin.

Cold : Plat.

Drawn backward, as if : Bell.

Exostosis : Ang; *Calc-f;* Hep.

Hard swelling : Anthx.

Immovable, A.M. in : Ther.

Motion, chewing : Cup.

loud : Plb.

sleep in : Calc.

Mouth opening Agg : Hep.

Necrosis : Merc-c; Pho.

Nodes, painful : Grap.

Sore : Aur.

Spasms : Tab.

Swelling :Kali-c; Lach; Pho.

beneath right : Ol-an.

Temples, to : Mang.

Thickened : Hecla.

Tension : Caus.

Throbbing : Lach; Nat-m.

biting Agg : Nat-m.

Toothache, with : Sil.

Twitching, trembling : Alu; Ant-t; Cadm; Carb-v; Cocl; Gel; Ol-an; *Pho.*

speak, attempting to, on : Cocl.

yawning while : Old.

Weak, eating,after : Bar-c.

feeling : Kalm.

ACHE : Merc; Thyt.

Bending head back Agg : Sars.

Sleep in, from Clenching : Merc-i-f.

ANGLES, Of : Ign; Merc; Phyt; Sang.

Behind : Chel; Colch; Sang.

Right : Radm.

BONES : Pho; Sil.

Caries : Cist; Pho; Sil.

BORING : Plat.

+ CLOSES, Tightly, disposition : Kob.

+ CLOSURE, Spasmodic : Dios.

CRACKING, Chewing, while : Lac-c; Nit-ac; Rhus-t.

Mouth, opening wide, on : Saba.

CRAMP : Kali-c; Plat; Tab; Ver-a.

Chewing, on : Ver-a.

DISLOCATION, Easy : Ign; Petr;

Rhus-t; Stap.

DROP : See Mouth open.

KEEPS Closed : Kob.

LOCKED, Clenched (Lock-jaw) : BELL; Cam; Cann; Cham; *Cic; Cup;* Hyd-ac; Hyo; *Hypr;* Ign; Merc; Merc-i-f; NUX-V; Op; Phys; Plat; Sec; Tab; Ver-a.

Emotional : Ign.

Grinding of teeth with :

Canth; Cic.

Morning : Ther.

New born, in : Amb; Cam.

Sunstroke, from : Glo.

PAINFUL : Caus.

PARALYSED, As if : Nux-m.

PERIOSTEITIS (Lower) : Calc-f.

SNAP, Shut: Bell; Cic; *Ign;* Lyss; Merc; Nux-v; Plat; Rhus-t.

STIFF : Ap.

Tired, and : Cham; Merc-i-f.

WAGGING : See Chewing motions.

JEALOUSY : Ap; Hyo; Ign; *Lach;* Lil-t; Pul; Stap.

HAPPY, Seeing others : Hell.

INSANE : Lach.

IRRATIONAL : Cocaine.

JELLY, BODY Were made of : Eupi.

JERKING PAIN : See under Pain.

JERKS (See convulsions) : *Bell;* Bor; Calc; Caus; Cic; Colch; Hyo; Hypr; Lyc; Meny; Merc; Nux-v; Plat; *Pul;* Rat;

Sep; Spig; Stan; Sul; Sul-ac; Tab; Tarn; *Val;* Zin; Zin-io.

CONVULSIONS, Before : Ars; Bar-m; Laur; Ver-v.

LIGHTNING, Like, head to foot : Hyd-ac.

MOTION Amel : Merc; Ther.

NIGHT, At : Zin.

PAIN, During : Colo; Ign; Lyc; Meny.

PAINFUL : Rhod.

PARALYZED, Part in; Sec.

RUN, Through whole body : Ign.

SIDE, Lain on : Cimi.

Not lain on : Onos.

SLEEP, On falling to : *Ars;* Cup; Ign; *Kali-c.*

SPINAL Origin: Thu.

TOGETHER : Ther.

JESTS JOKING : *Caps;* Cocl; Cof; *Hyo;* Kali-io; Lach; Op; Tarn.

JOINTS, AFFECTIONS In general : *Arn;* Bell; *Benz-ac; Bry; Calc;* Caus; *Cham;* Cimi; COLCH; Dros; Dul; Grap; Guai; Kali-bi; Kalm; Led; Lith; Lyc; *Mang;* MERC; Nat-m; Nux-v; Phyt; *Pul;* Radm; *Rhus-t;* Rut; *Sabi;* Sep; *Sil;* Stap; Stro; SUL.

ANKYLOSIS, Spurious, with : Kali-io.

ARTHRALGIA : Arg-m; Symp.

BROKEN, As if: Par.

.COLDS Agg : Calc-p; Rum.

CONSTRICTION, In : Anac; Aur; Grap; Nat-m; Nit-ac.

CRACKING, In Benz-ac; Cam; Cann; Caps; Caus; Fer; Kali-bi; Led; *Nit-ac*; PETR; *Rhus-t*; Rut; *Sul*; *Thu*.

Walking in open air Agg : Rut.

CRAMPS : Calc; Pho-ac; Plat; Sul.

CRUSTS, On: Sep.

DEEP, In: Cimi; Radm.

DEFORMED : See Arthritis Deformans.

DIGGING : Colch.

DISLOCATION Spontaneous : See Dislocation Easy.

DRYNESS : Canth; Lyc; *Nux-v*; Pul.

ERUPTIONS, On : *Ars-io*; Bor; Clem; Dul; *Grap*; Kre; Merc; Pho; Psor; *Ran-b*; SEP; Sul; Thyr.

+ FATIGUE : Stap.

+.GIVE Way, suddenly : Pho.

GLISTENING : Mang.

GRITTY Feeling : Con.

INFILTRATED : Mang.

LOOSE : Bov; Chel; Med; Pho-ac; Psor; Thu.

NODES, Hard, around: Form.

OEDEMA, About : Thu.

OIL, Lacking in, as if: Gnap; Lil-t.

PEG, As of a : Buf.

POWER, Loss of : Med.

QUAKING : Colch.

RED Spots, on : Bell; Stic.

RICE Bodies, in : Calc-f.

RUBBING, In : Con.

SKIN, Alternating, with : Stap.

SMALL: Act-sp; Benz-ac; *Caul*; Colch; Kali-bi; *Led*; Lith; Nat-p; Ran-sc; Rhod; Sabi; Sal-ac; Stic; Thu.

Blisters on : Nat-c.

Ulcers, on : Sep.

SORE, Bruised : Arg-m; Aur; Lapp; Pul; Sul.

SORES, Blisters : Ars; Bor; Lapp; Mez; Nat-c;Psor; *Sep*.

SPRAINED, Easily : Pho; Rhus-t.

STIFF, Little pain with: Pho.

STITCHES, In : *Ap*; Colch; *Hell*; *Kali-c*; Mang; *Merc*; *Rhus-t*; Sil; Tarx; *Thu*.

STRETCHES, Bends, or cracks : Caus.

SUPPURATING : Calc-hyp; Merc; Pho; Psor; Sil.

Skin around : Mang.

SWELLING, Pale (White swelling) : Ant-c; *Ars*; Colo; *Iod*; Kre; Merc; Pul; Rhus-t; *Sil*; Sul.

Fatigue, slight Agg : Act-sp.

Oedematous, fractures, after : Bov.

Shining red: Aco.

SYNOVITIS : Ant-t; Ap; Bry; Calc-f; Iod; *Pul*; *Sil*; Sul.

Chronic : Calc-f; Sil.

THICKENED : Spo.

TEARING, Very severe pain : *Arn*; *Chin*; Fer; *Guai*;

Hell; Hep; Merc; Old; *Pul;* RHUS-T; Stro.

TENSION, In : *Bry; Caus;* Led; Lyc; Nat-m; Pul; Seneg; Sep; *Sul.*

TUBERCULOSIS, Of : Ap; Calc; Calc-p; *Kali-c*; Kali-io; Pho-ac; Pul; Sil.

ULCERATED: Colo; Hep; Pho-ac; *Sep*; Sil.

WATER In (Hydrarthrosis) : Ap; Bry; Kali-io; Ran-b; *Sul.*

WEAK :Aco; Arn; Bor; Bov; Calc; Kali-c; Lyc; Mang; Merc; Pho; Psor; Rhus-t; Sep; Sul.

Dislocation, after : Rhe.

Exertion Agg : Pho.

Pregnancy, during : Murx.

Spasms, after : Rhe.

+ **JOURNEY** LONG, Ill effects : Cof.

+ **JOYLESS** : Card-m.

JOYOUS (See Cheerful) : Aco; Caus; *Cof;* Croc; Op.

HEADACHE, During : Ther.

MISFORTUNE, Others, from : Ars.

JUMP, TENDENCY, To : Agar; *Aur;* Croc; Stram; Tarn.

ANIMALS, Bed on, as if: Con.

BED Out of : Abs; Aeth; Bell; Cam; Chin; Hyo; Op; Stram.

Crawls on floor, and : Acet- ac.

BRIDGE, Crossing, whenn : Arg-n.

DREAM, In : Calc-f.

EPILEPSY, After : Arg-m.

EVERY Thing seems to : Ther.

HEIGHT, From : Arg-n; *Aur.*

RUNS, And Recklessly : Saba.

SUDDENLY, Pain, as from : Cina.

WINDOW, From : Aeth; Arg-m; *Aur;* Cam; Gel; Glo.

JUMPING AGG : Spig.

KELOID : *Flu-ac; Grap;* Nit-ac; Sabi; Sil.

KERATITIS : See Cornea, Inflammation.

KICKING : Bell; Lyc; Stram.

SLEEP, In : Bell; Sul.

KIDNEYS : *Ap; Ars; Berb;* CANTH; Helo; Kali-c; Merc-c; Polyg; Rhus-t; Samb; Scil; Scop; Solid; Stro; Terb.

RIGHT : Berb; Coc-c; Lyc; Nux-v; Oci-c; SARS.

LEFT: Chin; Colo; Merc; Par- b; *Zin.*

ABSCESS (Perinephritic) : Ars; *Canth;* Chin; Hep; Lyc; Pul; Sil; Sul-io.

ACHE : Helo; Phyt; Sep; Solid.

BLADDER, To : Arg-n; Nit-ac; Op.

BLEEDING : Merc-c.

BLOWING NOSE, Agg : Calc-p.

BREATHING Deeply Agg : Arg-n; Benz-ac.

BUBBLING : Berb; Med.

BURNING : Nat-m; Nux-v; Pho; Pho-ac; Phyt; Sabi; Sep; Terb .

COLIC : Berb; Canth; Colch;

Colo; Oci-c; Par-b; Polyg; Sars; Tab; Terb.

Glans, pressing Amel : Canth.

Haematuria, with: Oci-c.

Urination, profuse, Amel : Med.

CONGESTED : Aco; Ars;Canth; Kali-bi; Scop; Solid;Terb.

CONTRACTED : Dig; Nit-ac; Plb.

DANCING Agg : Alu.

DISTENDED : Helo; Solid.

EAR And *Eye* symptoms, with : Vio-o.

EPIGASTRIUM, To (left) : Thu.

FLOATING, Reflex symptoms, from : Bell; Ign; Stry-ar; Zin.

FLUTTERING : Brach; Chim.

FUNCTION, Defective : Solid.

HEAVY : Helo; Kali-bi.

INACTIVE : Benz-ac; Helo; Solid.

INFLAMMATION (Nephritis) : Aco; Ap; Arn; Bell; Benz-ac; Cann; CANTH; Fer; Hep; *Kali-chl*; Lyc; Med; Merc-c; Nit-ac; Oci-c; Pul; Rhus-t; Samb; Solid; Stro; *Sul*; Terb; Thu.

Bronchitis, with : Terb.

Cardiac and Hepatic affection, with : Aur; Calc-ar.

Cold, exposure, from : Kali-c.

Exanthemata, after : Hep; Terb.

Frequency, of : Gel; Kali-p.

Influenza, during : Eucal.

Injury, from : Kali-c.

Palpitation, with : Kali-ar.

Pregnancy, during : Helo; Merc-c.

Rheumatism, with: Radm; Terb.

Scarlatinal : Ars; Canth; Hell; Hep; Terb.

Slow : Merc-c.

Suppurative : Ars; *Canth*; Hep; Lyc; Merc; Polyg; Pul; Sil; Sul-io.

Toxemic : Crot-h.

Vomiting, with : Hell.

LAUGHING Agg: Cann.

LIFTING Agg : Calc-p.

LYING on Back, with knees drawn up Amel : Colch.

MOTION Agg : *Berb; Canth*; Chel; Kali-io.

Amel : Thu.

NUMB, Region of : *Berb*.

PRESSURE Agg : *Berb*; Canth; Colch; *Solid*.

Over : Thu.

SNEEZING Agg : Aeth; Bell.

SORE : Berb; Cadm; Grap; *Phyt;* Pul; Senec; Solid; Visc.

STANDING Amel : Berb.

STRETCHING Legs Agg : Colch.

TESTICLES, To : Dios; Op.

THIGHS, To : *Berb;* Ip.

THROBBING, Pulsation : Berb; Sabi.

URINATION, After Amel : *Lyc*; Med.

KILL DESIRE *To* (See Impulses
   Horrid) : Hyo; Iod.

   HERSELF Suddenly : Iod; Meli;
   Nat-s.

   THREATENS, to : Hep; Meli;
   Tarn.

KINDNESS Agg: See Sympathy
   Agg.

KISSES EVERYONE : Croc; Pho;
   Ver-a.

KLEPTOMANIA : Abs; Art-v;
   Cur; Nux-v; Tarn.

KNEADING BREAD or Making
   Similar motions Agg : Sanic.

KNEELING AND PRAYING : Ars;
   Stram.

   AGG : Cocl; Mag-c; Sep.

   AMEL : Aesc; Euphor.

   DIFFICULT : Tarn.

KNEES : Ap; Aur; Benz-ac;
   Caus; Chel; *Gel*; Kali-c;
   Led; Nat-m; Nux-v; Petr;
   Pul;Rhus-t; *Sep;* Sul.

   AIR, HOT, Through : Lach.

   ASCENDING Agg: Alu; Bad;
   Carb-v; Plb.

      And Descending Agg : Bad;
      Kali-c; Rut; Ver-a.

   + AURA,Begins : Cup.

   BANDAGED : Anac; Aur; Sil.

   BEND, Suddenly, standing
   when : Arn; Cup.

   BURNING, Below : Nat-s.
      In : Chel.

   CATCH, In : Nat-m.

   COLD : Agn; Ars; Carb-v;
   Lach; Pho; Sep; Sil.

      Bed in : Pho.

CLUTCHED, Bird's claws, by as
   if : Cann.

CONTRACTED : Caus; Guai;
   Nat-m.

CRACKING : Caus; Cocl; Con;
   Sul.

CRAMP : Calc; Colo; Terb; Zin.

DESCENDING Agg : Arg-m; Vera.

DRAWN UP, Involuntarily,
   walking while : Cup; Ign.

EFFUSION : Ap; Iod; *Rhus-t;
   Sul.*

ELBOW POSITION AMEL : See
   Lying Hands and Knees on
   Amel.

ERUPTIONS, On : Led.

GNAWING : Ran-sc.

HEAVINESS : Nux-v.

+ HOT, Nose cold : Ign.

HOUSE Maid's : Nat-m.

ITCHING : Sul.

   Pain, with : Mang.

JERKING : Pul.

JERKS, Absent : Cur; Oxyt;
   Sec; Sulfo.

   Increased : Lathy.

KNEELING Agg : Bar-c.

   Rising from Agg : Spig.

KNOCK : Arg-n; Caus; Colch;
   Con; Glo.

LARGE, As if : Merc.

NEURALGIA, Pressure Amel:
   Tarx.

NUMB : Colo; Merc-i-f;
   Nat-p; Plat.

   Scrotum, extending, to :
   Bar- c.

   Sitting Amel : Bar-c.

+ PARALYSED : Anac.

RESTLESS : Anac; Lyc; Rhus-t; Thu.

SHOCKS, Through : Pul; Val.
Falling, asleep, on : Agar; Arg-m.

SPREAD Apart : Lyc; Plat.

SPRAINED, As if : Elap.

TENSION : Caus; Nat-m.

THROBBING : Kali-c.

TOTTER, Bend and, while walking : Bry.
Ascending, on: Canth.
Descending Stairs : Sil.

+ Standing, when : Old.

TUBERCULAR : Calc; Iod; Lyc; Sul.

TWITCHING, In: Chin.

WALKING Agg : *Chel*; Led.

WEAK : Aur; *Cocl*; Con; Cyc; GEL; Mur-ac; Nat-m; Nat-s; Plb; *Sep*; Stap; Sul-ac.
Ascending stairs: *Con*; Kali-c; Rut.
Descending stairs : Gel; Kali-c; Rut.
Emission, after : Dios.
Kneeling, when : Tarn.
Knock together, as if they would : Agar; Cocl; Colch; *Nux-v*.
Lumbar ache, with : Kob.
Nausea, with : Bor.
Standing, when : Old.
Walking, while : Cocl; Colo.

KNIFE, Sight of AGG : Alu; Plat.

KNOT : See Ball.

KYPHOSIS : See Spine,
Curvature of.

LABIAE : See Vulva.

LABOUR PAINS (See Labour likepains, under Female organs) : Caul; Cimi; Gel; Kali-c; Kali-p; Pul.
BACK, In : *Gel*; Petr.
Downward : Nux-v.
CEASING, Weak : *Bell*; Cimi; Gel; *Kali-c*; Kali-p; Nat-m; *Op*; PUL; SEC.
Shivering, nervous with : Cimi.
EASING : Caul; Cimi; Vib.
ERUCTATIONS, With : Bor.
EXCESSIVE, Laborious, Violent : *Cham*; Pul; Sec; *Sep*.
FALSE : Bell; Calc; Caul; *Pul*.
FAINTING, Causing : Cimi; *Nux-v*; Pul.
INEFFICIENT : Caul; Cof; *Kali-c*; Nux-v; *Pul*.
+ IRREGULAR : *Caul*.
SPASMS, With : Caul; Caus; *Cham*; Gel; HYO; Ign; *Pul*.
UPWARDS, Going : Calc; Cham; Gel; Lach.

LACERATIONS : Calend; Stap.

LACHRYMAL DUCT : Ap; Fago; Hep; Merc-d; *Petr*; Plb; Sil; Stap.
Obstructed : Merc-d.
Pain, along : Fago.
Stricture : Arg-m; Hep; Nat- m; Sil.
FISTULA : Calc; Flu-ac; Nit- ac; Petr; Phyt; *Pul*; Sil.
Discharging on pressure

: Nat-m; Pul; Sil; Stan.

Eruptions, face on, with : Lach.

GLANDS : Bro; Saba.

INFLAMMATION : Iod.

LACHRYMATION : Ars; *Bell; Calc*; Caus; CEPA; Colch; EUPHR; Flu-ac; Ip; Kali-p; Kre; *Merc; Nat-m;* Nit-ac; OP; *Pho;* PUL; *Rhus-t;* RUT; Saba; Sil; STAP; Stram; SUL; Thu.

AFFECTED Side Agg : Lach; Nat-m; Nux-v; Pul; Spig.

AIR, Cold, from : Dig; Sanic.

Open Agg : Saba.

Amel : Phyt; Pru-sp.

BENDING, Head backward Amel : Seneg.

BITING : Como.

BRAIN, Affections in : Dig; Kali-io; Zin.

BREATHING, Deep, on : Grap.

CHILL, With : Saba.

COLD : See Tears.

Applications, from : Sanic.

COLDS, During : Carb-v; Cep; Euphr; Sang; Tell; Verb.

COUGH, With : Cep; Chel; Cup; Euphr; Grap; Nat-m; Pul; Saba; Scil.

Whooping : Caps; Grap; Nat-m.

DREAMS, During : Plant.

EATING Agg : Ol-an; Zin.

EYES, Closed, with : Spo. Closing, on: Berb. Opening, on : Kali-bi.

forcibly : Ap; Con; Ip; Merc-c; Rhus-t.

+ Using : Stro.

FEVER, During : Pul; Stram.

FIRE, Looking, at : Mag-m; Merc.

GUSHING : Am-c; Ip; Rhus-t.

HEADACHE, During : Ap; Ign; Mez; Plat; Pul.

HEART Symptoms, with : Am-c; Spo.

HOT, Scalding : See Tears.

LARYNX, Tickling in, from : Chel.

LAUGHING, On : Nat-m.

LIGHT, Bright, from : Dig.

LOOKING, Broad day light when : Mag-m.

Intently Agg : Chel.

LYING AGG : Euphr.

MENSES, During : Calc; Phyt; Zin.

MORNING, Early Agg : Calc; *Pul; Sul.*

MUSIC, Hearing : Grap.

NIGHT Agg : Ap; Nit-ac; *Zin.*

PAINS AGG : Chel; Cinb; Lach; Mez; Nat-m; Plant; Pul; Ran-b; Saba.

Throat, in : Sep.

READING, While : Am-c; Croc; Old; Seneg; Stro; Sul-ac.

ROOM, In Agg : Dig.

SNEEZING, With : Just; Nat-m; Saba.

SPASMS, Alternating, with : Alu.

Lids; Lower of, after : Rut.

SUN, in Agg : Bry.

Looking, at : Stap.

SWALLOWING ON : Arg-n.

TEARS Acrid : Ars; Caus; Colch; Euphr; Led; Merc-c; Sul.

Bloody, new born, in : Cham.

Brine, like : Bell.

Burning.hot : Ap; Ars; Cadm; Cedr; Chin; Euphr; Grap; Phyt; Plb; Pul; Rhus-t; Sul; Verb.

sun, looking at : Sang; Stap.

Cold : Lach.

+ Easy, sheds : Castr.

Itching : Ars; Senec.

Oily : Sul.

Sticky : Plat.

Suppressed : Sec.

Thick: Tarn.

Varnish mark, leave : Euphr; Grap; Nat-m; Petr; *Rhus-t;* Thu.

THROAT, Tickling in, with : Chel; Cocl.

WIND, In : Euphr; Pho; Pul.

WRITING, While : *Calc;* Ol-an.

YAWNING When : Ign; Nux-v; Saba; Stap.

LACK OF VITAL HEAT : See Cold AGG.

POWER, Of : See Control, Lack of.

LACTATION AFFECTIONS Of : Bell; Cham; Merc; *Pul;* Sep; Sil.

MILK Absent, scant : Agn; Alfalfa; BRY; *Calc;* Caus; DUL; LAC-C; *Lac-d;* LACT-V;

Lecith; PUL; Stic;Urt; *Zin.*

night watching from : Caus.

+ parturition, after : Urt.

Altered: Bell; Merc.

Bad, spoiled : Aeth; Bor; *Calc; Cham;* Merc; Sil.

Bitter : Rhe.

Bloody : Buf; *Cham; Phyt.*

Blue, thin : Lach.

Child refuses, mother's : Bor; Calc; *Calc-p;* Cina; Merc; Rhe; Sil; Stan.

Flowing : Calc.

as if : Dict; Kre; Nux-v; Pul.

Increased : *Bell; Bry;* Calc; Phyt; *Pul; Sabi.*

menses, before : Con.

+ Sour : Acet-ac.

Suppressed Agg : Agar; Hyo; Mill.

Thick : Bor; Kali-bi.

Weaning, after : Con; *Lac-c;* Pul.

Yellow : Rhe.

LAIN ON, PARTS AGG (See Pressure Agg and Pain goes to side lain on, under Directions) : Cimi; Grap; Mos; Nat-m; Phys; Tell.

LAMENTING : See Complaining.

LANCINATING : See Pain, Shooting.

+ **LARGER** APPEARS : Euphor.

LARYNX: Aco; *Arg-m; Bell;* Bro; *Caus;* Cep; Dros; Hep;

Iod; Kali-bi; LACH; Mang; Nux-v; PHO; *Pul;* Rum; Sele; *Spo;* Stan; Sul.

RIGHT : Agar; Kali-n; Pul; Stan; Stic.

LEFT : Caus; *Crot-h; Hep; Lach;* Rhus-t; *Sul-ac;* Thu; Til.

AIR, Hot, trachea, from : Rhus-t.

BENDING Backward Agg : Bell; *Lach;* Rum.

Amel : Hep.

BLOWING Nose Agg : Caus.

BURNING, Heat : Ars; Iod; Nit-ac; Rum; Sang; Seneg; Spo.

Coughing, when : Gel; Spo.

Hoarseness, with : Am-m.

CLOSED, Nearly, as if : Calc-f.

Salivation, with : Tarx.

COLD, As if, breathing on: Bro; Cist; Rhus-t.

Inspiration, hot expiration : Sul.

Shaving Amel: Bro.

CONSTRICTION, Spasm : Aco; *Bell;* Cup; Ign; Iod; *Mang;* Meph; Mos; Pho; Samb; Stram; Ver-a.

Auditory canal scratching, from : Sil; Sul; Tarn.

Singing Agg : Agar.

Sleep, during : Lach; Nux- v; Spo.

falling to, on : Kali-c; Lach.

Swallowing, on : Dig.

Talking, while: Dros; Mang.

Walking, Amel : *Dros.*

COUGHING Agg : Arg-m; Aru-t; Bell; Bro; Caus; Cep; Kre; Nux-v; Pho; Pul; Sul.

Amel : Asar.

CRAWLING : Con; Kali-c; Nat-m.

CRUMB, As if, in : Lach.

CUTTING : Arg-m; Manc; Merc-c; *Merc-cy;* Nit-ac; Vinc.

Coughing, on : *Cep;* Stap.

DOWNWARDS : Cham; Glo; Ip; Ver-a.

DRAWN, Backwards, thread with: Calc-ar.

In : Ap.

DRY : Bell; Con; Lach; Seneg; Spo; Sul; Thyr.

Singer's in : Sang.

Spot : Con.

EAR, To Left : Zinc-chr.

FISSURES, In : Buf.

FLAPPING Sensation : Lach.

FOREIGN Substance, sensation : *Bell;* Kali-c; Sang.

fever, during : Ip.

FOOD Drops into: Kali-c; Lach; Meph; Nat-m.

FULL, Singers, in : Sang.

FURRY : Pho.

GRASPS, The : Aco; Ant-t; Aru-t; Asaf; Cep; Dros; Iod; Naj; Pho; Spo.

Drinking, when : Aco.

HAIR, In : Naj; Sil.

HANGING, In : Lach; Pho; Spo.

LEAFLET, Trachea over, as if : Ant-t.

LIFTING Agg : Sil.

MOVEMENT, Up and Down: Lyc; Op; Stram; *Sul-io*.

Cough, with : Lach.

MUCOUS, In : Lyc; Pho; Seneg; Stan.

NUMB : Kali-br.

OEDEMA, Glotidis : Ap; Kali-io.

PAINFUL, Tender : Syph.

PARALYSIS : Caus; Lach.

PLUG, Wedge, Valve etc. : Lach; Pho; Spo.

Trachea, closing, as if : Mang.

POLYPUS : Berb.

PRESSURE, On : Chel.

RATTLING, In : Ant-t; Bro; Hep; Ip.

ROUGH, Raw : Carb-v; Caus; Mang; NUX-V; PHO; Pul; Rhus-t; Spo; Stan; Sul.

Talking, from : Arg-m; Tarn.

SINGERS Of : Aru-t; Fer-p.

SKIN As if, in : Pho.

SMOKE, Inhaled, as if : Bar-c.

STREAK : Caus; Ol-an.

SWALLOWING Agg : Spo.

TALKING, Singing Agg : Cep; Pho; Spo.

Amel : Rhus-t; Sele.

TEARING : Caps.

Coughing on : Cep.

Swallowing on : Ign.

THICKENED : Led.

TICKLING, In : *Aco; Ap;* Bro;

Caps; Cham; *Con; Ign;* Kali-bi; Lach; Lyc; Nat-m; Nux.v; Op; Pho; Psor; *Pul;* Rhus-t; RUM; *Sang;* Sep; Sil; Stan.

TOUCH Agg : Aco; Bell; LACH; *Pho; Spo;* Syph.

TRACHEA, Narrow, as if : Cist.

TUBERCULOSIS Of : Carb-v; Dros; Mang; Sele; Spo; Stan.

Cough and hoarseness, with : Stan.

TURNING Neck Agg : Lach; Spo.

UPWARDS : Stan.

VAPOUR, As of a : Ars.

VOCAL Cords, Nodes, on : Sele.

Oedema of : Lach.

Paresis, of : Kali-p; Lach; Ox-ac; Seneg.

Polypus, on : Thu.

Spasms of : Ip.

WEAK : Alu; Bar-c; *Caus;* Gel; Plb; Sul.

LASCIVIOUS : See Amorous.

IMPOTENT, But : Sele.

INSANITY : Hyo.

OGLING, Women on the street : Calad; Flu-ac.

PROSTATE, Enlarged, with : Dig.

LASSITUDE: See Inactive.

LAUGHING AGG : Aco; *Arg-m; Ars;* Aur; Bell; BOR; Cann; Carb-v; Chin; *Cof;* Dros; Kali-c; Mang; PHO; Plb; STAN; Sul; Syph; Tell.

ALOUD Agg : Calc-f.

EXCESSIVE Agg : Cof.

LAUGHS : Bell; Cann; Cic; Cof; Croc; Ign; *Hyo;* Nux-m; *Stram.*

+ ANGRY, Or : Lach.

ASTHMA, With : Bov.

AVERSE, To : Alu; Amb.

CAUSE, Without :Syph.

CHOREA, In : Caus.

CONTINUOUS : Cann.

CONVULSIONS, Before, during after : Caus.

Paroxysms, between : Alu; Plat.

CRIES, And by turns : Asaf; Bov; Cof; Croc; Ign; Mos; *Nux-m;* Samb.

+ Sleep, during : Caus.

EATING, After : Pul.

EVERYTHING, At : Nux-m.

FOOLISH : *Hyo.*

IMMODERATELY : Cann; Fer.

INVOLUNTARILY : Croc; Ign; Mang; Pho.

Pressure on spine, on : Agar.

Speaking, when : Aur.

Tears, with : Pho.

Yawning, after : Agar.

LOUDLY : Bell.

MENSES, Before : Hyo; Nux-m.

NERVOUS : Mos; Tarn.

NIGHT, At : Stram.

PECULIAR, To herself : Thyr.

REPRIMANDS, At : Grap.

SCREAMS, Then : Tarn.

SERIOUS Matters, over : Anac; Cann; Ign; Nat-m; Pho; Plat.

SEXUAL Excitement, with : Stram.

SLEEP, During : Alu; Caus; Hyo; Lyc; Stram.

SPASMODIC : Aur; Cup; Ign; Mos.

Asthma, with : Bov.

Epilepsy, after: Cup.

TITTERING : Buf.

+ TRIFLES, Over : Cann.

UNCONTROLLABLE : Cann; Caps; Mos.

WEEPS, And, by turns : Caps; Ign; Sumb.

WRONG, Time, at : Plat.

LAUNDRY WORK AGG : Sep.

LAX : See Relaxation.

LAYING HANDS ON PART *AMEL* : See Hands Laying on parts Amel.

LAZINESS (See Inactive, Indolent) : Ars; Caps; Chel; Chin; Lach; Nat-c; Nat-m; Nux-v; Sep; *Sul.*

LEAD AGG : See Drugs Abuse of.

LEAF, Valve, Skin, as of a : Alu; Ant-t; *Bar-c;* Fer; Iod; Kali-c; Kali-io; Lach; Mang; *Pho;* Saba; *Spo;*Thu.

LEANING Against a support AGG : Cimi; Hell; Nit-ac; *Samb;* Ther.

AMEL : *Carb-v;* FER; Gymn; Kali-c; Kali-p; Nat-c; Nat-m; Pho-ac; *Sep.*

HEAD, Sideways : Cina.

LEAN PEOPLE : See Thinness, Spare.

LEARNS EASILY : Cam; Cof; Lach; Pho; Plat.

POORLY, With difficulty : Agn; *Anac; Ars; Bar-c;* Calc; Calc-p; Carb-v; Caus; Con; Nat-m; Old; *Pho;* Pho-ac.

LECHEROUS LEWD (See Lascivious) : Flu-ac; Pic-ac.

OLD MEN : Dig.

LECTOPHOBIA : See Fear, Bed of.

LEECHES Application of AGG : Sec.

LEGS (Lower limbs) : Alu; *Ars;* Bell; *Calc;* CAUS; Grap; *Kali-c;* Lach; Led; LYC; *Mang;* Merc; Nit-ac; Nux-v; PUL; RHUS-T; Sep; SIL; SUL; Val; Zin.

RIGHT : Ars; Bell; Bry; Colo; Grap; Lach; Nux-v; Pho; Pul; Rhod; *Sars;* Sec; Sep. Motion involuntary : Cocl.

LEFT : Amb; Asaf; Calc; Cina; Con; Fer; Hep; Lyc; Nit-ac; Rhus-t; Sil; Stram; Sul.

To right : Mag-c.

Trembling : Cic.

ALTERNATING Between : Aco; Alo; Ars; BRY; Calc-p; Cham; Cic; Colo; Cup; Dios; Grap; *Kali-bi;* Kali-c; Kali-n; Lach; Lil-t; Mag-p; *Nat-m;* Nat-s; *Pul; Rhus-t;* Sep; Sil; *Sul.*

Arms, and : See Arms.

ACHING : Ars-io; *Eup-p;*

Gel Guai; Helo; Lil-t; Med; Nit-ac; Pic-ac; *Phyt;* Polyg; Rhus-t; Sul-ac; Sul-io; Vario.

Menses, before : Caul.

Night, at : Med.

Pregnancy, during : Ham.

BAND, About : Chin.

BATHING, Cool Amel : Aur; *Led;* Syph.

BED, Warmth of Agg : Merc; Syph; Ver-a.

BELONG, To him, not : See Not his own.

BELOW Knees : Am-c; Calc; Lyc; Phyt; Pul; Sep; Sil; Stap; Sul-io.

Burning : Nat-s.

Jerking : Dig.

BLOOD Rushes, to : Arg-m; Aur; Meph; Phel; Spo; Sul; Thyr.

BLOTCHY : Led.

BLUE : Nux-v; Ox-ac; Vip.

Menses, during : Amb.

BONES : Merc; Pho; Pul; Rut; Sil; Stap.

BRUISED, As if : Caus; *Eup-p;* Gel; Rhus-t; Rut.

BURNING : Ars; Crot-h; Nat-s; Pho-ac; Pic-ac.

CLAMMY : Lil-t.

COITION Agg : Calc; Nat-m.

COLD : Calad; Carb-v; Dig; Lac-c; Tab.

Chorea, in : Laur.

Clammy : Laur.

Day during, burn at night : Lathy.

Icy : Calc; Jat.

night, in bed : Lil-t.

Pains : Syph.

CRAMP : Cham; COLO; CUP; Kali-m; Med; Stro; *Sul*; Vip.

Extending Agg : Calc.

Pressing foot on floor Amel : Cup-ar; Zin-io.

CROSSES : Gel; Lil-t; Murx; Rhod; *Sep*; Thu.

CROSSING Agg : *Rhus-t*.

Amel : Ant-t; Lil-t; Murx; Rhod; Sep; Thu.

Impossible : Lathy.

DESCENDING Agg : Arg-m.

DOWN To feet, pain : Alu; Caps; Lyc; Pul; Rhus-t.

Burning : Pho-ac.

DRAWN Up : Arg-n.

DROPSY : Ant-t; Eup-p; Samb.

ELEVATING Amel (See Elevating Limbs AMEL) : Bar-c; Grap; Ham; Sep.

ELONGATED, As. if : Colo; Kali-c; Kre; Rhus-t; Sul.

EMACIATION : Abro; Nux-v; Rhus-t; Sele.

ERUCTATION Amel : *Pul*.

FEVER, In Agg : Pyro; *Rhus-t*; Tub.

FLEXES Changing position when : Hell.

FLOATING : Aco; Pho-ac; Spig; Zin-io.

FORMICATION : Calc; Nux-v; *Sec*; Sep.

FULNESS, Bursting : Ham; Vip.

Fever, during : Chin-s.

HANGING,Bed out of Amel : Ver-a.

HEAT, Flushes, of : Kob.

HEAVY : Alu; Calc; Gel; Kali- c; Med; Nat-c; Pho; Pic-ac; Pul; Rhus-t; Rut; Sul.

Ascending Agg : Med; *Nat-m*; Pho.

Exertion Agg : *Gel*; Pic-ac.

Feet glued to the floor : Pho.

Lead like, while walking : Med.

Painful : Bov.

Sitting while : Alu.

HOT Wind or wire darting through, as if : Dig.

IMMOBILE : Ox-ac.

INVERTED : Cic; Merc; Nux-v; Petr; *Psor*; Sec.

ITCHING : Agar; Calc; Caus; Mez; Rhus-t; Sil; Sul.

JERKING Up : Lach; *Lyc*; Myg.

Lying down, on : Meny.

Pain, with : Lyc.

LIFT Can not, when lying down : Lathy.

LONG, Too, as if, standing when : Kre.

MANY, As if : Pyro.

NOT His Own, as if : Bap; Coll; Op.

NUMB : Calc; Cup-ar; *Grap*; Kali-c; Onos; Ox-ac; Plant; Plb; Pul; Rhus-t; Tarn; Thyr.

Right : Cedr; Eup-p; *Kali-c*; Nux-m; Zin.

arm, left : Tarn.

Crossing on : Agar; Alu; Kali-c.

Menses, during : *Pul.*

One, other painful : Sil.

Sitting Cross legged, on : Alu.

Standing long Agg : Pul.

Walking, while : *Kali-n;* Rhus-t; Sep.

ONE, Shorter than other, as if, while walking : Cinb.

Motion constant, of : Bry.

OOZING, From, oedematous : *Grap;* LYC; Tarn-c.

PADDED, As if : Arg-n.

PARALYZED, As if : Cup-ar.

Dinner Agg : Tub.

PETECHIAE : Ap; Led; Solid.

PRESSES, Foot, floor to : Ign; Med; Zin-io.

PRESSURE Amel : Ars; Mag-p.

RED Hot wire : See Hot wind or wire.

RESTLESS : Agar; *Ars;* Carb-v; Kali-c; Med; Nit-ac; *Rhus-t;* Sul; *Tarn;* Tub; ZIN.

Menses, during : Lac-c.

Night, at : Ars; Caus; Med; Tarn.

ROTATION Agg : Bry; Cocl; Colo; Kali-c.

SEPERATED, As if, standing on : Pho.

SEVERED, Belonging to someone else : Op.

SHOCK, Electric : Caus.

SHOOTING Up : Guai; Nux-v.

SHORTENED, As if : Amb; Colo;

Mez; Old; Pho; Sep.

Numb, and : Merc.

STIFF, As if : Nux-v.

STOCKING, Elastic, covered with, as if : Pic-ac.

STOOL Agg : Ap; Sec; Ver-a.

STRETCH, Inclination to, or must : Cina; Sul-ac.

STRETCHING Amel : Med.

SWAYING To and Fro, while standing : Cyc.

SWEAT : Euphr; Mang; Petr; Pod.

Cold : Pul; Terb.

TENSION, Alternating anus, with : Kali-m.

TIED, Together, as if : Syph.

TINGLING : Grap; Kali-c; Lyc; Petr.

TREMBLING : Arg-n; Cimi; Lach; Nit-ac; Nux-v; Op; Plant.

Coition, after : Nat-p.

Walk, can scarcely : Cimi.

TWITCHING : Anac; Merc; Pho; Phys; Tarn.

Lying Agg : Meny.

ULCERS : Flu-ac; *Lach;* Sul-io.

Climaxis, at : Polyg.

Gangrenous : Rhus-t.

UNCOVERING Agg : Hep; Rhus-t; Sil; Thu.

VARICES : *Carb-v;* Caus; *Ham;* Lyc; *Pul; Zin.*

Inflammation, after : Calc-ar.

VEXATION, Felt in : Nux-v.

WEAK : Ars; *Cocl; Con;* GEL;

Mang; Nat-m; Nat-s; *Nux-m;*
Nux-v; Onos; Pho- ac; Plb;
Rhus-t; Sep; Sul; Tarn; Zin.

Back, sprain, from : Rut.

Descending Agg : Arg-m;
Sil.

ascending, and Agg : Rut.

Hips, spot between, from :

Phyt.

One, epilepsy, after : Cadm;
Pho.

Paralytic : *COCL;* Ruta Thu.

pregnancy durin g :
Agar;
Plb.

Parturition, after : Caus;
Rhus-t.

Rising, chair, from : Rut.

Sciatica pain, from : Grat.

Sitting down, when : Stan.

Smoking, from : Clem.

Uncertain : Mang.

Walking Agg : *Nux-m.*

WEATHER Changes Agg : Phyt.

WIND, Cool, blowing on, as if
: Lil-t.

WOODEN Sensation : Arg-n;
Ars; Rhus-t.

Walking while: *Kali-n;*
Thu.

LENS: Euphr; *Pul; Sil; Sul.*

CATARACT: *Calc;* Calc-f;
Calc-p; CAUS; Euphr;
Kali-m; Mag-c; Napth; Pho;
Sec; SIL; SUL.

Capsular : Am-m.

+ Incipient and progressive
: Chim.

Injuries, from : Con.

Lachrymation, with :
Euphr.

Menses absent, with : Lyc.

Ocular lesions, from : Tell.

Operations, after : Seneg.

Senile : Carb-an; Sec.

Women, in : Sec; Sep.

LEPROSY : Ars; Crot-h;
Hydroc; Sec; Sep; Sil; Sul.

LETHARGY : See Inactive.

LEUCOCYTHEMIA : See
Leukemia.

LEUCODERMA : Alu; Ars;
Ars-sul-fl; Calc-f; Merc;
Nat-c; Nat-m; Sele; Sep;
Sil; Sul.

LEUCORRHOEA : *Alu;* Ars;
Calc-s; Carb-an; Caus;
Grap; Hyds; Iod; Kali-c;
Kre; Med; MERC; *Nat-m;*
Nit-ac; Plat; *Pul;* SEP; Sil;
Stan; Sul.

AGG :Chin; Kalm; Kre;
Merc; Nat-m;Plat; Psor;
Sep.

AMEL : Carb-v; Murx; Phyt.

ACRID, Corroding : Agar; *Alu;*
Am-c; Ars; Bor; Caul; Con;
Fer; Flu-ac; Grap; Kali-bi;
Kali-io; *Kre;* Lil-t; Lyc;
Merc; Nit-ac; *Pho;* Pru-sp;
Pul; Rut; Sabi; Sang; *Sec;*
Sep; Sil; *Syph.*

Albuminous : Bor; Mez.

+ Children in : Cub.

Thighs and linen : Iod.

BLACKISH : Bur-p; *Chin;* Kre.

BLISTERING : Am-c; Kre; Med;

247

Pho.

BLOODY : Calc-s; Chin; Cocl; Murx; Nit-ac; Sep.

Menses, after : Chin; Zin.

instead of : Chin.

Stools, during : Murx.

Water : Calc; Kre; Mang; Nit-ac.

BLUISH : Amb.

BRINY : Sanic.

BROWN : Iod; *Lil-t; Nit-ac;* Sec; Ust.

Stains : Lil-t; *Nit-ac.*

BURNS, Hot: *Bor;* Calc; Calc-s; Hep; *Kre;* Lept; Lil-t; Pul; Sep; Sul.

Abdominal pain, after : Calc-p.

Watery : Hyds.

CLIMAXIS, At : Psor; Sang.

COITION, After : Nat-c; *Sep.*

Amel : Merc.

COLIC, After : Am-m; Calc-p; Con; Lyc; Mag-c; Mag-m; Sil; *Sul.*

CONSTANT : Am-m; Sec.

COPIOUS : Am-c; Ars; Asaf; Calc; Caul; Flu-ac; Grap; Hyds; Merc-i-r; Sep; Sil; Stan; Sul-io; Thu.

Menses, like: Alu; Caus; Kre.

Serum like discharge from anus and vagina : *Lob.*

DAY Only : Lac-c; Plat.

+ DAY time Agg : Alu.

DIRTY : Sec.

EXHAUSTING : Cocl; Frax; Senec; Visc.

FLATUS Passing Agg : Ars.

FLOWING Down, thighs : Alu; Lept; Lyc; Lyss; Onos; *Senec;* Syph; Tub.

Imperceptibly : Agn.

Warm water : Bor; Lept.

GIRLS, Little : Calc; Caul; Mang; *Merc;* Senec; Sep.

Acrid : Cub.

Infants : Cann.

Yellow : Merc-i-f.

GLAIRY : Pall.

GONORRHOEAL : Nit-ac; Pul; Sabi; *Sep.*

GREENISH : Asaf; Carb-v; Merc; Merc-i-r; Nat-m; Nat-s; Nit-ac; Sep.

Acrid : Merc-i-r.

Stains : Bov; Lach; Thu.

Water : Sep.

GUSHING : Calc; Grap; Kre; Lyc; Mag-m; Psor; Sil; Stan.

Cramp, with : Mag-m.

Sqatting, when : Cocl.

HEAD ACHE, with : Plat.

HONEY Coloured : Nat-p.

HOT : See Burns.

Water like : Bor; Hep; Lept.

ITCHING, Causing : Carb-ac; Helo; Hyds; Kre; Stap; Syph.

LABOUR Like pains, with: Dros; Kali-c.

+ LONG LASTING : Myr.

LUMPY, Curdy : Bor; Helo; Hep; Kali-c; Psor; Radm;

Sep; Sil.

Clear : Tarn.

LYING, While : *Pul.*

MAMMAE, Sore, with : Dul.

MASTURBATION, From: Canth; Plat; *Pul.*

MEAT Water, like : Kali-io.

MEMBRANOUS : Hep.

MENSES, Before : Bov; Calc; *Grap*; Kre; *Sep*; Sul-io.

And After : Grap; Pall; Sul-io.

After : Bov; Calc; Calc-p; *Grap; Kre;* Mag-c; Tab.

Between: Bor; Calc; Sep.

+ During : Iod.

Instead of : Ars; Cocl; Grap; Nat-m; Nux-m; Pho; Sep; Xanth.

Scanty, with: Calc-p; *Caus.*

Week One, after : Kalm.

MILKY : Calc; Fer; Lyc; *Pul;* Sep.

NIGHT Agg : Caus.

OFFENSIVE :Arg-m; Ars-io; Asaf; *Carb-ac;* Hep; *Kali-p;* Kre; Nit-ac; Nux-v;*Psor;* Sabi; Sec; Sep; Ust.

Forceps, delivery, after: Calend.

+ Purulent : Buf.

PERIODICAL : Lyc.

PILES, Suppression, from : Am-m.

PREGNANCY, During : Cocl; Kali-c; Kre; Sabi; Sep.

PUBERTY, At : Fer.

PURULENT : Hep; Kali-p;

Pru-sp; Sep.

RISING, Seat, from Agg : Plat.

SEROUS, Fluid : Tab.

SEXUAL Excitement, from : Canth; Hyds; Pul; Senec.

With : Ign.

SITTING, While : Ant-t.

SMELL, Cheese, old, like: Hep.

+ Fishy : Med.

Green corn, like : Kre.

Menses, like : Caus.

Sour : Hep; *Nat-p.*

Sweetish : Calc-p; Merc-c.

SQUATTING Agg : Cocl.

STAINS, Indelibly : *Bur-p;* Mag-c; Med; *Pulex;* Sil; Vib.

STANDING Agg : Lac-c.

STARCH Boiled, like: Bor; Fer-io; Nat-m; Sabi.

STICKY, Stringy: Alet; Hyds; *Kali-bi;* Nit-ac; Sabi; Tarn.

STIFFENS, Linen : Lach.

STOOL, After : Mag-m; Vib; Zin.

During : Fer-io; Sanic.

STOOPING Agg: Cocl.

STUBBORN : Mez.

THICK : Ars; Calc; Calc-s; Carb-ac; Hyds; Kali-bi; *Merc;* Murx; *Senec.*

Acrid: Bov; Hyds.

Creamy : Calc-p; Nat-p; Pul; Sec.

Profuse, as menses : Mag-s.

THIN, Watery : Fer; Grap; Lept; Lil-t; Nit-ac; Pru-sp;Pul.

+ TRANSPARENT, Imperceptible : Agn.

URINARY, Symptoms, with : Berb; Erig.

URINATING Agg : Am-m; Calc; Kre; Merc; Plat; Sep; Sil.

URINOUS : Ol-an.

VAGINA, Pressure in, with : Cinb.

WALKING Agg : Aur; Bov; Lac-c; Mag-m.

WASHING Amel : Kali-c.

WHITE : Alet; Bor; Calc-p; Grap; Merc; Nat-m;Sep.

Stains, linen yellow : Chel.

Turns, green : Nat-m.

YELLOW : Ars; Calc; Cham; Gel; Hyds; Kre; Merc-i-f; *Murx*; Sabi; Senec; Sep; Sul; Ust.

Stains : Agn; Carb-an; Chel; *Kre*; Nit-ac; Pru-s.

green : Bov.

LEUKEMIA : Ars; Ars-io; Bar-io; Bar-m; Benz; Nat-m; *Nat-ars; Nat-s*; Pho; Pic-ac; Thu.

SPLENIC : *Ceano; Nat-s.*

LEVITATION : See Floating, as if.

LEWD : See Lecherous, Lascivious.

LICE (Lousiness) : Lyc; *Merc; Ood*; Psor; Saba; *Sul.*

ITCHING OF : Led.

LICHEN : See under Eruptions.

LICKING LIPS AGG : Val.

TONGUE, with Amel : Mang.

LIE DOWN, INCLINATION, to : See Inactive.

BUT, Thereby Agg : Alu; Murx.

MUST : Ap.

WILL NOT, Sits up in bed : Kali-br.

LIENTERIA: See Diarrhoea after, eating, drinking.

LIFE + BURDEN Is : Alo.

SATIETY, Of : See Suicidal, disposition.

UNFIT, For : Sep.

UNWORTHY : *Nat-s*; Plat.

+ **LIFELESS BODY**, RESTLESS MIND : Bap.

LIFTED UP, Sensation : Hypr; Pho; Strop.

SLEEP, During: Strop.

LIFTING AGG (See Sprains and Strains): ARN; BRY; *Calc*; Calc-p; Carb-an; Caus;Con; Grap; Led; Nat-c; Onos; Pru-sp; Psor; *Pul; Rhus-t*;Sep; *Sil*; Stro; *Sul; Val.*

AMEL : Spig.

OVER AGG : Amb; Agn; Carb-v; Form; Grap; Lyc; Sep.

LIGAMENTS : See Fibroid Tissue.

LIGHT As IF, : See Floating.

BODY, Feels : Mez.

Onanism from or Hysterical : Gel.

LIGHT AGG : ACO; Aesc; Ap; Arg-n; *Ars*; Bar-c; BELL; CALC; Chin; *Con*; Dros; EUPHR; *Glo; Grap*; Hep; Hyo; Lac-d; *Lyc*; Mag-p; *Merc; Merc-c*; Nat-m; *Nat-s*; Nux-v; Op; *Pho*; Pho-ac; Pul; *Rhus-t*; Sang; SEP; *Sil; Stram; Sul.*

But cannot bear covering : Ap.

Little even : Lac-d.

AMEL, DARKNESS AGG : Am-m;
BELL; Calc; Cann; Carb-an;
Carb-v; *Gel*; Lyc; Plat;
STRAM; *Stro*; Val.

ARTIFICIAL, Fire Light AGG :
Bell; Calc; Caus; Con; Dros;
Euphr; Glo; Lyc; MERC;
Nat-m; Pho; Rut; Sep;
Stram.

Read, can not, in : Nat-m.

BLUE AGG : Tab.

BRIGHT, Bright objects AGG :
Canth; *Bell;* Buf; Stram; Thu.

GAS AGG : Caus; Glo; *Merc;*
Nat-c; Nat-p.

MOON : See under Moon.

REFLECTED AGG : Sep.

SNOW, From AGG : Ant-c;
ARS; Cic; *Glo*.

STAINED Glass from AGG :
Ant-c; Nat-s.

SUBDUED AGG : Nat-s.

SUN, AGG : *Ant-c;* Bell; Chin;
Euphr; *Glo;* Grap; Kali-bi;
Lith; *Nat-c;* Sele; Sul.

AMEL : Anac; Con; Crot-h;
Iod; Kali-m; *Plat;* Rhod;
Stro; Thu.

Blinds : Lith.

LIGHTNING: See Pain, Shooting.

+ AGG : Crot-h.

LIMBS UPPER : See Arms.

LOWER : See Legs.

ALTERNATING Between upper
and lower : See Arms.

BANDAGED : Chin; *Plat.*

BELONG To HER, did not: Agar;

Ign; Op.

BRITTLE : Radm.

CLAMMY : Cam; Carb-v; Pic-ac.

COLD : Calc-p.
Digestion, Affection of with
: Calc-p.
Moist : Stic.
Water, as if in : Led.

CONSTRICTION : Chin; Lyc.

CRAMP : Amb; Cimi; Ran-b;
Vip.

CRAWLING : Calc-p.

CROSSING AGG : See Crossing
Limbs.

DEAD, As if : Lyc.

DIARRHOEA, With: *Cup*; Jat; Sec.

DEEP Breathing Agg : Cann.

DETACHED (See Dislocated
Sprain, as if) : Hypr.

DOUBLE, As if : Petr.

DRAWING UP AGG and AMEL :
See under Drawing.

DRAWN Up Like hedge-hog :
Colo.

EATING AGG : Clem; Ind.
Amel : Nat-c.

ELEVATING AMEL : See
Elevating Limbs.

EMACIATED, Body plump, with
: Plb.

EYES Alternating, with : Kre.

FORMICATION : Lyc; Pho-ac;
Rhus-t; Sec; Stro; Tarn.
Menses during : Grap.

HANGING Down Agg : See
Hanging down limbs Agg.

HARD : Radm.

HEATED, Being Agg : Zin.

+ HEAVY : Ap.

HERPES, On : Manc.

+ IMMOVABLE : Ap.

JERKS : Phys.

   Cough, with : Stram.

   One, sleep in : Ant-t; Sul.

   Spasms, during : Sil.

LYING Agg : Kali-c.

NUMB : Aco; Ap; Calc-p; Echi.

   Left : Pul.

   One more, than other : Crot-h.

PARALYZED, As if : Thu.

RESTLESS : Tarx.

SHATTERED, As if : Mez.

SHORT, As if : Mez; Mos.

TOSSES, From side to side: Cina.

TOUCH Agg : *Chel;* Chin.

TREMBLING : Merc.

WEAK, Eating, after : Clem.

LINEA NASALIS: See Face Pale.

LINEAR PAINS : See under Pain.

LIPS : Ars; Aru-t; *Bell;* Bry; *Nat-m; Rhus-t;* Sep; Sil; *Sul.*

   UPPER : Bar-c; Carb-v; Kali-c; Sul; Zin.

   Cracked : Kali-c; Nat-m.

   Hair (in women): Ol-j.

   Heavy : Caus.

   Numb, as if : Cyc.

   Red : Ars-io; Calc; Nat-m.

   Retracted : Ant-t; Cam.

   Stiff : Euphr.

   Sweat, on : Kali-bi; Med; Rhe.

   Swelled : Bar-c; *Calc;* Hep;

Nat-m; Nit-ac; Psor; Sul.

   turned up : Merc-c.

   Twitching, Trembling : *Carb-v.*

   Weak : Card-m.

LOWER : Bry; Ign; Pul; Sep.

   Biting of, eating while : Benz-ac.

   Cracked : Sep.

   Centre : Pul.

   Crawling, bug, as if : Bor.

   Heavy, as if : Grap; Mur-ac.

   Numb : Glo.

   Red : Sep; *Sul.*

   Swelled : Asaf; Lach; *Merc;* Sep; *Sul.*

   as if : Glo.

   Tremble, eating, while : Arn.

ABSCESS : Anthx.

BLACK : Aco; ARS; *Chin;* Merc; Pho-ac; Ver-a.

   Blisters : Tub.

BLEEDING : *Aru-t;* Bap; Lach.

BLOATED : Mur-ac.

BLUE : Acet-ac; Ant-t; Arg-n; *Cam;* CUP; DIG; Hyd- ac; Lach; *Lyc;* Mos; *Nux-v;* Spo; Ver-a.

   Chill, during : Nat-m.

   Convulsions, during : Nux-v.

   Menses, during : Arg-n; Ced.

BROWN : Rhus-t.

BURNING : Am-m; Mur-ac; Saba; Thyr.

+ Fire like : Am-m.

Smoker's in : Bry.

Touched, when : Merc.

CANCER : Ars-io; Cic; Cist; Clem; Con; Cund; Hyds; Sil.

CHANGING Colour : Sul.

COLD Sores : See Herpes.

CORNERS, Cold : Aeth.

Cracked : *Aru-t; Cund;* GRAP; Mag-p; Merc-c; Mez; *Nit-ac;* Psor; Sil.

right : Merc.

Crusty Scaly : Grap; Merc; Nit-ac; Thu.

Droop : Agar.

Indented : Sil.

Inflammed : Sil.

Raw : Ant-c; Aru-t; Grap.

CRACKED : Ail; Alo; Am-m; ARS; *Aru-t;* Bap; BRY;Calc; Calc-p; Carb-v; Chin; *Grap;* Ign;Lach; Meny; Merc; Mur- ac; NAT-M; Pul; Rhus-t; Sep; Sul.

Middle : Calc; *Cham;* Hep; *Nat-m;* Pho; *Pul;* Sep.

CRAMPS : Ran-b.

CRAWLING, As of bugs: Bor.

CRUSTY, Scaly : *Ars;* Mur-ac; Nat-m; Pho; Pho-ac; *Rhus-t;* Sep; *Sil;* Stap.

DRAWN Up, Retracted: Ant-t; *Cam;* Nux-v; Phyt; Tab.

DROOP : Bar-c; Merc; Nux-v.

DRY : Alo; Am-m; Ant-c; Bry; Caus; Hyo; *Nux-m;* Pho; Pul; *Rhus-t;* Sul; Thyr; Ver-v.

EGG Albumin, on : Ol-an; Pho-ac.

EPITHELIOMA : Cic; Sep.

EVERTED (See Drawn up): *Ap;* Phyt.

Swollen : *Merc-c.*

FORMICATION : Bor.

Menses, during : Grap.

GLUED, Together : Cann; Stram.

HANG, Down : Ver-a.

HEAVY : Mur-ac.

HERPES, Vesicles on : *Ars;* Dul; Manc; NAT-M; Pho; *Rhus-t;* Sep; Sul-io.

Black : Tub.

Hard Small : Calc-f.

Inner Side : Med.

Menses, during : Sars.

ITCHING : Ap; Nit-ac.

JERKING, Twitching: *Carb-v;* Cham; Ol-an; Senec; Tell; Thu; Vip.

Cold air, in : Dul.

Convulsions, during : Sil.

Speaking, while : Arg-n.

Up. : Tell.

LICKING AGG : Val.

LICKS : Agar; Alo; Ars; Kre; Lyc; Nat-m; Phys; *Pul;* Stram.

+ MOISTENS, Thirst, without : Kre.

MOVE, Speaking, as if: Hell.

NEURALGIA : Ap.

NUMB : Aco; Crot-h; Nat m; Old.

OEDEMA : Ap.

PALE : Ars; Fer; Hyd-ac; Kali-ar; Med.

PEELING : Aru-t; Cham; Con; Kali-c; *Lac-c;* Nat-c; *Nat-m;* Nit-ac; Nux-v; Pul; Thyr.

PICKING, At : Ars; *Aru-t; Bry;* Hell; Kali-br; Nit-ac; Nux-v; Tarn.

POUTING, Thick : Bar-c; Calc; Grap; Merc; Nat-m; Psor; Syph.

Belly, big, with : Syph.

RED : Alo; *Ars;* Bell; Merc-c; *Sul;* Thyr; Tub.

RETRACTED : See Drawn up.

SALTY : Merc; Nat-m; Sul.

SCABBY : See Crusty.

SCARLET : Strop.

SHRIVELLED : Am-m; Ant-t.

SLIMY : Kali-io; Stram; Zin.

SMACKING, Of : Amy-n.

SORDES, On : *Ars;* Colch; Hyo; Pho; *Stram.*

SORE : Lyc; Mur-ac.

STICKY : Merc-i-r; Nux-m; Zin.

STIFF : Ap; Euphr; Kalm; Lach.

SWELLED : Ail; Ap; *Ars;* Aru-t; *Bell;* Bry; *Lach; Merc-c;* Nat-m; Nit-ac; Op; Sep.

THICKENED : Med.

TINGLING : Nat-m; Pic-ac.

TOUCH, Least Agg : Cadm.

TREMBLE, Eating, while: Arn.

Speaking, while : Arg-n.

TWITCH, Spasm : See Jerking.

ULCERATED : Bor; Stram.

VEINS, Distended : Dig.

VESICLES : See Herpes.

LITHEMIA : See Uric Acid Diathesis.

LIVELY : See Cheerful.

LIVER (Including Right Hypochondria) : *Aesc;* Alo; Am-c; Am-m; Ars; AUR; Bar-c; BELL; *Berb; Bry;* Card-m; CHEL; CHIN; Cocl; Colch; Dios; Gel; Hyds; Iris; KALI-C; LACH; Lept; LYC; *Mag-m; Merc; Nat-s;* Nit-ac; Nux-m; NUX-V; PHO; *Pod;* Rhe; Sang; *Sep;* Sul; Ust.

ABSCESS : Bell; Bry; *Hep;* Lach; *Merc-c;* Nux-v; Pul; Rut; Sep; *Sil;* Ther.

Forming, as if : Laur.

ANGER Agg : Cocl.

ARM. Right, and : Bry; Iris.

ATROPHY : Aur; Calc; Hyds; Laur; Pho.

Acute yellow : Pho.

Nutmeg : Laur; Lyc.

BACK, Of : Arn; Bor; Calc; Echi; Kali-bi; Lept; Rhus-t; Thu.

BACKWARD, Extending to Scapulae : Berb; *Chel;* Dul; Lept; Merc; Myr; Sep.

Right, to : Aco; Aesc; Aral; *Bor; Calc;* CHEL; Dios; Grap; *Hyds;* Kali-bi; *Lyc;* Mag-m; *Nat-m.*

cutting : Hyds.

Left, to : Dios; Dul; *Lept;* Myr.

BALL, Lump, in : Aesc; Bar-c.

Below : Arn; Bor; Echi;

Gel; Lach; *Nat-s;* Thu;
Ver-a; Zin.

Hard, in: Nux-m.

BREATHING DEEP Agg : *Bell;*
Hep; Nat-s; Ptel; Sele; Ther.

Amel : Ox-ac.

BURNING, Heat : Alo; Aur; *Lach;*
Lept; Merc; Myr; Stan;
Ther.

Stool, after : Stan.

BURSTING : Bry; Lept; Nat-s.

CANCER : Chel; Choles; Hyds;
Myr; Ther.

Early : Senec.

Jaundice, with : Myr.

CIRRHOSIS : Card-m; Cup;
Hep; Hyds; Mur-ac; Pho;
Sul.

Boils, with : Nat-p.

Hypertrophic : Merc-d.

COUGHING Agg: Bry; Chin-s;
Dros; Eup-p; Hep; Kali-c;
Kali-c; Nat-s.

CRAMP : Canc-f; Mag-m;
Phys.

Menses, during : Buf.

CUTTING : Berb; Dios; Hyds;
Lach; Thyr.

DEEP, In : Lach.

DOWNARDS : Chel.

ENLARGED, Swelled : Alo;
Chin; Chio; Lach; *Lyc;*
Mag-m; *Merc; Nat-s;* Nux-v;
Sele; Sep; Tarx; Vip; Zin.

Cardiac affections with :
Mag-m.

Children, in : Calc-ar;
Nux-m.

+ Chronic : Mang.

+ Hard and Sore : Zin.

Pain, anger, after : Cocl.

+ Spleen, with : Iod.

EPIGASTRIUM, To : Lach;
Mag-m.

EYE Symptoms, with : Con.

GRIPING : See Cramp.

HARD, Small, as if: Ab-c.

HEART symptoms, with (See
Heart with Liver symptoms,
with) : Myr.

HEAVY : Bry; Mag-m; Nat-s;
Pho-ac; Ptel.

Aching : Phyt.

HIPS, To : Vip.

INDURATED, Hard : Ars; Chin;
Dig; *Grap;* Iod; Laur;
Mag-m; Pho; Rat; Tarx.

INFLAMMATION : Aco; Ars; Bell;
Chel; Lyc; *Mag-m;* Nat-s;
Nux-v.

JARRING Agg : Lach; Nat-s.

LAUGHING Agg : Psor.

LEUCORRHOEA Amel : Phyt.

LUNG Symptoms, with :
Card-m; Chel; Hyds.

LYING, Back on Amel : Hyds;
Mag-m; Nat-s.

Right side, on Agg : Chel;
Dios; Hyds; Kali-c;
Mag-m; Merc.

Left side, on Agg : Arn;
Bry; Card-m; Mag-m;
Nat-s; P*ul;* Sep.

Painful side, on Amel : Bry;
Ptel; Sep.

MENSES Agg : Pho-ac.

NAVEL, To : Berb; Dul; Lept; Myr; Sep.

NIPPLE, To (R) : Dios.

OCCIPUT, To: Kali-c; Nux-v; Sep.

PRESSURE Agg : Bell; Bry; Carb-v; Card-m; Chin; Hep; Lach; Lyc; *Merc;* Pho; Sele.

Amel : See Lying on painful side.

RASH, Over : Sele.

RUBBING And Shaking Amel : *Pod.*

SHOULDER, To : Kali-c; Nux-v; Sep; Vip.

Right : Kali-bi; Med.

Top of, and : Crot-h.

SNEEZING Agg : Psor.

SORE, Tender : Aur-m; *Bell; Bry;* Carb-v; Chio; Dig; Iod; Iris; *Kali-io; Lach;* Lept; *Lyc; Mag-m; Merc;* Mur-ac; NAT-S; *Nux-v; Pod.*

Menses, with : Pho-ac.

Vomiting, during Agg : Pod.

SPINE, To : Lept; Mag-m; Sil.

SPOTS : See Chloasmae.

STICKING : Berb; Calc; Chel; Con; Lept; Mag-m; Merc; *Nux-v;* Ran-b; Sele; Sep.

TENSION : Chel.

THROBBING : Crot-h; Lapp.

URTICARIA, With : Canc-fl; Myr.

UTERINE Symptoms, with : Mag-m.

WALKING Agg : Hep.

+ LIVES, OWN WORLD, In : Bell.

LIVID : See Blue.

LOAD : See Heaviness, Weight.

+ **LOAFS** : Sul.

LOATHING : See Aversion.

HERSELF : Lac-c.

LOCHIA ACRID : Kre.

+ AFTER Pains, with : Xanth.

BLOODY, Child nurses, when : Sil.

DARK : Kre; Sec.

GREEN : Lac-c; Sec.

OFFENSIVE, Foul : Echi; Kali-chl; Kali-p; *Kre; Sec.*

PROTRACTED : Carb-ac; Caul; Chin; Nat-m; Sec; Senec; Tril.

Limbs, numb, with : Carb-an.

+ SCANTY : Nux-v; Radm.

SUPPRESSED : BRY; Hep; Hyo; Mill; *Pul;* Pyro; *Sul.*

Cold, from : Cimi; Pyro.

Emotions, from : Cimi.

+ Fright, from : Op.

LOCK-JAW : See Jaws, Locked, clenched.

LOCOMOTOR ATAXIA : *Alu;* Nux-m; Onos; Pho; Plb; Sec; Sil; Sul; Thal.

EATING Amel : Nat-c.

LOINS : Canth; Plb; Rhe; Thu; Zin.

BURNING : Bar-c.

HOLLOW : Pall.

STICKING : Berb; Plb.

LONELY : See Forsaken.

LONGING : See Craving.

LOOKED AT AGG : ANT-C; Ant-t; *Ars;* Cham; *Cina;*

Nat-m; Pul.

LOOKING AROUND AGG : Calc; *Cic;* CON; Ip.

ALL Sides, on : Kali-br.

BED, About, to find something : Ign.

BRIGHT, Shining objects, at AGG : *Bell;* Canthl; Hyo; *Lyss*; Mur-ac; Stram.

CONSTANTLY In one direction : Bro; Hyo.

DISTANT Objects, at AGG : Dig; Euphr; Rut.

AMEL   : Bell.

DOWN AGG : Arg-n; Bor; Calc; Kali-c; Kalm; Old; *Pho; Spig; Sul.*

AMEL   : Saba.

ECLIPSE, At AGG   : Hep.

EITHER WAY, Right or Left AGG : *Con;* Spig.

EVERY Body at her : Meli.

FLOWING Water, at AGG : See Moving things.

INTENTLY AGG (See Reading AGG) : Cina; Mur-ac; Old.

AMEL   : Agn; Petr.

KNIFE, At : See knife.

LONG, Anything at AGG : Aco; Aur; Nat-m; Rut; Sep; Spig.

AMEL : Dig; *Nat-c;* Saba.

MIRROR, In AGG   : Kali-c.

MOVING Things, Flowing Water etc. AGG : Agar; BELL; Bro; Canth; *Con; Fer;* Hyo; Jab; Lyss; Stram; Sul.

OTHERS, In distress AGG :

Tarn.

OVER A Large surface AGG (See Agarophobia) : *Sep.*

POINT, At One AMEL : Agn.

RED Objects, at AGG : Lyc.

REVOLVING Objects, at AGG : Lyc.

SHINING Objects, at : See Bright objects.

SIDEWAYS AGG : *Bell;* Merc-c; Old.

AMEL   : Chin-s; Old; Sul.

On all   : Kali-br.

SKY, At; reason without : Bov.

SNOW, at AGG : Ap.

STARING AGG (See Stares) : Cina.

STRAIGHT Forward AGG : Old.

AMEL : *Bell;* Old.

THROUGH Sharp spectacles, as if : Croc.

UPWARDS AGG : Ars; CALC; Chel; Cup; *Pho; Pul;* Saba; Sang; Sele; Sil; Thu.

High Buildings at AGG : Arg-n.

Walking in open air AGG : Arg-n; Sep.

WHITE Objects, at AGG : Ap; Ars; Cham; Lyc; Nat-m; Tab.

Yellow spots   : Am-c.

WINDOW, Out of AGG : Cam; Carb-v; NAT-M; Ox-ac.

For hours   : Mez.

LOOSE, As if : *Am-c;* Bar-c; Bov; Carb-an; Caus; Chin; Croc; Hyo; *Kali-c;* Kali-m; Laur; Med; Nat-s; NUX-M;

Nux-v; Psor; RHUS-T; Sec; Sul-ac; Thu.

OPEN, And : Sec.

LOOSE LAX : See Relaxation.

LOQUACITY : Agar; Aur; Cann; Cimi; Cocl; Cup; *Hyo; Lach;* Meph; Op; Par; Pod; Pyro; Sele; *Stram;*Ver-a; Ver-v.

BUSINESS Of : *Bry;* Hyo.

CHANGING Quickly from one subject to another : Amb; Cimi; *Lach;* Stram; Val.

CHILL, During : Pod; Zin.

COUGH, After : Dros.

EXCITED, When : Mar-v; Sele.

FEVER, During : Lach; *Mar-v;* Pod; Tub; Zin.

HILARITY, With : Ther.

INCOHERENT, Rambling : Amb; Arg-n; Bry; Cimi; Hyo; *Lach;* Mar-v; Onos; Pho; Pod; Rhus-t; Sele; Stram; Tub.

   Headache, during : Bar-c; Lach; Stram.

MENSES, During : Stram.

PRECOCIOUS (Child) : Strop.

RAPID Questioning : Aur.

SWEAT, With : Calad; Cup; Sele.

LOSS OF VITAL FLUIDS AGG : See Discharges Agg.

LOUSINESS : See Lice.

LOVE DISAPPOINTMENT, Unhappy, pangs : Ant-c; Aur; Cact; Calc-p; Cimi; Cof; Hell; *Hyo;* Ign; Iod; Lach; *Nat-m; Pho-ac;* Tarn; Ver-a.

EXALTED : Ant-c.

SICK : Til.

LOWER LIMBS : See Legs.

LUMBAGO : See Lumber Back, Pain.

LUMBAR BACK (See Back) : *Aesc;* Alu; ANT-T; Arg-m; *Ars;* Bar-c; *Berb;* Bry; CALC; Canth; *Caus;* Chin; *Cimi;* Dul; Eup-p; Grap; *Kali-c;* Led; *Nux-m;* NUX-V; Pho; Pul; RHUS-T; Sanic; SEP; Solid; *Sul; Vario;* Zin-ar.

AFFECTED, By everything : Kali-c; Sep.

BLOWING Nose Agg : Calc-p; Dig.

BREAKING, Broken : Aesc; *Bell;* Eup-p; Kali-io; *Lyc; Nat-m;* Pho; Rut; Senec.

BURNING : Aeth; Pod; Terb.

   Spot : Pho.

CHEST, To : Berb; Sul.

CHILL, Starts, in : Gel; Hyo; Lach; *Nat-m;* Stro; Sul.

COITION Agg : Kob.

COLDNESS : Bry; Canth; Dul; *Eup-p;* Gel; *Lach;* Merc-c; Rhus-t; Sanic; Sul.

   Coughing Agg : Carb-an.

COMPRESSION : Aeth; Caus; Thu.

   Tight band, as from a : *Pul.*

COUGHING Agg : Aco; Kali-bi; Nit-ac.

CRACKING : Sec; Sul.

   Walking, while : Zin.

CRAMPS : Ant-c;*Caus; Chin.*

Buttock, and : Caus.

CRUSHED, As though : Berb; Chin.

DAMP Cloth, around as if : Lathy.

DISLOCATIVE Pain: Eup-p; Lach.

DOWN Legs : Kali-c.

EMACIATION : Plb; Sele.

EXERTION Agg : Agar; Calc-p; Zin-ar.

FLATUS, Passing Amel : *Lyc*; Pic-ac; Rut.

FORWARD, In: *Berb;* Cham; *Kali-c*; Kre; SABI.

Around pelvis: Sabi; Sep; Vib.

GROINS, To: Pho; Sabi; Vib.

HEAVY : Cimi;Pic-ac; Rhus-t.

Hips, down thighs : Cimi.

HOT, IRON, As if : Act-sp; Alu; Cann; Grap.

Clothes, as if, on fire : Ars-io.

ILIAC Crest, to thighs : Berb.

INJURY, After : Kali-c.

JARRING Agg: Thu; Zin-ar.

LAME (See Weak : Berb; Gel; Kali-io; *Lach*; Ox-ac; *Pho*; *Rhus-t*; Sul.

LEUCORRHOEA Gushing Amel : Kre.

LIFTING Agg: Ant-t; Med.

NUMB : Aco; Ap; *Berb;* Grap; Lapp; PLAT; Sil.

OPERATIONS After : Berb.

PAIN (Lumbago) : *Aesc;* Ant-t; Bell; Berb; Bry; Caus; *Dul*; *Grap;* Kali-bi; *Led*; Mur-ac;

NUX-V; Ox-ac; RHUS-T; Sec; Sele; *Sep; Sul.*

Amel, rising on in *A.M.* : Fer.

Coughing Agg : Carb-an.

Diarrhoea with : Bar-c; Kali-io.

Efforts, Repeated at rising : Aesc.

Exertion Amel : Radm.

Head ache, alternating with : Alo.

Leucorrhoea, with : Gel.

Menses, during : Am-c; Cimi; Lach; Nux.m; Pul; Sul.

Motion, least Agg : Buf; Chin; Lyc.

Night, only : Fer.

Sick, feeling, all over with : Solid.

Urination, frequent, with : Sep.

Vertebra, broken, as if : Grap.

Vertex and occiput, with : Radm.

PARALYTIC : Cocl; Kali-c; Sep.

Labour, difficult, after : Nux-v.

PRESSURE Amel : Dul; Kali-c; Nat-m; Rhus-t; Rut; Sep.

PUBES, To : Pho; Sabi; Vib.

PULLED, Down, from, as if: Visc.

RADIATING, From : Bap; Berb; Laur; Sep.

RAISES, With the help of arms

: Buf; Hyds.

RAW, As if : Nat-c.

RENAL Diseases, in: Calc-ar; Senec; Solid; Visc.

RESTLESSNESS : Bar-c; Calc-f.

Flatus passing Amel : Bar-c.

SHORT, Tense : Am-m; Berb.

SITTING Agg: Agar; Arg-m; Berb; Kob; Rhus-t; Val; Zinar.

Bent, Agg : Kali-io.

Amel : Ran-b.

Down, when Agg : Zin.

SLEEP Agg : Am-m.

SNEEZING Agg : Con; Sul.

STANDING Agg : Con; Psor; *Val;* Zin; Zin-ar.

STIFF : Bar-c; Caus; Lach; *Rhus-t.*

Thighs can not raise : Aur.

STITCHES : Agar; Berb; *Bry;* Colo; *Kali-c;* Lyc; Pul; Sul.

Coughing Agg : Nit-ac.

STOMACH, To : Sul.

STOOLS Agg : Bar-c; Caps.

STOOPING, Prolonged Agg : Dul.

STRAIGHTEN, Can not : Kob.

SWEAT : Naj; Sil.

Menses, before : Nit-ac.

THIGHS, Raising Agg : Aur.

THROBBING : Bar-c; Lac-c; Sep; Sil.

TOUCH Agg : Cimi; Lil-t.

TREMBLING : Benz-ac.

UPWARDS, From : Radm.

URINATION Amel : Nat-s.

UTERUS, To : Nat-m.

VERTEBRAE, Of : Kre; Stan; Zin.

Dislocated or as if : Sanic.

Gliding over each other as if : Sanic.

WALKING Agg : Aesc; Murx; Psor; Sep.

Amel : *Arg-m;* Kob; Radm; *Sep.*

Impulse, to, with : Murx.

With cane pressed across the back Amel : Vib.

WEAKNESS : Ars; Calc; Calc-s; Cocl; Nat-m; Pic-ac; Pul; Rhus-t; Sele; Sep; Sul; Zin.

WIND, As of a : Sul; Sumb.

LUMP : See Ball.

LUMPS, LUMPY Effects : Aeth; Alu; Alum; Ant-c; Calc-s; *Grap;* KALI-BI; Kre; LYC; *Merc; Merc-i-f;* PLAT; Rhus-t; Sep; Sil; Stan.

PAINFUL : Kali-io.

LUNGS : See under Chest.

LUPUS : See Cancer of Skin.

LYING AGG : Adon; *Amb;* Ant-t; Ap; Arn; ARS; AUR; Bell; *Caps; Cham; Con;* Dros; Dul, Euphor; *Fer; Hyo;* Kali-c; *LYC,* Lycps; *Meny;* Merc; Nat-s; Pho; *Plat;* PUL, RHUS-T; Rum; *Rut; Samb;* Sang; Sep; Sil; Stro; Tarx; Verb.

AMEL :Am-m; Asar; Bell; BRY; *Calc;* Cham; Colo; Fer; Form; Ign; Mang; *Nat-m;* Nit- ac; NUX-V; Pic-ac; Pul; Rhus-t;Sep; *Scil;* Sil; Stan.

ABDOMEN, On AMEL : Acet-ac;
BELL; Calc-p; Chel; Chio;
Cina; COLO; Elap; Eup-p;
Lach; Lept; MED; Nit-ac;
Par; Pho; Phyt, *Pod; Psor;
Sep;* Stan; Thyr.

ALL Troubles AMEL : Mang.

BACK, On Agg : *Aco;* Am-m;
Arg-m; *Ars;* Cact; *Caus;
Cham; Colch; Colo; Cup;*
IGN; *Iod; Kali-n;* Merc-i-f;
Nat-s; NUX-V; *Op;* PHO; Pul;
Rhus-t; Sep; Sil; Spig; *Sul;*
Zin-ch.

AMEL : Am-m; BRY; CALC;
Colch; Dig; *Merc-c; Pul;
Rhus-t;* Rut; Sang.

Flat Amel : Dig.

Head elevated, with : See
Reclining.

Jerks the head
backward, while : Hypr.

Knees, drawn up and
spread apart with : Plat.

Thighs and, flexed on
abdomen : Stram.

BED In AGG and AMEL : See
Bed lying in AGG and
AMEL.

BENT Amel : See Bending
Forwards Amel.

BOARD, On, as if : Bap; Sanic.

CURLED Up, one side, on : Bap.

FACE, On AMEL : Hypr.

HANDS And KNEES on AMEL
: Con; Eup-p; Euphor;
Lach; Med; Par-b; Sep;
Tarn.

HARD Surface on AMEL :

Kali-c; *Nat-m;* Rhus-t;
Sanic; *Sep;* Stan.

HEAD High, with Amel :
Ant-t; Ap; Aral; *Arg-m;*
ARS; Bell; Cact; Caps;
Chin; *Con;* Gel; Glo; *Hep;*
Kali-c; KALI-N; Lach; *Pul;*
Samb; Sang; Spig; Spo.

HORIZONTAL Position Amel:
Ap; Arn; Bell; Con; Laur;
Psor; Spo; Tab; Ther; *Ver-v.*

ICE On, as if : Lyc.

KNEES, On, body bent
backwards, with : Nux-v.

LEGS, Crossed, with, uncross
can not : Bell; Ther.

Spread apart : Hell.

ON ONE SIDE, one person,
other side, other person, as
if : Pyro.

PAINFUL Side, or affected part,
on AGG : See Pressure AGG.

PAINLESS Side, on AGG : BRY;
Cham; Chin; *Colo;* Flu-ac;
Ign; Nat-s; PUL; Rhus-t;
Sec; *Sep.*

QUIETLY AMEL : Bry; Psor.

RECLINING, On Back AMEL :
Gel; Kalm; Led; Sang; Thyr.

SIDE, On AGG : ACO; ANAC;
Arg-n; Bar-c; BRY; Calad;
CALC; CARB-AN; Cina;
Con; Fer; Ign; Ip; KALI-C;
Kre; *Lyc;* Merc; Merc-c;
Nat-s; Par; PHO; Pho-ac;
PUL; *Rhus-t;* Seneg; SIL;
STAN; Sul; Thu.

AMEL : Anac; *Cocl;* Lept;
NUX-V; Pho; Sep.

Right **A**GG : Alu; Am-c; Am-m; *Arg-n;* Benz-ac; Bor; Caus; Iris; Hyds; Kali-c; Kalm; Lycps; *Mag-m;* Mag-p; MERC; *Nux-v; Pho;* Rum; Spo; Stan; Sul-io.

AMEL : Am-c; Ant-t; Naj; Nat-m; Pho; Sep; Sul; Tab.

contents, body, of, were dragged to that side : Cinb.

head high, with **A**MEL : Ars; Cact; Spig; Spo.

Left **A**GG : Aco; Am-c; Ap; *Arg-n; Bar-c; Bry;* Cact; *Carb-an;* Colch; Dig; Ip; Kali-c; Lil-t; Lyc; Naj; *Nat-c;* Nat-m; Nat-s; *Par;* Petr; PHO; Ptel; PUL; *Sep;* Sil; *Sul; Thu;* Tub; Vib; Zin-io.

AMEL : Ign; Lil-t; Mur-ac; Nat-m; Phyt; Sang; Stan.

STRANGE Position in **A**MEL : See Attitude Bizarre.

UNCOMFORTABLY, As if : Lept; Psor; Pul; Rhus-t; Sil; Sul.

Aching of body, from : Lapp.

WET Surface, Floor, on or sitting on moist ground **A**GG : Ars; Calc; Caus; Dul; *Nux-v;* Rhod; Rhus-t; Sil.

LYMPHANGITIS (See Skin, Red streaks) : Ap; Bell; Buf; Lach; Merc; Pyro; Rhus-t.

LYMPHOID TISSUE : *Radm.*

LYPOTHEMIA : See Mental exhaustion, from Grief.

MADDENING : See Besides himself, Shrieks with Pain in head.

MADNESS : See Insanity.

MAGNETISED, DESIRES, To be. : *Calc;* Lach; *Pho; Sil.*

MAGNETISM AMEL : Calc; *Cup;* Lach; *Pho;* Sil.

MALAR BONES : *Ars-io; Aur;* Colo; Glo; *Kali-bi;* Kali-io; Mag-c; Mez; Ol-an; Old; Sep; Stan; Stap; Stro; Thu; Tub; Verb.

ACHING, Sore: Ars-io; Aur; Glo; Merc-i-r; Phyt; Tub; Verb.

BORING : Thu.

EXOSTOSES : Aur.

NEURALGIA : Stan.

Night Amel : Cimi.

Running, about Amel : Bism.

NUMB : Plat; Sep.

PULLED, Up : Ol-an.

STITCHES : Par.

TENSION, Across : Ver-v.

TUMOURS : Mag-c.

MALARIA : See Fever, Intermittent.

MALE (Genital) **O**RGANS, in general : Agn; Arg-n; Aur; Cann; Canth; Cinb; CLEM; Con; *Grap; Lyc;* MERC; NIT-AC; *Nux-v;* Plat; PUL; *Rhod; Rhus-t;* Spo; Stap; *Sul; Thu.*

ACHING, Can not sit still : Syph.

BRINY Odour, coition after : Sanic.

BURNING : *Calc; Canth;* Sul-ac.

Coition during: Kre.

COLD : *Agn;* Caus; Gel; *Lyc;* Sabal; Sul.

DROPSICAL : Grap.

ERECTION, Of: See Erection.

ERUPTIONS : Crot-t; Grap; Petr; Rhus-t.

FLACCID : *Agn;* Calad; *Dios;* Gel.

Coition, during : Nux-v; Pho-ac; Sul.

Suddenly : Grap; Lyc; Nux-v.

FORMICATION : *Plat; Sec;* Tarn.

GRASPING, Fumbling : Aco; Bell; Buf; Canth; HYO; Merc; Stram; Zin.

HEAVY : Nat-c; Psor.

HOT : Spo.

ITCHING : Calc; Caus; Plat; Rhus-t.

NUMB : Grap.

ODOUR, Stinking : Nat-m; Sars; Sul.

PAINFUL : Arg-n; Arn.

Coition, during : Arg-n.

SHRIVELLED : Ign; Lyc.

SPOTS, Yellow, brown, on : Kob.

SWEAT : Aur; Flu-ac; Sele; Sep; Thu.

Offensive : Sul.

Oily, pungent : Flu-ac.

SWELLED : Arn; Rhus-t.

Dropsical : Grap.

TINGLING : Alu.

UNEASY, Feeling : Kali-c.

MALICE, HATRED : ANAC;
Cham; Cup; Led; Lyc; Nat-m; Nit-ac; NUX-V; Stram; Tarn.

PERSONS, Who had offened him : Aur; Nat-m.

Who do not agree with him : Calc-s.

MALIGNANCY : Ail; Am-c; Ars; Crot-h; Lach; Nit-ac; Tarn-c.

MALINGERING : Arg-n; Bell; Plb; Saba; *Tarn;* Ver-a.

MAMMAE : Bell; Bry; Carb-an; Cham; *Con;* Hyds; Iod; Lac-c; Merc; Oci-c; Phel; *Pho; Phyt;* Sabal; Sil; Urt.

RIGHT : Ign; Kali-bi; *Phel;* SIL.

Below : Carb-an; Caus; Chel; CIMI; *Grap;* Laur; Lil-t; Merc-i-r; *Pho Sul;* Ust.

+ Jumping alive, as if Croc.

Scapula, to : Merc.

LEFT : Bor; Bov; *Lil-t; Lyc; Phel.*

Arms to fingers : Ast-r.

Below : Ap; Bry; Bur-p; Cimi; Pho; Sul; Ust.

Pain, cough, with : Mos.

+ drawn back, as if : Croc.

dysmenorrhoea, with : Caus.

head, to : Glo.

jumping : Croc.

meals, after : Rum; Stro.

menses, at : Grap.

between : Ust.

Scapula to : Como.

Swollen, hard : Cist.

ALTERNATING Sides : Pul.
  Teeth, with : Kali-c.
ABDOMEN, To : Phel; Sang.
  Hot water, running, from : Sang.
ABSCESS : Hep; Merc; Pho; Phyt; Sil; Sul.
  Threatening in old cicatrices : Acet-ac; *Grap; Phyt.*
ACHING : See Sore, Painful.
  Nursing Amel : Phel.
ARMS, To : Lith.
AXILLA, To : Bro.
BACKWARD : CROT-T; Laur; Lil-t; Til.
  Left : Form.
  Drawn : Croc.
BALL, Below : Hura.
BARES : Cam.
BURNING : Cimi; Laur; Sul.
  Below, right : Aeth; Pho.
    left : Laur; Mur-ac; Rum.
  Motion Amel : Ars.
CAKING, Milk of : Nux-v.
CANCER : Ast-r; Aur-m; Bad; Bro; Buf; Con; Cund; Grap; Hyds; Merc; Pho; Sil.
  Itching, with : Sil.
  Stitches in shoulders and uterus, with : Clem.
+ Swelling of, axillary glands, with : Goss.
CHILLINESS, In : Cocl; Guai.
CICATRICES, Old : Carb-an; *Grap; Phyt.*
  Suppurating : Sil.
COLD : Cocl; Med.

Agg : Sabal.
Left : Nat-c.
  coughing, while : Nat-c.
CONGESTED : Aco; Ap; Fer; Pho.
  Milk with, insanity in :

  Bell; Stram.
COUGHING Agg : Con.
CRAMP : Plat.
CRAWLING (left) : Ant-t.
  Cold : Guai.
DWINDLED, Emaciated : Ars-io; Bar-c; Cham; Chin; *Cof;* CON; Fer; IOD; *Kali-io;* Nat-m; Nit-ac; *Nux-m;* Sabal; Sec; Sil.
  Lump hard, small, painful with : Kre.
  Ovaries, with : Bar-c.
EMPTINESS, After child nurses : Bor.
ENLARGED, As if : Calc-p; Cycl; Sep.
ERUPTION : Caus; Psor.
  Herpes, nursing women, in : Dul.
ERYSIPELAS : Ap.
EVERYTHING, Affects : Phyt.
FINGERS, To : Ast-r; Lith.
FISTULA : Pho; Sil.
FLACCID : Con; Iod.
FLOWING Milk, as if, in : Dict; Kre; Nux-v; Pul.
HARD, Indurated : Ast-r; Bry; *Carb-an;* Cham; Con; Grap; Phyt; Plb; *Sil.*
  Menses, absent, with : Dul.

+ Nodes : Ast-r; Nit-ac.

Small and, colic, during : Plb.

HEAD, To : Lac-ac.

HEAVY : Bry; Chin; Iod; Lac-c; Phyt.

HYPERTROPHY : *Calc*; Chim; *Con; Phyt.*

Climaxis, at : Sang.

INFLAMED (Mastitis) : Bell; Bry; Hep; Phyt; Sil; Sul.

INNER Side arms, to fingers : Ast-r.

ITCHING : Alu; Caus; Con.

Warm getting, on : Aeth.

JERKS : Croc.

LARGE : Chim.

MENSES, Before Agg : Bry; Calc; *Con*; KALI-M; LAC-C; Lyc; Ol-an; *Phyt*; Pul.

During Agg : Con; Helo; Lac-c; Merc; Murx; Phel; Pho; Phyt; Zin.

MILK Present, Absent menses with : Bell; Bry; Calc; Lyc; Pho; Pul; Rhus-t; Sabi; Stram.

Boys, in : Merc.

Flowing in, as if : See Flowing.

Increased : Aco.

+ Insanity, during : Bell; Stram.

Menses, during : Calc; Merc; Pall; Pul; Tub.

Menses instead of : Merc.

+ Painless gathering from not nursing : Nux-v.

Virgins, non-pregnant women in : Asaf; Bur-p; Cyc; Lyc; *Merc*; PUL; Tub. Urt.

NEURALGIA, Left : Sumb.

NIGHT Agg : Buf.

NODES, In : Bels; Calc-f; *Carb-an; Con*; Crot-t; Lyc; *Phyt*; SIL; Tub.

Black points on skin, with : Iod.

Girls puberty, before : Pul.

+ Hard, burning : Lyc.

Knots in axilla, with : Merc-i-f.

+ Milk, secretion, of with : Chim.

Movable, tender, moving arms Agg : Calc-io.

Old : Chim.

Painful, old fat men, in : Bar-c.

Skin, on : Iod.

Soft, tender : Kali-m; Pul.

Touch Agg : Ars-io.

Walnut like, males in : Bar-c; Calc-p.

NUMB : Grap.

NURSING Agg : Phel.

OUTWARD, Dartings : Arg-m; Clem; Ol-an.

Menses, during : Grat.

PRESSES HARD, hand with : Cimi; Con.

RADIATING, From : Phyt.

RIVET Or Bullet feeling of, in region : Lil-t.

SHIVERING Over: Cocl; Guai.

SHOOTING : Polyg.

SHOULDER, To, between : Phel.
Left : Sang.

SHUDDERING In, with goose
flesh : Guai.

SMALL, Undeveloped : Iod; Lyc;
Nux-m; Onos; Sabal; Sul.
One, than other : Sabal.

SORE, Painful : Arn; Bell; Bry;
Calc; Cham; *Con;* Helo;
Kali-m; LAC-C; Lyc; Med;
Merc; Onos; Phyt; Pul;
Sabal; Sil; Syph.

Axillary glands enlargement,
with : Lac-ac.

Bath cold Agg : Sabal.

Climaxis, at : Sang.

Dysmenorrhoea, with :
Canth; Sars.

Infants : Cham.

Menses, at the begining of
: Tub.

absent, with : Dul; Zin.

during or other time :
Grat; Med; Murx; Syph.

Pregnancy, during :Calc-p.

Rubbing, hard Amel : Radm.

Sneezing Agg : Hyds.

+ Stooping, when : Grat.

Urination Agg : Clem.

Yawning Agg : Mag-c.

STITCHES : Ap; Carb-an; *Con;*
Nit-ac; Sil.

Dysmenorrhoea, with : Caus.

Nursing, when : Calc.

SUCKLING, While Agg: Ant-t;
Bor; Bry; Crot-t; Lac-c; Lil-t;
Phel; Phyt; *Pul;* Sil.

Amel : Phel.

Cramps : Cham.

Pain in opposite : Bor.

SWELLED : *Bell;* BRY; Con;
Helo; Hep; *Pho;* PHYT;
PUL; *Sil;* Sul; Urt.

As if : Calc-p.

Bath cold Agg : Sabal.

Climaxis, at : Sang.

+ Inguinal glands, with :
Oci-c.

Lancinating pain : Aeth.

Leucorrhoea, with : Dul.

Menses after, secretion of
milk, with : Cyc.

instead of : Dul; Rat.

Milk, secretion of, with :
Asaf; Cyc; Tub.

Weaning, after: All-s; Pul.

THROBBING : Bor.

TINGLING : Sabi.

TUMOURS : See Cancer,
Nodes.

ULCERATION : Hep; Phyt; Sil.

UTERUS, With : Sil.

WARTS : Castr-eq.

MANIA : See Insanity.

MONO : Ign; Sil.

KLEPTO : See Steals.

MARASMUS (See Emaciation)
: Abro; Bor; Iod; Mag-c;
Nat-m; Nux-m; Sanic; Syph.

FEEDING And Medicines, in
spite of : Mag-c.

GLANDS, Enlarged with :
Ther.

INFANTS, Bottle fed : Nat-p.

MARRIAGE, IDEA OF, Seemed

unendurable : *Lach;* Nux-v;
Pic-ac; Pul.

DISSOLVE, Must : Flu-ac.

PREPARATION, Of : Hyo.

THAT HE is married : Ign.

THOUGHT Of Amel : Orig.

MASSETERS : Hyd-ac; Ign.

CONTRACTED : Meny; Merc.

CRAMP : Cocl; Cup; Hyd-ac;
Stram; Stry.

STIFF, Hard : Ign.

MASTITIS : See Mammae,
Inflammation.

MASTODYNIA : See Mammae,
Sore.

MASTOID CARIES : *Aur;* Caps;
Flu-ac; *Nit-ac;* Sil.

INFLAMMATION : Aur; Calc-p;
Canth; *Caps;* Fer-p; Hep;
Lach; *Pho;* Sil.

NECK, To : Lith; Mur-ac.

OPERATIONS, After : Caps.

MASTURBATION, DISPOSITION
To (Males) : Anac; Buf; Con;
Lach; Orig; Plat; Sep; Stap; Ust.

FEMALES (See Males): O*rig;*
Tub.

Children due to pruritus
vulvae: *Calad;* O*rig;* Zin.

Menses, during: Zin.

ILL EFFECTS, Of, AGG : Arg-m;
Arg-n;CALC; Carb-v; CHIN;
Cocl; *Con;* Dios; Gel; Lach;
Lyc; Merc; *Nat-m;* Nat-p;
Nux-v; Orig; Pho; PHO-AC;
Pic-ac; Plat; Pul; Sele; *Sep;*
STAP; SUL; Ust.

INVOLUNTARY : Cam.

PUBERTY, Before : Plat.

MAXILLARY JOINTS : Bell;
Ign; Merc; *Rhus-t;* Thu.

CRACKING, Chewing when:
Nit-ac; Rhus-t.

CRAMP : Bell; Spo.

DISLOCATION, Easy : Ign; Petr;
Rhus-t; Stap.

Laughing Agg : Tab.

TIGHT, On chewing or
opening mouth : Alu.

MEAN (See Avaricious): Sul.

MEASLES : ACO; Ars; *Bry;*
Cam; Cof; Dros; Euphr;
Fer-p; *Kali-bi;* Kali-m; Pho;
PUL; Stic.

COMPLICATIONS or Sequelae of:
Ant-c; *Ant-t;* Ars; *Bry;*
Cam; Carb-v; Cup-ac; Dros;
Kali-c; Pul; Sul; Zin.

HAEMORRHAGIC : *Crot-h;* Fer-p.

RECEDING : *Bry;* Pho; Pul;
Rhus-t

UNDEVELOPED : Bry.

MEAT WATER Like : See
Discharges, Meat water.

MEATUS AGGLUTINATION, Of
: Cam; Cann; Cup; Med;
Nat-m; Petros; Thu.

Morning : Pho; *Sep;* Thu.

BURNING : Berb; Sul.

Clothes rubbing Agg :
Chin.

CRACKS : Nat-c; Nit-ac.

CUTTING : Zin.

DROP, Clear, morning : Pho.

Green : Merc.

Urinating, before : Berb.

Yellow : Flu-ac.

ERUPTIONS, About : Caps.

EVERTED : Caps.

HARD : Cann.

INFLAMMED : Cann; Sul.

ITCHING : Amb; *Caus; Coc-c;* Petros.

PAINFUL : Canth.

Women : Lac-c; Sars.

POUTING : Cann; Sul; Thu.

RED : Merc; *Sul.*

STITCHING : Nit-ac.

ULCERS : Merc-c; Nit-ac.

MEDICINE ABUSE Of : See Drugs, Abuse of.

OVERACTS Without curing : Cup; *Mar-v; Pho-ac.*

REFUSES, To take : Calad; Cimi; Hyo.

SENSITIVE, To : Cup; Nux-v; Pul.

High potency : Nit-ac.

THINKING Of it Agg : Asaf.

WANT of Susceptibility to : Carb-v; Laur; *Mos;* Op.

MEDULLA : *Aco;* Agar; Cup; Naj; Ver-v.

MELANCHOLY (See Sadness) : Ant-t; Ars; Calc; Castr;Cup; Grap; Helo; Hypr; *Lach;* Nux-v; Plb; *Pul;* Sul; Ver-a.

BROODING : *Aur.*

DEATH, Fear, of, with : Cup.

EYES, Closed, with : Arg-n.

FINANCIAL : Mez; Psor.

+ INTERNAL Grief, from : Am-m.

PARTURITION, After : Anac.

PUBERTY, During : Hell.

RELIGIOUS : Kali-p; Mez; Psor.

MEMBRANE : See Mucous and Serous Membranes.

MEMORIES DISAGREEABLE

Recur : Amb; Am-c; Benz-ac; Calc; Cham; Hep; Hyo; *Lyc; Nat-m;* Nit-ac; Pho; Psor; Sep; Sul; Thu.

OLD Grievances, of : Glo.

MEMORY (AFFECTED in General) : ANAC; Arn; Aur; *Bar-c;* Bell; *Calc;* Cann; Con; Hell; HYO; *Lach;* LYC; *Merc;* NAT-M; NUX-M; Op; *Pho-ac;* Rhod; Stap; Sul; Syph.

ACTIVE : BELL; *Cof; Hyo; Lach; Op.*

BAD, Weak : Aco; Amb; *Agn;* ANAC; *Arg-m; Arg-n; Ars;* Art-v; *Bar-c;* BELL; Buf; CALC; Caus; Cocl; Colch; *Con;* Crot-h; Glo; Guai; Ham; Hell; Hep; *Hyo;* Kali-br; *Kali-p; Lach;* Laur; *Lyc;* Med; *Merc;* Nit-ac; *Nux-m;* Onos; Petr; *Pho;* Pho-ac; Plat; Plb; *Sep; Stap;* Syph; VER-A; *Zin.*

Faces, events, names, for : Syph.

remembers past events : Syph.

Naming objects, for : Chin-s.

Vexation Agg : Am-c.

What he is doing or done : Cic; Nat-m; Nux-m.

Suddenly from pain, right, etc. : Am-c; Anac; Arg-n; Bell; Hep; Laur; Nux-m;

Pall; Pru-sp; Pul.

LOST : BELL; *Cic;* HYO; VER-A.

Objects, naming for : Chin-s.

Past life : Nux-m.

MENIERE'S. DISEASE : Arn;
Benz-ac; Caus; Cheno; *Chin-s;*
Eucal; Kali-m; Nat-sal; Radm;
Sal-ac; Sil; Tab; Thyr.

SEA SICK, As if : Tab.

MENINGITIS : See Cerebro-
spinal axis.

MENOPAUSE : See Climaxis.

MENSES BEFORE AGG : Bov;
Calc; Calc-p; Cimi; Cocl;
Cup; KALI-C; LACH; *Lyc;*
Nat-m; PUL; *Sep;* Spo; *Sul;*
Ver-a; Vib; *Zin.*

AMEL : Murx.

Queer, feeling : Bro.

AT START Of AGG : Aco;
Calc-p; *Hyo;* Jab; Kali-c;
Lac-c; Lach.

AWKWARD during : Alu.

BEFORE AND AFTER AGG : Bor;
Calc; Fer; *Grap;* Kali-m;
Kre; Lac-c; Lach; Lil-t;
Mag-c; *Nat-m;* Pall; Thu.

DURING AGG : Aco; AM-C;
ARG-N; Bov; Castr; Caus;
Cham; Cimi; Cocl; GRAP;
HYO; Ign; Kali-c; Lac-c;
M*ag-c;* MAG-M; Nux-m;
Nux-v; PUL; Sec; *Sep;* Stap;
Sul; Thu; *Zin.*

AMEL : Cyc; Kali-c; *Lach;*
Mos; Murx; Senec; *Zin.*

AFTER AGG : Bor; Carb-an;
Grap; Kre; Lac-c; Lach;
Lith; Lyc; *Nux-v;* Sep; Tarn.

Old symptoms of AGG :
Nux-v.

DISTURBANCES, of (In general)
: Aco; BELL; *Calc; Cham;*
Cocl; Fer; *Grap;* Ip; *Kali-c;*
Kre; Lach; Mag-c; Nat-m;
NUX-M; Nux-v; Pho; Plat;
PUL; *Sabi;* Sec; Sep; *Sul.*

ABDOMEN, Pressure on Amel
: Mag-c.

ABSENT, Suppressed
AMENORRHOEA : Aur; Bell;
Cimi; *Con;* Cup; Cyc; *Dul;*
Grap; Hell; Helo; *Kali-c;*
Lac-d; Lach; *Lyc;* Nat-s;
Pho; PUL; *Senec;* Sep;
Sil; Sul; Tub; Xanth.

Abdomen, bloated, with :
Apoc.

Asthma, with : Spo.

Bath, from: Nux-m.

Careworn, tired, women,
in : Ars.

Cause without : Ust.

Chagrin, from : Colo.

Cold, from : Hell; Senec.

Concomitants, with :
Senec; Ust.

Dancing, excessive, from :
Cyc.

Deafness, with : Nat-c.

Diabetes, in : Uran-n.

Dropsy, with : Ap; Apoc;
Kali-c; Senec.

Emigrants, in : Bry; *Plat.*

Emotions, from : Cimi.

Foot sweat, suppressed,
from : Cup.

Fright, from : Op.

Functional : Senec.

+ Girls, young : Senec.

Grief, from : *Ign.*

Hands putting in cold water from : Lac-d.

+ Indignation, from : Stap.

Jaundice, with : Chio.

Liver, affections, with : Lept.

Love, disappointed, from : Hell.

Mammae, scirrhus of, with : Bro.

Milk in breast, with : Pho; Rhus-t.

Months, for : Lyc; Sil.

Neuralgic pain, in

body with : Kalm.

ophthalmic, with : Euphr.

+ Puberty of : Ap; Sep.

Rheumatism, with : Bry; Cimi; Lach; Rhus-t.

Suddenly : Aco.

Tuberculosis, in : Solid; Ust.

Weaning, after: Sep.

Wet getting feet, from : Pul; Rhus-t.

ACRID: Kali-c; Lach; Nit-ac; Sil; Stram.

AMMONIACAL : Lac-c.

BATHING Amel: Kali-c.

BETWEEN, Periods : Amb; Bov; Calc; Cham; Ham; Helo; Hyds; Ip; Lyc; Mang; Pho; Rhus-t; Sabi; Sil.

Day time, only : Ham.

Sexual excitement, with : Amb; Sabi.

BLACK : Chin; Croc; Cyc; Ham; Helo; Kali-m; Kali-n; Lach; Mag-p; Plat; Pul; Ust; Xanth.

A.M. only : Carb-an.

Sticky: Coc-c.

BLADDER Symptoms, with : Canth; Erig; Sabal.

BREATHING, Difficulty with: Flu-ac.

BROWN : Bap; *Bry;* Carb-v; Iod; Thu.

BURNING, Hot : Arn; *Bell;* Kali-c; Kre; Sabi; Sul.

Like fire : Lac-c.

Lying, cease when : Scil; Sil.

CHILDBIRTH, After : Tub.

CHOLERIC Symptoms, with : Am-c; Sil.

CLOTTED (See Discharges lumpy) : Am-c; Apoc; Bell; Calc; Calc-p; Chin; Coc-c; Cyc; Ip; Kali-m; Kre; Lach; Mag-m; Med; Murx; Pul; Sabi; Zin.

Dark : Am-c; Bell; Cham; Coc-c; Croc; Med; Sabi; Vip.

Fluid, blood, with : Apoc; Bell; Sabi; Sec; Ust; Vip.

Gelatinous, bright blood with: Laur.

Serum, and : Lyc; Ust.

Urinating, while : Coc-c.

COITION Agg : See Female affections, Coition after.

COLD Bath Agg : Ant-c.

COLLAPSE, At : Merc.

COPIOUS, Profuse,Excessive :
Apoc; *Ars; Bell;* Bov; *Calc;*
Calc-p; Cham; *Chin;* Cocl;
Croc; Cyc; Erig; *Fer;* Ham;
Helo; Ip; Kali-n; Kre;
Mag-m; Med; *Mill;* Murx;
Nat-m; Nux-m; NUX-V;
PHO; *Plat;* Rat; SABI; *Sec;*
Senec; *Stram;* Tril; Ust;
Vinc; Zin.

Abortion, after : Ust.

Bathing Amel : Kali-c.

Climaxis, during : Apoc;
Aur-m; Calc; Lach; Sep;
Sul; Tril; Vinc.

long, after : Vinc.

Clots, large with : Apoc;
Coc-c; Murx; Zin.

Dancing, after: Croc; Cyc.

Erotic, Spasms with : Tarn.

Faintness, with : Ip; Tril.

Forceps delivery, after :
Calend.

Icy coldness of body, with
: Sil.

Labour, hasty, after : Caul.

+ Labour like pains : Alet.

Mania, with: Sep.

Moon, new and full Agg :
Croc.

Nausea, with : Apoc; Caps;
Ip.

+ Night Agg : Bad.

Obstinate, continuous :
Nux-m; Vinc.

Old Maids : Mag-m.

Short duration : Lach; Plat;
Sil; Thu.

Tenesmus of bladder and
rectum, with : Erig.

Urination, hot, with : Fer.

+ Vomiting, with : Ver-a.

+ Widows, young : Arg-n.

Women young, in : Kali-br.

Sedentary habits, of : Colo.

CURETTING Agg : Bur-p; Nit-ac.

DAY Only : *Caus* Cof; Cyc;
Ham; PUL.

DELAYED, In Girls at puberty :
Ap; Caus; Grap; *Kali-c;*
Lac-d; *Lyc;* Mang; Nat-m;
Pul; SENEC; Sep; Sul.

Feels disturbed, if slightly
: Flu-ac.

Mammae undeveloped,
with : Lyc.

Milk, drinking much, from
: Lac-d.

DIARRHOEA Agg : Am-m; Bov;
Castr; Kre; Mag-c.

EARLY : *Amb;* Ars; BELL; Bor;
Bov; CALC; Calc-p; Carb-an;
Carb-v; Caul; CHAM; *Cocl;*
Cyc; *Fer;* Fer-p; *IP;* Kali-c;
Lac-c; Mag-m; Mag-p; *Mang;*
Nat-m; Nux-m; NUX-V; *Pho;*
PLAT; Rat; *Rhus-t; Sabi.*

+ Black clots, preceded by
Blindness : Dict.

Profuse, and : Alet; Kali-c;
Sep; Stan; Ver-a; Xanth.

Scanty, and : Alu; Lept;
Nat-m.

EVENING, Only : Coc-c; Cof;
Phel.

EXERTION Agg : AMB; Bov;
Calc; Erig; Kre; Nit-ac; Tril.

EXHAUSTION : Alu.

FAINTS, At : *Ip; Lach;* Nux-v; Sep.

FEARSOME : Nat-m.

FEEL Like coming: Carb-an; Lil-t; Mos; Onos; Pho; Pul; Senec; Vip; Zin-chr.

Diarrhoea with : Kali-io.

Frequently : Plat.

Uterine symptoms, with : Kali-c.

FEVER, Septic Agg : Pyro.

FOUL : Bell; Bry; Carb-v; Croc; Helo; Kali-p; Kre; Sabi; Syph.

Putrid meat, like : Alu-sil; Cham;Lachn; Med; Psor; Syph.

GREEN : Grap; *Lac-c*; Med; Pul; *Sep;* Tub.

GRIEF, Brings on: Ign.

GUSHING (See Haemorrhages - gushing) : Ip; Lac-c; Pho; Sabi.

Tip toe standing on : Cocl.

+ Wakes her from sleep : Coca.

HEART Symptoms, with : Cact.

HOT : See Burning.

INDELIBLE : Bur-p; Calc-s; Mag-c; Mag-p; Med; Pulex.

INKY : Kali-n.

INTERMITTENT,Reappearing : Amb; Arg-n; Bov; Coc-c; Fer; Ham; *Kre; Lach;* Mang; Nux-v; Pho; Pul; Saba; Sabi; Sil; Ust.

Abortion, after : Plat.

Blood. black : Elap.

Daytime, only : Ham.

Girls young, in : Polyg.

Interval of one day : Ap.

Old Maids, in : Mag-m.

Parturition, after : Acet-ac.

Sexual excitement, with : Amb; Sabi.

Sometimes stronger, sometimes weaker : Saba.

Women, childness or young widows, in : Arg-n.

IRREGULAR : Cimi; Cocl; Con; Ign; Iod; Kali-p; *Nux-m; Sec;* Senec.

In time and amount : Cimi; Coc-c; Ign; Nux-m; Plat.

Palpitation, with : Phys.

ITCHING, Causing : Petr; Sul; Tarn.

JOINTS, Pain, with : Sabi.

JOLTING, From : Ham.

LACTATION, During : Calc; Calc-p; Pall; Sil.

LATE : Caul; *Caus;* Con; Cup; *Dul; Grap; Kali-c;* LACH; *Lyc; Mag-c; Nat-m;* Nux-m; PUL; Saba; *Sep, Sil;* SUL; Vib.

First menses : See Delayed.

Scanty, and : Kali-c; Sep; Vib.

LEUCORRHEA, With : Kre; Sep.

LIFTING Agg : Kre.

LUMBAR Pain with : See Pain,

Lumbar Back.

LYING, Ceases, on : Cact; Caus; Lil-t; Sabi.

Back, on Agg : Cham.

More, on : Kre; Mag-c; Pul.

MAMMAE AGG (See Mammae) : Bry; Calc; Lac-c.

MEMBRANOUS : Bor; Cham; Cyc; Lac-c; Mag-p; Phyt; Vib.

Puberty, at : Cham.

MENTAL Excitement Agg : CALC; Tub.

MOLASSES Like : Mag-c.

MONTH, Alternate : Bur-p; Syph.

MOON Full or New Agg : Croc.

MORNING More : Bor; Bov; Carb-an; Sep.

Rising, on : Mag-c.

MOTION Agg: Croc; *Erig;* Helo; *Ip;* Sabi; Sec.

Amel : Bov; Cyc; Kre; Mag-c; *Sabi.*

Only, during: Cact; Caus; *Lil-t;* Manc; Nat-s; Sec.

NIGHT Only : Am-c; Am-m; Bov; Coc-c; Mag-c; Mag-p; Nat-m.

NURSING Agg : *Pall;* Pho; Sil; Vip.

OFFENSIVE : See Foul.

+ ONE Hour or Day : Euphr.

PAINFUL, Dysmenorrhoea : Bell; Cact; *Calc;* Calc-p; Caul; CHAM; *Cimi;* Cocl; Con; Cup; Dios; *Grap;*

Kali-c; Lyc; Med; Nux-m; Plat; PUL; Psor; Sep; SUL; Tub; Ver-a; VIB; Xanth; Zin-val.

Abortion, after : Senec.

Barren women, in : Phyt.

Bending back Amel : Lac-c.

double must : Op.

Blood. black. with : Elap.

gray, serum like : Berb.

Blotches, all over, body with : Dul.

Climaxis, at : Psor.

Colic, after : *Kali-c.*

Convulsions, with: Caul; Nat-m.

Emotions, from : Cham.

Eructations, with: Vib.

Fainting, with : Kali-s; *Lap-a;* Lyc; Nux-m.

Feet, pressing against support, Amel : Med.

Few drops of blood, with : Castr.

First day : Gnap; Lach.

Flatulence, with : Vib.

Flow Amel : Mag-p.

scanty, with : Caul; Gnap; Grap.

Frightful : Tub.

Gnawing : Thyr.

Jerks, with : Plat.

Lying, back on, with legs stretched Amel : Sabi.

Hard pillow, over Amel : Mag-m.

Mental excitement Agg : Calc.

More flow, more pain :
Cann; *Cimi;* Pho; Tarn;
Tub.

pain less flow. : Lach.

No relief, in any position :
Xanth.

Over whole body : Nux-v;
Xanth.

Prolapsus, with : Ver-a.

+ Retracted nipples, with :
Sars.

Sexual desire, with: Cham.

Shrieks, with : Plat.

Strangury, with : Ver-v.

Sweat, cold, after : Castr.

Thighs, down : Cham; Chel;
Cimi; Kali-c; Rhus-t; Sep;
Zin-val.

Urination, frequent, with :
Med.

Washing Amel : Kali-c.

PALE : *Fer; Grap; Nat-m.*

PREGNANCY, During: Asar; Cham;
Cocl; Croc; Ip; Kali-c; Lyc;
Nux-m; Pho; Rhus-t; Sabi;
Sec.

PRESSURE Abdomen, on Amel :
Mag-c.

Back on, while sitting Amel
: Kali-c; Mag-m.

PROTRACTED, Too, long : *Calc;*
Carb-an; Carb-v; *Cup;* Fer;
Kali-c; *Lyc; Mill; Nat-m;*
NUX-V; Pho; *Plat;* Psor; Pul;
Radm; Rat; Rhus-t; Sabi;
Sec; Senec; Sil; Vinc; Vip.

Labour, hasty after : Caul.

Replaced by smarting
leucorrhoea : Pho.

Scarcely recovers from
one, when another
begins : Bur-p.

Sexual desire, with :
Kali-br.

PUBERTY, Before : Calc;
Cina; Sabi; Sil.

PUTRID, Meat like : Lachn;
Syph.

RECTUM, Symptoms, with :
Erig.

RETURN, Old women, in:
Calc; Plat.

SCANTY : *Am-c;* Calc-p; *Con;*
Cyc; *Dul; Grap; Kali-c;*
Lach; Mag-c; Mang;
Nat-m; Pho; PUL; Seneg;
Sep; SUL.

Dispnoea, with : Arg-n.

SEMEN, Odour like, strong :
Stram.

SERUM, Like, gray : Berb.

SHORT : Am-c; Lach; PUL;
Sul.

Leucorrhoea, bloody,
followed by: Radm.

One day only : Alu; Ap;
Arg-n; Euphr; Radm;
Sep.

appear at the interval
of : Ap.

hour : Euphr; Psor.

few : Val.

SHREDDY : Phyt.

SITTING Agg : Mag-m.

Amel : Kre.

SKIN Symptoms, with : Bor;
Carb-v; *Dul; Grap;* Kali-c;
Mag-m; *Nat-m;* Sang;

Sars; Sep; Stram; Ver-a.

STAIN Indelibly : See Indelible.

STANDING Agg : Am-c; Cocl; Mag-c; Psor.

Tiptoe on Agg : Cocl.

STOOLS During, after Agg: Hep; Iod; Lyc; Murx.

Hard, from : Amb; Lyc.

STOOPING Amel : Mag-c.

SUPPRESSED : See Absent.

Agg : Aco; Bry; Caul; Cimi; Cup; Glo; Hell; Lyc; Mill; Mos; Pho; Pul; Senec; Sil; Sul.

TARRY : Kali-m; Mag-c; Mag-m; Mag-p.

THROAT Agg : Bar-c; Calc; Gel; Lac-c; Mag-c; Sul.

URINARY Symptoms, with : Berb.

VICARIOUS (See Discharges Vicarious) : Bry; Fer; Grap; LACH; Pho; *Pul*; Sec; Senec; Sul; Ust; Zin.

WATERY, Thin : Aeth; Alum; Dul; Fer; Goss; Nat-m; Pul; Ust.

WEEKS, Every two : Bov; Bro; Calc-p; Cean; Lyc; Mag-c; Pho;Tril.

Three : Fer-p.

MENTAGRA : See under Eruptions.

MENTAL ALTERNATIONS : See Alternations.

DEPRESSION : See Sadness.

EXERTION AGG : Agar; Anac; Arg-m; *Arg-n; Aur;* CALC;

Calc-p; *Ign*; Kali-p; *Lach*; Lyc; *Nat-c; Nat-m;* NUX-V; Pho; Pho-ac; *Pic-ac*; Pul; Rhus-t; Sele; *Sep; Sil;* Stap; *Sul.*

EXHAUSTION, Prostration (See Brain fag) : *Agar; Anac;* Arg-m; Aur; *Bar-c;* Con; Cup; Kali-p; Lach; *Lyc;* Nat-c; Nat-p; Nit-ac; NUX-V; *Pho;* PHO-AC; PIC-AC; *Plb;* Pul; Sep; Sil; *Stap; Sul;* Tab.

Grief, from : Ign; Nux-m.

Menses, after : Alu.

MERCURY ILL EFFECTS, Of : See under Drugs Abuse of.

MESENTERY : Bar-c; Calc; Iod; Sul-io; Tub.

METALLIC TUBE, Breathes through as if : Merc-c.

METASTASIS (See Alternating States) : Abro; Carb-v; Cup; Pul.

MILK Suppression, from : Agar.

MICTURITION : See Urination.

MIGRAINE (See Head, One sided Symptoms) : Chio; Gel; Ip; Kali-bi; Lac-d; Nat-m; Nat-s; Onos; Psor; Rob; *Sang;* Spig; Sil; Ther.

+ CEREBRAL Origin : Stan.

FACE, Pale with : Amy-n; Ars.

+ NAUSEA, Vomiting, with: Ip.

PROLONGED : Cyc; Lac-d.

POLYURIA With : Ol-an.

SLEEPY, Before : Sul.

SUNSET Amel : Lac-d.

+ VOMITING Amel : Stan.

MILDNESS : See Placid.

MILIARY : See Eruptions, Miliary.

MILK : See under Lactation.

AGG AND AMEL : See under
Food.

CRUSTS : See Head, External.

LEG : See Phlegmasia Alba
Dolens.

MILKY : See under Dischagres.

MIND, AFFECTIONS OF, In
General : *Aco; Ars;* Aur; BELL;
Bry; *Calc;* Cham; Chin; HYO;
Ign; LACH; Lil-t; *Lyc;* Nat-c;
Nat-m; NUX-V; Op; *Pho;*
Pho-ac; Plat; PUL; Sep; STRAM;
Sul; Val; *Ver-a.*

ACUTE : *Cof; Op.*

Weakness, physical, with :
Sil.

ADMONITION Agg : Bell; Pall;
Plat.

ANGER, Suppression of Agg :
Ign; Lyc; *Stap.*

ANTICIPATIONS : See Anticipations.

BLANK : Cor-r; Hell; Stan.

CHILDISH, Body grows : Buf.

DIARRHOEA Amel : Cimi.

DIGESTIVE, Affections, with :
Arg-n.

EATING, Little Amel : Bell;
Tarn.

EVENING Amel : Tarn.

EXERTION Physical Agg : Plb.

Amel : Calc; Iod; Tarn.

EYES, Closing Agg: Carb-an;
Mag-m.

Amel : Kali-c; Zin.

+ FICKLE : Bism.

FILTHY : Merc.

HEART Alternating with :
Lil-t.

LAUGHING Agg : Ther.

LEUCORRHOEA, Appearing
Amel : Murx.

MENSES, Before Agg : Stan.

Amel : Cimi.

During Agg : Nat-m; Stan;
Stram.

Suppressed Agg : Plat.

NARRATING Her symptoms
Agg : *Calc;* Pul.

NOSE Blowing Amel :
Kali-chl.

PAIN Agg : Cham; Sars; Ver-a.

RHEUMATISM Agg : Cimi.

SHAVING Agg : Calad.

SOLES, Rubbing Amel : Chel.

STOOLS Amel : Bov; Cimi;
Nat-s.

SYPHILIS Agg : Asaf; *Aur;*
Hep; Lach; Merc; Nit-ac;
Phyt.

+ TENSION : Mos.

+ TRANQUIL, Haemorrhage
with : Ham.

UTERUS, Alternating with :
Arn; Lil-t.

VACANT : Am-c.

WAKING On Agg : Calc;
LACH; *Lyc;* STRAM; Zin.

WALKING In Open air Agg:
Glo; Nux-m; Petr.

WASHING Face Amel : Ars;
Pho.

Feet Agg : Nat-c.

WEAK, Spasms after : Sec.

YAWNING Amel : Bry.

MINER'S DISEASE : Carb-sul; Card-m; Nat-ar.

COAL : Sul.

MISCARRIAGE : See Abortion.

MISCHIEVOUS: Anac; Calc; Cann; Nux-v.

MISDEEDS OF OTHERS AGG : Colch; *Stap.*

MISERABLE : Flu-ac; Grap; Iod; Kre; Saba; Sep; Stan; Tab; Zin.

MAKES Himself, by brooding over imaginary wrongs and misfortunes : Naj.

MISERLY : See Avaricious.

MISFORTUNE : See Fear of Future.

CONSOLATION, Refuses for his own : Nit-ac.

OTHERS of Agg : Colo.

MISTAKES Of Speech etc : Alu; *Calc; Chin;* Grap; Hep; Kali-br; Lac-c; LYC; Nat-c; *Nat-m;* Nux-v; Sep; Thu.

+ CALCULATING : Am-c.

+ READING : Sep.

WRITING In : Am-c; Hypr; Lach; Lyc; Sep; Thu.

+ Omits words : Benz-ac.

MOANING, GROANING : Aco; Bell; *Bry;* Cann; Cham; *Cic;* Grap; Kali-c; Mang; Merc; *Mur-ac;* Zin.

ANXIOUSLY : Calad.

BREATH, Every, with : Bell.

CHILDREN : Lach; Mill.

+ CONTINUOUS : Kre; Mang.

FEVER, In : Arn; *Pul.*

HEAD, Holds and vomiting when : Cimi.

IMPULSE, To : Grap.

INVOLUNTARILY : Alu; Cham.

LOUDLY, Persistent : Mur-ac.

Sleep, in : Calad.

MENSES, During : Ars.

After : Stram.

PAIN, With : Eup-p; Sil.

SLEEP, In : Aur; Carb-an; Lach; Pod; Stan.

MOBILITY : Cam; Croc; Stram.

MOCKERY : *Lach;* Nux-m; Tarn.

MOISTNESS, INCREASED : See Discharges, Increased.

MOLASSES, Like : See Discharges, Molasses like.

MOLLITIS OSSIUM : See Bone, Curvature.

MONOMANIA : Ign; Sil.

MONS VENERIS : Nat-m; Rhus-t; Sil.

ERUPTIONS : Sil.

ITCHING : Eup-p.

MONTH : See Day, Every 28th.

MOODS CHANGING : See Changing Moods.

MOON LIGHT AGG : Ant-c; Sep; *Sul;* Thu.

AMEL : *Aur.*

BLINDNESS : Bell.

MOON PHASES, FULL MOON Etc. AGG : ALU; Bry; CALC; CINA; Cup; *Lyc;* Nux-v; *Pho;* Saba; SIL; Sul.

AGG and AMEL : Clem; Phel;

Tarn.

EVERY ALTERNATE, Full AGG :
Syph.

NEW AGG : Caus; Cup; Kali-br;
Nux-v; Rhus-t; Saba; Sep;
Sil.

FIRST QUARTER AGG : Ars; Bry;
Nat-m.

FULL AGG : Bov; Calc; Cina;
Grap; Nat-m; *Pho;* Psor;
Saba; Sep; Sil; Sul.

INCREASING AGG : Thu.

LAST QUARTER AGG : Lyc; Sep.

WANING AGG : Daph.

MORAL PERVERSIONS: *Anac;*
BELL; Buf; HYO; Nux-v; Op;
Pho-ac; *Plat;* STRAM; Tarn;
VER-A.

+ SENSE Blunted : Cocain.

MORBID : Stap.

MORBUS COXARIUS : See Hip
Joint, Tuberculosis of.

MORNING AGG : See under Time.

ONE DAY, Evening other day :
Eup-p; Lac-c.

MOROSE AND SULLEN : Anac;
Aur; Bry; Lyc; NUX-V; Pul;
Sang; Sil; Sul-ac; Tab; Tub.

MORPHINISM : Avena; Nat-p;
Passif.

MORTIFICATION, CHAGRIN,
VEXATION And AGG From : *Aco;*
Alu; Am-m; Anac; Aur-m; Bell;
Bry; Caus; Cham; *Colo;* Gel;
Ign; Lyc; Merc; NAT-M; *Nux-v;*
Op; Pall; *Petr;* Pho-ac; Plat;
Stap; Ver-a; Zin.

MOTION : See Gait.

ABSENT *: Bry;* Cocl; Gel;

Hell; Rhus-t.

AGILE : See Active.

+ ANGULAR : Agar.

AUTOMATIC : See Automatic
Acts.

AVERSE, to : Aco; Ars; Bell;
BRY; *Calad;* Calc; Calc-s;
Caps; Chel; *Guai; Lach;*
Nat-m; NUX-V; Rut; Sil;
Sul.

Seated. after being : Kali-p.

DIFFICULT : Bell; *Bry;* Caus;
Lyc; Petr; Rhus-t; *Sep.*

DISORDERLY : Stram.

Paralytic parts, of : Merc.

ERRATIC : Tarn; Ver-v.

EXAGGERATED : Agar; Ign.

GRACEFUL : Pho; Stram.

INCESSANT, But walking Agg
: Tarn.

IRREGULAR : Agar.

OSCILLATORY : Agar; Elap;
Stram.

RHYTHMIC : Elap; Stram.

SIDE, One, only : Stro.

TUMULTUOUS: Aco; Glo; Tab.

+ UNCERTAIN : Agar.

MOTION, WALKING Etc.
(See alsoWalking) AGG :
Aesc; *Arn;* BELL; Bism;
BRY; Calad; *Calc;* Calc-s;
Caus; Chel; Chin; *Cocl;*
COLCH; Colo; Con; Guai;
Kali-c; Kalm; *Led;* Merc;
Nat-m; Nit-ac; NUX-V; Pho;
Phyt; Pic-ac; Pod; Pyro;
Radm; Ran-b; Rhus-t; Sabi;
Sep; SIL; SPIG; Stan; *Sul;*
Sumb; Tab; Tarn; Tril; Tub;
Vib; Zin-ch; Zin-val.

AMEL (Rest AGG) : Ant-t; *Arg-n; Ars; Aur;* CAPS; *Con;* Cyc; DUL; EUPHOR; *Fer; Flu-ac;* Gel; Helo;Iod; Kali-c; *Kali-io;* Kali-s; Kre; Lil-t; *Lyc;* Mag-c; Mag-m; Merc-c; PUL; Pyro; *Rhod;* RHUS-T; *Saba; Samb; Sep; Sul;* Tarn; *Tarax; Val;* Zin.

AFTER AGG : *Agar;* ARS; *Cann; Pul;* RHUS-T; SEP; Spo; *Stan;* Sul-ac; *Val.*

AIR Open Agg : Ars; Caus; Cocl; Mag-p; Nux-v; Sele; Spig; *Sul.*

  AMEL : *Alu; Arg-n;* Dios; *Flu-ac;* Iod; *Kali-io;* Kali-s; Lil-t; Lyc; Mag-c; Mag-m; *Pul; Rhus-t.*

ARMS, Of AGG : See Arms, Motion, Agg.

BEGINNING AGG, Continued AMEL : *Amb;* Anac; *Calc-f;* Caps; Con; Euphor; Fer; Ign; Kalm; Kob; Lyc; Pho; *Pul;* Radm; RHUS-T; Sep; Syph.

DISTANT Parts of Agg : Ap; *Bry;* Cocl.

FEET, Of AMEL : Ars; Rhus-t; *Zin.*

GLIDING AMEL : Nit-ac.

RAPID, Violent etc. AGG : *Ars; Bry;* Sil; Sul; Symp.

  AMEL (Running Dancing etc.): Am-m; *Ars;* Aur-m; Bro; Bur-p; Flu-ac; Grap; Ign; Nit-ac; Scop; *Sep;* Stan; Sul-ac; Tarn; *Tub.*

SLIGHTEST AGG : *Bry;* Buf; Cadm; Latro; Lob; Ther.

SLOW, Gentle AMEL : Agar; Alu; Amb; *Aur;* Caus; Colo; FER; Glo; *Kali-p;* Mag-m; PUL; Sumb; Syph; Tarn.

SUDDEN AGG : Cocl; Fer; Kali-c.

  AMEL : Rhod; Saba.

WRONG AGG : Bry; Lyc.

  AMEL : Am-m.

MOTTLED, PATCHY : AIL; Ars; Bap; Bell; *Carb-v;* Con; *Crot-h;* Glo; Kali-bi; Kali-m; LACH; Led; Lil-t; Manc; *Nat-m; Nux-v;* Ox-ac; Pho; Rhus-t; Sars; Syph; *Thu;* Ver-v.

MOULDY : See Musty

  FORMING Body over, as if : Sil.

MOUNTAIN CLIMBING AGG : *Arn;* Ars; Coca.

MOUTH AFFECTIONS in General : See Throat.

  AGG And AMEL : See Throat.

  ABOUT : Ars; Bry; Cina; Kali-n; *Kre;* Nat-m; Rhus-t; Sep; Stap; *Sul.*

  Bluish : *Cina;* Cup; Ver-a.

  Cobweb : Rat.

  Eruptions : Kali-m.

    coryza during : Mez.

    pimples : Ant-c; Ast-r.

  Muscles, seem contracted : Gel.

  Pale : Aru-t; Bell; Cic; Cina; Merc-c; Stram.

  Sweat : Rhe.

  Trembling, Twitching : Ign; *Op;* Senec; Thu.

Yellow : Nux-v.

ANGLES Droop : Agar.

Jerks, pain, with: Tell.

APHTHAE (See Ulcers) : Ant-c; *Ars; Bap; Bor;* Caps; Carb-v; Kali-bi; Kali-chl; Kali-m; Lach; Med; MERC; Merc-c; Mur-ac; Nux-v; Plb; Rhus-t; Sanic; *Sul; Sul-ac;* THU.

Chewing gum, from : Merc.

Children : Bor; Merc; Sul-ac.

Diarrhoea, lienteric, with : Hell.

Eye affections, with : Bro.

Mother's, nursing : Bap; Hyds.

Pregnancy, during : Kre.

Small and sore : Med.

Sour and salty food, after : Bor.

Suckling, of : Bap.

BITTER : Menis; Zin.

BLEEDING : Chin; Crot-h; Hep; Pho.

BROWN-RED : Lyc.

BURNING, Heat, Raw, smarting : ARS; *Aru-t; Bell; Bor;* Cham; Iris; Manc; Med; Mez; Sang; Sul; Sul-io.

Cold, not Amel by : Merc.

Sneezing, with : Ver-v.

Thirst, with : Hypr.

BURNT, Scalded, as if : Iris; Mag-m; Pul; Sep.

CLAMMY : Bell; Dios; Lach; Onos.

CLOSE, Can not, at night : Chim.

Desire to keep : Kob.

COLD : Ars; Cam; Carb-v; Kali-n; Tell; Ver-a.

Corners : Aeth.

COVERS It: Am-c; Arg-n; Cor-r; Cup; Ip; Kali-bi; *Lach;* Rum; Thu.

CRACKED : Cocl; Pho; Pho-ac.

Corners : Cund; Mez.

CRAWLING : Zin.

CRUSTS : Myr

DISTORTED : Con; Dul.

DRAWN To left : Pho; Ver-v.

+ One side, to : Dul.

DRY : *Aco; Ars;* BELL; Berb; Bry; Chin; Lach; Lyc; *Merc;* Mur-ac; Nat-m; Nux-m; *Nux-v; Pho; Pho-ac;* Rhus-t; *Sep;* Stram; Stro; *Sul;* Sul-io; Tub; Ver-a; Ver-v.

Anterior : Ars; Bry; Nux-v.

But no thirst : Ap; Bry; Calad; Cocl; Kali-c; Lach; Lyc; NUX-M; *Nux-v; Pul;* Spig.

Chewing, food, on : Thu.

Chill, during : Petr.

Cough, with, as if : Phyt.

Food seems too, while eating : Calad; Chin; Fer; Ign; Kali-io; Ox-ac; Raph.

Posterior : Mez; Thu.

Rinse, must : Cinb.

Saliva increased, with : Alu; Aral; Colch; Kali-c; Lyc; Mag-m; *Merc;* Nat-m; Plb.

Scraping : Seneg.

Sleep, in : Nux-m.

Wakes, from sleep : Cinb.

+ Water, no amel : Chio.

EATING Amel : Benz-ac.

FINGERS In, Children put : Calc; Cham; *Ip.*

FOAM, Froth : Bell; Cham; Cic; Cup; *Hyo;* Ign; Laur; Sec; Stram; Ver-v.

Chill, Shaking, during : Ther.

Constant, chewing, from : Asaf.

Milky : Aeth.

Reddish, Bloody : Crot-h; Ign; Lach; Sec; Stram.

Talking, while : Lac-d.

White, rises from

throat continuously : Mag-m.

Yellow green : Sec.

FOOD Escapes from, during chewing : Arg-n.

FURRED, As if : Ther.

GANGRENOUS : Lach.

Children, in   : Ars.

GRASPS, At : Sil.

GREASY : Iris; Ol-an.

Rancid : Euphor.

HAIRY Sensation, in : Ther.

HERPES In, after sea-bathing : Zin.

HOT, As if : Hypr.

INDURATION Inside, cheek : Caus.

INFLAMMATION : Kali-chl; Merc; Nit-ac; Petr.

ITCHING : Merc; Phyt; Rhus-t.

LOOSE Skin, in   : Phys.

MILK Covered with, as if : Kali-io.

MOTION Of, as if talking : See Talks to himself.

Sucking, as of : Bell.

MUCOUS, Adhesive : Myr.

Foul : Myr; Rhe.

Sleep after: Rhe.

NUMB : Bap; Bar-c; Bell; Bov; Kali-br; Mag-m; Stro; Ther.

Prickling, with : Nat-p.

ODOUR From, bad breath : See Breath, Offensive.

OPEN, Hangs, Jaws drop : *Ail;* Ars; Bap; Bar-c; Carb-v; Colch; Gel; Hell; Hyo; *Lach; Lyc;* Merc-c; Mur-ac; Naj; Nat-c; Op; Rhus-t; *Sul;* Zin.

Can not, or difficult : Caus; *Lach;* Merc-c; Nux-m; Pho.

Convulsions or epilepsy before : Buf.

during : Cup.

Involuntarily : Ther.

Night, at : Chim.

Rapid succession, in : Myg.

Remains, yawning after : Ant-t.

can not close : Ther.

sleep, during : Nat-c.

OPENING AGG : Aru-t; Bry; Caus; Cocl; *Lach; Merc;* Merc-c; Nux-v; Pho; Saba; Spig.

AMEL : Mez.

PEPPERY : Coca.

PINS, Needles, full of, as if :

Spig.

PLATE Of Teeth Agg : Alum; Bor.

RAW : See Burning.

RINSING Agg : Coc-c.

SALT Water, in : Carb-an; Verb.

+ SCALDED, As if : Ver-v.

SLEEP, After : Rhe.

STICKY (See Clammy) : *Aesc;*
Berb; *Caps;* Chel; KALI-BI;
Kali-c; Lach; Merc; Myr; Pul;
Rhus-t; Tub.

SWELLED : Kali-chl; Merc; Nit-ac.

TONGUE, Protruding Agg: Cist.

TUMOURS : Calc; *Lyc; Nit-ac.*
Painless : Calc; *Nit-ac.*

TWISTS, Face, with : Lyc.
Side, one to, when speaking
: Cub.

TWITCHES : Op.

ULCERS (See Aphthae): *Ars;*
Iod; Kali-io; Lach; Mur-ac;
Nit-ac; Phyt.
Extending from mouth, to
intestines : Terb.

VARICOSE Veins : Thu.

VESICLES : Ars.
Burning : Ars.

WARM, Biting in, sneezing on
: Ver-v.
Unusually : Cimi; Croc.

WIPE, Must : Kali-bi; Sec.

YELLOW : Plb.
Red : Lyc.

MOVEMENTS : See Motion.

MUCOUS COLITIS : See Stool
Mucus and Colitis Mucous.

MUCOUS MEMBRANES : Aco;
Ant-t; Ap; *Arg-n; Ars; Bell;*
Bor; *Bry;* Caps; Cep; *Cham;*
Dul; Eucal; Euphor; Hep;
Hyds; Ip; Kali-bi; Kali-c;
Merc; Nux-v; Pho; *Pul;* Rum;
Saba; Sang; Scil; Senec;
Seneg; *Stan; Sul;* Syph;
Terb; Thu.

DARK : Aesc; Bap; Carb-v;
Ham; Lach; Merc-i-r; Mez;
Pho.

DRY : Alu; *Bell;* Bry; Caus;
Kali-c; Nux-m; Sang; Stic.

PALE : Ars; Chin; Fer; Kali-c;
Mang; Pho.

PATCHES : Arg-n; Lach;
Merc-i-f; Nit-ac; Phyt; Pul.

RAW : Aru-t; Nux-v.

RED Bright : Aco; Bell; Canth.

SECRETION, Altered : See
Discharges, Mucous,
altered.

SHRIVELLED : Bor.

SPONGY : Caps; Phyt.

ULCERATED : Arg-n; Ars;
Hyds; Kali-io; Kre; Merc-c;
Nit-ac; Phyt; Sil; Sul-ac.

VESICLES : Ap; Bor; Canth;
Carb-v.

WRINKLED : Ars Elap; Merc.

MUDDLED : See Confusion.

MUMPS (See Parotids) : Bell;
Cham; Con; Jab; Lach;
Merc; Phyt; Rhus-t; Sil.

FEVER, Without : Kali-m.

+ LIMITS, Duration of : Jab.

MEASLES, After : Dul.

METASTASIS, Mammae to :
Pul.

Testes, to : Ars; Carb-v; *Pul*; Rhus-t; Stap.

+ RIGHT, Side : Kali-bi.

SEPTIC : Anthx; Lach; Syph.

TYPHOID Fever, in : Mang.

MUSCAE VOLITANTES : See Under Vision.

MUSCLES : Agar; Anac; Arn; Ars; BELL; BRY; *Calc;* CAUS; Cimmi; Cocl;Con; *Eup-p;* Gel; Hell; Hyo; Kali-c; *Mur-ac;* Nux-v; RHUS-T; Sec; Til; Val; *Ver-a;* Zin.

+ ABSCESS, Deep : Calc.

+ ACHING : Bap.

ATROPHY : Ars; Calc; Caus; Plb; Thall; Thu.

Progressive : Crot-h; Kali-p; Mang; Pho; Phys; Plb; Ver-v.

BELLY, Of : Cimi; Thu

+ CONTROL, Uncertain : Caus.

CRAMPS : Anac; Bell; *Cacl;* Cina; *Con; Cup; Lyc;* Merc; *Nux-v; Plat;* Sep; Tab.

+ HEAVY : Bap.

+ INCREASED ability to exercise, without fatigue : Flu-ac.

INDURATED: Calc-f; Sil.
Neuralgia, after : Bry.

JUMPING : Colch; Dios; Hyds; Pul.

KNOTS : Cup; Phyt; Senec; Syph.

LAX, Flabby : *Aeth;* Ant-t; Calc; Caps; Carb-ac; *Chin;* Cocl; Colch; *Gel; Lyc;* Mur-ac; Pho; Pho-ac; Stram; Sul.

OBEY Feebly : Anac; Ast-r; Gel; Hell; Phys;Tarn.

+ RIGIDITY : Phys.

SHORT : See Contractions.

SORE, From dancing etc. : Cimi.

STIFF : Terb.

STITCHES, Burning, in : *Ap;* Asaf; Cocl; Glo; Mez; Nux-v; Rhus-t; Stap; Sul-ac; Thu.
Pressive, in : Sars.

TENSE : Aco; Lach; Nit-ac; *Nux-v;* Pho; Sep.

UNDEVELOPED : Nat-m.

UNDULATING : Asaf.

WEAK (See Weaknes) : Calc; Cimi; Cocl; Gel; Kali-c; Phys; Radm; Sil; Sul-ac; Ver-v.

MUSIC AGG : Aco; Amb; Buf; *Calc; Cham;* Croc; Dig; Grap; Kre; Lyc; Med; *Nat-c;* Nat-m; NUX-V; *Pho; Pho-ac;* Sabi; SEP; Sumb; Tarn; Tub; Vio-o.

AMEL : Aur; Tarn.

MENSES During Agg : Nat-c.

SAD Amel : Mang.

MUSTY, MOULDY : Bor; Crot-h; Mar-v; Rhus-t; Sanic; Stan; Stap; Thu; Thyr.

MUTINISM Of Childhood : Agrap; Lyc.

MUTTERING : See Delirium, Muttering.

HIMSELF, To: Tarx.

MYOPIA : See Vision, Near sight.

MYXOEDEMA : Ars; *Thyr..*

NAEVI : See Birth Mark.

NAGGING : Lyc; Nux-v; Plat.

NAIL : See Plug.

NAILS : Ant-c; Grap; Merc; *Sil; Sul;* Thu; Ust.

AROUND : Psor.

BASE : Calc-p; Caps.

BITES : Aco; Ars; Aru-t; Cina; Lyc; Med; Senec; Stram.

BLOOD, Oozing, from : Crot-h.

BLUE : Aur; Chin; Dig; Nit- ac; *Nux-v;* Ox-ac; Sil; *Ver-a.*

BRITTLE, Crumbling : Alu; Clem; Flu-ac; Grap; Lept; Merc; *Psor;* Scil; Senec; Sil; Sul; Thu.

BURNING : Sars.

CORNER, Of : Lach.

+ CRIPPLED : Sep.

CURVED : Nit-ac.

Consumption, in : Med; Tub.

CUTTING : Petr; Sars.

DEFORMED, Thickened etc. : Alu; Ant-c; Calc-f; Flu-ac; *Grap;*Saba; Sep; *Sil;* Sul; Syph; Thu.

DEPRESSED : Med.

DISCOLOURED : Grap; Nit-ac; Thu.

EDGE Of : Calc-p; Radm.

FALLING : Grap; Hell; Scil; Sil; *Ust.*

FLY, Off : Pyro.

FOLD, Remains attached to the growing : Osm.

GNAWING : Alu; Berb; Lach; Lapp.

GREY : Merc-c.

GROW, Quickly : Flu-ac.

Do not : Ant-c; Radm.

Interrupted : Kali-s.

HANG NAILS : Calc; *Nat-m;* Nat-s; Rhus-t; *Sul.*

HYPERTROPHY : Calc-f; Laur.

INGROWN : Flu-ac; *Grap;* Hep; *Mag-p-aus; Mar-v;* Nit-ac; *Sil;* Sul-io.

Pain, motion Amel : Mar-v.

KNOTTY : Laur.

LOOSE, As if : Ap; Pyro; Ust.

PAINFUL : Caus; Grap; Merc; Nit-ac; Sil; Sul.

PRICKING, Under: Elap.

RIBBED : Flu-ac; Thu.

Transversely : Ars.

RUN AROUND : See Fingers, felon.

SCALING : Alu.

SOFT : Lept; Plb; Thu.

SPLITTING : *Ant-c;* Flu-ac; Lept; Rut; Scil; *Sil;* Thu.

SPOTTED : Nit-ac; Sil.

White : Alu; Nit-ac; Sil.

THICK : See Deformed.

THIN : Lept.

TINGLING, In: Colch.

Under . Nat-3.

ULCER : Sil.

UNDER : Alu; Berb; Bism; Sars; Sep.

Growth : Ant-c.

Irritable feeling: Am-br.

Splinter : Calc-p; Coc-c; Flu-ac.

YELLOW : Con; Nit-ac; Sep; Sil.

NAKED WANTS, To be : Bell; *Hyo;* Pho; Sec; Tarn.

NAPE : See Under Neck.

NAPS AMEL : See Sleep Short Amel.

NARCOTICS Agg : See Under Drugs, Abuse of.

NARRATING Her Symptoms AGG : Calc; Cic; Mar-v; Pul.

NARROW : See Forced through, narrow opening.

NASO-PHARYNX (Posterior-nares) : Cinb; Elap; Hyds; *Lyc; Merc; Merc-c;* Merc-i-r; *Nat-c; Nat-m;* Pho; Rum; Sep; *Spig; Stap;* Sul; Ther; Thu; Zin-io.

BLEEDING : Cor-r; Spig.

DISCHARGES, From : Arn; Coc-c; Cor-r; Mag-c; Nat-c; Phyt; Syph; Ther.

Bloody : *Hep;* Saba; Tell.

Drips : Cep; Hyds; Merc-c; Spig.

Lumpy : Calc; Cimi; Mar-v; Merc-c-f; Sep; Syph.

Sticky : Caps; Kali-bi.

DRY : Rum.

EXPANSION, Sensation of : Flu-ac.

FOOD, Sensation of : Nit-ac; Sil.

HOT, Dry : *Aco;* Aesc; Lyc; Sep; Zin-io.

ITCHING : Ail; Kali-p; Nux-v; Ran-b.

LUMP, As of, a : Aesc; Cist; Hyds; Kali-bi; *Lach;* Mar-v;

Nat-m; Pho; Sep; Spig; Stic; Sul; Zin.

MUCUS Drops, into : Cinb; Cor-r; Lith; Med.

RAW, Sore : Aco; CARB-V; Kali-n; Sep.

STUFFED, Up : Elap.

NATES : See Buttocks.

NAUSEA : AETH; ANT-C; *Ant-t;* Arg-n; ARS; Bell; BRY; *Carb-v; Cham;* Chin; COCL; *Colch; Cup; Dig;* Dul; Hell; *Hep; Ign; Ip;* Kali-c; Lac-d; Lob; *Lyc;* Nat-m; *Nit-ac; Nux-v;* Petr; *Pho; Pul; Rhus-t;* Sang; *Sep;* Sil; *Sul;* Sul-ac; Tab; Val; VER-A; Zin.

ABDOMEN, Felt in: Cimi; Polyg.

ALCOHOLISM, From : Cimi.

AMOROUS Caresses, from : Ant-c; Sabal.

ANUS, Burning in, with : Kali-bi.

ANXIETY, with, Deathly : Ant-c; Ant-t; Cocl; *Crot-h; Ip;* LOB; Pul; *Tab.*

ASCENDING Rapidly, on : Glo.

CHEST, Felt, in : Ant-t; Calend.

CHILL, With : Cocl; Echi; Eup-p; Kali-m; Sul-ac.

COFFEE Agg : Caps.

Amel: Alet:

COITION, During : Saba; Sil.

After : Kali-c; Mos.

Thought of : Sep.

COLD, When : Cadm; *Cocl;* Hep.

CONCOMITANT, As a : Nat-s.

CONTINUOUS : IP; Iris; *Nux-v;* Sil; Vib.

+ Eating Amel : Vib.

CONVULSIONS, Before : Hyd-ac.

COUGH, During : Ip; Kali-p; Pul.

CROWD, In : Sabi.

DEATHLY : See Anxiety, with.

DESCENDING Agg : Nat-s.

DIARRHOEA, With : Cist.

DINNER Amel : Alet.

DREAM, In : Arg-m.

DRINKING, After: Calc; Cocl; Pul.
Amel : *Bry;* Lob; Pho.
Ice water Amel: Calc.

DROWSINESS, With : Apoc.

EAR, Felt in: Dios.

EATING AMEL: Arg-n; Fago; Lac-ac; Mez; Phyt; Radm; Sang; Sep; Vib.
While : Ver-a.

ERECTION, With : Kali-bi.

ERUCTATION, During: Cimi; Kali-c; Nit-ac.
Amel : Caus; Kali-p; Lac-c; Rum.

+ EXCESSIVE, Vanishing of sight, with : Crot-t.

EXCITEMENT, After : Kali-c.

EYES, Closing Agg : Lach; Ther.
Amel : Con.
Using Agg : Jab; Pul; Sars; Sep; Ther.

FAINT Like : Cocl; Lach; Nux-v.

FASTING, While : Calc; *Lyc.*

FATTY, Food Agg : Dros.

FEVER, During: Nat-m.

FISH, After : Nat-m.

FLATUS Passing Agg : Ant-t.
Amel : Bell.

FOOD : See Odour.
Thought of Agg : Cocl; Colch; Mos.
eaten, of : Sars.

FRUITS Agg : Ant-t; Ip.

HAWKING Agg : Stan.

HEADACHE During : Ant-c; Caus; Cocl; Con; Ip; Iris; Sang; Stro.
Trembling of body, with : Bor.

HEAD, Felt in : Colch.

HEAT Of body, with : Kali-bi.

HICCOUGH, With : Lach.

HOT Drinks Amel : See Warm drinks.
Stove, near Agg : Laur.

HUNGER Agg : Ign; Petr; Val; Ver-a.

ICE Creams, from: Rhus-t.
Drinks, from : Laur.

+ INDIGESTIBLE Things, Amel: Ign.

ITCHING, With, before urticaria : Sang.

LIPS, Touching on : Cadm; Nux-m.

LOOKING Moving objects, at : Asar; Cocl; Ip; Jab.
One object, at steadily : Ther.

LYING Side, on Amel: Ant-t; Nat-m.
Right side, on Agg : Bry; *Cann;* Crot-h; Iris; Sang; Sul-ac.

MENSES Agg : Bor; Cocl; Grap; *Nux-v*; Symphor.

After : Crot-h.

Profuse, with: Caps.

MIDNIGHT, After : Ran-sc.

At : Fer.

MILK Amel : Chel.

MORNING : Calc; Carb-v; Cimi; Grap; Lac-ac; Med; *Nux-v*; PUL; *Sep*.

Early : Lob.

continues whole day : Cact.

MOTION, Least Agg : Tab; Ther.

NIGHT Agg : Carb-an; Lob.

NOISE, From : Ther.

NOSE, Blowing Agg : See Sneezing.

ODOUR, From any : Vario.

Food, of, cooking etc. Agg : Ars; Cocl; COLCH; Dig; Ip; Merc-i-f; Sep; Stan; Vario.

Of his own body : Sul.

OPERATION On Abdomen, after : BISM; Stap.

PAIN, During : Cadm; Chel; Ip; Kalm; Sep; Spig.

Abdomen, in, from : Colo; Nux-v.

PALPITATION, With : Arg-n; Bro; Myg; Sil.

PESSARY in Uterus, from : Nux-m.

PREGNANCY, During : Asar; Cimi; Kre; Lac-ac; Mag-m; Nux-v; Sep; Stap; Tab.

PRESSURE, Abdomen, on : Tub.

Downward in intestine with : Agn.

Forehead, in : Alet.

Neck, on : Cimi.

Painful spot, on : Nat-m.

Spine, on : Cimi.

Throat, on : Lach.

PRICKLING, All over, with : Lob.

PUTTING Hands in warm water : PHO.

QUIET Amel : Cadm.

RECTUM, Felt in : Rut.

RENAL, Origin, from : Senec.

RESPIRATORY Symptoms, with : Lob.

RINSING Mouth, on : Bry; *Sep*; Sul-ac.

ROOM, Closed, in : Lyc; Nat-c; Tab.

SALIVA, Swallowing on : Colch.

SALT, Thinking of : Nat-m.

SEWING, While : Lac-d; Sep.

SHIVERING, With : Kali-m; Sul-ac.

SINGING, While : Ptel.

SLEEP, Before going, to : Lach.

SMOKING Agg : Carb-an; Clem.

Amel: Sanic.

SNEEZING, While: Hell; Lach; Sang; Sul.

SOUR Things Amel : Arg-n.

SPEAKING Agg : Ther.

SPITTING Agg : Led.

STANDING Amel : Tarx.

STOMACH, Felt in : Cocl; *Ver-a*.

STOOL, Loose, after : Aco.

Amel : Terb.

Urging, with : Dul.

STOOPING Amel : Petr.

STOVE Near : Laur.

SUDDEN Eating, when: Rut.

SUN, Heat of, Agg: Carb-v.

SWALLOWING, Empty, on: Colch.

Preventing : Arn.

SWEETS Agg : Arg-n; Cyc; *Grap;* Ip; Merc.

THINKING, Hard, when: Bor.

Food, about, he has eaten : Sars.

THROAT, Felt, in : Aral; Cyc; Mez; Pho-ac; Stan; Val.

Dryness, with : Cocl.

TREMBLING, With : Ars; Bor; Plat.

UNCOMFORTABLE : Ars-io.

+ UNCOVERING Amel : Tab.

URINATION Agg : Dig.

Amel : Nat-p.

URTICARIA, Then : Sang.

VISION, Dim, with: Myg.

+ VOMITING And Purging, with : Ver-v.

VOMITING Does not Amel : Dig; Ip; Sang.

Amel : Phyt; Pyro.

WARM Drinks Amel : Phyro; Ther.

WASHING, While : Bry; Ther; Zin.

WATER, From: Apoc; Ars; Calc; Ver-a.

Iced Agg : Lach.

Amel : Calc.

WAVES, In : Ant-t.

WORM, Rising in throat, as if

with : Spig.

YAWNING, While : Arn; Nat-m.

NAVEL AND REGION : Bry; *Colo;* Dios; *Dul;* Ip; Kre; Lept; Nux-v;*Pho-ac; Rhus-t*; Spig; *Ver-a;* Verb.

ACHING, Headache, with : Lept.

BACK, To : Plat.

BLADDER, Alternating, with : Terb.

BLEEDING From, In new born : Abro; *Calc-p.*

BLOATED : See Inflated.

BREAST, To : Pall.

BUBBLING : Aeth; Hypr.

BURNING : ACO; Bov; Kali-io; *Lach;* Lyc; Phyt; Plb; Sep.

Oesophagus, to : Hyd-ac.

CRAMP, Colic : Chio; *Colo;* Dios; Ip; Nat-s; Rhod; Senec; Stro.

Directions to, all, stool Amel : Senec.

CREEPING : Rum.

CUTTING : Colch; *Colo;* Dul; Ip; *Nux-v*; Ver-v.

Breathing Deep Agg : Mang.

Leucorrhoea, with : Am-m; Sil.

Stools Amel : Benz-ac.

DRAWN, In : Chel.

EMPTY : Flu-ac; Kob.

ERUPTIONS, About: Dul.

Eczema: Sul.

FESTERS : Abro; Calc-p;

Nux-m.

FLATUS Amel : Mag-c.

+ GROINS, To : Ver-v.

HARD : Pul.

HERNIA : See under Hernia.

HUNGER, Felt, in: Val.

INFLATED : Calc; Phys.

LUMP At. as if : Kre; Nux-v; Rhus-t; *Sep;* Spig; Verb; Zin.

Behind : Ran-sc.

Falling to back, from : Laur.

Hard, below : Bism.

MOISTURE, At: Calc-p.

+ MOST Painful, children with worms : Spig.

MOTION, As of, expiration, on : Card-m.

PELVIS, To : Pall; Rum; Sep.

POUTING : Dul.

PROUD Flesh: *Calc;* Kali-c; Nat-m.

RADIATING, from : Benz-ac; Senec.

RECTUM, To : Alo; Ars; Crot-t; Dios; Fer-io; Lyc.

Navel to : Colo; Lach.

RED : Phys.

Streak, curved above : Par.

RETRACTED : Calc-p; *Plb;* Pod; Pul; Stan; Tab; Ver-a; Zin.

Colic, with : Nat-c.

RUMBLING : Tarx.

Pinching, and : Strop.

SICKENING Pain, Stools, after : Pho-ac.

SITTING Agg : Symp.

SORE : Nux-m; Phys; Thu.

STOOLS Agg : Lept.

Ame : Senec.

SUPPURATING : Pho.

SWELLING, Painful : Caus.

THROBBING : Kali-c.

TURNS and Twists :Plat.

TWISTING, At : Cina; Verb.

ULCERATION, New born: Ap.

Above : Ars.

Infants : Petr.

URINE Oozing, from : Hyo.

UTERUS, to (See Pelvis to) : Ip.

YELLOW Discharge, gonorrhoea suppressed from : Nat-m.

NEAR SIGHT: See Vision Near.

NECK AND NAPE : Aco; Bar-c; *Calc;* Cimi; Gel; *Nux-v;* Phyt; Pul; Rhus-t; Sanic; Sep; Sil; Stap; Tub.

ABSCESS : Sul-ac.

ACHING : *Bry;* Chin; *Cimi; Gel;* Guai; Hyds; Kali-p; Kalm; *Lach;* Lachn; Lil-t; Lyc; Lyss; Onos; Par; *Phyt;* Sil; Ver-v.

Nape : Cocl; Gel; Pho-ac; Pic-ac; Stro.

ALTERNATING Sides : Calc-p; *Pul.*

ARMS, To :*Kalm; Lach*; Nat-m; Nux-v.

ASCENDING From nape : Meny; Sul.

BENDING Head, forward AGG : Cimi; Lyss; Radm.

BLOW, As of : Naj.

BLOWING Nose Agg : Kali-bi.

BLUISH Nape : Lach; Rhus-t.

BLUISH : Kali-io; Sil; Sul; Sul-io.

Nape : Pic-ac; Sul.

BOILS : Kali-io; Su;

Nape : Pic-ac; Sul.

BREATHING Deeply Agg: Chel.

BROWN : Sanic.

+ BUBBLING : Lyc.

BURNING, Heat : Lach; Merc; Pho-ac.

Swallowing when : Petr.

CARBUNCLE : Lach; Sil.

CHEWING Agg : Form.

CHLOASMAE : Caul; Sanic.

Greasy : Lyc; Petr.

CLOTHES Agg (See Clothes pressure about neck Agg) : Caus.

COLD : Con; Sil; Spo.

Icy, Nape : Chel.

CONSTRICTION, As of a band : Bell; Glo; Lach; Nux-m; Sep; Spo.

Cord, as from : Chel; Spo.

CONTRACTED, Rigidly : Ran-b.

Speaks by moving shoulders up and down : Ran-b.

CRACKING : Chel; Cocl; Nat-c; Petr; Sul.

CRAMP : Calc-p; Cic; Cimi; Naj; Phyt; Plat; Spo; Ver-v.

Nape : Hyd-ac; Nux-v.

CURVATURE : Calc; Syph.

CUTTING : Kali-bi.

CYSTS, Both sides, on : Bro.

DRAFT, Air On Agg: Calc-p; Hep; Lach; Merc; Psor; Sanic; Sil; Stro.

DRAWING : Chel; Cimi; Thu.

EMACIATED : Calc; Lyc; Mag-c; NAT-M; Sanic; Sars.

ERUPTION : Arn; Sil; Sul-io.

EXERTION Agg : Arg-n; Calc; Lil-t; Sep.

Mental Agg : Par; Zin.

FACE, To : Kalm.

FINGERS, To : Par.

FORMICATION : Nux-v; Sec.

FULL: Glo.

GARGLING Agg : Form.

GNAWING : Nat-s; Thu.

HAND, Motion of Agg : Cimi.

Seized, by, as if : Grat.

HAWKING Agg : Form.

HEAD Could not support, as if : Fago.

HEAVY : Par; Rhus-t.

Nape : Meny; Nux-v; Par; Rhus-t.

INJURY, Concussion: Mez.

ITCHING : Alu; Nat-m; Sul.

JERKING, Muscles, in: Aeth; Colo; Sep.

Convulsions, before : Buf.

LAME Nape (See Weak) : Zin.

LARGE, Too, as if : Kali-c.

LEFT, Head or Shoulder, to : Spig.

LIFTING Agg: Calc.

LOOKING Up Agg : Grap.

NEURALGIA : Hyds.

NUMB : Chel; Plat.

PRESSING : Bell; Par; Pho.

PRICKLING : Carb-an.

PULSATION : See Throbbing.

RED : Bell; Crot-h; *Grap;* Pho; Rhus-t; Ver-a.

SHORT : Alu; Bell; Cic; Cimi; Syph.

Nape : Ign; Nat-m; Tub.

SHOOTING : *Nat-m;* Sul-ac.

SHOULDER, And : Crot-t; Guai; Lachn; Stic; Sul; Ver-v.

Right : Nux-v; Zin.

SITTING Erect. Amel : Radm.

SNEEZING Agg : Am-m; Arn.

Amel : Calc.

SORE : Nat-s; Pho-ac; Sil; Stic.

SPONDYLITIS : Pho-ac.

STANDING Amel: Radm.

STIFF : Agar; Anac; Arg-m; Bar-c; *Bell;* Bry; Calc; Chel; *Caus;* Cimi; Glo; Ign; *Kali-c;* Lach; Lachn; Lyc; Mag-c; *Merc;* Merc-i-r; *Nit-ac;* Nux-v; Pho; Phyt; Rhus-t; Sep; Sil; Spig; Stic; Sul; Tub.

Back, down : Anac.

Bending head forwards Agg : Kali-bi.

Cracks, moving when : Petr.

Headache, with : Sil.

One side : Colo; Guai; Stic.

right : Agar; Caus; Nat-m.

temples, to : Chel; Spig.

left : Bell; Carb-an; Chel; Colo; Glo; Guai; Kre; Lyc.

spine, with: Adon.

temples, to : Spig.

yawning, on : Nat-m.

STOOLS Amel: Asaf.

+ STRING Around (See Constriction) : Chel.

SWALLOWING Agg : Calc-p; Colch; Zin.

Amel: Spo.

SWEAT : *Calc;* Chin; Lach; Mang; *Pho-ac;* Sanic; STAN; *Sul.*

Cold, Nape: Con.

SWELLING, Nape : Bar-c.

Fatty : Am-m.

TEMPLE, Cold : Chel.

Right, to : Chel.

Left, to : Spig.

TENSE : Con; Sep; Sul; Tub.

Numbness, with : Plat.

THICK Growing : Con; *Iod;* Pho.

Talking, while : Iod.

THROBBING, Pulsation : Ap; *Bell;* Op; Pyro; Spig; Ver-v.

Menses, before: Nit-ac.

during : Nit-ac; Ver-v.

TOUCH Agg : Lach.

TUMOURS Cystic : Bro.

Fatty : Bar-c; Thu.

Malignant : Calc-p.

TURNING Agg : *Bell;* Bry.

UNCOVERING Amel : Sars.

UNEASY, Nape : Aeth.

VEINS, Swollen : Op.

VERTEBRAE, Crack: Chel; Ol-an.

sore : Ham.

VERTEX, To : Kalm.

WEAK, Tired: Abro; *Aeth ;*
Ant-t; Bap; Calc-p; Caul;
Cocl; Nat-m; Par; PLAT;
Sanic; Sep; Sul; *Ver-a;* Ver-v.

Headache, with : Fago.

falls, forwards: Nux-m.

Then, stupor : Hyo; Zin.

WRINKLED, Skin : Sars.

WRITING Agg: Carb-an; Lyč;
ZIN.

WRY, Torticollis : *Bell;* Cimi;
Dul; Glo; Hyo; Lachn; Lyc;
Nux-v; *Pho; Rhus-t.*

Right : Cup; Lyc.

Left : *Bell; Lyc*; Nux-v; *Pho.*

Chronic : Bar-c.

Shock, from : Nux-v.

Throat, sore, with : Lachn.

YAWNING Agg : Cocl; Nat-s.

NECROSIS (See Bones) :
Calc-io; Radm.

NEEDLES: See Pain, Stitching.

COLD *: Agar;* Ars.

HOT (See Hot, Iron) : Ars; Lith;
Ol-an; Vesp.

NEGLECTED, HIS Duty, he has
: AUR; Ign; *Lyc.*

APPEARANCE, His own: Coca.

HE is : *Arg-n,* PALL.

NERVOUS PATIENTS, Nerves
etc. : *Aco;* Arg-n; Asaf; Aur;
Bell; Bor; Castr; Caul; *Caus;*
Cham; *Chin;* Cimi; *Cocl; Cof;*
Con; Cup; *Hyo;* IGN; Iod; Jab;
Kali-p; LACH; *Lil-t;* Mag-c;
Mag-m; Mag-p; Merc; *Mos;*
Nat-m; Nit-ac; Nux-m; NUX-V;
Pho; Pic-ac; Pru-sp; PUL;
Sabal; Senec; Sep; SIL; Stap;

Stic; *Stram;Sul; Tarn*; Ther;
Thyr; Vib; Visc; Zin; Zin-val.

ACTIVITY *:* Vio-o.

COUGHING, when : Cimi.

DISORDERS, Suppressed
eruptions, from : Asaf.

PARALYSIS : Pru-sp.

PROSTRATION, Neurasthenia :
Agar; Ars; *Calc*; Gel; Ign;
Kali-p; *Lach;* Lecith; Lyc;
Nat-m; Nux-v; Ol-an;
Onos; Pic-ac; Pho; Plat;
SEP; SUL; Vio-o.

Grief, from : Phys.

Prostatic : Thu.

Sexual : Calad; Onos;
Sabal; Stap.

Unmarried persons, of :
Agn.

Urinating, when : Cimi.

NETTED : See Birth-mark.

NETTLE RASH : Dul; Urt.

NEURALGIA : See Pain.

BRACHIAL : Kalm; Terb; Ver-a.

Cervico : Chel; Nux-v.

CARIES, From: Stap.

+ CILIARY : Mez; Pru-sp; Rhod.

+ COFFEE, Abuse of : Grat.

COITION After (male) : Ced.

COLDNESS, Along nerve, with
 : Terb.

CRURAL : Stap.

DIAPHRAGMATIC : Stan.

INJURY, From : Hypr.

INTERCOSTAL *:* See
Pleurodynia.

LUMBO-ABDOMINAL : Aran.

MENSES During : Amy-n;
Aran.

Suppressed from : Kalm.

OPERATION, Surgical, after :
Cup.

ORBITAL : See Orbits.

PALPITATION, With : Lach.

PARALYTIC Weakness and
trembling with : Kalm.

PERIODICAL : Cact.

PERIPHERAL : Arg-n.

PHRENIC : Bell.

PRODROME, As a : Nux-v.

SEPSIS, From : Crot-h.

SHINGLES, After : Caus; Dol;
Kali-chl; Kalm; Mez; Plant;
Pru-sp; Ran-b; Vario; Zin.
Touch Agg : Petr.
Amel : Zin.

STUMP, Of : Am-m; Arn; Asar;
Cep; Hypr; Pho-ac; Stap;
Symp.
Breathing, deep Amel :
Pho-ac.

SUBSCAPULARIS : Terb.

SUPPRESSED Agg: Stan.

VEINS, Pressure from
distended : Sec.

NEURASTHENIA : See
Nervous Prostration.

NEURITIS INJURY, After : Cep;
Hypr; Stram.

MULTIPLE : Ars; Bov; Con;
Morph; Stro; Thal; Vip.

NUMBNESS, And tingling with
: Bov.

OPTIC : Plb.

RETROBULBAR : Chin-s; Iodf.

TOUCH Amel : Sang.

+ **NEUROMA** : Cep.

NEVER WELL Since : Carb-v.

ABORTION : Sec.

BURNS : Caus.

CHEST Affections : Sul.

CLIMAXIS : Lach.

DIPHTHERIA : Lac-c; Phyt; Pyro.

INFECTIOUS Diseases: Psor.

INFLUENZA : Gel.

PNEUMONIA : Kali-c.

+ PUBERTY : Pul.

SEPTIC Fever : Pyro.

TYPHOID : Carb-v; Mang; Psor;
Pyro.

NEVUS: See Birth Mark.

NEW ALL Objects seem : Hell;
Stram.

CANNOT, Do anything: Agar.

GROWTH : See Growth, New.

NEWS BAD : See Bad News.

GLAD : See Joy.

NIBBLING : See Appetite,
Nibbling.

NICTALOPIA : See Night
Blindness.

NIGHT : See under Time.

BLINDNESS : Bell; *Chin*; Hell;
Lyc; Nux-v; Phys; Stram.

MARE, Terrors : See Awakes,
Fright, Night terrors from.

SEES, Better, at : Fer.

SWEATS, Phthisis, of : Ars;
Bry; Calc; Carb-v; Chin; Fer;
Pho; Pho-ac; Samb; Sep; Sil;
Stan; Sul.
First Sleep, in : *Ars*.
after : Lach.
All night : Pho.

Amel : Kali-io.

Awaking on : Samb.

WATCHING AGG (See Sleep loss of AGG) : Caus; *Cocl*; Cup; *Nit-ac*; Sele; Zin.

NIPPING : See Twinges.

NIPPLES : *Arn*; Cham; Grap; Lyc; Pul; Rat; *Sul*.

LEFT : Nat-s; Pyro; Rum.

Under : Ascl; Rum.

palpitation, with : Ascl.

ABSCESS : Merc; Sil.

AIR, From : Cyc.

BACKWARD, From : Crot-t; Phel.

Left : Sul.

Nursing, when : Crot-t.

BLEEDING : Buf; Ham; Lyc; Merc; *Sep;* Sil; Sul.

BLOODY Water, from : Lyc; Phyt.

BURNING : Agar; Grap; Lyc; Sil; *Sul.*

Left : Senec.

+ Look angry, pregnancy during : Alu.

Sore, and : Pho.

COLD : Med.

CRACKED : Aesc; Carb-an; Cast-eqi; *Caus;* GRAP; PETR; *Phyt;* Rat; SARS; Sep; Sul.

Herpes, around with: Caus.

Nursing women : Hyds.

CRAWLING : Sabi.

CUTTING,Scapula, to (Male) : Tell.

DEFORMED : Merc.

DRYNESS : Cast-equi.

ERECT : Lach.

EXCORIATED : Arn; *Caus; Flu-ac; Phyt;* Sul.

GLANDULAR, Swelling, about : Merc-c.

HANGING : Cast-equi.

HOT : Pho.

INDURATED, Hard : Bry; Calc; Carb-an; Merc.

INFLAMMATION : Cadm; Cham; Pho; Sil.

INVERTED : See Retracted.

ITCHING : Grap; Onos; Petr; Sep; Sul.

Menses, during : Hep.

Pimples, around : Psor.

Voluptuous : Sabi.

MEALY, Covering, on : Petr.

MILKY Water, from (right) : Bur-p.

NEURALGIA : Plant.

NUMB : Sars.

OOZING : Med.

OUTWARD Going, pains : Berb; *Bry;* Gel; Kali-bi; Lapp; Lyc; Mez; *Ol-an;* Spig; Stan.

RED : Psor.

RETRACTED, Inverted : Con; Grap; Hyds; Lach; *Nat-s;* Phyt; *Sars;* Sil; *Thu;* Tub.

Dysmenorrhea, with : Sars.

SCAPULA, To : Crot-t.

SORE, Tender : Arn; Bap; Caus; Crot-t; Flu-ac; Ham; Helo; Lach; Lyc; Med; Pho; Pyro; Sil.

Constantly : Lac-c.

Menses, during : Helo.

Touch of clothing Agg : *Cast-eq;* Con; *Crot-h;* Helo;Oci-c.

Under : Sang.

STITCHES : Con; Nat-m.

Breath deep Agg: Con; Ign.

Walking Agg : Con.

SWELLING : Merc-c.

Glandular, about : Merc-c.

Right : Flu-ac.

ULCERATION : Cast-eq.

WHITE, Spot in centre : Nux-v.

NIPS : See Pain Twinging.

NODES : *Ant-c;* CALC; Carb-an; Caul; Caus; Cinb; Dul; *Grap;* Guai; Iod; Kali-s; Lach; Lyc; Mag-c; Mez; *Pul;* Rhod; Rhus-t; Rut; Sars; Sil; Stap; *Sul;* Ther.

+ GOUTY, Sore : *Sars.*

HARD : Mag-c.

Burning : Hep.

Joints, around : Form.

Painful : Phyt.

Red, sore : Petr.

RED : Med.

SHIN, Bones, on : Cinb.

SITE Of an old boil : Lyc.

NOISE AGG (Sensitive to) : Aco; Asar; BELL; Bor; CHIN; Chin-ar; *Cof;* Con; Kali-c; *MAG-C;* Mag-m; *Nit-ac;* NUX-V; Op; *Sep; Sil;* Tarn; *Ther;* Tub; Zin.

AMEL : Grap.

BELL, of AGG : Ant-c.

LABOUR Pains, during: Cimi.

MENSES, During : Kali-p.

PENETRATION AGG : *Asar;* Bar-c; Chin; Cocl; Con; Fer; Iod; Lept; Lil-t; Lyc; Manc; Mur-ac; Sabi; *Ther.*

RATTLING, Shrill AGG : Calc; Nit-ac.

SLIGHTEST AGG : Asar; Buf; Calad; Cof; Fer; Nux-v; Op; Sil; Ther.

But not loud : Bor.

Greatly accentuated : Bad.

STRIKES, Painful part : Ther.

SUDDEN AGG : Bor; Calad; Cocl; Nat-c; Nat-m.

TALKING Of several persons AGG : Petr.

WATER, Splashing of AGG : Bro; LYSS; NIT-AC; Stram.

+ **NOISE** EVERY, Hears in sleep : Alum.

NOISY : Aco; Bell; Cham; Cic.

NOMA : See Cancer, Cancrum oris.

NOSE : Aco; Aescl; Alu; *Ars;* Aur; Calc; Grap; Hep; Hyds; Ign; Iod; KALI-BI; *Kali-io;* Lyc; *Merc;* Merc-i-f; *Nat-m;* Nit-ac; Nux-v; Pho; PUL; Saba; *Sep;* SIL; Spig; *Sul;* Zin-chr.

ONE SIDE : Am-m; Hep; Ign; Nux-v; Pho; Phyt; *Saba;* Sinapl Sil.

Right : Con; Mar-v; Spig.

hot swollen, coryza in : Merc-i-r.

Left : Carb-v; Nat-m; Rhod; Sep.

Alternating, between :
Kali-io; Lac-c; Lach; Mez;
Nux-v; *Pho*; Phyt; Rhod;
Sinap; Sul.

ACHING, In : Dul.

ACNE : Ars.

AIR, Open Amel : Aco; *Cep;*
Hyds; Iod; Nux-v; *Pul;* Tell.

Feels cold, in : Hyds.

Inspired Agg : See Air
inspiring Agg.

feels cold : Lith.

ALAE : See Nostrils.

BEHIND : Merc-c.

BLEEDING (See Epistaxis) : *Pho;*
Vip.

BLOWING AGG : See Blowing
Nose Agg.

Lumps, of : Merc-d.

Painful, on : Mang.

Tendency for : Am-m; Bor;
Hyds; Kali-bi; Lyc; Mang;
Mar-v; Stic.

but no relief : *Kali-bi;* Lach;
Mar-v; Psor; *Stic.*

BOILS, Small, painful inside :
Ap; Tub.

BONES : Aur; Kali-bi; *Merc*
Pho; Rhus-t.

Caries : Aur; Nit-ac.

Painful : Aur; Hep; Kali-bi;
Rhus-t; Sil.

+ Two loose bones rubbing
together as if : Kali-bi.

BORING Into, with fingers
PICKING at, ITCHING : Anac;
Aru-t; Aur; Carb-v; Caus;
CINA; Hep; Lyc; Mar-v; Merc;

Nat-m; Nat-p; Pho; *Pho-ac;*
Saba; *Sil;* Spig; Stro; Sul; Thu;
Zin.

Brain symptoms, in : Cina;
Sul.

BRIDGE : Pho-ac; *Sep;* Thu.

Bones : Kali-bi; Rhus-t.

Painful : Cinb; Thu.

Squeezing : Chio; Lachn.

BROWN, Across : *Carb-an;*
Lyc; Op; Sanic; SEP; Sul;
Syph.

BUBBLING Sensation : Sars;
Sul.

BURNING, Sore : Led.

Inspiring, cool air, on :
Aesc.

Throbbing : Kali-io.

CANCER, Flat : Euphr.

CATCHES, Of passing
strangers : Merc.

COLD : Ap; Arn; *Cam; Caps;*
Carb-v; Lac-c; Meny;
Murx; VER-A.

Agg : Sul.

Inspiration, during : Cor-r.

Knees, hot with : Ign.

Sores : Ars.

CONGESTION, High blood
pressure from : Iod.

CRACKED : Aru-t; Carb-an.

CRAWLING, Formication :
Mar-v; Merc; Nat-m; Ran.b.

Blows and hawks, to
relieve : Ran-b.

until tears flow : Cham.

CRUSTS, Scales from : Alu;
Aur; Bov; GRAP; *Kali-bi;*

Kali-c; Merc; Nit-ac; SEP;
Stic; Sul; *Thu*; Zin-chr;
Zin-io.

Bloody : Thu.

CUTTING : Kali-bi; Nit-ac.

DESQUAMMATION : Carb-an.

DIRTY : Med; Merc.

DISCHARGES, Acrid : *Ars;*
Ars-io; Aru-t; Hyds; Merc;
Merc-c; Nit-ac.

Bluish : Am-m; *Kali-bi.*

Burning, hot : Aco; Ars-io;
Cep; Iod; Nat-m; Pul.

Changing : Stap.

Cold : Ambros; Ichthy;
Kali-io; Lach.

Coryza, without : Agar; Terb.

Cough Agg : Agar; Lach;
Nat-m; Nit-ac; *Scil*; Sul;
Thu.

Crusts : See Crusts.

Bloody : Stro.

Dark : Cinb; Merc-d.

Dinner after : Tromb.

Dripping : Am-c; *Ars;*
Ars-io; Aru-t; Calc; *Cep*;
Eup-p; Euphr; Grap;
Kali-io; Nit-ac; Nux-v;
Pho; Rhus-t; Saba; Scil;
Sul; Tab.

diphtheria, in : Nit-ac.

Eating on : Carb-an;
Clem; Nux-v; Plb; Sanic;
Sul; *Tromb.*

Expectoration, with : Sabal.

Fish-brine : Elaps; Thu.

Frothy : Merc; Sil.

Glutinous : Hep; *Kali-bi;*

Merc-c.

Grey : Amb; Lyc.

Green : Ars-io; Kali-bi;
Kali-io; Lac-c; Merc;
Nit-ac; Pul; *Sep.*

blood streaked : Pho.

strains pillow, sleep in :
Lac-c.

Gummy : Sumb.

Gushing fluids : Agar; Dul;
Euphr; Flu-ac; Hyds;
Kali-bi; Lach; *Nat-c*;
NAT-M; Pho; Scil; Sele;
Thu.

morning : Scil.

Lips, upper, reddening :
Ars-io.

Lumpy : Alu; Cinb; KALI-BI;
Mar-v; Merc-d; Pho; Sele;
Sep; Sil; Solid; Zin-io.

Musty : Nat-c.

Night : Lac-c; Nat-s.

Offensive : See Ozena.

Orange coloured : Pul.

Purulent : Aur; *Calc*; Con;
Hep; LACH; *Merc; Pul;*
Zin-chr.

Reading aloud, when :
Verb.

Salty : Aral; Cimi; Nat-m.

Singing, when : Cep.

Stool, during : Thu.

Talking, while : Kali-bi;
Nat-c.

Urinous odour : Pul.

Watery, Coryza, without :
Agar; Terb.

Yellow-green : Kali-bi;

Kali-c; Merc; Ther.

stains pillow at night : Lac-c.

watery, suddenly : Plant.

DRY : Ars; Ars-io; Bar-c; *Bell*;
Bry; *Calc*; Carb-v; GRAP;
Kali-bi; *Lyc*; *Nat-m*; *Nux-m*;
Pho; Saba; *Samb*; *Sep*; SIL;
Sinap; Spo; *Stic*; *Sul*; Thu;
Thyr; Zin-io.

As if : Petr; Sil.

Breathe, through mouth,
must : Meli.

Indoors : Nux-v; Thyr.

Painful : Grap.

Sensation, blowing nose on
: Bar-c.

DYSPNOEA (See Obstruction)
in : *Ars*; Kre; Lach; Merc;
Pho; Pul; Saba; Sul.

EARS, To : Elap.

Swallowing Agg : Elap.

ECZEMA : Cist.

ERUPTION, On (lower) : Caus.

EXCORIATED : ARS; Ars-io;
Aru-t; Caus; *Cep*; Gel; Grap;
Iod; Kali-io; Kre; *Merc*;
Merc-c; Nat-m; Nit-ac;
Nux-v; Pho; Sinap.

EXTERNAL : *Aur*; Carb-v; Caus;
Kali-c; *Merc*; Nat-c; Pho-ac;
Pul; *Rhus-t*; Sep; Spig; Sul.

Heat, burning : Agar; Saba.

Itching : Carb-an; Caus;
Cina; Saba; Sul.

Pimples : Carb-an.

FACE Ache, with : Spig.

FLOWS, Obstruction, with : Ars;
Aru-t; Bry; Calc; Kali-bi;
Lach; Merc; Nux-v; Onos;

Pul; Sil.

Coryza without : Agar; Terb.

FOREIGN Body, Plug, as if in
: Psor; Rut; Sep.

Upper, part, in : Am-m.

FOETOR, Foul : See Ozoena.

FULLNESS : Bap; Kali-io.

HARD : Carb-an; Kali-c.

HEAT, Burning : Ars; Carb-an;
Chin; Kali-io; Merc; Sang;
Sil.

Fever, in : Arn.

Sneezing, when : Como.

HEAVY : Kali-bi; Merc; Phyt.

Stooping, on: Am-m; Sil.

Weight, as if, hanging :
Kali-bi.

HOT : Saba.

Water flowing from, as if
: Aco; Gel.

ITCHING : See Boring with
Fingers.

Child starts out of sleep,
and rubs : Lyc.

Eating, when : Jatr; Lach.

Menses, after : Sul.

Pharynx, to : Rum.

Rubs constantly : Cina.

+ Violent, rubs : Arg-n.

LIQUIDS, Food return
through, swallowing
when : Arut-t; Cocl; Gel;
Kali-per; Lac-c; Lach;
Lyc; Merc; *Pho*; Sul-ac.

LYING Agg : Pul.

NUMB : Aco; Bell; Vio-o.

Epistaxis, with : Aco; Bell;
Med.

One side : Nat-m.

OBSTRUCTED : Ars; Ars-io;
ARU-T; Aur; *Calc;* Caps;
Carb-v; Caus; Con; *Grap;*
Hep; *Kali-bi;* Kali-c; *Lyc;*
Mang; *Mar-v;* Med; *Nat-c;*
Nat-m; NIT-AC; NUX-V;
Pho; Pul; *Samb; Sil.*

Air open Amel : Kali-c;
Pho; Pul; Sul.

Alternately : Lac-c; Pho;
Phyt; Rhod; Sul.

lachrymation, with : Bor.

Blood pressure, high from
: Iod.

Blow, desires to : Am-m.

Breathes through mouth :
Am-c; Kali-c; Lyc; Mag-c;
Mag-m; Nux-v; Samb.

adenoids, removal after
: Kali-s.

Children in (snuffles) :
Amb; Am-c; Apoc; Aur;
Kali-bi; *Lyc;* Med; *Nux-v;*
Osm; Pho; *Samb; Syph.*

+ new-born : Nux-v.

Chronic : *Calc;* Con; Sars;
Sele; Sil; Sul.

obstinate : Sars.

years, for : Sars.

Diphtheria, in : Kali-m;
Lyc; Merc-cy.

Fluent discharge, with :
Aru-t.

Foetid, discharge with :
Aru-t.

Fresh air, in : Dul.

High, in : Nat-m.

Hot wet application Amel

: Dul.

Lachrymation with : Bor.

Lying Agg : Bov; Caus;
Nux-m.

Menses, before : Mag-c.

Night, at : Amb; Am-c; Lyc;
Nux-v; Zin-io.

Pus, with : Calc; Lyc; *Sil.*

Room, in Amel : Dul.

Speaking, reading aloud
while : Kali-bi; Mar-v; Sil;
Verb.

Stooping, on : Agar.

ODOURS, In : Calc; Pul; Zin-chr.

Eggs, rotten : Meny.

Fishy : Thu.

Remains for a long time :
Dios.

Sweetish : Nit-ac.

OILY : Hyds; *Iris.*

OPERATIONS, After : Fer-p.

PAIN, In: Aur; Grap; Hep;
Kali-bi; Kali-io; Merc; Pul;
Sil.

Saddle : Cinb; Thu.

PARCHMENT Sensation, as if :
Kali-bi; Sul.

PEELING : Nat-c; Nat-m; Nit-ac;
Pho.

PINCHED : Cam; Kali-bi; Lyc;
Spo.

As if : *Kali-bi;* Spo.

Blue, and : Ver-v.

PLUG : See Foreign body.

POINTED : Ars; Cam; Nux-v;
Ver-a.

Point, cracked : Alu.

POLYPUS : Cadm; CALC;

Kali-bi; *Mar-v*; Merc-i-r; Pho; *Sang*; Thu; Zin-chr.

PRESSURE Of glasses AGG : Arg-n; Chin; Cinb; Con; Cup-ar; Flu-ac; Kali-bi; *Merc*; Pho.

PRICKLING, Tears, with : Nat-p.

PULLED, As if : Nat-c.

PULLS, Strangers, of : Merc.

PULSATION : Ars; Kali-io.

RAW (See Excoriated) : Aral; Aru-t; Caus; Nat-m.

RED : Agar; ALU; Ap; *Aur*; Bell; *Calc*; Cann; *Caps*; Carb-an; Chel; Iod; Kali-io; *Lith*; Merc; Nit-ac; Pho; Rhus-t; SUL; Lapp.

Across : Lapp.

Anger, from : Vinc.

Knobby : Aur.

Pimples, on : Kali-c; Lach; Psor.

white : Nat-c.

Swollen : Lith; Mag-m.

Young women : Bor.

ROOT And ABOVE : Aco; Ars; Calc; Chio; Cimi; Cup; Gel; *Hep*; *Hyo*; Ign; Iod; Kali-bi; Kali-io; Merc; Par; Pho; *Pul*; Sang; Sars; Stic;

Abscess : Pul.

Cramp : Mang; Plat.

Fullness, stuffy : Stic.

+ Heaviness : Bism.

Jerks, suddenly : Hyo.

Painful : Hep; Kali-bi; Ther.

vomiting, after : Dig.

Pressure : Cinb; Sep; Stic; Zin.

epistaxis with : Rut.

Pulsation : Kali-bi.

Sore : Ant-t; Nit-ac.

operation, after : Fer-p.

Swelling : Sars.

Tension : Ant-t; Cep; Kali-bi; Kali-io.

Twitching : Hyo; Mez.

ROSACEAE : Carb-an;Kali-io; Rhus-t; Sars.

RUM BLOSSOM : Agar; Lach; Led.

SENSITIVE To inspired air : Aco; Aur; Bro; Cam; Cimi; Cist; Cor-r; *Ign*; Med; Nux-v.

SEPTUM, Boil : Anthx.

Crusts : Thu.

Deviated : See Obstruction.

Perforated : Kali-bi; Kali-io; Merc; Merc-c; Sil; Syph.

Sore : Kali-bi.

Ulcers : Aur; Kali-bi; Sil.

SHINY : *Pho.*

SINUSES : Cinb; Hyds; Kali-bi; Kali-io; Lach; Merc; Pho; Syph.

Burning, throbbing : Kali-io.

SMOKE, As if, in : Bar-c.

SNUFFLES : See Obstruction, in Children.

SUNKEN : Aur; Psor.

SWEAT, About : Rhe.

On : Rut; Tub.

cold : Chin.

SWELLED, Thick : Ap; Arn;

Aur; *Bar-c;* Bell; *Calc;*Caus;
Hep; Iod; *Kali-c;* Kali-io;
Lyc; *Merc;* Merc-c; Nat-c;
Pho; Pho-ac; Pul; Rhus-t;
Sars; *Sep; Sul;* Zin.

Knobby : *Ars; Aur.*

Shiny : Bor.

SYPHILITIC : Aur.

TENSION : Aco; Ham; Kali-io;
Petr; Senec; Thu.

Skin, in : Petr; Pho.

TINGLING, In : Arn; Saba.

Cobweb, as from : Bro.

Spreading to whole body :
Saba.

TIP : Carb-an; Carb-v; Caus;
Sep.

Abscess, Boil : Aco; Am-c.

Cold : Alo; Ap; Calc-p; Med.

Cracked : *Alu.*

Drips, water : Rhus-t.

Eruptions : Aeth.

pimples : Caus.

Hot : Caps.

Itching : Med; Petr; Sil.

Knobby : Aur.

Numb : Gel; Vio-o.

Painful : Cist.

Red : Nit-ac; Rhus-t.

drunkards, in : Agar;
Lach; Led.

Scurfy : Nit-ac.

Sensitive : Rhus-t.

Shiny : Bell; Pho; Sul.

Sore : Bor; Cist; Lith.

Swelling : Bry; Caus; Chel.

Tremulous, Twitching : *Bry;*
Chel.

Tumour : Carb-an; Sul.

TWITCHING : *Amb;* Am-c; Aur;
*Calc; Chel; Con; Hyo;
Kali-bi;* Nat-m; Phys; *Plat.*

ULCER : Ars; Merc; Nat-m; Pul.

Menses, instead of : Euphr.

UNEASY, Feeling around : Ail.

WARTS, On : Caus.

WEATHER, Changes Agg : Ars.

WINTER Agg : Am-c; Ars; Sul.

WRINKLED, Skin : Cham.

YELLOW, Across : Sep.

NOSTALGIA : See Home-sick.

NOSTRILS, Alae (Wings) : Lyc;
Thu.

AGLUTINATED : AUR; Lyc.

+ BLACK : Ant-t.

CRACKS : Ant-c; Merc; Thu.

CRUSTS : Ant-c; Bor.

DARK, Sooty : Ant-t; Colch;
Crot-h; Hell; Hyo.

DILATED : Ant-t; Ars; Cup;
Hell; Iod; Lyc; Spo.

As if : Iod.

DIRTY : Merc.

DRAWN, In : Aeth; Cina.

+ ECZEMA : Ant-c.

GUMMY : Bor.

HAIR, In : Kali-bi.

ITCHING : Syph.

MOTIONS, Flapping : *Ant-t;*
Ars; Bap; Bell; Bro; *Chel;*
Cup; Diph; *Lyc; Pho;* Pyro;
Rhus-t; Spo; Sul-ac; Zin.

Palpitation, with : Lyc.

Snoring, with : Diph.

SORE : Ant-c; Nux-v.

WATER, Hot, flowing as if : Gel.

WHITE : Stram.

+ WIDE, Apart, as if : Iod.

NOTHING *Ails,* Him, says : Ap; Arn; Iod; Op.

SEEMS, Right : Phys.

NUMBNESS Insensibility: ACO; *Anac;* Ap; *Aran;* Ars; Berb; Cadm; Carb-v; Caus; Cham; COCL; *Con;* Crot-h; Diph; Gel; Glo; GRAP; Hyo; *Kali-c; Kalm;* Lapp; LYC; Mag-c; Med; Nat-m; Nux-m; Nux-v; *Old; Op; Pho; Pho-ac;* Pic-ac; *Plat; Plb;* PUL; Radm; RHUS-T; *Sec; Stram;* Sul-io; Tarn; Tell; Thu; Xanth; Zin.

AFFECTED Part, of : *Cham;* Cocl; *Con; Kali-n;* Led; Lyc; Old; PLAT; Plb; Pul.

BAD NEWS, After : Calc-p.

BRAIN, Affections, in : Flu-ac.

COLDNESS, With : Plat; Sumb.

DIAGONAL : Thyr.

EPILEPPSY, Before: Buf.

EXTREME Heat or Cold, to : Berb.

GENERAL, Whole body: Acet-ac; Ascl; Bar-m; Ced; Chel; *Kali-br;* Ox-ac.

Headache, during : Ced.

Lying, on : Zin.

Morning : Amb.

GRASPING Objects Agg : Cocl.

INTERNAL : *Gel;* Op; *Plat.*

LOWER Half : Spo.

LYING Down Agg : Zin.

ONE SIDED : Ars; Caus; Chel;

Nat-m; Pho; *Pul.*

Right : Caus; Elap; Naj.

Left : Ars; Sumb; Xanth.

PAIN, From : Asaf; Cham; *Colo;* Gnap; Hypr; Kalm; Mez; Nat-m; Plat; Pul; Rhus-t.

PART Lain, on (See Side lain on Agg) : Am-c; Arn; Calc; *Carb-v;* Chin; Mag-c; Nat-m; *Pul; Rhus-t;* Sil.

Not lain, on : Flu-ac.

PARTIAL, Single parts : Aran; Bar-c; Cadm; Carb-an; Cocl; Croc; Grap; Kali-c; Kali-n; Lyc; Merc; Plat; Pul; Rhus-t; Sil.

PLACES, Changing : Raph.

PRICK, Pain, Heat, etc. : Kre; *Plb;* Thu.

PRICKLING, With : Tarn.

RADIAL Nerve, along : Pho-ac.

SPINAL Affections, in : Flu-ac.

SPOTS In : Amb; Buf; Lyc; Plat; Sul-io.

STRETCHING Part Agg : Old; Radm.

ULNAR Nerve, along : *Aran.*

UPPER Half : Bar-c.

WAKING, On : Aran; Cham.

WOODEN Feeling : Kali-n; Petr; Thu.

NUTRITION AFFECTED : Abro; BAR-C; *Bor;* CALC; *Calc-hyp;* CALC-P; *Grap;*

Lac-c; LYC; NAT-M; Sanic; SIL.

NYMPHOMANIA : See Female, Sexual desire, violent.

OBESITY :Am-m; *Ant-c;* Bell; Buf; CALC; CAPS; *Fer; Grap;* Kali-bi; Lac-d; Lith;Phyt; Pul; Rum; Seneg; Sul; Thyr.

ATROPHY, Limbs of, with : Plb.

BODY Fat, Legs thin : Am-m.

OLD People : Bar-c; Kali-c.

OBSCENE : See Lecherous.

OBSTINATE : See Stubborn.

SAYS, There is nothing the matter with him : Ap; ARN.

OCCIPUT : Bell; *Bry;* Calc; *Carb-v;* Chin; CIMI; Cocl; GEL; Ign; Nat-s; *Nux-v;* Onos; *Petr; Phyt;* Sep; SIL; Sul; Vario; Ver-v; Zin; Zin-ar.

RIGHT : Bell; Chel; Sang.

LEFT : Kali-bi; Lyc; Nat-m; Nux-v; *Onos; Sep;* Spig; Sul.

ACHING, Waves, in, spine from : Crot-h.

AIR COLD, on Agg : Sanic.

ALTERNATING Sides: Sep.

ASCENDING Through: Arg-n; *Bell; Calc;* Carb-v; *Cimi;* GEL; *Glo; Kali-bi;* Lac-c; Lach; Lil-t; Onos; *Par;* Petr; Pho; Saba; SANG; Sep; SIL; *Spig;* Sul; Ver-v.

Warm water, as if : Glo.

BAND, Constriction : Arg-n; Grap.

Sensation, of : Grap.

BATHING, Cold Amel : Calc-p.

BENDING Backwards Amel : Cocl; Murx.

BLOW On, as if : Ap; Bap; Bell; Cimi; Crot-h; Kali-m; Lach; *Naj;* Tab; Tarn; Zin.

BONE Sinks, marasmus in : Mag-c.

BURNING, Heat : Aur; Med; Pho; Zin.

BURSTING : Gel; Lach.

COLD : Calc-p; Chel; Dul; Pho.

CONFUSION, In : Amb.

COUGHING Agg : Fer; Pul.

CUTTING : Sul.

Night : Syph.

DEPRESSION, At : Calc-p.

DOWNWARD : Calc-p; Pho; Pic-ac; Val; Zin.

DRAWING : Arn; Bry.

EMPTY : Stap; Sul.

ENLARGED, Swelled, as if : Bry; Cocl; Dul; Med.

ERUPTION : Caus; Sil; Sul.

EXERTION Agg : Onos.

EXTERNAL : Carb-an; *Carb-v; Petr; Sil.*

EYES, To : Med; Sars.

EYE Strain Agg : Onos.

FINGER Pressing, as if : Meph.

FORMICATION : Sep.

FORWARD, From : Sang; Sil.

Right, to : Bell; Gel; Sang; Sil.

Left, to : Arg-n; Cimi; Lach; Lil-t; *Spig;* Thu.

HAND, Putting on Amel : Murx.

HEAT : See Burning.

HEAVY : BELL; Calc; *Carb-v;* CHEL; Kali-m; Merc-i-r; Mur-ac; NAT-M; *Petr; Pic-ac.*

Looking intently Agg : Mur-ac.

Sitting bent, while : Con.

Waking, on : Lach.

LEGS, Weak with : Zin.

LYING On Agg : Bry; Cact; Carb-v; COCL; Kali-p; Nux-v; PETR; Pho; *Sep*; Spig.

NOSE, Root of, to : Sars.

NUMB : Flu-ac; Kali-br; Stap.

Prickling : Ox-ac.

Spine, down : Phys.

OPENS And SHUTS: Cocl.

PILLOW On, Agg : Buf; Glo.

PRESSURE, Outward : Aesc; Calc; Gel; Sul.

PUPILS Dilated, with : Ver-v.

SCREWED, As if : Onos.

SHOCKS : Pho.

SHOULDER, To : Kali-bi; Onos; Stic.

SINCIPUT, To : Senec.

SORE, Bruised : Cimi; Eup-p; Gel; Nux-v; Pru-sp; Stap.

SPRAINED, As if : Amb.

STOOLS Amel : Asaf.

SWEAT, On : Sanic.

SWOLLEN : Bar-c.

TENSION : Lyc.

THROBBING, Pulsating : Bell; Bry; Cann; Lyc; *Pho; Sep.*

Hot if, Agg : Lyc.

Night Agg : Lyc.

Standing Amel: Cam.

Stools, during : Ign.

TWITCHING : Mag-m; Spig.

ULCER : Sil.

UNEASY : Aeth.

UP And DOWN, from : *Onos;* Sep.

VISION, Dim, with : Ver-v.

VOMITING Agg : Ip.

OCCUPATION AMEL (See Active AMEL and Busy when AMEL) : Cup; Hell; Ign; Kali-br; Merc-i-r; Nat-c; Nux-v; Pip-m; *Sep.*

OCCUPATIONAL Diseases : Arn; Caus; Gel; Mag-p; Nux-v; Pic-ac;Sil; Zin.

ODOURS, Smells (See also Sensitive, Nausea) AGG : Ars; Aur; Bell; Cof; COLCH; Eup-p; Grap; Ign; Lyc; *Merc-i-f;* Nux-v; Op; Pho; Saba; Sang; SEP; Stan; Sul; Ther; Vario.

CAMPHOR AGG : Kali-n.

DIRTY Clothes AGG : Carb-an.

EGGS Of AGG : Colch.

FISH, Of AGG : Colch.

Smells, foul : Par.

FLOWERS AGG : Cep; Grap; Lac-c; Nux-v; Pho; Saba; Sang.

FOOD, Of cooking etc : See under Food.

FOUL AGG : Anthx; Kre; Pyro.

Bread, to : Par.

Milk : Par.

Remains for a long time : Dios.

Sensitive, to : Par.

IMAGINATIONS Of : See under Smell, Illusory.

MICE, Of AGG : Saba.

MUSK, Of AMEL : Mos.

PEACH, Skin of AGG : Cep.

SOUR AGG : Alu; Dros.

STOOLS of AGG : Dios; *Sul.*

STRONG AGG : Anac; Cof; Sele.

SWEET, Agreeable *A*GG : Arg-n; Aur; Nit-ac; Sil.

TAKES Away, her breath: Pho-ac.

TOBACCO AGG : Bell.
Addicted, though : Lob.

WOOD AGG : Grap.

OEDEMA : See Dropsy.

AFFECTED Part, around : Crot-h.

ANGIO-NEUROTIC: Agar; *Ap;* Ars; Hell; Hep; *Rhus-t;* Urt.

INJURY, After : Bels.

JOINTS OF, Fractures, after : Bov.

NEONATORUM : Ap; Carb-v; Dig; Lach; Sec.

RED : Ap; *Como.*

SACCULAR : Ap; Ars; Kali-c.

SPRAIN, After : Bov.

SUDDEN : Kali-n.

OESOPHAGUS, BUBBLING, In : Chel.

BURNING : Canth; *Merc-c;* Pho; *Sang;* Ver-v.
Eating Agg : Pho.
Pregnancy, during : Hell.
Typhoid, in : Ars; Bell; Bry; Nux-v; Pho; Rhus-t; Sul.

CHOKING: Cact; Ign; Kali-c; Merc-c.

CLUCKING, In : Cina.

COLD : Meny.

Hot and/ or ascending –All-s.

CRAMP, Eructation, on : Colo.
Palpitation, with : Colo.
Swallowing, on : Op.

CUTTING : Vinc.

+ DISTENDED, As if : Hypr; Op; Ver-a.

+ DRINKING Water, runs out side, as if : Ver-a.

DRINKS, Roll audibly : *Laur.*

DRY : Cocl; Lach; Mez; Naj; Sep; Sul.

FOOD, Feels, going through : Alu.
Lodged in, as if : Ars; Barc; Calc; Caus; Chin; Gel; Kali-c; Pul.
whole length : Alu.

FOREIGN Body in, as if : Gel; Lyc.

GURGLING In, drinking while : Ars; Hyd-ac.

HOT Risings, fright, after : Hypr.

INFLAMMED : Ars; Rhus-t; Ver-v.
Corrosive things, swallowing, from : Rhus-t.

INJURY, Fish bone etc. Agg : Cic.

LUMP, In : Chel; Pod.
Hard : Lyc.

PARALYSIS : Con; Elap;Hyd-ac.

ROUGH : Nat-c.

SPASM, Constriction : Asaf; *Bap;* Bar-c; *Bell; Ign;* Lach; Laur; Merc-c; *Naj;* Nux-v; Ran-b; Ver-v.
Can swallow liquids only : *Bap;* Bar-c; Plb.

Food, suddenly arrested, then falls heavily in stomach : Elap.

SPLIT, As if, eructation, on : Coca.

SPONGY : Elap.

STRICTURE : Am-m; Ars; Bap; *Bar-c*; Cic; Cund; Kali-c; Nat-m; *Pho*; Stro; Zin.

Old : Pho; Zin.

OFFENDED EASILY : Anac; Ars; Calc; Caps; Cocl; Ign; Lyc; *Nux-v*; Pall; Plat; *Pul*; Sars; Sep; *Stap.*

+ AT EVERYTHING : Colo.

OFFENSIVENESS, FOETOR : Ail; Arn; *Ars*; Asaf; *Bap*; Bry; Carb-ac; Carb-an; *Carb-v*; Con; Crot-h; Grap; Hep; Kali-chl; Kali-p; Kre; LACH; Med; *Merc*; Mur-ac; Nit-ac; Osm; Pho; Pod; PSOR; Pyro; Rhus-t; Sabi; Sec; Sep; *Sil*; Sul; Sul-ac; Tell; Thu; Tril; Ust.

BODY, Of : Bap; Guai; Hep; Kali-io; Kali-p; Med; Nit-ac; *Psor*; *Pyro*; Sep; Sil; Stan; *Sul*; *Syph*; Thu.

Can not wash it off : Lac-c; Med; Psor.

Cheese, old, like : Sanic.

Menses, during : Psor; Stan.

Unclean : Guai.

Urinous : Ust.

OIL APPLICATION OF AMEL : Euphor.

OILY : See Greasy.

OLD AGE, SENILITY : Amb; Ant-c; Arn; Ars; AUR; BAR-C; Caps; Carb-an; Carb-v; Chin; *Con*; Flu-ac; Hyds; KALI-C; LACH;

LYC; Nit-ac; OP; Pho; Sanic; Sars; Scil; *Sec*; Sele; Seneg; Sil; Sul; Sul-ac; Sumb; Syph; Tub; Ver-a.

ATHELETS : Coca.

EARLY, Premature : Amb; Arg-n; Bar-c; Berb; Con; Flu-ac; Kali-c; *Lyc*; *Sele*; Sumb.

LOOK : See Face.

MAIDS : Bov; Cocl; Con; Lil-t; Mag-m; Plat.

MEN : Sabal.

ONANISM : See Masturbation.

ONIONS, SMELL, like : Bov; Kali-io; Kali-p; Lyc; Petr; Tell.

ONYCHIA : See Fingers, Felon.

OPENING AND **SHUTTING,** As if: *Cact*; Calc; CANN; *Cimi*; COCL; Cup; Glo; Lil-t; *Lyc*; Sep; Spo; Tarn.

OPERATIONS, SURGICAL, (See Injuries) After AGG : Arn; Bels; Calen; Cep; Echi; Ham; Hypr; Pho-ac; Rhus-t; Stap; Stro; Sul-ac; Zin.

+ ABDOMINAL : Bism.

ADHESIONS, After : Calc-fl; Sil.

FISTULA, After : Calc-p.

ORIFICES, On : Colo.

SKIN is drawn tight over the wound : Kali-p.

STONES, For : Mill.

OPISTHOTONOS (See Tetanus) : Abs; Ign; Stram; Ver-v.

DIARRHOEA, After : Med; Ver-v.

ORBITS : *Ap*; Asaf; Aur; Bar-c;
Cinb; Kali-bi; Merc; Merc-i-f;
Mez; Rhus-t; Spig; Syph; Val;
Zin-s.

CELLULITIS : Phyt; Rhus-t.

HERPES, Around : Hep.

NEURALGIA, Of : Ars; Ced;
Chin-s; Kali-bi; Kalm;
Nat-m; Spig; Stan.

Coition Agg : Ced.

Screaming and
unconsciousness, with :
Kali-cy.

Testes, of, with : Lycps.

ORDEALS : See under Fear.

ORGASMS : See Waves.

SEXUAL, Easy : Stan.

ORIFICES, AFFECTIONS Of
: *Aesc*; Alo; *Bell; Caus*; Grap;
Ign; Kali-c; Lach; Lyc; *Merc*;
Mur-ac; Nat-m; NIT-AC;
NUX-V; Pho; Pod; Rat; *Sep*;
Sil; SUL.

CRACKED : Nit-ac.

RED : Alo; Nit-ac; Pyro; Sul.

SWELLED : Nit-ac.

OSCILLATIONS : See Eyes,
and Movements.

OSTEOMALACIA (See Bones
softening): *Iod*; Merc-c;
Pho-ac.

OSTEOMYELITIS : Arn; Calc;
Pho.

OVARIES : AP; *Bell;* Canth;
Colo; Guai; LACH; Lil-t;
Lyc; Mag-p; Pod; Pul; Sabal;
Stap; THU; Ust; Zin-val.

RIGHT : Bell; Lyc; Pall; Pod.

Lying on, Side, Amel : Ap.

LEFT : Arg-m; Lach; Thu;
Ust; Zin.

+ Heart, to : Naj.

Lying on, side, Amel :
Kali-p; Pall.

ALTERNATING Between (See
Genitals Alternating) :
Cimi; Colo Lac-c; Lil-t;
Onos; Ust.

ATROPHY : Bar-m; Con; *Iod.*

BACK, To, right : Rum.

BALL, Like a heavy, right :
Carb-an.

BED, Turning, in Agg : Lyc.

Warmth of Agg : Ap; Merc.

BENDING Back Amel : Lac-c.

BREAST, To : Lil-t; Murx; Senec.

With : Sabal.

BURNING (R) : Ust.

COITION After Agg : Ap; Plat;
Stap; Syph.

CONGESTED : Ap.

CONTINENCE Agg : *Ap;* Kali-br.

CUTTING : Con.

Coition, during : Syph.

CYSTIC : Ap; Apoc; Arg-m;
Aur; Bov; Form; Kali-br;
Iod; Lyc.

DRAWING : Med.

FEET, Moving Amel : Ars.

HEAD, With : Sabal.

HEAVY : *Ap*; Plat; Sep.

HYDATID, Of : Buf.

INDURATED, Hard : Ap; Bro;
Con; Grap; Lach.

INFLAMMED : Ap; Bell; Lyc;
Merc; Pho; Pod; Sabi.

INSUFFICIENCY, Of : Lecith.

LEFT, Heart, to : Bro; Cimi;
Lac-c; Lach; Lil-t; *Naj;* Sul;
Vib.

LIMBS, To : Lil-t.

MENSES, Before Agg : Thu.

+ Checked, suddenly : Aco.
During and after Agg: Zin-val.

NUMB *: A*p.

PAINFUL : Naj.
Love sick girls, in : Ant-c.

PARTURITION, After : Lach.

PINCHING : Plat.

PRESSURE Agg : Stap.
Amel : Med.

PULSATIONS : Bell; Cact; Lach;
· Onos.

RAISING, Arms Agg : Ap.
Legs Agg : Lyc.

SEXUAL, Desire during Agg :
Kali-br.

SHOULDER, To : Pod.

SITTING Bent Agg : Ars.

SORE *:* Ap; *Lil-t;* Sep.
Rectum, with : Onos.
Uterus, with : Ust.

STOOPING Agg : Ap.

STRETCHING Legs Agg : Pod.
Amel : Plb.

SWELLED, Enlarged : Ap; Bell;
Con; Lach; Lil-t; Lyc.

TEARING : Plat; Thu.

THIGHS, To : Colo; Grap; Lil-t;
Pod; *Stap;* Ust; Xanth; Zin-val.

TUMOURS : Ap; Lach; Lyc;
Pod.

+ UTERUS, To : Iod.

OVEREXERTION : Bov.

OVERLIFTING : See under
Lifting Agg.

OVERPOWERED, As if (Under
Superhuman Power) : Anac;
Lach; Naj; Op; Plat; Thu.

+ **OVERSTRAIN** MENTAL,
PHYSICAL : Cocl; Con.

+ **OVERSTUDY** : Nat-c; Sele.

+ **OVERUSE** *:* Arn; Con.

OXALURIA : See under Urine,
Oxalic acid, Containing.

OZOENA : Asaf; AUR; CALC;
Grap; *Hep; Kali-bi;* Kali-io;
Merc; Nat-c; Nit-ac; Nux-v;
Psor; PUL; Sep; Sil; *Sul;*
Syph; Ther.

ACRID *:* Lyc; Mag-m.

CRUSTY : Mag-m.

MENSES, During : Grap.

SYPHILITIC : Aur; Hep; Nit-ac;
Sil.

PAIN, NEURALGIA, in general
: ACO; ARS; BELL; *Bry; Caus;
Cham;* Chin; Cimi; Cof;
COLO; Dios; Gel; Hypr; IGN;
Iris; Kali-bi; Lach; *Lyc; Mag-c;
Mag-p; Merc;* Nat-m; *Nux-v;*
Pho; *Psor,* Pul; Ranb; *Rhus-t;*
Rum; *Sang; Spig;* Stan; *Sul;*
Sul-ac; Thu; *Ver-a;* Verb.

ABSENCE, Of (In affections
which are usually painful)
: Am-c; Ant-t; *Hell;* OP;
STRAM.

ACHING : Agar; Arn; *Bap;*
Bels; Bry; Carb-v; *Chin;*

Cimi; Dul; Echi; Erig;
Eup-p; Gel; Hyo; Ign; Kalm;
Lach; Lapp; Lept; Merc-i-f;
Nux-v; *Onos; Phyt;* Pyro;
Radm; Rhus-t; Rut; Terb;
Vario; Ver-v.

Heavy : Carb-v.

ASSOCIATED *:* See Synalgia.

BEARING Down : See Pressing.

BEGINS On one side, goes to
other and there Agg :
Arg-n; Fer; Iris; Lac-c; LYC;
Mang; Nat-m; Tub.

Sleep, in : Nit-ac.

disappears on waking :
Sul-ac.

BITING, Raw, Smarting :
ARG-M; Aru-t; Berb; Calc;
Canth; Carb-v; CAUS; Cist;
Euphr; Flu-ac; *Grap; Hep;*
Hyds; *Ign;* Iod; Kre; *Lach;*
Led; *Lyc;* Meli; *Merc;* NUX-V;
Nit-ac; Ol-an; Petros; *Pho;*
Polyg; *Pul;* Ran-sc; Sang;
Sep; Stap; Stan; *Sul; Sul-ac;*
Zin.

Burning : See under Burn-
ing.

Internal : Bro; Carb-v;
Nux-m; *Nux-v;* Pho; Sang.

BORING, Grinding : ARG-N;
Asaf; *Aur; Bell;* Bism;
Colo; Dios; Hep; Lach;
Mag-p; Med; *Merc; Mez;*
Plat; Plb; *Pul; Ran-sc;*
Spig; Xanth; *Zin;* Zin-chr.

BREAKING, Broken: *Arn;* BELL;
Calc; Calc-p; Chel; *Cocl;*
EUP-P; Grap; Guai; *Lyc;*
Merc; Nat-m; Nux-v; Pho;

Ran-b; Rhus-t; *Rut;*
Sil; Sul; *Thu;* Val.

BRUISED, Soreness : *Ap;* ARN;
Aur; *Bap; Bell;* Bels; *Bry;*
Canth; *Carb-v; Caus; Chin;*
Chio; Cimi; *Con;* EUP-P;
Gel; Ham; Hep; Hypr; Kalm;
Lach; Lapp; *Lith; Mill; Nit-*
ac; NUX-V; Ol-an; Onos;
Plant; Pho; Phyt; *Pul; Pyro;*
Ran-b; RHUS-T; RUT; SIL;
Sul; Terb; Til.

+ Body all over : Gamb.

+ when touched : Mang.

Coition, after : Sil.

Deep : Mang.

Excessive exertion, as if,
from : Chel; Clem.

Internally : Bels; Cann; Pul.

Menses, during : Nat-c.

scanty, with : Carb-v.

Pains, after : Aco; *Arn;*
Chin; *Cimi;* Gel; Glo;
Grap; Mez; Onos; *Plat;* Sele;
Tell.

Parts, bleeding : Arn; Fer.

lain, on : Arn; Nux-m;
Pyro; Rut.

Spots : *Arn;* Glo; *Kali-bi;*
Lith; Merc; Pho; Ran-b;
Saba; Sul.

blows, fall, as from : Lith.

trifles, every from : Terb.

Waist, about : Visc.

BURNING : See Burning.

Hot irons : See Hot Irons.

Stinging : See Stinging,
under burning.

BURSTING, splitting : Act-sp;
BELL; BRY; Calc; Caps;
Carb-ac; *Chin;* Eup-p; *Glo;*
Ham; *Ign;* Kali-m; Lac-c;
Lept; Lil-t; Lyc; *Merc;* NAT-M;
Nux-v; Ran-b; Rat; Sani;
Sep; *Sil;* Spig; Stan; Sul;
Thyr; *Vip.*

CAN NOT Stand : See Sensitive,
and Besides himself.

COME AND GO : See Fleeting.

COLD : Arn; Med; Syph.

COLICKY : See Cramp.

CONSTRICTING : See Constriction.

CRAMPS, Griping, Colic : Agar;
Bell; Cact; CALC; Caus;
Cham; Cocl; COLO; CUP;
Dios; Dul; *Grap;* Hyo; *Ign;*
Lach; *Lyc;* Mag-m; Mag-p;
Nit-ac; NUX-V; *Plat;* Plb;
Rhe; Scop; Sec; Sil; Stan;
Stap; SUL; Ver-a; Ver-v; Vib.

Coition Agg : Colo; Cup;
Grap.

Every where : Hyd-ac; Old.

Exertion, prolonged on:
Mag- p.

Menses, after : Chin; Cup; Pul.
with: Mag-m.

Nursing Agg : Cham.

Pains, after : Sec.

Paralysis, then : Tab.

Radiating over whole body
: Dios; Lyc; Nux-v.

Stiffness, then : Sec; Sele.

Transfixion : Cup.

CUTTING : Aco; BELL; Bry;
Calc; Calc-p; Calc-s; *Canth;*
COLO; *Con;* Dios; Hyo;

KALI-C; Kali-m; Lyc; Merc;
Nat-m; Nit-ac; *Nux-v;*
Petr; Plant; Polyg; Pul;
Rat; Sabal; Sil; *Sul;* Tell;
Ver-a; Zin.

Smarting : Canth.

Squeezing : Thu.

DARTING : See Shooting.

DRAWING : Arn; *Bry; Carb-v;*
Caus; Cham; *Chel;* Chin;
Cimi; Colo; Grap; Kali-bi;
Kali-c; Lach; Lil-t; Lyc;
Merc; Nit-ac; Nux-v; Pul;
Rhod; RHUS-T; Sep; Sil;
Sul; *Val.*

EXTEND, Original site, from :
Ther.

FINE : See Pain, Stitching,
Needle like.

FITS And STARTS, In : Bar-m;
Cup; Mez.

FLEETING, Come and Go :
Nit-ac; Nux-m; Pall; Phyt;
Potho; Sabal; Stro; Tell;
Val.

Attacks repeated in : Bell.

+ FLESH, Torn from body as
if : Nit-ac.

FLUID, Forcing its way, as if,
with : Coc-c.

GNAWING, Eating Festering :
Agn; Am-m; Berb; Bry;
Cham; Colo; Grap; Guai;
Ign; Kali-s; Kre; *Lach;*
Lyc; Mag-m; Nat-s;
Nit-ac; Old; Ox-ac; *Pho;*
Plat; PUL; *Ran-sc;*
Rhus-t; Rut; Sec; Sep;
SIL; Spo; Stap; Sul; Sul-ac;

Thu; Ver-a; Zin-chr.

Burning : Rut.

Grinding : Zin-chr.

GOES To side lain, on : Ars;
Bry; Calc; Kali-c; Merc;
Nux-v; Pho-ac; PUL; Sep; Sil.

Not lain, on : Bry; Cup;
Flu-ac; Grap; Ign; Kali-bi;
Pul; Rhus-t.

Parts, recently lain, on:
Pul.

GIRDLE : Lach; Sul.

GRADUALLY INCREASE, Decrease
etc. : See Directions of
Symptoms.

GRINDING : See Pain, Boring.

GROWING : See Growing Pains.

HACKING Like Hatchet :
Am-c; Ars; Aur; Clem;
Kali-n; Lyc; Pho-ac; Rut;
Stap; Thu.

HEAT Agg : Tab.

+ INSENSITIVE, To : Bap.

ITCHING, Alternating, with :
Stro.

JERKING : Asaf; Bell; Calc;
Caus; CHIN; Ign; Kali-c;
Meny; Nat-m; Nit-ac;
NUX-V; PUL; Rhus-t; Sil;
Sul; Tarx; Thu; Val.

Part affected : Merc.

Shock, sudden from : Pod.

LABOUR : See Under Labour.

LIGHTNING : See Shooting.

LINEAR : Bell; Buf; Caps;
Caus; Cep; Fago; Ox-ac;
Pyro; Syph; Tell.

MADDENING: See Besides,
himself.

MANY : Med; Mez; Naj; Rum.

NAIL, Clavus : See Plug.

NEEDLE, Like : See Pain,
Stitching.

NERVES, Along : Terb.

NIPS : See Twinging.

OPERATIONS, After : Hypr.

PARALYTIC : See Paralysis.

PARALYZED Parts, in : Agar;
Ars; Cact; Caus; Cocl;
Kali-n; Latro; Plb.

PECKING : Chin; Rut.

PERSISTENT : Syph.

PIERCING : Ap; Mill; Nat-s.

PINCHING : See Squeezing.

suddenly, As if : Arg-n.

PRESSING, Bearing down :
Agar; Ap; Bell; CANTH;
Castr; Cimi; Con; LIL-T;
MERC-C; Nat-m; NUX-V;
Pall; Pho; Plat; Pul;
Rhus-t; Rut; SEP; Sil;
Stan; SUL; Thyr.

Blunt, instrument, as
from : Lith.

Coldness, with : Sec.

Inward : Anac; Plat; Stan.

deep, with as if instrument
: Bov; Ign; Ver-a.

Outward : Asaf; Bry; Cimi;
Pul; Sul.

Together : Asar.

PRICKLING : Aco; Ap; Bry; Ham;
Kali-p; Lob; Lyc; Nat-m;
Nat-p; Plat; Ran-sc; Rhus-t;
Sul; Symp; Tarn; Urt; Ver-v;
Xanth.

All over : Lob.

Numbness, with : Tarn.

PULLING : See Drawing.

QUICK : See Shooting.

RADIATING : See under Directions.

RAGING : Led.

RAWNESS : See Biting.

RHEUMATIC : See Rheumatism,
Joints.

SHIFTING : See Wandering.

SHINGLES, Before : Stap.

SHOCKS In : Cina; Zin-chr.

SHOOTING, Darting, Quick,
Lightning : Aco; *Agar;* Alu;
Arg-n; Ars; BELL; *Berb;*
Cimi; Colo; Cup; Dios; Fer;
Hyd-ac; Hyo; Hypr; Kali-bi;
Kali-c; Kali-m; Kalm;
Mag-c; Mag-m; *Mag-p; Mez;*
Nit-ac; Nux-v; Ox-ac; Paeon;
Plb; Pru-sp; Radm; Ran-b;
Rhus-t; Rum; Sabi; Sep;
Spig; SUL; Tell; Xanth; Zin.

Burning : Sul-ac.

Laming : Colch; Iris.

SLEEP, Felt in : Nit-ac.

Waking Amel : Sul-ac.

SMARTING : See Biting.

SORE : See Bruised.

SPLINTER : See Stitching,
Needle like.

SPOTS, In : See Spots, under
Pain Bruised.

SQUEEZING, Pinching,
Compression : Alu; Anac;
Ant-t; Asar; Bels; Berb; Bry;
Cact; Calc; Carb-v; Cimi;
Cocl; COLO; Grap; Ign; Kali-io;
Kalm; Meny; *Merc; Nat-m;*
Nat-s; Nit-ac; Old; PLAT;
Rut; Stap; Thu; Val; Verb; Zin.

STICKING : See Stitching,
Needle like.

Point, one to : Merc.

Smarting : Stap.

STINGING : Aco; AP; *Ars;* Berb;
Bry; Kali-c; Lyc; Merc;
Nit-ac; *Pho;* Pul; Sabal;
Sep; SIL; *Sul;* Ther; Zin.

Burning : See Burning,
Stinging.

STITCHING :Aco; Ars; Asaf;
Bell; Berb; Bor; BRY;
Caus; Colch; KALI-C;
Kali-m; Kali-s; Led; Merc;
Nit-ac; Pul; Ran-b; *Rhus-t;*
Sep; *Sil;* Spig; Strop; SUL;
Symp; Zin-chr..

Crawling : Arn.

Jerky : Cina; Nux-v.

Motion, impeding : Zin-chr.

Needle like, Fine Splinter
: Agar; Alu; Ap; ARG-N;
Ars; Bry; Caps;Cep; HEP;
Kali-bi; *Kali-c;* Nat-m;
NIT-AC; Paeon; Rhus-t;
Saba; SIL; Sul; Syph;
Tarn; Val; Ver-a.

Tensive : Spig.

Wounds, healed, in : Symp.

STRANGLING : Caps; Sul; Val.

STUMPS,In (after operation)
: Am-m; Arn; Asaf; Cep;
Hypr; Pho-ac; Symp.

SYMPATHETIC (See Synalgia)
: Tarn.

TAKES The BREATH Away :
See Respiration, Pain Agg.

TEARING, Very Severe,
Violent : Aco; Anac; *Arn;*

Ars; Bell; Bry; *Calc;* Caps; *Carb-v; Caus;* Cham; *Chin;* Colch; Con; Kali-c; *Lyc; Merc;* Nat-c; *Nit-ac; Nux-v; Plat; Pul; Rhod;* RHUS-T; Sep; Sil; Stap; Stro; Sul; Vip; Xanth; Zin.

Paralytic : Carb-v; Chin; *Kali-c; Stap.*

Pressive : Carb-v; Stan.

Stitching, Prickling : Anac; Calc; Colch; Guai; Led; Mang; Merc; Pul; Stap; Thu; *Zin.*

Twitching, Jerking : Chi ; *Pul.*

THROBBING, Pulsating : See Pulsation.

TREMBLING and paralytic weakness, with : Kalm.

TUGGING, Pulling : See Drawing.

TWINGING, Nips : Am-m; Laur; Mos; Plb.

TWISTING : Ars; Bell; Calc; Cina; *Colo;* DIOS; Ign; *Nux-v;* Pul; Rhus-t; *Sil;* VER-A.

ULCERATIVE : See Gnawing.

UNDULATING : Anac; Asaf; Colo; Zin-io.

VIOLENT : See Tearing.

VOLUPTOUS : Lach.

WAKENED, By : Aco; Ars; Chin; Kali-c; Lach; Nux-v; Sil; Sul.

WANDERING, Shifting : Arn; Berb; *Caul;* Cimi; Colch; Cup; Fer; KALI-BI; Kali-n; Kali-s; Kalm; *Lac-c; Led;* Mag-p; Merc-i-r; Nux-m;

Plant; Pru-sp; PUL; Rhod; Rhus-t; Rum; Sil; Thu; Zin-chr.

Rheumatic : Merc-i-r.

Suddenly : Amb; Arn; Colch; Radm; Rhod.

Zigzag : Rhod.

PAIN DURING AGG : Ars; Cham; Cimi; Colo; Ign; Lyc; Nat-c; Onos; Rhus-t; Sars; Sep; Thu; Ver-a.

PAINLESSNESS : See Numbness and Pain, Absence of.

PALATE : *Aur;* Bell; Crot-h; *Merc; Nux-v;* Pho.

HARD : Bell; *Nit-ac;* Nux-v; *Pho.*

Cancer : Hyds.

SOFT : Merc.

Rim : Merc-i-f.

Ulcer, eating, uvula : Hep.

ABSCESS : Pho.

APHTHAE : Agar; Bor; *Kali-bi;* Sars.

BLEEDING : Crot-h; Lach; Pho.

BLUISH, Red : Aco; Ap; Cham.

BURNING : Cam; Mez; Polyg.

CHEWING Agg : Bor.

CRAWLING : Ars; Carb-v; Pho; Polyg; Ran-b; Sil.

DRY : Nux-m; Pho; Pho-ac; Sul; Ver-a.

EXCORIATED : Caus.

GREASY : Asaf; Card-m; Kali-p; Ol-an.

HAIR, On : Kali-bi.

HEAT : See Burning.

INDURATED : Mez; Phyt.

ITCHING : Aru-t; Kali-p;

Mar-v; Merc; Mux-v; Pho; Polyg; Saba; Stry.

Ear, with: Mar-v.

NODE : Asaf; Mang.

NUMB : Bap; Ver-a.

OEDEMA : Ap; Kali-io.

PRESSING : Carb-v.

RAW, Sore : Aru-t; Bell; Caus; Iris; Lach; Merc; NIT-AC; Nux-v; *Pho;* Phyt.

SCALDED, As if : Sang; Sanic.

SHRIVELLED : Bor; Cyc.

SKIN, Loose, on : Phys.

STIFF : Crot-h; Grat; Nat-m.

SWELLED : Arg-m; *Lach;* Sul.

VESICLES : Mag-c; Nat-s.

WHITE : Fer; Merc; *Nat-p.*

WRINKLED : *Bor;* Pho.

YELLOW, Creamy : *Nat-p.*

PALMS : Anac; Grap; Petr; Ran-b; Sele; Spig.

ABSCESS : Ars; Cup; Flu-ac; Sul; Tarn-c.

CONTRACTIONS, In : Caus; Grap; Guai; Nat-m; Ver-a.

CRACKS : Calc-f; Kre; Merc-c; Merc-i-r; Ran-b; Rhus-t; Sul.

Moist : Merc-i-r.

CRAMPS : Naj; Sabi.

DESQUAMATION : Elap; Grap; Rhus-t; Sep; Sul.

Tender, and, as if : Mer-c.

DRY : Ars; *Bism;* Cham; Diph; Lyc; *Nux-m;* Rhus-t; Sul.

Crusts : Sele.

ECZEMA : Sul; Vario.

GNAWING *(L)* : Ran-sc.

HOT, Burn : *Ap;* Crot-h; Diph; Ip; Lach; Med; Ol-j; Pho; Rhus-t; Sang; Stan; *Sul.*

Climaxis, at : Sang.

Flushes, in : Phys.

Soles, and : Bism; Lil-t; Lyc; Petr; *Pho;* Sang; Stan; Sul.

Washing Agg : Rhus-t.

ITCHING : *Anac;* Fago; Kre; Ran-b; *Sul;* Tub.

Jaundice, in : Ran-b.

Night, at : Anac.

MOIST, Sweaty : Cratae; Dul; Ign; Naj; Nux-v; Sep; Sil; Sul; Vio-o.

Clammy : Anac.

Cold : Con.

Cough, with : Naj.

Putting them together, when : Rhe; Sanic.

Warm. : Ign.

NODES : Caus; Rut.

PEELING Of skin : See Desquamation.

PRICKING, Grasping, when : Rhus-t.

PSORIASIS : Petr; Pho; Sele.

RED : Flu-ac.

SORE : Rhus-t.

STIFF, Writing, while : Kali-m.

VESICLES : Anthx; Buf; Kali-c; Kre; Merc.

WARTS, On : Anac; Dul; Nat-m; Rut; Sul.

WASHING Agg : Rhus-t.

WITHERED : Diph; Sang.

YELLOW : Chel; Sep.

Ascites, with : Chel.

PALPITATION : See under Heart.

PANARIS : See Fingers, Felon.

PANCREAS : Chio; Con; Iod; *Iris*; Merc; *Pho; Spo.*

CANCER : Calc-ar.

INDURATION: Bar-m;Carb-an.

PANNUS : Arg-n; Aur-m; Hep.

PAN OPHTHALMITIS : Hep; Rhus-t.

PARADOXICAL: *Ign.*

PARALYSIS (Paralytic Pain) : *Ant-t*; Arn; *Ars*; Bell; Carb-v; CAUS; Chin; *Cocl*; Colch; Con; Dul; *Gel*; Hell; Helod; Hyo; Kali-p; *Lach*; Lyc; Mang; NUX-V; *Op*; Phys; PLB; RHUS-T; Sang; Sec; Sil; Stap; Sul; Verb; Zin-ph.

AGITANS: *Agar*; Ant-t; *Arg-n*; Bar-c; Buf; Con; *Gel*; Hyo; Kali-br; Lil-t; Lol-t; Mag-p; Mang; MERC; Nux-v; Phys; Plb; Rhus-t; Stram; Zin.

APOPLEXY, After : *Arn; Bell;* Cocl; Lach; Nux-v; Pho; Stan; Zin.

ASCENDING : Ars; Con; Mang; Ox-ac; Pho; Pic-ac; Vip.

COLD Bathing Amel : Caus; Con.

COLDNESS, of Parts, with : Caus; Cocl; Dul.

Icy : Ars; Dul; Grap; Nux-v; *Rhus-t.*

body of, with : Bar-m.

CONTRACTION Of limbs, with : Ars; Cheno; Old; Sec; Val.

CONVULSIONS, Then : Tarn-c.

CRAMPS, After : Tab.

DESCENDING : *Bar-c*; Merc; Zin.

DIPHTHERITIC : Ap; Arg-n; Caus; *Cocl*; Diph; Gel; Lac-c; *Lach; Rhus-t.*

EMACIATION, Rapid, of part, with : Sec.

EMOTIONS, From : Gel; Ign; Lach; Nat-m; Stan; Stram.

EPILEPSY, After : Cur; *Hyo.*

EXTENSOR, Muscles, of : Alu; Ars; Cocl; Crot-h; Cur; *Plb.*

FLACCID : Plb.

FLEXOR, Muscles, of : Caus; Mez; Nat-m.

FORMICATION, with : Cadm; Pho; Sec.

GENERAL, of Insane : Cann; Crot-h; Pho; Phys; Stram.

GRADUAL : Caus; Syph.

HAEMORRHAGE, With : Plb.

HEAT, In paralyzed part, with : Alu; Pho.

HYPERAESTHESIA Of well side : Plb.

HYSTERICAL: Arg-n; Asaf; Cham; Cocl; *Ign;* Nux-m; Pho; Plb; *Tarn;* Val.

INFANTILE : Bung; Calc; Caus; Gel; Kali-p; Lathy; Plb; Vip.

Dentition, during : Kali-p.

Paresis, after : Old.

INFECTIOUS Diseases, after : Caus.

INTERNAL, Sense of : *Lyc;* Nat-m; Pho.

LIMBS, of : Agar; Alu; Buf; CAUS; COCL; Nux-v; Plb; Rhus-t; Rut; Sec; *Sil;* Sul.

One arm or one leg only : Bothr.

Sensation, of : Grap.

walking, while : Rhus-t.

LOCALIZED, Single parts, Organs : *Ant-t;* Bar-c; Bell; CAUS; Dul; Gel; Hyo; Nux-v; *Op;* Pho; Pul; Sec; Sil; Sul.

MOISTNESS, With : Stan.

MOTION, Disorderly, with : Merc.

MUSCLES, Isolated, of : Cup.

NUMBNESS, With : Sec.

ONE SIDE : See Hemiplegia.

PAIN, From : Nat-m.

With : Cadm.

PAINLESS : Cann; *Cocl; Con; Gel; Hyo; Lyc;* Old; Plb; RHUS-T.

PARAPLEGIA : Agar; *Arg-n; Ars;* Bap; Mang; Nat-m; NUX-V; Plb; Rhus-t; Rut; Sec; Sul; Thal; Vip.

Atrophy, with : Ars.

Diphtheria, after : Ars.

Exertion, after : Nux-v; Rhus-t.

Fever, after : Rhus-t.

Hunger, with : Cina.

Hysterical : Cocl; Ign; Tarn.

Parturition, after : Caul; Caus; Plb; *Rhus-t.*

Progressive : Mang.

Rigidity of muscles, with : Chel.

Sensation, of : Aesc; Aur.

Sexual excess, after : Rhus-t.

Spastic : Gel; Hypr; *Lathy;* Nux-v; Sec.

Vaccination, after : Ars.

PSEUDO-HYPERTROPHIC : Cur; *Pho;* Thyr; Ver-v.

RHEUMATISM, After : Bar-c; Chin; *Fer; Rut.*

RUNS Forward, when attempting to walk : Mang.

SEXUAL Excess, from : Nat-m; Rhus-t.

SPASMS, After : Cocl; Cup; Cur; Elap; Hyo; *Sec;* Stan; Vib.

Then : Tarn.

With : Nux-m.

SPHINCTERS, Of : Gel.

SPINE, Diseased, from : Med.

SUPRESSIONS, After : *Caus;* Hep; Lach; Sul.

Foot sweat, after : Colch.

TINGLING of affected part, with : Cann.

TOUCH, Sensitive to : Plb.

TREMORS, After : Plb.

TWITCHING : Stram.

TYPEWRITERS : Stan.

TYPHOID,In : Agar; Lach; Rhus-t.

UNILATERAL : See Hemiplegia.

PARAPLEGIA : See under Paralysis.

PARCHMENT LIKE : Anac; *Ars;* BAR-C; Calc-f; Lyc;

Petr; Sil; Sul.

PAROTIDS (See Mumps): Calc-f; Cham; Iod; Merc; Phyt; Pul.

ENLARGED, Ear Affections, in : Ail Sil.

+ FISTULA : Calc.

HARD, but warm : Bro.

HYPERTROPHY, Mumps, after: Sul-io.

SWOLLEN : Carb-an.

PAROXYSMS, Repeated (See also Convulsions and Relapses) : *Agar; Ars; Bell; Calc; Caus;* CHAM; *Chin;* COCL; COLO; Cup; *Dios;* Gel; Ign; Lach; MAG-P; NUX-V; Plat; Plb; Pul; SEP; Stan; Sul; Tab.

PASTY : See Sticky.

PATCHY : See Mottled.

PATELLAE : Bell; Con.

BURSA, Enlarged, over : Sil.

DISLOCATED, As if : Gel.

Upstairs, going, on : Cann.

GURGLING : Asar.

HYGROMA : Arn.

PAIN, Impeding walking : Nit-ac.

PLUG Under : Cham.

PULSATION : Spig.

PECKING, Hacking: See under Pain.

PEDICULOSIS : See Lice.

PEDUNCULATED : See Fungus Growth.

PEELING Of SKIN : See Desquamation.

PEEVISH, PETULENT : Aco;

Am-c; *Ant-c;* Ant-t; Aur;*Calc;* Calc-p; Caps; *Cham;* CINA; Clem; Cocl; Cop; Kali-c; Lyc; Old; Rat; Stap; Sul; Syph; Zin.

CHILDREN, Old person : Sul.

PELLAGRA : Ars; Bov; Gel; Hep; Sec.

PELVIS AROUND : Sabi; Sep; Vib.

BONES, Painful, sitting on : Carb-an.

Loose, as if : Murx.

CELLULITIS : Pyro.

DISORDERS : Med.

HEAVY :Alo; Gnap; Helo; Lil-t; Pall; Tarn; Vib.

Dragging,dysuria, with : Lil-t.

+ Standing Agg : Pall.

MENSES, Amel : Vib.

+ ORGANS, Upside down: Vib.

PERITONITIS : Pall.

SORE Spot. pressing on, something, as if : Murx.

Above : Ver-v.

THIGHS, To : Thyr; Vib.

THROBBING : Jab.

PEMPHIGUS : See under Eruptions.

PENIS : Arn; *Cann;* Canth; Clem; Dul; *Merc;* Thu.

ABSENT, As if : Coca.

ATROPHY : Ant-c; Arg-n; Berb; *Ign; Lyc;* Stap.

BUBBLING : Grap; Kali-c.

Erection, during : Kali-c.

BURNING : Mez; Spo.

Coition, during : Clem; Kre.

COLD : Agn; Lyc; Onos; Sul.

Small, and : Agn; Lyc.

+ CONDYLOMATA, head of: Sep.

CONSTRICTION : Kali-bi.

By string, as if : Plb.

CONTRACTED, Small : Ign.

DRAWING : Iod.

ECZEMA, Back of : Alum; Radm.

ERECTIONS : See Erections.

FLACCID : Agn; Lyc.

FORMICATION : Sec.

GANGRENE : Canth; Lach.

INDURATION, old men, in : Berb.

INJURY : Mill.

ITCHING : Caus; Plat.

JERKING, Sleep in : Cinb.

LONG, As if : Calad.

NEEDLES At : Asaf.

NEURALGIA : Tab.

NUMB : Merc.

OEDEMA : Rhus-t.

PULSATION : Cop; Ign.

RED, Spots on : Caus.

RETRACTED : See Contracted.

RIGID, Tenesmus, with: Thu.

SENSITIVE : Tab.

STIFF, Emission, after : Grat.

SWELLING : Arn.

Hard, dorsum : Sabi.

Lymphatic vessels, along : Merc.

Painless : Mez.

TWITCHING : Thu.

+ UPWARDS, Bends : Berb.

VESICLES : Crot-t; Nit-ac.

WARTS : Ant-t; Med; Thu.

PERCEPTION, CHANGED
(Mental or Visual) : Aco; Arg-n; *Ars*; Bar-c; BELL; Calc; *Cann*; HYO; Kali-br; Lac-c; *Lach*; Merc; Nux-m; Op; Pho; Pho-ac; Plat; Pyro; STRAM; Sul; Ver-a.

PERFORATION : Kali-bi; Merc; Merc-c; Sil; Tub.

+ **PERICARDIUM. EFFUSION** : Ascl.

+ HYDRO : Colch.

+ INFLAMMATION: Colch.

PERINEUM : Agn; Alu; Carb-an; Carb-v; Chim; Cyc; Ol-an; Paeon; Sanic; Sul.

ABSCESS : Crot-h; Hep; Merc; Sil.

Anus in and around, as if : Cyc.

BALL, Lump : Cann; CHIM; Kali-m; *Ther*.

Sitting, on, as if : Chim.

BURNING : Rhod.

Coition, after : Sil.

BURSTING : Sanic.

Stools, after : Sanic.

DRAWING : Cyc; Kali-bi.

ERECTION, During : Alu.

ERUPTIONS : Petr; Sul.

Herpes : *Petr*.

EXCORIATED : Lyc.

FISTULA : Thu.

FULLNESS : Chin.

GENITALS, To : Bov.

HEAVY, Weight : *Con*; Med; Ther.

INJURY, Penetrating : Symp.

ITCHING : Petr; Sul.

  Stools, after : Tell.

LACERATED : Stap.

MOIST : Carb-an; Carb-v;
  Paeon; Thu.

PAIN : Caus.

  Coition, after : Alu.

  Erection, during : Alu.

PENIS, To : Phyt.

PINCHING : Pul.

PRESSING : Berb; Cyc; Ol-an.

PULSATION : Caus.

RECTUM, To : Bov.

SITTING Agg : Cyc.

STITCHING, And Extending to
  penis : Calc-p.

STOOLS Agg : Sanic.

SWELLING, Suture of : Thu.

TUBERCLE : Thu.

WALKING Agg : Cyc.

WRIGGLING : Chel.

PERIODICITY, PERIODICALLY,
  in General AGG : Alu; Aran;
  Arg-m; ARS; Cact; *Ced;* CHIN;
  Chin-ar; *Chin-s; Eup-p; Gel;*
  Hep; *Ip;* Kali-c; Lach; Lyc;
  NAT-M; Nit-ac; *Nux-v;* Pul;
  Rhus-t; Sep; Sil; Spig; Sul;
  Tarn.

  AT THE SAME HOUR AGG :
  Ant-c; Aran; Ars; Bov;
  Ced; Chin-s; Cina; Ign;
  Lyc; Nat-m; *Saba;* Verb;
  Tarn.

  Neuralgia, every day :
  Kali-bi.

  EXACT : Aran; Ars; Ced; Chin-s;

  Nat-m; Tarn.

  YEARLY AGG : Am-c; *Ars;* Crot- h;
  Echi; Elap; Lach; Lyc; Naj;
  Psor; Rhus-t; Tarn; Urt; Vip.

  Half : Lach; Sep.

PERIOSTEUM : See under
Bones.

PERISTALSIS, REVERSED
: Asaf; Elap; Nux-v; Rhus-t;
Ver-a.

PERITONITIS : See Abdomen,
Inflammation.

PERSECUTION, IDEAS Of :
Anac; *Chin;* Con; Cyc; *Dros;*
Hyo; Lach; Thyr.

PERSEVERE CAN NOT : Alu;
Asaf; Bism; Grat; Lac-c;Lach;
Nux-m; Nux-v; SIL; Sul.

PERSPIRATION : See Sweat.

PERVERSITY WITH TEARS
(Children) : Bell.

PETECHIAE : See Ecchymosis.

PETIT MAL : See Epilepsy;
Monor.

PETULENT : See Peevish.

PHAGEDENA, Slough : ARS;
Carb-v; Caus; Chel; Crot-h;
Hep; *Lyc; Merc;* Merc-c;
Merc-cy; Mez; NIT-AC; *Petr;*
SIL; *Sul.*

PHANTASY : See Imaginations.

PHARYNX, BURNING : Bell;
Carb-v.

  Menses, during : Nat-s.

  CHRONIC Conditions : Aesc;
  Cinb; Rum; Sep.

  DRY : Bell; Nux-m.

  FISSURED : Elap; Kali-bi.

GLISTENING : Ap.

INFLAMMED : Bell; Merc.

SCRAPING : Mez; Sang.

TICKLING : Stic.

+ TIGHTNESS, Of, to stomach : Alu.

PHILOSOPHER : Sul.

PHIMOSIS, PARA PHIMOSIS : Ap; Canth; Colo; Guai; *Merc*; Merc-c; *Nit-ac*; Rhus-t; Thu.

FRICTION, From : Arn.

PHLEBITIS : See Blood Vessels, Inflamation.

PHLEGMASIA ALBA DOLENS (White Milk Leg): Ap; Ars; Bell; *Bry*; CALC; Ham; *Lach*; Lyc; Merc; *Pul*; *Rhus-t*; Sul; Vip.

FORCEPS, Delivery, after: Cep.

TOUCH Agg : Crot-h.

PHLYCTENAE : See Conjuctiva.

PHOTOMANIA : See Light Amel.

DELIRIUM, With : Calc.

PHOTOPHOBIA: See Light Agg.

CHRONIC ·: Aeth.

INFLAMMATION, Without : *Con*; Hell.

MASTURBATION, After : Cina.

OPERATIONS, After : Stro.

SPRING, Season, in : Kob.

WARM ROOM Agg : *Arg-n*.

PHTHISIS : See Consumption.

PHYSICAL EXERTION AGG : See Exertion, Physical Agg.

PHYSOMETRA : See Vagina, Flatus, from.

PIANO PLAYING AGG (See Fingers,

Working, with AGG) : Nat-c; Sep.

BODY, Heaviness of, after : Anac.

PICKING : See Carphology.

PIECES, IN : See Duality.

PIERCING : See Under Pain.

PILES, HAEMORRHOIDS : AESC; ALO; Ars; Carb-an; Carb-v; *Caus; Coll; Grap; Ham; Kali-c; Lach*; Lyc; Merc-i-r; MUR-AC; NIT-AC; NUX-V; Paeon; Pho; Pul; Sep; SUL.

ALTERNATING, With : Abro; Coll; Sabi.

BATHING Cool, Amel : Alo; Bro; Kali-c; Nux-v; Rat.

Warm, or Agg : Bro.

BLEEDING : Am-c; Bar-c; Caps; Coll; *Fer*; Hypr; Kali-c; Nat-m; *Pho;* Pho-ac; Psor; *Pul;* Sabi; Sep; Sul.

Amel : Aesc.

+ Easy : Nit-ac.

Flatus, passing, while : Pho.

Menses, during : Am-c; Am-m.

Removal, after : Nit-ac.

Slight, exhausts : Hyds.

Stools, during : Am-c; Ham; Nat-m; Pho.

after : Am-c.

Walking, while : Sep.

BLIND : Aesc; Nux-v.

+ Smarting: Led.

BLUISH : Aesc; *Carb-v; Lach;* Mur-ac.

Bunch Of Cherries, like : Alo;
Calc; Dios; Mur-ac.

+ Burning : Caps.

Bursting : Ham.

Chronic : Aesc; Coll; Merc-i-r;
Nux-v; Sul.

Climaxis, During Agg : Aesc.

Cough Agg : Caus; Ign; *Kali-c;*
Lach.

During Agg : Coll.

Dysmenorrhoea, After : Cocl.

Foul, Offensive : Carb-v;
Med; Pod.

Hot Application, Heat Amel
: *Ars;* Lyc; Mur-ac; Petr; Pho;
Zin.

Large, Impeding stools :
Caus; Paeon; Sul-ac.

+ Ulcerated : Paeon.

Leucorrhoea, Suppressed
Agg : Am-m.

Lifting Agg : Rhus-t.

Lying Agg : Pul.

Menses Agg : Am-c; Lach.

Milk Agg : Sep.

Moisture, Oozing, from :
Calc-p; Sul-ac.

Operations, After Agg : Coll;
Croc.

Painful : Mur-ac; Nit-ac;
Paeon; Stap.

Stand can-not : Plant.

Parturition, After : Kali-c; Lil-t.

Pendulous : Nit-ac.

Pregnancy During : Mur-ac;
Sep.

Protruding : Abro; Alo; Am-c;
Calc; Kali-c; Mur-ac; Sep;
Sul; Zin.

Bleeding, with : Lach; Lept.

Flatus, passing, while :
Bar-c; *Mur-ac;* Pho.

Lying, when : Pul.

Menses, during : Pul.

Stool, after : Am-c.

during : Calc-p; Rat; Sil.

preventing : Caus; Sul-ac;
Verb.

Urination, during : *Bar-c;*
Kali-c; Mur-ac.

Walking Agg : Am-c; Sep.

Reflex, From : Coll.

Riding Amel : Kali-c.

Sitting Agg : Caus; Grap; Thu.

Amel : Calc; Ign.

Sneezing Agg: See Cough
Agg.

Standing Agg : Caus.

Stepping, Wide Agg : Grap.

Sticking : Sep.

Cough, during : Ign; *Kali-c;*
Lach; Nit-ac.

Stricture, From : Bap.

Suppressed Agg : Coll; Lycps;
Mill; Nux-v; Sul.

Thinking, Of it Agg : Caus.

Touch Agg : Bell; Caus;
Mur-ac; Rat; Sul; Thu.

Ulcerate : Carb-v; Sil; Zin.

Urinating Agg: Kali-c.

Walking Agg : Aesc; Bro;
Carb-an; Caus; Mur-ac;
Sep; Sul; Zin.

Amel : *Ign.*

White : Carb-v.

PIMPLES : See Eruptions.

PINCHING : See Pain, Squeezing.

AMEL : Ap; Ars.

PINING : *Aur; Lyc*; Nat-m; Pho-ac; *Tub.*

PINK EYE : Euphr.

PINWORMS : See under Worms.

PITCHY : See Discharges, Tarry.

PLACENTA ADHERENT, Retained : Canth; Hyds; Ign; *Pul*; Sabi; Sec; Sep; *Habitual*; Hyds.

PREVIA : Erig; Ip.

SEPTIC : Sec.

PLACID, TRANQUIL : Ap; Arn; Chin; *Hell; Op; Pho;* PHO-AC; SEP; Stap; Sul.

ANGER, After : Ip.

PLAGUE : Ars; Crot-h; Ign; Lach; Pho; Pyro;Tarn-c.

PLAINTIVE : Crot-h.

PLETHORA, FULL BLOODED : *Aco;* Aur; BELL; Bry; Calc; *Fer;* Hyo; Kali-bi; Lyc; Nat-m; *Nux-v;* PHO; *Pul;* Sep; Sil; *Sul.*

PLEURISY : See under Chest.

PLEURODYNIA : Aco; Arn; Ascl; Bor; Bry; Chin; Cimi; Fer; Fer-p; Lach; Nux-v; Pul; Ran-b; Saba; Sul.

PLICA POLONICA : Grap; Vinc; Vio-o.

PLUG, Nail, Wedge, Clavus : Agar; *Anac;* Arn; Asaf; *Cof;* Hep; *Ign;* Lith; Mos; *Plat; Ran-sc;* Rat; *Rut;* Spo; Sul; *Sul-ac;* THU; Val.

BLUNT : Rut; Sul-ac.

ROUGH : Rut.

PNEUMONIA : See under Chest.

POISON, FEARS : See under Fear.

POISONED, FEELING : Lac-c; Lach; Naj; Vip.

POLLUTIONS : See Seminal Emissions.

POLYPI (See Fungus Growth) : Calc; Calc-p; Coc-c; Con; Form; Mar-v; Pho; Sang; Stap.

POLYURIA : See Urine, Profuse.

POMPOUS, IMPORTANT : Bell; Calc; Cup; *Lyc*; Pho; PLAT; *Ver-a.*

POPLITAE :Bell; Con; Mez; Nat-c; Nat-m; Onos; Pho.

ACHING : Mez.

BENDING Knee Agg : Calc-p; Chin; Rhus-t.

BUBBLING, Heels, to : Rhe.

CONTRACTION : Caus; Guai; Nat-m; Tell.

EXCORIATION : Amb; *Sep.*

EXTENDING Leg Agg : Carb-an; *Rhus-t.*

FIBROIDS, Recurrent : Calc-f.

HEEL, To : Alu.

ITCHING: Lyc; Mez; Sep; Zin.

MOTION Agg : Nat-c; Plb.

NUMB : Onos.

PAINFUL : Caus; Lyc; Nat-c; Phys; Radm.

SITTING Agg : Berb.

STANDING Agg: Grap; Par; Rum.

STIFF : Caus.

Stooping, on : Sul.

SWEAT, On: Bry; *Carb-an;* Con; Dros; Sep.

SWELLING : Mag-c.

WEAKNESS : Val.

POSITION, AWKWARD, Strange : See Attitude, Bizarre.

CHANGE Of AMEL : See Change of Position Agg and Amel.

ODD AMEL : Rhe.

REST, CAN NOT, in ANY : Lyc; Pip-m; Ran-b; Rhus-t; Sanic; Sul; Syph; Xanth. Sleep, during : Caus.

WRONG, In, AGG : Ars; Bry; Lyc; Tarx.

POWER, HIGHER, Under, as if : Anac; Lach; Naj; Thu.

LACK, Of : See Control.

Therefore powerless : Anac.

WILL, Of : Op.

PRAISE AMEL : Pall.

PRAYING : Ars; *Aur;* Bell; *Pul;* Stram; *Ver-a.*

PRAYS, CURSES, Shrieks, in turns : Ver-a.

PRECOCIOUS : Lyc; Merc.

LOQUACIOUS (Children) : Strop.

PREGNANCY, CHILD-BED affections of or since AGG : *Aco;* Alet; Arn; Bell; *Bry;* Calc; Caul; Cham; Cimi; Cocl; Con; *Gel;* Helo; Ign; Ip; *Kali-c; Kre;* Mag-c; Nux-m; NUX-V; Plat; PUL; Pyro; *Rhus-t;* Sabi; Sec; SEP; Stram; Sul; Tab; Ver-a; Vib.

ABDOMEN, Lying on Amel :

Pod.

BILIOUS Complaints, during : Chel.

FALSE : *Caul;* Croc; Nux-v; *Thu.*

FEVERISH Restlessness, during last month : Colch.

ITCHING : Sabi; Tab.

LATE : Bell.

+ LOOKS, As if : Vario.

STRANGE, Notions, desires : Lyss.

TOXAEMIA, Of : Kali-chl.

+ TROUBLES, Many, during : Pod.

WALK About, must at night : Rat.

PREMONITION : See Fear of Future.

PREPUCE : Ap; Calad; *Merc;* Rhus-t.

BURNING : Nit-ac.

COLD : Berb.

CRACKED : Hep; Merc; Sep; Sul; Sul-io.

ERUPTIONS : Nit-ac.

EXCORIATION : Merc.

Coition : Calen.

Easy : Nat-c.

+ GANGRENE : Kre.

+ HAEMORRHAGE : Kre.

HARD, Like leather : Sul.

HERPES, On : Pho-ac; Sars.

INFLAMMATION : Cinb; Merc.

ITCHING : Caus; Cinb; Con; Ign; Nit-ac; Petr; Rhus-t.

NUMB : Berb.

OEDEMA : See Swelling.

PHIMOSIS : See Phimosis.

RED, Scurfy, spots on : Nit-ac.

RETRACTED :Calad; *Nat-m.*

RUBBING, Slight Agg : Cyc.

SCURF, Inside : Caus.

SLOUGH : Thu.

SWELLING : Calad; Cinb; Merc;
Nit-ac; Rhus-t; Thu; Vesp.
Itching, with : Vio-t.

THICKENED : Lach.

ULCERS : Aur-m; Merc; Merc-c.

VARICES : Ham; Lach.

WARTS : Cinb; Sep; *Thu.*

PRESBYOPIA : See Vision,
Far Sight.

PRESENTIMENTS : See Fear
of Future.

PRESSING : See Pain Pressing.

PRESSURE AGG (Lying on
Painful side or affected side
AGG) : Aco; *Agar;* Ap;
Arg-n; Ars; *Bar-c;* Bell; Bry;
Calad; Calc; Carb-v; *Cina;*
Dros; *Hep;* IOD; Kali-c;
Kali-io; LACH; Laur; Lil-t;
Lyc; Mag-c;Mag-m;Merc-c;
Nat-s; Nux-m; *Nux-v;* Pho;
Pho-ac; Psor Rut; Saba; SIL;
Spo; Tarn; Tell; Ther; Thu;
Vib; Zin-chr.

AMEL (Lying on Painful or
Affected side **A**MEL) : Am-c;
Arg-n; BRY; Calc; Caps;
Castr;Cham; Chel; *Chin;*
COLO; *Con;* Cup-ar; Dios;
Dros; IGN; Lil-t; *Mag-m;*
Mag-p; *Meny;* Nat-c; *Plb;*
Pul; Pyro; *Rhus-t;* Sep; Sil;
STAN; Vib.

BOOTS, Shoes, of **A**GG : Bor;
Paeon.

CLOTHES Of **A**GG : See Clothes,
Pressure *Agg.*

HARD Over Edge **A**GG : Rut.

AMEL : Bell; *Chin;* COLO;
Con; Ign; *Lach;* Mag-m;
Meny; Nux-v; Psor; Samb;

Sang; Stan; Zin.

HAT, Cap, of **A**GG : Carb-v;
Nit-ac; Sil; Val.

OPPOSITE SIDE On **A**GG :
Vio-t.

PAINLESS Side on **A**GG : See
under-lying, on Painless
Side Agg.

SHARP : Ign.

SIMPLE, Sense of : Bell; Bry;
Lach; Lyc; *Nat-m;* Nit-ac;
Nux-v; Pul; Sep; Sil; Stan;
SUL.

SPINE, On **A**GG : Agar; Arn;
Bell; *Chin;* Kali-c; *Phys;*
Sep; SIL; Ther.

STEADY **A**MEL : Nit-ac; Spig.

SUPPORT, And **A**MEL : Murx.

PRIAPISM : See Erections,
Painful.

PRICKINGS : Crot-h; *Nit-ac.*

PRICKLING : See under Pain.

PRICKLY HEAT : Ant-c; Urt.

PRIDE, ARROGANCE : Lil-t; Lyc;
PLAT; Sul; *Ver-a*

OVER WEENING : Grat.

WOUNDED : Pall; Plat; Ver-a.

PRIM : Plat.

PRODROME : Chel; Chin;
Corn; Eup-p.

PROFANITY : ANAC; Lil-t; Lyc;
Nit-ac; Stram; Tarn; Ver-a.

PROLAPSE, FALLING : Alo;
Arg-m; Arg-n; Aur; *Bell;* Bor;
Calc; Gel; Helo; *Ign;* Kali-cy;
Lach; Lil-t; *Merc; Mur-ac;*
Nat-m;Nux-v; Pall; Pho; Plat;
Pod; *Pul; Rhus-t;* Sep; Stan;
Sul.

PROPHYLACTICS CATHETER
Fever : Cam-ac.

C**HOLERA** : Ars; Cup-ar; Ver-a.

D**IPHTHERIA** : Ap; Diph;
Merc-cy.

E**RYSIPELAS** : Grap.

H**AY** FEVER: Ars; Kali-p; Psor.

H**YDROPHOBIA** *: Bell;* Canth;
Hyo; Lyss; Stram.

I**NFLUENZA** : Eucal.

I**NTERMITTENT** Fever : Ars;
Chin-s.

L**ABOUR,** Pains, false : Caul.

M**EASLES** : *Aco;* Ars; Pul.

M**UMPS** : Triof.

P**LAGUE** : Ign.

P**US** Infection : Am.

Q**UINSY** : Bar-c.

S**CARLET** Fever : Bell; Eucal.

V**ARIOLA** (Small-Pox) :
Maland; Vacci; Vario.

W**HOOPING** Cough : Dros;
Vacci.

Y**ELLOW** Fever : Ars.

PROPORTION SENSE OF,
Disturbed : Agar; Calc;
Cann; Onos; Plat; Stram.

PROSOPALGIA : See Face,
Pain.

PROSTATE GLAND : Ap;
Bar-c; Chim; CON; Crot-h;

Dig; Lyc; Med; Par-b; Pho;
Polyg; PUL; *Sabal; Sele;*
Sep; Solid; *STAP;* Sul; THU.

A**BSCESS** : Sil.

B**ALL,** Sensation on Sitting :
Chim; Sep.

B**URNING** : Caps.

C**ANCER** : Crot-h.

C**OITION** Agg : Alu; Cep; Psor.

E**MISSION** of Prostatic fluid
(Prostatorrhea) : Con; Lyc;
Pho-ac; SELE; *Sep;* Stap.

Cause, without : Zin.

Easily discharged, with
even passing flatus :
Mag-c.

Emotions, from : Con.

Fondling women : Agn;
CON.

Lascivious thoughts, with
: Con; Nit-ac.

Sitting, while : Sele.

Sleep, in : Sele.

Stools, with : Con; Hep;
Nat-c; Nux-v; Pho-ac;
Sele; Sep.

difficult, with : Nit-ac;
Pho-ac; Sil; Sul.

Talking to a young
lady, while : Nat-m; Pho.

Tobacco Agg : Daph.

Urination, After : Hep;
Nat-c; Sul.

Walking, while : Sele.

E**NLARGED** : Apoc; *Bar-c;*
Calc; Cann; Chim; *Con;*
Dig; Med; Ol-an; Par-b;
Pic-ac; *Pul;* Sabal; Senec;
Sil; Ther.

As if : Ther.

Piles, with : Stap.

Pressure, Perineum in, with : Berb.

Senile : Bar-c; Dig; Fer-pic; Sabal; Sele.

HARD, Indurated : Con; Iod; Senec; Sil; *Thu.*

As if : Senec.

HEAVY : Med.

INFLAMMED : Ap; Aur; Chim; Fer-pic; Pul; *Sabal;* Solid; *Thu.* Suppresed gonorrhoea, from : Merc-d; Nit-ac; Thu.

MASTURBATION, Complaints, after : Tarn.

PULSATION, Painful: Polyg.

RECTAL Troubles, with: Pod.

SORE : Chim.

STITCHES, Urging to stool, or urination, with : Cyc.

Walking, when : Kali-bi.

SWELLED : Chim.

As if : Senec.

URETHRA, Extending, to : Stap.

URINATION Agg : Lyc; Polyg; *Pul.*

WALKING Agg : Cyc; Kali-bi.

PROSTATORRHOEA : See Prostate Gland, Emissions of.

PROSTRATION : See Weakness, and Nervous.

PROTRUSION, Also Sense of Internal Parts as Eyes, Hernia etc. : *Aco;* Aur; *Bell; Cocl;* Fer; *Glo;* Hyo; Iod; LACH; *Lyc;* Lycps; NUX-V; Op; Spig; Stram; Sul-ac.

PROUD : See Pride.

PROUD FLESH (See Fungus Growth) : Alu.

PRURIGO : See Itching.

PRURITIS SENILIS : See under Itching, Old People, in.

PRYING : Sul.

PSORA : Ars; Bar-c; *Calc;* Grap; Hep; Iod; Merc; Pho; *Psor;* Sil; *Sul;* Tub.

PSORIASIS : See under Eruptions.

PTERYGIUM : Cann; Rat; Sul; Tell; Zin; Zin-s.

CORNEA, Over : Nux-m.

PINK : Arg-n.

PTOMAINE POISONING : ARS; Carb-v; Crot-h; *Cup-ar;* Kre; Lach; Pul; Pyro; *Ver-a.*

PTOSIS : See Prolapse, and Eyelids heavy.

PUBERTY AND AFFECTIONS of YOUTH : *Ant-c;* Bell; *Calc-p;* Caus; Cimi; Croc; Fer; *Fer-p;* Guai; Hell; Kali-br; *Kali-c;* Kali-p; *Lach;* Nat-m; PHO; Pho-ac; PUL; Senec; Vio-o.

DRIED and Wrinkled girls : Alu.

SLOW, Girls, in : Calc-p.

PUBES, BACKWARD To Lumbar Region, from : Calc; Pho; Sabi.

ACHING, over, menses during : Radm.

GURGLING : Scil.

PLUG, Wedge, Weight between Coccyx and : Alo; Cact; Sep.

PULSATION, Constant, behind

: Aesc.

PUDENDUM Urine Burns :
Caus; Scop.

ITCHING : Amb.

Menses before : Grap.

during : Hep.

PULSATION : Pru-sp.

PUERPERAL SEPSIS (See
Blood Sepsis) : Arn; Ars;
Echi; Lach; *Lyc; Op;* Pho;
Pul; Pyro; RHUS-T; Sec;
SUL.

LOCHIA. Suppressed, from : Lyc;
Sul.

PUFFINESS (See also
Swelling) : Ap; ARS; Bov;
CALC; Caps; *Fer; Flu-ac;
Kali-c;* Kre; Led; Lith; Med;
Nat-c; Nux-m; Op; Pho; Phyt;
RHUS-T; Rum; Rut; Ust.

PULLED UP : Ol-an.

PULSATION, THROBBING : Aco;
Ast-r; BELL; *Bels;* Bry; *Calc;*
Chin; Coc-c; Fer; GLO; Jab;
Kali-c; Kre; Lach; Lil-t; Meli;
Nat-m; *Pho;* Polyg; PUL; *Sep;*
Sil; Strop; Sul.

ARTERIES, In : Bell; Chin; Glo.

Carotid : Pru-sp.

Large, in : Iod.

FEVER, In : Urt.

Sudden : Pyro.

GENERAL, All over body : Aco;
Alu; Amb; *Ant-t; Bell;* Calc;
Calc-hyp; *Carb-v;* Fer;
GLO; *Grap; Kali-c; Kre;*
Lach; Lil-t; Lyc; Nat-m;
PHO; PUL; Sang; Sele;
Sep; Sil; Sul; Ver-v; Zin.

Breath holding Agg : Cact.

Eating Agg : Sele.

Sleep, preventing : Sele.

Sweat, with : Jab.

HARD : Asaf.

+ LOCALISED : Am-m.

LYING Agg : *Glo;* Sele.

MOTION Agg : Sil.

NUMBNESS, With : Glo.

ODD Places, in : Cact.

PAINFUL : Aco; Am-m; *Bell;
Fer; Ign;* Polyg; Sep.

Wandering : Polyg.

SINGLE Parts in : Kali-c;
Mur-ac.

SITTING Agg : Sil.

VEINS, In : Glo.

VIOLENT : Sabi.

PULSE, CHANGEABLE Variable
: Cina; Dig; Laur; Naj.

DICROTIC : Gel; Kali-c.

FAST : See Rapid.

FLOWING : Fer-p; Gel; Syph;
Ver-v.

FLUTTERING : Nux-v.

FULL : Aco; *Ant-t;* Bell; Berb;
Bry; Calc; Canth; Chel;
Colo; Dig; Fer; FER-P; *Gel;
Glo;* Grap; Hep; *Hyo;*
Kali-n; Merc; Mez; *Nux-v;*
Op; Pho; *Ran-sc; Spo;
Stram; Sul;* VER-V.

Right : Kali-chl.

Strong, and : Aco; Bell; *Bry.*

Weak, and : *Fer-p;* Gel;
Ver-a.

HARD : Aco; Am-c; *Bell;* Berb;
Bry; Canth; Chel; Chin;

Colch; Colo; Fer; Grap;Hep;
Hyo; Ign; Iod; Mez; *Nit-ac;*
Nux-v; Pho; Plb; Sil; Stram;
Sul.

Cord like : Tab.

Single Beats : Aur; Cact;
Lach; Lil-t; Zin.

IMPERCEPTIBLE : Aco; Carb-v;
Colch; Cup; Sil; Tab; Ver-a.

Almost : Aco; Cam; Gel.

INTERMITTENT : Adon; Ars;
Carb-v; Chin; *Dig;* Kali-c;
Lycps; Merc; Mur-ac;
Nat-m; Pho-ac; Sec; Sep;
Spig; Tab; Terb; Ver-a.

Every third beat : Mur-ac;
Nat-m; Nit-ac.

third or fourth beat : Cimi.

third to seventh beat : Dig;
Mur-ac.

fourth beat : Calc-ar;Nit-ac.

Long interval, exciting fear
of death : Nux-m.

IRREGULAR: Aco; Adon; Ant-c;
Ars; CACT; Cann; *Chin;* DIG;
Fer; Glo; *Kali-c;* Lach; Myr;
NAT-M; *Op;* Pho-ac; Sec;
SPIG; Stram; Strop; VER-V.

Forceps delivery, after :
Cact.

LARGE : Aco; *Fer-p;* Lycps;
Manc; Pho; Syph; *Ver-v.*

RAPID, Quick, Fast : ACO; Adon;
ANT-T; Ap; Arn; ARS; Aur;
BELL; Bry; Coll; Con;
Crot-c; Cup; Dig; Fer-p; Gel;
Glo; Iod; LACH; Merc;
Nat-m; NUX-V; Op; PHO;
Pho-ac; Pyro; *Rhus-t;* Sil;

Spig; *Spo;* Stan; Stram;
SUL; Thyr; VER-V; Zin.

Eating Agg : Lyc.

Eveniong Agg : Lyc.

Morning, in : Ars; Grap;
Sul.

Out of all proportion, to
temperature : Lil-t;
Pyro; Thyr.

Tumultuously : Aco
Amy-n; Lycps.

sweat, with : Coca.

SHARP : Rhus-t.

SLOW: Berb; Cann; Cic; Cup;
DIG; Gel; *Kalm; Myr;* Naj;
Ol-an; Op; Scil; Sep;
Stram; *Ver-v.*

Day, during : Grap.

Hard : Scil.

Heart beat, violent with :
Ver-v.

Neuralgia, with : Kalm.

Puberty, at : Dig.

Rapid, Alternately : Chin;
Dig; *Gel;* Iod; Strop.

than heart beat : Dig;
Kali-n; Spig.

Sinks to 40 beats : Cann;
Naj; Plb.

Vertigo, with : Ther.

SMALL : *Aco; Ars;* Cam;
Carb-v; *Cup;* Dig; Guai;
Hell; *Rhus-t;* Scil; Sec; Sil;
Stram; Strop; *Ver-v.*

Left : Kali-chl.

SOFT : Ant-t; Carb-v; Cup;
Dig; *Fer-p; Gel;* Lach;
Mur-ac; Op; Stram; Syph;

Terb; *Ver-v.*

SYNCHRONIZE, Does not, with heart : Lycps.

TEMPERATURE, Discordant : Pyro.

THREADY : Ars; *Calc*; Colch; Tab; Terb; Ver-a.

TREMULOUS : Ant-t; Calc; Cimi; Kalm; Naj; *Spig.*

UNEQUAL : Agar; Hyd-ac; Ign; Kali-chl; Op.

VENOUS : Glo.

WEAK : Aco; *Ant-t; Ars;* Aur; Berb; Cam; *Carb-v;* Cimi; Colch; Crot-h; Gel; Kali-c; Kalm; Lach; Laur; Merc; *Mur-ac;* Naj; *Pho-ac; Rhus-t;* Ver-a.

PUNCTURED WOUNDS (See Injuries) : Led; Plant.

PUPILS ADHERENT : Nit-ac.

CONTRACTED : Aco; *Chel;* Cocl; Jab; *Op;* Sep; Sil; Sul; Thu; *Ver-a.*

DILATED : Agn; Ail; Arg-n; BELL; Bro; Buf; CALC; Chin; Cina; Gel; *Hyo;* Mang; Op; Sec; Spig; Stram; Ver-v.

Contracted and Alternately : Bar-c; Hell; Lach; Phys; Strop.

Convulsions, before : *Arg-n;* Buf.

One : Nat-p.

Reading Agg : Pho-ac.

INSENSIBLE To Light Fixed : Arn; *Bell; Cup;* Hyo; OP.

IRREGULAR : Aur; Dig; Merc; Sul.

LIGHT, Not Reacting: Carb-v.

MOBILE : See Dilate and Contract, alternately.

UNEQUAL (One smaller than Other) : Colch; Hyo; Tarn.

PURGATIVES Agg : See under Drug, Abuse, of.

PURGING AMEL : Abro; Nat-s; Zin.

WITH VOMITING : See Vomiting with Purging.

PURPLE : See Bluish.

PURPURA : See Ecchymosis.

PURSUED, As IF : Anac; Hyo; Kali-br; Lach; Rhus-t; Stram.

ANIMALS, By : Nux-v.

PUS (See Discharges) ACRID : Ail; *Ars; Bels;* Bro; Echi; Euphr; Gel; *Kali-iol; Nit-ac;* Ran-b; Saba; Sanic; Sars; *Sul.*

AIR BUBBLES, In : Sul.

BLOODY : Calc-s; Merc; Nit-ac; Pho; Rhus-t.

BURROWING (See Fistulae): Arn; Asaf.

FOUL, Offensive : *Ars;* Asaf; Bap; Calc-f; *Carb-v;* Hep; *Lach;* Led; Mag-m; Nit-ac; Pho; *Psor; Pyro;* Sep; Sil; *Sul:* Syph.

Asafoetida like : Carb-v.

GREEN : Sec; Syph; Tub.

HAIR, Destroying : Bels; Lyc; Merc; Rhus-t.

PLUGS, Of : Kali-bi; Nit-ac.

PROFUSE : Ars; Asaf; *Calc;* Dul; Hep; Kali-io; *Merc;* Nat-m; Nux-v; Pul; Sep;

Sul.

SALTY : Iod; Kali-io.

SCANTY : Aco; *Bry; Hep;* Lach; Sil.

SLIMY : Merc.

SOUR : Sul.

SUPPRESSED: *Bry;* Dul; *Lach;* Pul; Sil; Stram; *Sul.*

TENACIOUS : Bor; Coc-c; Con; Hyds; Kali-bi.

THICK : Arg-n; *Calc-s;* Euphr; *Hep; Kali-bi; Pul;* Sanic.

THIN : Ars; *Asaf;* Caus; *Flu-ac;* Mag-m; Merc; Nit- ac; Pho; *Sil; Sul.*

UNHEALTHY : Asaf; Hep; Merc; Pho; *Sil.*

YELLOW : Calc-s; Euphr; Mag-m; Mez; Pul; Sanic.

Bloody : Arg-n; Hep.

Green: Ars-io; Kali-bi; *Kali-s; Merc;* Pul.

WATERY : Asaf; *Merc; Sil.*

PUSHED, DOWN : Lyc; Psor.

FORWARD : Fer-p.

PUSTULES : See Eruptions, Pustulating.

PYEMIA (See Blood Sepsis) : Ars-io; Chin; Lach; Pho; Pyro.

PYELITIS : Berb; Calc-s; Kali-s; Merc-c; Hep; Rhus-t; Sul-io; Terb.

COMA, With : Bap.

PYLORUS CONSTRICTION : Chin; Nux-v; Pho.

CANCER : Acet-ac; Grap.

RELAXATION : Fer-p; Pho.

WALL, Indurated : Sil.

PYORRHOEA : See Gums, Suppuration.

PYREXIA : See Fever.

PYROSIS : See Waterbrash.

QUALMISHNESS : Ars; Caus; Nat-s; Sul.

QUARRELSOME (See Abusive) : Rat; Rut; Ver-v.

HIMSELF and his familywith : Kali-c.

QUESTIONS, SPEAKS In, continuously : Aur.

QUICK PAINS: See Pains, Shooting.

TO ACT : Cof; Ign; Lach.

QUIET AMEL : *Bry;* Cadm; Colch; Nux-v.

QUININE ILL EFFECTS : See under Drug Abuse.

QUINSY : See Tonsils, Suppuration.

QUIVERING : Agar; *Asaf; Bell; Con;* Hyo; Kali-c; Mez; Nat-c; Stram; *Sul;* Tarn; Thyr;Tub; Zin.

ALL OVER : Lyss.

Vertigo, followed by : Calc.

LYING, While : Clem.

RADIATING : See Directions.

RADIUS BROKEN : Gymn.

RAGE (See Delirium Maniacal) : Ap.

RAGS ARE SILK or Beautiful, thinks : Sul.

BODY TORN INTO, As if : Phyt.

RAINS, WHEN AGG : Aran; Plat.

RAINY Season agg : See Dampness Agg.

Amel : See Air, Dry Clear *Agg.*

RAISING Arms agg : See under Arms.

U**p A**gg *: Aco;* Bell; *Bry;* Cadm; Cham; Cocl; Fer; Ign; *Merc-i-f;* Nat-m; Nux-v; Op; Pho; *Phyt;* Pul; Rhus-t; Sil; Sul; Ver-v; Vib.

Amel : Am-c; Ant-t; Aral; *Ars; Calc;* Dig; Glo; Kali-c; *Samb; Sep.*

RANCID, Taste, Odour etc. : Alu; Carb-v; *Pul;* Tell; Thu; Val.

RANULA : Amb; Calc; Flu-ac; Merc; Mez; Nit-ac; *Thu.*

Chewing, Talking Agg : Mez.

RASHNESS: See Reckless.

RATS Sees (See also Vision Illusions, of) : Aeth; Ars.

RATTLING : Am-m; ANT-T; Cact; Calc-s; *Chin; Cup;* HEP; IP; Kali-s; Lob; *Lyc;* Op; Scil; Sil; Sul; Ver-a.

RAW : See Pain, Burning.

Scratches, Himself : Aru-t; Psor.

RAWNESS, Feeling : Meli; Nux-v.

RAYNAUD'S Disease : Ail; Ars; Cact; Fer-p; Sec.

REABSORBENT : See Absorbent, Action.

REACHING High agg : Sul.

REACTION, Lack of, Poor: Aeth; *Amb; Am-c; Ant-t;*

Calc; Caps; Carb-v; Castr; Con; CUP; Dig; Fer; Gel; Hell; Hyd-ac; Kali-bi; *Laur; Med;* Mos; Old; OP; Pho-ac; PSOR; SUL; SYPH; Tarn; Ther; Tub; Val; ZIN.

Genito-urinary, Sphere, in : Senec.

Violent : Bell; *Cup; Nux-v;* Zin.

READING, Eye strain, **A**gg : Arg-n; *Calc;* Cina; Con; Croc; Kali-c; Lil-t; *Lyc;* Mang; Naj; NAT-M; Onos; Pho; Pho-ac; Phys; Radm; Rhod; Rhus-t; RUT; *Seneg;* Sep; Sil; Sul.

All Symptoms, of **A**gg : Carb-ac.

Aloud agg *:* Amb; *Carb-v;* Pho; Sele; Verb.

Amel *:* Nat-c.

Difficult, Light, artificial in : Nat-m.

Fine Print, difficult : Cadm; Mang; Meph; Nat-c.

more distinctly : Cof.

Someone, After her : Mag-m.

RECKLESS, Rashness (See Boldness) : Aur; Cic; Tub.

RECLINING Amel : See under Lying.

RECOGNIZE, Does not, his relatives : Bell; Hyo.

Children, Her own : Acet-ac.

RECOVERY, Despair Of : See Despair.

RECTUM : Aesc; Alo; Calc; *Ign;* Lyc; Mag-m; *Merc-c;* Nat-m; *Nux-v;* Pho; *Pod;* Rut; Sep; *Sul.*

ABSCESS (Peri-rectal) : Calc-s; Rhus-t; Sil.

ACHING : *Aesc*; Coll; Grap; Lyc; *Rat.*

ANKLES, To : Alu.

BALL, As if, sitting on : Cann.

+ BALL, Big, as if in : Sul-ac.

BLADDER (Urinary) With : Amb; *Canth;* Caps; Erig; *Merc-c;* Lil-t; Pyro; Sabi.

BLEEDING (See Piles) : Bism; Rat.

Clots, large: Alu; Alum.

Constant in drops, no blood with stool : Kob; Pul.

Flatus, passing on : Pho.

Menses, during : *Am-m;* Grap; *Lach.*

Piles, removal after : Nit-ac.

Standing Agg : Crot-h.

Stools, after : Echi.

hard, from : Flu-ac; Kali-c; *Nat-m;* Tub.

soft, with : Hep.

Walking, while : Alu; Crot-h; Sep.

Women, old : Psor.

BORING : Bry.

BURNING: *Ars;* Caps; Carb-v; Cep; Iris; Kali-c; Lyc; Merc; Stro; Sul.

Cold application, Amel : Alo; Kali-c; Terb.

Continuous : Kali-c; Lyc.

Pregnancy, during: Caps.

Pressure Amel : Kali-c.

Standing Agg: Crot-h; Lach.

Stools, after Amel : Ver-v.

+ Stools, during and after : Am-m.

Urination, After: Nit-ac; Rhus-t.

CANCER : Alum; Laur; Phyt; Rut; Sang.

CHILLINESS, Stool, before : Lyc.

COITION Agg : Caus; Merc-c; Sil.

COLD, Passing flatus or stool during : Con.

CONSTRICTION, Spasm : Caus; IGN; LACH; Lyc; *Merc-c;* NIT-AC; *Nux-v;* Op; Plb; Rat; Sep; Sil.

Itching, alternating, with : Chel.

Lying Amel : Mang.

Standing Agg : Arn; Ign.

Stools, during : Nat-m; Nit-ac; Plb; Rat; Sil.

after : Colch; Ign; Lach; Nit-ac.

hard, from : Fer.

preventing : Lyc.

Urination, during : Caus.

Uterine, Cancer, from : Kre.

Walking, preventing : Caus.

COUGHING Agg : Ign; *Lach;* Nit-ac; Tub.

CRAWLING (See Anus): Sul.

CUTTING : Alu; Nux-v; Sil.

Diarrhoea, during : *Ars.*

Flatus or passing stools, Amel : Canth.

Standing Agg : Lach.

DRAGGING, Heavy : Aesc; Alo.

DRY : Hypr; Nat-m.

ELECTRIC, Shock, stool, before : Ap.

ENEMA, Water of, escapes : Syph.

FAECES, Remained, as if, in : Grap; Lyc; *Nat-m;* Nit-ac; *Sep;* Ver-a.

FISTULA (See Anus) : Calc-p; *Sil;* Sul.

Pulsating : Caus.

Vagina, and : Thu.

FLUID, Dark, from: Med; Merc-i-f.

FULLNESS : Aesc; Alo; Ham; NIT-AC; *Sul.*

Urination, frequent, with : Fer-pic.

GENITALS, To : Chin; Lil-t; Rhus-t; Sil; Zin.

HEAT, Glowing : Cep.

HEAVY : See Dragging.

HOT Applications Amel : Rat.

ITCHING : See Anus.

LAUGHING Agg : Lach.

NARROW : Nat-m.

NEURALGIA : *Plb.*

+ NUMB : Caus.

ORANGE Coloured, fluid, from : Kali-p.

PAIN, Continuous : Kali-chl; Nit-ac; Phyt.

Diarrhoea, in : Kali-chl.

Long, after stool : Aesc; Agar; Alo; Alum; Am-c; Am-m; Calc; *Colch;* Grap; *Ign;* Mur-ac; Nit-ac; Paeon; Rat; Sil; Stro; Sul.

PAINFUL, Knife sawing up and down : Aesc.

PARESIS, Piles removal, after : Kali-p.

PARTURITION, After : Gel; Pod; Rut.

PASSING Out, something, as if : Lept.

PLUG, Lump : Anac; Cann; Crot-t; Kali-bi; *Lach;* Lil-t; Nat-m; *Plat;* SEP; Sul-ac.

Menses, during : Sil.

Stool, before: Lach.

not amel, by : Sep.

Urination,urging, with : Lil-t.

POCKETS : Polyg.

POLYPUS : Kali-br.

PRESSED, Asunder, as if : Op.

PRESSING Down, on: Crot-t; Pod; SUL.

PRESSURE On Navel Agg : *Crot-t.*

Amel : Kali-c.

PROLAPSED : *Alo;* Ap; Calc; Coll; Gel; *Ign;* Lyc; Merc; *Mur-ac;* Nux-v; Pho; *Pod;* Radm; Rut; Sep.

Acute : Ars; Bell.

Bleeding, from : Ars.

Contracted : Mez.

Coughing, on : Caus.

Diarrhoea Agg : Dul; Merc; Nux-v; Pod.

Easy, straining, without : Grap; Kali-c; Rut.

Flatus, passing : *Mur-ac;* Val.

Mental excitement from : Pod.

Paralysis, with : Plb.

Parturition, after : Gel; Pod.

Pregnancy, during : Pod.

Replacing, difficult : Mez.

Sitting Agg : Ther.

Smoking on : Sep.

Sneezing, on : Pod.

Stool, after : Merc; Mez.

before : Pod; Rut.

during : Ign; Lyc; Pod; Sep.

urging, with : Rut.

Straining without, easy :
Grap; Kali-c; Rut.

Urinating, while : Mur-ac.

Vomiting, while : Mur-ac;
Pod.

Walking, after : Arn.

Washing Body, Amel : Arn.

SHOOTING : Ign.

SNEEZING Agg : Lach.

SORE, Sensitive, smarting:
Bell; Carb-v; Grap; *Mur-ac;*
Nit-ac; Onos; Pul; Radm; Sul.

Ovaries, with : Onos.

STANDING Erect Agg : *Petr.*

STICKS, Burr, Splinter : AESC;
Caus; Grap; Hell; Iris; Nit-ac;
Nux-v; *Rat;* Sanic; Sul.

Flatus passing Amel : Colo;
Mag-c.

Menses, during : Ars.

Vomiting, on : Agar.

STOOPING Agg : Caus; Rut.

Amel : Chel.

STRICTURE : Rut; Syph.

Piles, from : Bap.

TEARING : Tub.

TENESMUS (See Constipation)
: Erig; *Merc-c.*

Dysentery, after : Calc.

Stools, during and after
Amel : Ver-v.

TENSION : Sil.

TESTES, To : Sil.

THIGHS, To : Alum.

THROBBING, Pulsation : Lach.

TINGLING : Carb-v; Colch.

ULCERS : Cham; Sil.

UPWARD, In : Grap; *Ign;* Lach;
Pho; *Sep;* Sul.

URGING, Constant, not for
stool : Lach.

URINATING Agg : *Mur-ac;* Val.

VOMITING Agg : Mur-ac; Pod.

WRISTS, Alternating with :
Sul.

RECURRING : See Relapses.

**RED, REDNESS (Skin, Discharges
etc.)** : ACO; *Ap; Arg-n;* BELL;
Bry; Cham; Chin; Jab; Lach;
Meli; *Merc; Nux-v;* Op; Pho;
Rhus-t; Sabi; *Sang;* Sep;
SUL.

BLUISH, Dark : Bap; Phyt;
Rhus-t.

BODY, Whole : Op.

FIERY : Bell; Cinb; Med;
Stram; Sul.

ORIFICES : See Orifices.

+ PARTS, Become PALE : Fer.

ROSY : Ap; Pyro; Sil.

SPOTS : Merc; Pic-ac; Rhus-t;
Stic; Sul.

Blood : Cor-r; Pho.

Elevated : Mang.

Fiery : Med.

Pink : Colch.

Small, body, all over : Scil.

Wine : Coc; *Sep.*

STREAKS : Bell; Bry; Buf; Myg; Pyro.

TURN, White : Bor; Hell; Merc; Val.

Yellow or green : Con.

REELING, TOTTERING,Staggering, Feeling (See Gait): Ars; Bell; Bry; Caus; Gel; Ign; *Lach*; Nux-v; Op; Rhus-t; Stram; Sul; Ver-a; Ver-v.

COITION, After : Bov.

REGURGITATION : Aeth; Ant-c; Ant-t; Arn; Asaf; *Bry*; Carb-v; Chin; Fer; Fer-p; Lach; Merc; NUX-V; PHO; Pho-ac; *Pul*; Sars; *Sul*; Sul-ac; Vario.

ASTRINGENT : Merc-c.

BITTER : Lyc; Nat-c.

Food : Lyc; Nat-s.

COUGHING After : Raph.

EATING, Immediately, after : Mag-p.

Hour, after : Aeth.

FLUIDS, Of : Asaf; Kali-bi; Pul; Sul-ac.

Painless, Diphtheria in : Carb-ac.

INGESTA, Of : Bry; *Pho;* Pul.

MILKY : Sep.

MOUTHFUL, By : Fer; *Pho.*

MUCOUS, Of : Hyds.

Frothy : Sep.

SALTY : Kali-c.

SOUR : Mag-c.

STOOPING, While : Pho.

VEXATION, After : Fer-p.

WALKING, While : Mag-m.

WANTS, To : Vario.

WATERY : Ap.

RELAPSES, RECURRENCES, Attacks, recurrent (See also Paroxysms repeated) : Aco; Ars; Bar-c; Bar-m; Bell; Chin; Colo; Cup; Dios; Hep; Kali-io; Lyc; Mag-p; Mez; Nat-m; Pho; *Psor;* Sul; Tub; Val; Verb.

EASY : Asaf; Cup.

RELAPSING FEVER : See under Fever.

RELAXATION, FLABBY Feeling (See Inactive) : *Aeth;* Alet; Alo; *Ant-t;* Ars; Bov; *Calc;* Caps; CAUS; Chin; Cocl; *Colch;* GEL; Grap; Hell; *Hyo;* Lob; LYC; *Mag-c;* Merc-cy; MUR-AC; Nat-c; Nat-m; Op; PHO-AC; Seneg; Sep; *Spo;* Ver-a.

AMEL : Tarn.

INTERNAL : *Calc;* Kre; SEP.

RELIGIOUS, IDEAS, Minded : *Ars; Aur;* Hyo; *Lach;* Lil-t; Lyc; Pul; *Stram; Sul;* VER-A; Zin.

CHILDREN, In : Ars; Calc; Lach; Sul.

INSANITY : Nat-c; Stram.

+ MANIA : Anac.

MELANCHOLY : Kali-p; Meli.

+ SALVATION, Despair of : Ver-a.

SEXUAL EXCITEMENT, Alternating with : Lil-t; *Plat.*

WANT, Of, Feeling : See Godless.

REMITTENCY : Gel.

REMITTENT FEVER : See Under Fever.

REMORSE : See Guilt, Sense of.

COMPLAINTS, From : Arn.

TRIFLES, About : Sil.

RENDING : See Pain, Shooting.

REPEATED: Lach; Lyc; Stan; Zin.

SAME ACTION : Cheno.

REPENTENCE, ILL EFFECTS, Of : Arn.

REPRIMANDS AGG : Colo; *Ign;* Op; Stap.

LAUGHS, At : Grap.

REPROACHES, HIMSELF : Aur; Cyc; Kali-br; Stram.

OTHERS : *Aco; Ars;* Chin; Mez; *Nux-v.*

REPUGNANCE TO EVERYTHING : Ant-c; Merc; Pul.

REPUTATION, LOSS OF AGG : Kali-br.

RESERVED : Lyc; Nat-m.

+ ANGER : Stap.

DISPLEASURE : Aur; Ign; Ip; Nat-m; *Stap.*

RESPIRATION AFFECTIONS, In General : Aco; *Ant-t; Ap;* ARS; *Bell;* Bry; Carb-v; Cup; Dig; Dros; Grind; Hep; Ip; *Kali-c;* LACH; Lob; *Lyc;* Nat-s; OP; PHO; PUL; Ran-b; *Samb;* SPO; Stan; SUL; Tarn; Vib.

ABDOMINAL : *Ant-t.*

AIR, Open Agg : Psor.

Amel : Ant-t; Ap; Nat-m; Pul;

Sul.

ANXIOUS : ACO; Ars; Bar-m; Chel; *Ip;* Nat-m; *Pho;* Pru-sp; *Pul;* Ran-b; *Scil;* Sec; Spo; *Stan.*

ARMS Apart Amel : Lach; Laur; Nux-v; Psor; Spig; Tarn.

Exertion, Amel : Nat-m.

Motion of, Raising Agg : Am-m; Berb; Lach; Spig; Tarn.

ARRESTED : See Difficult.

Children, lifted on being : Bor; Calc-p.

Coughing or drinking, on : Anac.

ASCENDING Amel, Walking on level ground, Agg : Ran-b.

Stairs Agg : Iod; Merc.

ASTHMATIC : See Asthma.

BACK Touching Agg : Adon.

BENDING, Backwards Agg : Cup; Psor.

Head, backwards Amel: Hep; Lach; *Spo;* Ver-a.

BREATHE, AGAIN Can not : See under Breathe.

CARDIAC (See Difficult) : Cratae; Strop.

CHEYNE-STOKES : Bell; Carb-v; Coca; Grind; Op; Sul; Sul-ac.

CHOKING : See Difficult.

CLOTHING Agg : Ars; Chel; Lach.

COITION, Emission Agg : *Amb;* Ced; Dig; Pho; Stap.

Desire for, with : Nat-c.

COLIC Agg (See Pains during AGG) : Arg-n; Berb.

CONSUMPTION, In: Carb-v; Ip; Pho.

COUGH Agg : Am-m; Ant-t; Ars; Cup; *Dros;* Ip; Just; Merc-cy; Naj; Nux-v; Op; *Pho;* Stan;Tarn; Tub.

Alternating, with: Ant-t.

Before : Ant-t; Caus.

COVERING Nose or Mouth Agg : Arg-n; Cup; Lach.

DEEP :Arg-n; Aur; *Bry;* Calc; *Caps;* Carb-v; Coca; Hep; IGN; *Ip; Lach;* Lil-t; Nat-s; *Op;* Pho; Plat; *Sele; Sil;* Sul.

Breath, wants : Arg-n; Aur; Bro; Bry; Cact; Calc; Caps; Cup; Dig; Hyd-ac; *Ign; Lach;* Lil-t; Mos; Nat-s; Op; Sele; Sul; Xanth.

Agg : Thu.

Amel : Caps; Sul.

Enough, cannot get: Aur; Crot-t; Lach; Pru-sp; Radm.

Excites, cough: Arg-n; Bro; Bry.

Inability to take : Strych.

Yawns to force it down: Pru-sp.

DIFFICULT, Suffocating Choking : Aco; Anac; *Ant-t;* Ap; ARS; *Bro; Bry;* Cact; Carb-v; Caus; Chel; Chin; *Chlor;* Cina; Crot-t; *Cup;* Cup-ar; Fer; *Hep; Ign; Iod;* IP; Kali-ar; *Kali-c; Kali-io;* Kali-m;

LACH; Laur; Lob; Lyc; Meph; Merc-c; *Naj;* Nat-m; *Nat-s;* Nux-m; *Op; Pho;* PUL; Rum; *Samb;* Scil; Sele; SPO; *Stan;* SUL; *Sumb;* Tarn; *Ver-a;* Ver-v; Vib.

Anger from, Adults : Ran-b.

children : Arn.

Ankles, swelling around with : Hep.

Athletes, aged, in : Coca.

+ Breathing deep Agg : Thu.

+ Coition, Agg : Stap.

+ Consumption, in: Carb-v; Ip; Pho.

Coryza, with : Ars; Ars-io; Calc; Ip; Nit-ac; Pho; Sul.

Crowd, in : Arg-n.

+ Crowded room, in: Lil-t.

Diseased condition of distant parts not involved in respiration : Berb; Pul.

Dropsy, in : Eup-pur.

Epilepsy, before : Am-br.

Exhalation (See exhalation AGG*):* *Chlor;* Kali-io; Med; Meph; *Samb.*

Eyes, closing on : Carb-an.

Falling down, on : Petr.

Flatulence, from : Arg-n; Zin.

Formication, preceded by : Cist.

Fright, from : Samb.

+ Gastric Pain, with : Arg-n.

Haemoptysis, with : Arn.

Hiccough, with : Aeth.

Inhalation : Bro; Caus; Samb.

Itching, with : Saba.

Knocked down, when: Petr.

Labour pain, each, with : *Lob.*

Lips, redness of, with : Spig.

Menses, after : Am-c.

   during : Colo.

Metrorrhagia, with: Flu-ac.

Motion, rapid Amel: Lob.

Nausea with : Ip; Kali-n.

Nervous : *Arg-n*; Ars; Carb-an; Lob; Mos.

Nose felt, in: See Nose, Dyspnea, in.

  itching, after : Saba.

Pregnancy, during : Vio-o.

Pricking, with : Lob.

+ Sitting up, Agg : *Lauro.*

Sleep, falling to, on : Bap; Dig; Grap; *Grind; Lach; Op.*

  after : Sep.

Sneezing Agg : Naj; Pho.

  with : Ars-io; Pho.

+ Standing Amel : Sep.

Sweat, with : Bap.

Ulcer, with : Kali-n.

Uremia, with : Solid.

Uterine displacement, from : Nit-ac.

Vertigo, with : Kali-c.

+ Wakes him : Am-c.

Yawning Agg : Bro.

DRAWING Shoulders back Amel : Calc; Calc-ac.

DUST Agg : Ars-io; Bro; Dul; Nat-ars; *Poth; Sil.*

EATING Agg: Kali-p; Lach; Nat-s; *Pho;* Pul; Zin-val.

  Amel : Amb; *Grap;* Iod; Med; *Spo.*

EMPHYSEMA Agg : Am-c; Sars.

EPIGASTRIUM, or, Stomach, from : *Ars;* Chin; Cocl; Guai; Lach; Nat-m; *Pho;* Rhus-t; Sul.

ERUCTATIONS Amel : Amb; Ant-t; Aur; *Carb-v;* Mos; *Nux-v.*

EXERTION Agg : Ars; Calc; Coca; Ip; Lach; Lob; Lyc; Lycps; Nat-m; Spo.

  Least Agg : Calc; Con; Kali-c; Nat-s.

EXPECTORATION Amel: *Ant-t;* Aral; Grind; Hypr; Ip; Lach; Sep; Zin.

EYES, Closing Agg: Carb-an; *Carb-v.*

FANNED, Wants to be : Carb-v; Med; Naj.

GASPING : Ap; Carb-v; Cor-r; Hyd-ac; Kali-n; Latro; Laur; Lob; Lyc; Meph.

  Chorea, with : Laur.

  Haemorrhage, with : Ip.

  Spasms, before, during, after : Caus; Laur.

HANDS, Using on : Bov.

HANG Down Legs Amel : Sul-ac.

HEART Symptoms or pain with : Cact; Carb-v; *Kalm;* Spig; Spo; Strop; Sumb; Tarn.

  And ovarian troubles with : *Tarn.*

And urinary troubles with : *Laur;* Lycps.

HEAT, With or overheated Agg : Ap; Kali-c.

HEAVY : Glo; Ver-v.

HISSING : See Whistling.

HOLDING, Something to Amel : Grap.

HOT : See Breath Hot.

HUMID AIR Agg : Aur; Bar-c; *Nat-s.*

HYSTERICAL (See Nervous) : *Arg-n;* Ars; Nux-m; Val.

INJURY,From : Petr.

INSPIRATION Double : Led.

IRREGULAR : Ail; BELL; *Cup;* Dig; Hyd-ac; Op; Sul.

ITCHING, With : Saba.

JERKY : Bell; *Ign;* Laur; Ox-ac; Tab.

KNEELING Amel : Caus.

KYPHOSIS, In : Aco; Ant-c; Asaf; Aur; Bar-c; Bell; Bry; Calc; Cam; Cic; Clem; Colo; Dul; Hep; Ip; Rhus-t; Rut; Sabi; Sep; Sil; Stap; Sul; Thu.

LAST Breath, cease as if : See Breathe again can not.

LAUGHING Agg : Aur; Cup.

LIGHT : See Shallow.

LIPS, Red, with : Spig.

LONG : Lil-t.

LOUD, Noisy : Calc; CHAM; *Chin;* Kali-bi; Lach; Pho; *Samb;* SPO; Sul; Ver-a.

LYING Agg : Ap; Ars; Carb-v; Grap; Kali-c; Lob; Tub.

Amel : Calc-p; Chel; Dig;

Hell; Kali-bi; Laur; Nux-v; *Psor;* Terb.

Back on Agg : Lyc.

Amel : *Cact;* Kalm.

Head low, with agg : Ap; Cact; Chin; Kali-c.

Side on Agg : Ars; Pul.

Amel : Alu.

right Amel : Naj; Spig.

head high with Amel : Cact; Spig; Spo.

left Agg : Merc.

Amel : Castr.

MOTION Agg : Ars; Bry; Calc; Chin; Kali-c; Spig; Spo; Stan.

Amel : Arg-n; Aur; Bro; *Fer;* Lob; Pho; Pul; Samb.

Quick Agg : Merc.

NIGHT Agg : Ars; Kali-ar; Lach; Naj; Ox-ac; Pho; Samb; Sul; Vib.

Mid night Agg : Ars; Fer; Grap; Samb.

ODOUR Agg : Ars; Pho-ac; Sang.

OPPRESSED : ACO; Am-c; Ap; Apoc; ARS; Ars-io; *Bell; Bry;* Cact; CARB-V; Chin-s; Colch; *Cup;* Fer; *Ign;* IP; Kali-c; Kali-m; Nat-s; Nux-m; *Nux-v;* Op; PHO; PUL; Sele; Seneg; *Sep;* SUL; Tub; *Ver-a.*

Epilepsy, before : Am-br.

Fever, during: Bov; Kali-c.

Room, crowded, in : Lil-t.

Spasms, alternating with : Ign.

Talking Agg : Caus.

Walking rapidly Agg : Meli.

PAIN, During Agg : *Ars*; Bry; Carb-v; Cocl; Kalm; Nat-m; Pru-sp; *Pul;* Ran-sc; Sep; Sil; Sul.

Gastric Agg : Arg-m; Arg-n; Berb.

PAINFUL : Bry; *Ran-b.*

PALPITATION, With : Aur; Kalm; Mer-i-f; Pul; Spig; Ver-a.

PANTING : Bry; Calad; *Ip; Nit-ac;* Pho; Stram; Ver-v.

Reading, when : Nit-ac.

Running rapidly, as from : Hyo.

Stooping on : Nit-ac.

PUFFING, Stertorous : Am-c; Cheno; Naj; Op.

QUICK : ACO; Ant-t; Ars; *Bell;* Bry; *Carb-v;* Chel; *Cup;* Gel; Ip; *Lyc; Pho; Sep;* SUL.

RATTLING : Am-c; ANT-T; Apoc; Ars; Cact; *CAarb-v;* Caus; Chin; *Cup;* Dul; HEP; IP; Kali-s; Lob; *Lyc;* Pho; Pul; *Scil; Seneg;* Sil; Stan.

But no expectoration : *Ip; Lob.*

Cold drinks Agg : Pho.

READING Agg : Nit-ac.

RUNNING Amel, Slow motion Agg : Sep.

SHALLOW : *Bell;* Chin; *Laur;* Nux-m; *Pho.*

SHRILL : Bell; Gel; Ign; Mos.

SHORT : See Difficult.

SIGHING : Bry; Calad; Calc-p; Carb-v; Dig; IGN; Ip; *Lach;*

Op; Sec; Sele; *Sil;* Stram.

Cough, after : Led.

Leucorrhea, with : Phys.

Sleep, in : *Aur;* Calc.

Unconsciousness, with: Glo.

SINGING, When Agg : Arg-m.

SITTING Erect Amel : Aco; *Kali-c;* Lach; Laur; Lyc; Nat-c; Seneg; Terb.

Head bent forward on knee, with Amel : Kali-c.

SLEEP Falling to, on Agg (See also Difficult) : Am-c; *Ars;* Cadm; Carb-v; Gel; *Grind;* Kali-c; *Lach;* Pho; Spo; Sul; Tab.

SLOW : Bell; Hyd-ac; *Op;* Ver-v.

SMOKE, Vapour, Fumes, as of : Ars; Bar-c; Bro; Chin; *Ign;* Lach; Lyc; Pul.

SNEEZING Agg : Naj; Pho.

Amel : Naj.

With : Ambro; Ars-io; Pho.

SNORING : Hyo; Merc-c; Nat-m; Op.

Adenoids, removal after : Kali-s.

Children, in : Mez.

SOBBING : See Sighing.

SPINE, Pressing on Agg: Chin-s.

STANDING Amel : Bap; Cann; Sil; Spig.

STOMACH, From : See Epigastrium.

STOOL Amel : Poth.

STOOPING Agg : Calc; Nit-ac; Sil.

STOPS, Coughing or Swallowing on : Anac.

SUMMER Agg: Arg-n; Syph.

SWALLOWING Agg : Bell; *Bro*; Calc; Cup.

SWEAT, With : Samb.

TALKING Agg : Lach; Spo; Sul; Thu.

Amel : Fer.

Fast Agg : Caus.

TONGUE, Red, with : Mos.

UNEQUAL, Intermittent : Ant-t; Nit-ac; Op.

URINATING Agg : Chel; Dul.

WATER, Standing in Agg : Nux-m.

WET WEATHER Agg : Aran; Nat-s.

WHISTLING, Hissing, Wheezing : Ars; Aur; Caus; Chin; Hep; Ip; Kali-c; Kali-io; *Samb*; Seneg; Spo; Stram.

YAWNING Amel : Croc.

RESPONSIBILITY, INABILITY To realize: Flu-ac.

UNUSUAL Agg: Aur.

REST *AGG*: See Motion, Amel.

CAN NOT, IN ANY POSITION : *Lyc*; Pip-m; Ran-b; Rhus-t; Sanic; Sul; Syph; Xanth. Sleep, during : Caus. When things are not in proper place : Anac; *Ars*.

RESTLESSNESS *ANXIOUS* : ARS; *Calc*; Cimi; Iod; Kali-ar; Kali-c; Merc; Nat-c; Pho; *Tarn*.

Lying down Amel : Mang.

GENERAL, Physical : ACO; Anac; *Ap*; Arg-n; ARS; Bap; *Bell*; Calc; Calc-p; Cam; *Cham*; *Cimi*; Cina; *Cof*; Colo; Cup; *Fer*; HYO; Lyc; Mag-p; Mar-v; MERC; *Pho*; Plb; Pul; RHUS-T; Sec; SEP; Sil; Stap; Stram; *Sul*; TARN; Val; Vib; *Zin*.

AFTERNOON Agg : Bor.

+ ALONE, When : Pho.

+ BUSY : Ver-a.

COMPELLING, Rapid walking : Arg-n; *Ars*; Tarn.

+ CONSTANT Walking : Pru-sp.

CONVULSIONS, Before: *Arg-n*; Buf.

After : Oenan.

EXERTION, Least, Agg: *Merc*.

EYES, Closing on, at night : *Mag-m*; Sep.

HANDS, Clutching, tightly Amel : Med.

INTERNAL : Ars; Rhus-t; Sil.

MENSES, Before : Kre; Sul.

SITTING, While : Lyc.

SLEEP, Loss of, from : Lac-d.

SUNLIGHT Agg : Cadm.

THUNDERSTORM, Before : Psor.

TOSSING About, in: Aco; Ars; Bell; Cham; *Cof*; Cup; Fer; Rhus-t; Tarn.

WALKING, Air open, in, Amel : Lyc; Pul.

+ WEEPING, With : Rhod.

WORKING, While : GRAP.

FDCRETCHING AND GAGGING
: Bell; Bry; Cham; Colch;
Dros; Eup-p; *Ip; Nux-v;* Phyt;
Pod; Pul; Rhus-t; Sul; Tab;
Ver-a.

AGG From : Asar.

CONSTANT : Pod.

COUGHING, When : Cina; Hep;
Nit-ac; Stan.

DYSPNOEA, From : Am-c.

EATING, When : Ver-a.

Amel : Ign; Nat-c.

EMOTIONS, From : Op.

EMPTY : Asar; Sec.

+ Agg, all Symptoms : Asar.

EPILEPSY, Before : Cup.

EXPECTORATING, When : Carb-v;
Sil; Tarn.

FOOD, Thought, of : Merc-cy.

HAPPY SURPRISE, From : Kali-c.

HAWKING Agg : Arg-n; Nux-v.

MENSES, During : Pul.

STOOL, Diarrhoea, during :
Arg-n; Cup; Pod.

SWALLOWING, Empty, On : Grap.

VIOLENT : Phyt.

+ Before, vomiting : Cham.

VOMITING, After : Colch.

WARM Drinks Amel: Ther.

YAWNS, Then : Tell.

RETENTION SENSE, Of : Tell.

RETICENT : See Taciturn.

RETINA, ANAEMIA : Lith.

ANAESTHESIA, Looking at
eclipse, from : Hep.

DETACHMENT, Of : *Aur;* Dig; *Gel;*
Naph; Pho.

EMBOLISM, Central Artery of :
Op.

EXUDATION : Kali-m.

HAEMORRHAGE: Arn; Bothr;
Crot-h; Ham; *Lach;* Led;
Pho.

+ HYPERAESTHESIA: Ox-ac.

IMAGES, Retained, too long
: Gel; *Jab; Lac-c;* Nat-m;
TAB; Tub.

INFLAMMATION : Aur; Merc;
Merc-c; Plb; Sul.

Albuminuric : Gel; Merc-c;
Pho.

pregnancy during : Kalm.

Diabetic : Sec.

Eyes, overuse from : Sul.

Haemorrhagic : Merc-c.

Pigmentary (Retinitis

Pigmentosa) : Nux-v; Pho.

INJURIES : See Haemorrhage.

OEDEMA : Ap; Kali-io.

THROMBOSIS, Degeneration
: Ham; Pho.

RETINITIS: See Retina,
Inflammation.

RETRACTION DRAWN BACK
: Ast-r; Cic; Clem; Crot-t;
Cup; Hyds; Lach; *Merc;*
Nat-m; Nux-v; Op; Par; *Phyt;*
PLB; Sars; Sil; Thu; *Zin.*

REVENGEFUL, SPITEFUL :
Calc; Lach; Nat-m; Nit-ac;
Nux-v.

REVERBERATIONS : See
Noises in Head, also
Hearing Illusory Sounds.

REVERY : See Dreaminess.

RHEUMATISM (See Joints)
: Aco; Arn; Ars; *Bell;* Benz-
ac; BRY; *Caus;* Cham; Chel;
Colch; Fer-p; Form; Kali-io;
Kalm; Led; *Lyc; Merc;* Med;
Phyt; PUL; Rhod; RHUS-T;
Sang; Sars; Stic; *Sul;* Thu.

+ **A**CUTE **A**RTICULAR : Tub.

ALTERNATING, With: Kali-bi;
Lapp; Urt.

Mental Symptoms, with :
Cimi.

Urinary, affections, with :
Benz-ac.

ASTHMA, With : Benz-ac.

CHRONIC, Rigidity, with : Ol-j.
Ankylosis, with : Kali-io.

COLD **A**MEL : Am-c; Guai; *Led;
Pul; Sec.*

DIARRHOEA, After : Abro; Cimi;
Dul; Kali-bi.
With : Dul.

DYSPEPSIA, With : Nat-c.

ERUPTIONS, With : Dul.

GONORRHOEA, Checked, from
: Thu.

HIVES, With : Urt.

HOT WEATHER, Heat Agg :
COLCH; Kali-bi; Kali-s; Rhod.

INABILITY To move limbs :
Abro.

KIDNEY Affections, with :
Radm; Terb.

PARALYTIC : Colch.

RECURRENT : Nat-s; Senec.

TONSILITIS, After : Echi; Guai;
Lach; Phyt.

RHUS POISON : Rhus-t.

RHYTHMIC : Agar; Lyc; Stram.

RIBS ALONG : Ap.

BALL, Round moving to and
from, as if : Cup.

BELOW : Ap; Chin; Sul; Terb.
Balls, round : Cup.

DISLOCATED, Broken, as if :
Agar; Caps; Kali-bi; Naj;
Petr; Psor; Stram.

EXOSTOSIS : Merc-c.

FIFTH and Sternum, right :
Mag-c; Thu.
Left : Ox-ac.

FLOATING : Benz-ac.
Right : Berb.
undulating pain, along :
Amy-n; Arg-n.

LAST, Left : Arg-n.
Boil, near : Arg-n.

LUNG, Sticking to, as if :
Kali-c.

NEURALGIA, Lower left : Arg-m.

PLUG Between: Anac; Aur;
Caus; Cocl; *Lyc; Ran-sc;
Ver-a.*

SORE : Carb-v.

STEPPING Agg : Rat.

UPWARDS, From : Ap.

RICKETS: *Calc; Calc-p;* Kali-io;
Pho; Sil; Sul.

+ **RIDICULED**, IS BEING : Bar-c.

RIDING ON HORSE BACK (See
Jarring) **A**GG : Ars; Bell; Bor;
Bry; Grap; Lil-t; Mag-m; Rut;
SEP; Sil; Spig; *Sul-ac;* Val.

AMEL : Bro; Calc; Lyc; Tarn.

CAR, In **A**GG and **A**MEL : See
Car Sickness.

RIGIDITY : See Stiffness.

RINGING NOISES : See Hearing, Illusory Noises.

RINGWORM : See Eruptions.

ALL OVER, the body: Psor; Ran-b.

RISING, ARMS, Uses for :Hyds.

EFFORTS At : Aesc; Agar; Petr; Rut; Sul.

SITTING, Seat from AGG : Aesc; Agar; Ant-t; Berb; BRY; Calc; *Caps; Caus; Con*; Kali-bi; Led; *Lyc; Nat-s;* Petr; PHO; *Pul; Rhus-t;* Rut; Sep; *Spig;* Stap; SUL.

AMEL : Kob; Rut.

Bed from Amel : See Bed.

Body feels heavy, sore : Spig.

STOOPING, From AGG: Lyc; *Pho;* Pul.

THEN FALLING : See Directions, Up and Down.

TURNS, To right, when : Kali-c.

RIVET FEELING : Lil-t; Sul.

ROAMING, ROVING : Lyss; Nux-v.

AIMLESS : Ver-a.

ROARING : See Head, Noises in, and Hearing Illusory Sounds.

ROBUST HABIT : Aco; Asaf; Bell; Caps.

EMACIATING, Suddenly : Samb.

ROCKING AGG : *Bor;* Carb-v; Cocl; Thu.

AMEL: Carb-an; Cham; Cina; Kali-c; *Merc-c;* Pul; Pyro; Rhus-t; Sec.

To and Fro : Bell; Hyo.

ROLLING, ROLLS on the floor

: Calc; Cic; *Op;* Paeon; Tarn.

OR TURNING Over, as if : Am-c; Ars; BELL; Cact; Crot-h; Cup; Gel; *Grap;* Kali-c; LACH; Lyc; Pho; Pul; Rhus-t; Saba; SEP; Tarn.

FILTH, In his own : Cam.

SIDE To SIDE : Am-c; Ars; Lach; Tarn.

ROMANTIC : Cocl.

+ SENSITIVE GIRLS : Cocl.

ROOM IN AGG : See Air Open Amel.

AMEL : Chin; Cocl; Tarn.

CLOSE AGG : Amy-n; Just; Lil-t; Med; *Tub;* Vib.

FULL OF PEOPLE AGG : Arg-n; Lil-t; Lyc; Pho; Plb; Sep.

LIGHTS Many, with AGG : Nux-v.

SHUT AGG : Arg-n; Lac-d.

TOO MANY, Things, in AGG : Phys.

ROSEOLA: See under Eruptions.

ROTATION AGG : Bry; Cocl; Colo; Kali-c.

ROUGH, SCRATCHY, As of a rough body : Aesc; *Alu;* Amb; Am-m; Arg-n; *Berb;* Kal-bi; Mang; Naj; Nat-m; *Nux-v;* Par; Pho; *Phyt;* Rut; *Sul.*

RUBBING, STROKING AGG : *Anac; Con; Old; Pul; Sep; Stro;* Sul.

AMEL : *Calc; Canth;* Cina; *Cup; Dros;* ag-p; Merc; Mos; NAT-C; Ol-an; Pall; (Calc-f; Carb-u; Graph;)

PHO; PLB; Pod; Rhus-t; Rut; Sep; Sil; Tarn; Thu; Val; Zin; Zin-v.

ABDOMEN AMEL : Nat-s;Pall; Pod.

CLOTHES, Of AGG : Old.

GENTLY AGG : Mar-c.

AMEL : Crot-t; Form; Dios; Lil-t; Lyss; Med.

HAND, Warm, with AMEL : Lil-t.

HARD AMEL : Med; Radm.

SOLES AMEL : Chel.

TOGETHER, As if : Cocl; Kali-bi; Sul.

RUBELLA: See under Eruptions.

RUDE : See Insolent.

RUMBLING : See Abdomen, and Roaring under Hearing, illusory sounds.

RUNNING : See Creeping as of Animals; and Motion Rapid.

BACKWARDS : Bry.

BETTER, Than walking : Tarn.

FORWARDS, Trying to walk when : Mang.

IMPULSE, For : Iod; Orig; Ver-a.

Menses, before : Lach.

RECKLESSLY, Room, in: Saba.

RUNS ABOUT (See Escape) : Hyo; Stram; Ver-a.

MENSES, Before: Lach.

RUN ROUND : See Fingers, Felon.

RUPIA : See under Eruptions.

RUSTY : See Brownish.

SACRUM And REGION : Aesc;

Agar; Gel; Grap; Hep; Hypr; Mur-ac; Pul; Rhus-t; Sep.

BREATHING Agg : Merc.

BRUISED : Aesc; Rut.

BURNING : Kre; Pho; Pod; Terb.

COLD, Icy, near : Arg-m; Benz-ac; Dul.

COUGHING Agg : Bry; Chel; Tell.

CRAWLING : Grap.

DAMP Cloth, on : Sanic.

DRAGGING : Helo.

Buttocks, to : Helo.

EXOSTOSES : Rhus-t.

FEET, To : Kali-m; Kob.

FORCEPS Delivery, after : Hypr.

HEAVY, Weight : Arg-n; Chin.

Genitals, in, with : Lob.

Sitting, while : Rhus-t.

LAUGHING Agg : Tell.

LEUCORRHOEA Agg : Aesc; Psor.

Amel : Murx.

LYING Agg : Berb.

Amel : Agar.

MENSES, At start of Agg : Asar.

Before Agg : Nux-m; Sabi; Spo.

Instead, of : Spo.

NUMB : Calc-p; Grap.

Legs and : Calc-p; Grap.

PARALYSED, As if : Pho.

PARTURITION, After : Hypr; Nux-v; Pho.

+ PILES, Due to : Abro.

PRICKLING : Mez.

PULSATING : Nat-m.

RIDING, Car in, Agg : Nux-m.

SENSITIVE To touch of clothes : Lob.

SITTING + Agg : Rhod.

Erect Agg : Lyc.

SOLID, As if : Sep.

SPRAINED, As if : Ol-an.

STANDING, Erect Agg : Petr.

STOOLS Pressing, at Agg : Tell.

STOOPING Agg : Kali-bi.

SWEAT, Cold, on : Plant.

THIGH Into, right : Colch; Tell.

Left : Kali-c.

TOUCH, Slight Agg : Lob.

URINATING Agg : Grap; Sul.

+ UTERINE, Disease from : Sep.

WEAK : Pho; Sep; Sil.

WOOD, Stretched Across, as if : Nux-m.

SADNESS, LOW SPIRITS, Mental Depression : Abro; Aco; *Ars*; AUR; Calc; CARB-AN; Caus; Cham; *Chin; Cimi;* Colch; Gel; GRAP; Helo; IGN; Iod; Kali-br; Kali-io; *Kali-p;* Lac-c; Lac-d; *Lach*; Lept; Lil-t; *Lyc; Med;* Merc; Mill; Murx; *Mur-ac;* NAT-C; NAT-M; *Nat-s;* NIT-AC; Plat; PSOR; PUL; *Rhus-t;* Sele; Sep; STAN; Sul; Syph; Tarx; Thu; Ver-a; Zin; Zin-ph.

CAUSELESS : Nat-m; Pho; Sars; Stap; Tarn.

CHILDREN, In : Ars; Calc; Lach.

CLIMAXIS, At : Manc.

COITION Agg : Nat-m; Sep; Sul.

COMPANY, Society Agg : Euphr.

Amel : Bov.

+ CONFIDENCE, Lack of : Old.

CONTINENCE Agg : *Con.*

DOMESTIC Affairs, over : Sep.

EATING Agg : Grap; Nux-v.

Amel : Tarn.

ELATION, Alternating with : Cof; Senec.

EMISSION, From : *Nux-v;* Pul.

ENJOYS : Ign; Nat-m.

+ EVERYTHING Viewed, in Bad light : Alu.

FEAR, From : Sec.

FLATULENCE, With : Scop.

FLOWERS, Smell of, from : Hyo.

GIRLS, Puberty before : Ars; Hell; Lach.

+ GRIEF, From : Nux-m.

HAPPY, On Seeing others : Cic; Helo.

HEALTH, One's over : Sep.

HORRID : Syph.

INDIFFERENCE, Alternating with : Sep.

JOY, Alternating, with : See Elation, Alternating.

LIGHT, Subdued Agg : Nat-s.

LOVE, Unhappy, from : Dig.

MASTURBATION Agg : Con; Nat-m; *Pho-ac;* Plat.

MENSES, Before : Nat-m; Pul; Stan.

Suppressed : Con.

MUSIC Agg : *Aco;* Dig; Nat-p; Nat-s; Sabi.

Distant Agg : Lyc.

Sad Amel : Mang.

PAIN, From : Sars.

PARTURITION, After : Thu.

PERSPIRATION, During : Con.

PREGNANCY, In : Lach; Nat-m.

PUBERTY, At: Ant-c; *Hell*; Manc; Nat-m.

   Girls, before : Ars; Hell; Lach.

SAD Stories, from : *Cic.*

SEXUAL Erethism, with : Manc.

   Loss of power, from : Spo.

SOCIETY : See Company.

STERILITY, From : Aur.

SUNSHINE Agg : Stram.

SYMPATHY Agg : Con.

THUNDER Storm Amel : Sep.

TRIFLES, About : Dig; Grap.

WAKING, On: Alu; Coc-c; Lach.

WALKING Only while : Pho-ac.

WEEP, Can not : Am-m; Gel; *Nat-m*

   Amel : Dig; Med; Pho.

SALIVA : Merc; Sul.

ACRID : Aru-t; Kre; Merc; Merc-c; Merc-i-f; *Nit-ac.*

BITTER : Ars; *Chel.*

BLOODY : Buf; Crot-c; Mag-c; Merc; NIT-AC; *Pho*; Rhus-t.

   Menses, before : Nat-m.

   Sleep, during : Rhus-t.

   Taste, disgusting, with : Kali-io.

     sweetish, with : Kali-io.

BLUE : Plb.

COLD : Asar; Bor-ac; Cist.

CONVULSIONS, With : Bar-m; Kali-bi; *Oenan.*

COTTONY : See Frothy.

DARK : Merc-d.

DIMINISHED, Scanty : *Bell*; Kali-bi; Merc-c; Nux-m; Nux-v; Pho; Stram; Sul; *Ver-a.*

DRIES On Palate and Lips, Becomes tough : Lyc.

EGG, White of, like : Calad; Jab.

FOUL, Foetid : Iod; Lach; Manc; MERC; Merc-d; *Nit-ac*; Petr.

   Hot : Daph; Saba.

FROTHY, Cottony, Foamy : Ap; Bell; *Berb*; Caul; Dul; *Ign*; Iod; Kali-m; Lach; *Nux-m*; Ol-an; Pho; Pho-ac; Pic-ac; *Pul*; Sabi; Spig.

GREEN : Grap; Sec.

GUSHES, Of : Carb-v; Ign; Nat-m.

   Suddenly : Ign; Nat-m.

   Colic, with: Led.

INCREASED (Salivation): Am-c; Aru-t; Bar-c; Bor; *Dig; Dul*; Flu-ac; Ip; *Iris*; Kali-c; Lyss; *Manc;* MERC; Merc-c; Merc-i-r; Nat-m; *Nit-ac; Nux-v*; Pho; *Pul*; Ran-b; RHUS-T; Stram; VER-A.

   Accompaniment, as a : Lob.

   Colic, with : Led.

   Coryza, with : Kali-io.

   Cough, with : Am-m; Lach; Thu; Ver-a.

   Dark, putrid : Merc-d.

   Dentition, during : Helo.

   Diarrhoea, with : Rhe.

Diphtheria, during : Lac-c.

Dryness, with : Calad; Lyc; *Merc*; Nat-m.

Dyspnoea, with : Lob.

Headache, with : Epiph; *Merc*; Nat-s.

Heat, all over, with : *Cic.*

Hiccough, with: Lob.

Hunger, with: Lob.

Larynx, pressure on, as if, with : Tarx.

Menses, before : Pul.

during : Merc; Nux-m; Phyt; Pul; Pulex

after : Ced.

Nausea, with : Lob.

Nauseous, taste, with : Sul.

Night, sweetish taste : Cham.

Pain, colic etc. Agg : Cocl; Epiph; Gran; Helo; Led; Mang; Merc; Pho; Plant; Rhe.

Paralysis, in : Mang.

Pregnancy, in : Ant-t; Cof; Helo; Kre; Lob; Zin-s.

Retching, with : Lob.

Sleep, during : *Bar-c*; Cup; Ign; Ip; Lac-c; Lach; MERC; Nit-ac; *Pho; Rhus-t*; Syph.

Sneezing, with: Flu-ac.

+ Spit, desire to : Cocl.

Oily : Aesc; Cub.

Onion, Odour of : Kali-io.

Pasty : Lach.

Ropy: Coc-c; *Iris;* Saba; Sul.

Salty : Ant-c; Cyc; Sanic; Ver-a.

Water : Verb.

Soapy (See Frothy) : Bry.

Sour : Con; *Ign.*

Sticky : Bell; *Kali-bi; Lach;* Plb.

Stooping, When : *Grap.*

Swallow, Must: Ip; Merc.

Sweet : Canth; *Cham;* Iris; Pho; Plb; PUL.

Disgustingly : Canth.

Meals, after : All-s.

Talking, While : Iris; Lach; Mang.

Viscid, Thick : Chel; *Cimi;* Dul; Glo; *Kali-bi; Lach;* Lyc; Lyss;Merc; Merc-c; Nux-m; Phys.

A.M. in: Glo.

Dribbles : Stram.

Watery : Cyc; Sul-ac.

Yellow : Gel; Manc; Merc; Merc-c; Phyt.

Blood, As from: Gel.

SALIVARY GLANDS : Calc-f; Cham; Iod; Merc; Nit-ac; Phyt; Pul.

SALIVATION : See Saliva, Increased.

SALPINGITIS : See Fallopian Tubes.

Serum or Pus, escapes from uterus : Sil.

SALT Agg : See under Food.

SALTY, Saltiness : *Ars;* Calc; Carb-v; Flu-ac; Grap; Iod; Kali-io; *Lyc;* MERC; Merc-c; Nat-c; Nat-m; *Pho; Pul;* Sanic; *Sele;* SEP; Tell.

SALVATION : See Religious

Ideas.

SAND AS IF : Ap; Ars; Berb; Bov; Cist; Coll; Thu.

SARCASM, SATIRE : Ars; *Lach.*

SARCOCELE : *Aur;* Calc; Iod; Merc-i-r; Pul; Rhod; Spo.

I**NDOLENT** : Tarn.

SARCOMA : See under Cancer, and Fungus Growth.

C**UTIS** : Calc-p; Sil.

SATYRIASIS : See Sexual Desire (males) increased.

SAWING, AS IF: Aesc; Bro; Hypr; Pho; Spig; Spo; Sul; Syph; Tarn.

SCABIES : See Eruptions, Itch Like.

SCABS: See Crusts.

SCALDED : See Burnt, as if and Burns.

SCALES: See Desquammation.

SCALP: See under Head, External.

SCAPULAE (And Region) : Chel; Chin; Dul; Kali-c; Kre; Merc; Rhus-t; *Sep;* Tell.

R**IGHT** : Bry; *Chel;* Ol-an; Pod; Rum.

L**EFT** : Cimi; Zin-ch.

B**ETWEEN**: Am-m; Ars; Calc; Calc-p; Caps; Helo; Nit-ac; Pho; Rhus-t; Sep.

Aching : Carb-ac; Helo; Rhus-t; *Sep;* Sul.

breathing, impeding: Calc.

Air, blowing, on : Caus; Hep.

Broken, as if: Crot-c; Lil-t;

Mag-c; Nat-m; Plat; Ver-a.

Burning : *Ars; Lyc;* Med; *Pho;* Rob; Sul.

Coldness : Ars; *Caps;* Caus; Nat-c; Pyro.

icy : Am-m; Lachn. *Sep.*

Colic, with : Am-c.

Cramps : Grat; Pho; Ver-a.

motion, during : Ip.

Cutting : Canth; Nat-s; Zin.

Epigastrium, to: Bry.

Eructation Amel : Zin.

Fluttering : Cup.

Heart, to : Bry; Sul.

Heaviness : Calc; Chin; Gran; Lach; *Nux-v;* Rhus-t.

Lump : Chin; Lyc; Mag-c; Nux-v; Rhus-t.

Numb : Bry.

Soreness : *Chin;* Cimi; Ham; Hypr; *Pho;* Sep.

spot, in (R) : Berb; Chel.

Sprain : Am-m.

Stitches : Lac-c; Nit-ac; Petr.

Swallowing Agg : Kali-c; Rhus-t.

Throbbing : Plant; Sul.

Weakness: Agar; Alu; *Ap;* Bur-p; *Cocl;* Kali-io; *Nat-m;* Radm; Raph; Sars; Sul-ac.

A**CHING** (R) : Ol-an.

A**DHERENT** : Ran-b.

B**ORING**, Left : *Aur;* Dig; Hypr; Meny; Mez; Nat-c; *Pho-ac;* Rut; Spig.

B**REATHING** Agg : Am-m.

BRUISED, Right : Calen; Kali-c; Kre.

BUBBLING, At : Lyc.

+ Beneath : Scil.

BURNING : Bar-c; Echi; Med; Merc.

Right : Lycps.

Left : Med.

CRAWLING, Left : Med.

Right : Hep.

CUTTING : Lac-c; Med; Spig.

Edge, of : Ran-b.

FINGERS, Using Agg : Ran-b.

FORWARD, From : Bar-c; Pho; Sul.

Right : Merc.

Left : Mez; Pho; Ran-b.

heart, to : Bry.

ITCHING, Left : Caus.

LUMP, Left : Pru-sp.

PRESSURE Amel : Ol-an.

SORE : Ham.

Inner edge (L) : Ran-b.

THROBBING, Left : Mag-m.

UNDERNEATH : Calc; *Gel*; Merc; Myr.

Right : Chel; Colo; Pod; Rum.

hot ache : Lycps.

Left : Cratae; Gel.

burning : Echi.

buzzing : Kali-m.

Bubbling : Scil.

Chilly, cold : Cam.

SCARLATINA : See under Eruptions.

SCARLET : Am-c; Bell; Croc;

Merc.

SCARS : See Cicatrices.

+ REMAINING After Eruptions : Kali-br.

+ UNSIGHTLY : Carb-an.

SCIATICA : Ars; Bry; Buf; COLO; Dios; Grap; Ign; Iris; Kali-bi; Kali-c; Mag-p; *Nux-v;* RHUS-T; Rut; Sele; Sep; Sul; *Tell;* Zin.

ASCENDING : *Led;* Nux-v; Rut.

ATROPHY, Of parts, with: *Calc*; Caus; Ol-j; Plb.

BED, Turning in Agg :Nat-s.

BLOWING Nose Agg : Grap.

BORING : Lach.

BROWN, Spots, with : Sep.

COUGHING Agg : *Caps;* Caus; Sep; *Tell.*

Alternating, with : Stap.

CHRONIC : Ran-b.

DAY, During Amel : Rut.

DEEP, Pain : Kali-bi; Rut.

DESCENDING : Am-m; Rut.

FEET, Tender, with: Mag-p.

FLEXING Leg Amel : Ars; Gnap; Kali-bi; Kali-io; Val.

Abdomen, on Amel: Colo; Glo; Gnap.

FORMICATION, With : Gnap.

HANG Down, Leg Agg : Val.

Over Sides of Bed Agg : Ver-a.

HEAT Agg : Fer; Guai; *Led;* Merc; Visc.

Amel : ARS; Lyc; *Mag-p;* Rhus-t.

HEELS, Localized, in : Sep.

INJURY, After : Arn; Hypr.

JARRING Agg : *Bell*; Nux-m; Tell.

KNEES, To : Ind.

LAUGHING Agg : Tell.

LIMB, Gives way, pain with : Grat.

LYING Agg : Gnap; Kali-io; Nat-m; Rut; Tell.

Amel : *Am-m*; Bry; Dios.

Back, on Amel : Pho.

Painful side on Agg : See Pressure Agg.

Right side on Amel : Pho.

MENTAL Exertion Agg : Mag-p.

MOTION Least Agg, Must lie still : Colo; Lach.

MOVE, Must : Bry; Caus; Lyc; Mag-c; *Rhus-t;* Val;Zin-val.

MUSCLES, Jerking with : Kali-c.

NUMBNESS, With : Aco;Caus; Cham; Colo;Grap; Phyt; Rhus-t.

Burning, with : Dios.

OTORRHOEA, With : Visc.

PAIN, All over the body, with : Petr.

PREGNANCY Amel : Sep.

PRESSURE Agg : Kali-bi; Kali-c; *Kali-io; Lyc; Rhus-t.*

SHOOTING Pain: Aco; *Colo*; Iris; Mag-c.

SITTING Agg: *Am-m*; Bell; Hypr; Ind; Lept; Lyc; Val.

Chair, in Amel : Gnap.

Prolonged Agg : Hypr.

Rising, from Agg : Nat-s.

SNEEZING Agg : Fer; Sep; Tell.

SPINE, Painful with : Petr.

SPRAINED Agg : Tell.

STANDING Amel : Bell; Mag-p; Stap; Tell.

STEPPING, Agg : Gnap.

STOOLS, Agg : Rhus-t.

STOOPING Agg : Tell.

STRETCHING Limbs, standing while Agg : Val.

SUDDEN, Soreness with : Sele.

SUMMER Agg : Xanth.

Amel : Ign.

TOUCH Agg : CHIN; *Chin-s;* Cof; *Lach*; Plb; Visc.

UNCOVERING Agg : *Mag-p;* SIL.

URINATION Amel : Tell.

UTERINE : Bels; Fer; Gnap; Merc; *Pul;* Sep; Sul.

VERTEBRAL Origin: Nat-m; Sil.

WALK, Must : Ars; Sep; Sul.

Amel : Val.

WETTING, After : *Dul; Rhus-t.*

WINTER Agg : Ign.

YAWNING Agg : Zin.

SCIRRHUS: See under Cancer.

SCLERODERMA : Radm; Thyr.

SCLEROSIS: Aur; Aur-m; Bar-m; Plb.

CORONARY : Aur.

DISSEMINATED : Acet-ac; Arg-n; Ars; *Hyo-hydr.*

MULTIPLE : Arg-n; Bar-m; Crot-h; Lathy; Plb; Tarn.

SCLEROTITIS : Ars; Merc-c; Spig; *Thu.*

SCOLDING : See abusive.

AGG : Agar; Stap; Tarn.

ANGRY, Being without : Dul.

HERSELF : Merc.

SCOOPED OUT (Cupped) : Thu; Vario.

SCORBUTIC SYMPTOMS : Am-c; Carb-v; Kali-m; *Merc*; Mur-ac; *Nux-v;* Stap; Sul.

SCORCHED : See Burnt, as if.

SCORN : See Contemptuous.

SCORPIONS SEES : Op.

SCRAPED, As if : Bro; Dros; Nux-v; Pul; Sul; Ver-a.

SCRATCHES, HANDS, With : Stram; Tarn.

DESIRE, To : Arn.

HIMSELF, Raw : Aru-t; Psor.

LIME OF the WALLS : Arn; Canth.

SCRATCHING AGG : *Anac; Ars*; Asar; Caps; Grap; Kali-c; Lach; Old; PUL; RHUS-T; SUL.

AMEL : *Asaf; Calc; Cyc; Mur-ac; Nat-c; Pho;* Rut; *Sul.*

SCRAWNY: Calc-p; Nux-m; Rat; Sec.

SCREAMS: See Cries.

SCREWED TOGETHER : Aeth; *Colo;* Elap; Naj; *Onos;* Ox-ac; Sars; Stro; Zin.

SCROFULA (Psora of childhood) : Bar-c; *Calc*; Calc-p; Cist; Hep; Iod; Lyc; *Merc; Sil; Sul.*

ERETHISTIC: Calc-p; Psor; Tub.

TORPID : Calc; Sul.

SCROTUM : Arn; *Crot-t; Petr*; Rhus-t; Sul.

BLUE : Ars; Mur-ac; Pul.

BUBBLING : Stap.

COLD : Berb; Caps; Merc. Shrivelled, and : Caps.

ELEPHANTIASIS : Sil.

ERUPTIONS, On : Grap; Hep; Petr.

Eczema : Alum; Crot-t; Pho-ac.

EXCORIATED : Ars; Hep; Polyg; Sil; Sul.

Between, and thighs : Lyc; Merc; Nat-c; Petr.

FISTULA : Spo.

HEAT, Burning : Calc; Chel; Spo.

INDURATED : *Rhus-t; Sul.*

ITCHING : Rhod; *Sul.*

+ Perineum, and : Sars.

Spots : Sil.

Voluptuous : Anac; Stap.

MOISTURE : Cinb; Petr; Rhod; Sul.

Between, and thighs : Hep.

Spots, on : Sil.

NODULES, Hard, Brown, on : Nit-ac; Syph.

NUMB, Knees, up to : Bar-c.

OEDEMA : Ap; Ars; Colch; Flu-ac; Grap; Rhus-t.

SCALY : Calc.

SENSITIVE : Stap.

SHINY : Grap; Merc.

SPOTS : Sil.

SWEAT : Ign.

Cold : Plant.

+ Strong smelling : Dios.

+ Warm, profuse : Gel.

SWELLING : Rhus-t.

   Painless : Mez.

THIN : Pyro.

WRINKLED : Rhod.

SCURFS : See Skin, Scaly.

SCURVY : See Scorbutic Symptoms.

SEA AGG : *Ars*; Bro; Mag-m; Nat-m; Nat-s; *Rhus-t; Sep;* Syph.

AIR AMEL : Bro; Med.

BATHING AMEL : Med.

SEARCHING ON THE **F**LOOR : Ign; Plb; Stram.

SEASICKNESS : See Car Sickness.

FEELING, Of : Tab.

NAUSEA, Without : Kali-p.

SEASONS, CHANGE Of : See Change of Temperature.

AUTUMN, SUMMER etc. : See Different Headings.

SECRETIONS : See Discharges.

SECRETIVE : Dig; *Ign;* Lyc; Nat-m.

SEDENTARY LIVING **A**GG : Alo; Asar; NUX-V; *Sul.*

BURNING, Spots, from : Ran-b.

SEEING : See Looking.

ALIVE Things : Cocl.

FACES : Amb; *Bell;* Calc; *Op;* Tarn.

   Mirror, in, except his own

     : Anac.

IMAGINARY Objects : Med.

OTHERS In Misery AGG : Tarn.

SAME Person, in front and behind Euphor.

THINKS, Someone else is, for him : Alu.

SELF, ACCUSATION : Hell; Op; Stram.

ANGRY, With : Ign.

ANTAGONISM : See Antagonism.

CENTERED : Senec.

CONTEMPT : Agn; Aur.

CRITICISM : Aur.

CONFIDENCE, Want of : *Anac;* Arg-n; Ars; *Lyc;* Old; Pic-ac; *Sil;* Ther.

KNOWS Not, what to do, with her : Stan.

LOATHING : Lac-c.

ODD, At : Anac; Bar-c; Cann.

OVER ESTIMATION of : Cic.

PITY : Agar; Nit-ac.

REPROACHES : See Reproaches.

TORTURE : *Aco; Ars;* Bell; *Lil-t;* Plb; Tarn; Tub.

SELFISH : Agar; Ars; Pul; Senec; Sul; Tarn.

SEMEN, BLOODY : Canth; Caus; Flu-ac; Merc; Led; Lyc; Petr; Pul; Sars.

COLD, Coition during : Nat-m.

DRIBBLING : Calad; Pic-ac; Sele.

HOT : Agar; Calc; Tarn.

ODOURLESS : Sele; Sul.

OFFENSIVE : Thu.

   Pungent : Lach.

   Urine, stale like : Nat-p.

THICK : Sabal.

WATERY : Led; Nat-p; Sele; Sul.

SEMINAL DISCHARGE, Failing, Coition, during : Calad; *Grap;* Lyc; Lyss; Psor.

DIFFICULT : Lach; Zin.

PAINFUL : Cann; Canth; Sabal; *Sul.*

Cutting : Con.

PREMATURE, Too quick : Agar; Agn; Calc; Carb-an; Chin; *Grap; Lyc;* Pho; Sele; **ZIN.**

During coition, followed by roaring in head : Carb-v.

SEMINAL EMISSION (Nightly) : Bar-c; Bor; Calc; *Chin; Con;* Dig; Dios; *Fer; Gel;* Kali-p; Lyc; Nat-c; Nat-m; Nat-p; Nux-v; PHO; PHO-AC; Plb; *Sele;* Sep; Stan; Stap; Sul.

AGG (See Coition Agg and Masturbation Agg) : Kob.

AMEL : Calc-p; Lach; Zin.

AFTERNOON, Sleep : Alo; Ther.

ATONIC : Dig.

AWARE, Without being : See Involuntary.

CARESSING or Frolicking with woman, while : Arn; CON; Gel; *Pho;* Sars; Sele; Sul.

COITION, After : Am-c; *Nat-m;* Pho-ac.

DIARRHOEA, During : Ars.

DREAMS, Without : Anac; Arg-n; Dios; Guai; Pic-ac.

+ Lascivious : Pho-ac.

Urination of, after : Merc-i-f.

Vivid, with : Vio-t.

ERECTION, Feeble, with : Sele.

Painful, then : Grat; Kali-c.

Without : Dios; Gel; Grap; Kob.

EROTIC : Scil.

EXERTION, Over, from : Fer.

FREQUENT : Nux-v;Pho-ac; Stap.

Old man, in : Bar-c; Caus; Nat-c.

INVOLUNTARY : Dios; Ham; Nat-p; Sele; Sep.

LEANING The back, against anything, on : Ant-c.

+ **N**IGHT, Every : Ust.

OLD Symptoms Agg : Alu.

PAIN or Colic, during : Plb.

PAINFUL : Kali-c; Nat-c; Sabal.

SPASMS, With : Art-v; Grat; *Nat-p.*

STOOLS, During : Sele; Vio-t.

Difficult, with : Petr.

Straining, when : Ol-an.

URINATION, After : Daph; Kali-c.

VERTIGO, During : Sars.

VOLUPTUOUS : Vio-t.

Thrill long after : Sele.

WOMEN, Caressing when : See Caressing.

In the presence of : *Nux-v;* Salix; *Ust.*

SEMINAL VESICLES : Merc; Pul.

SENILITY : See Old Age.

SENSES, SPECIAL, ACUTE : Aco; Ars; Asar; Bell; Cimi; *Cof;* Lyss; Nux-v; Op; Pho.

BLUNT, DULLED : Anac; Bell; *Calc;* Caus; Gel; Hell; Hyo; Laur; Lyc; Merc; *Nat-m;* Nit-ac; Nux-m; Pho; PUL; *Sil; Sul.*

PERVERTED : Arg-n; Op.

VANISHING, As if (See Fainting) : Alu; Calc; Cann; Carban; *Cup; Plat;* Stram.

Pains, from : Plb.

SENSITIVE (Susceptible to Noise; Light, Pain, Odour, Touch,Trifles etc.) : *Aco; Amb;* Arg-n; Arn; Ars; *Asaf;* Aur; BELL; Bor;*Cham;* CHIN; Chin-s; Cic; Coc-c; *Cof;* Colch; Croc; Cup; Fer; Gel; *Hep;* Hyo; *Ign;* LACH; Lyc; Lyss; Mag-c; Mang; *Mar-v;* Med; Nat-m; *Nit-ac;* NUX-V; Paeon; *Pho; Plat;* Plb; Psor; Pul; Ran-b; Sep; *Sil;* Sul; Sul-io; Tarn; Tell; Terb; *Ther;* Tub; Val; Vip; *Zin.*

DIFFUSED, Affected Part around : Kali-io.

EVERYTHING, To : Sul-io.

MORBIDLY *: Stap.*

WHAT, Others, say about her, to : Stan; Stap.

SENSORIUM, *DEPRESSED* : Bap; *Hell;* Pho-ac; Pyro; Rhus-t.

SENTIMENTAL (See Dreaminess) : *Ant-c; Ign.*

DIARRHOEA, During : Ant-c.

MENSES, Before : Ant-c.

TWILIGHT, In : Ant-c.

SEPERATED, AS IF (See

Duality) : Agar; Arg-n; Calc p; Cocl; Daph; Dul; Hypr; *Psor;* Sabi; Sep; Stram; Tril; Ver-a.

SEPSIS : See Blood Sepsis.

ADYNAMIC : Elap; Pyro.

SEPTICEMIA (See Blood Sepsis) : Ars; Carb-v; Crot-h; Lach; Pyro.

+ SERIOUSNESS, ALTERNATING with **B**UFFONERY : Sul-ac.

SEROUS MEMBRANE : Aco; Ap; Ars; BRY; CANTH; Colch; *Hell;* Kali-c; Lyc; Ran-b; Seneg; Scil; Sil; Sul.

SEWING AGG : See Fingers Working, with.

AMEL : Lach; *Nat-m.*

SEXUAL AFFECTIONS, Disturbances in General : Agn; Bar-c; Calc; CANTH; Chin; *Con;* Grap; *Lil-t;* LYC; *Nux-v;* PHO; Pho-ac; Pic-ac; Plat; Sele; *Stap;* Stram; Sul.

DESIRE (Males) Decreased, Weak : Agn; Bar-c; CAUS; Grap; Kali-bi; Kali-br; *Lyc;* ONOS; *Pho-ac;* Sabal; Sil; Stap; Sul.

Abnormal, From Agg : Lyss.

+ Absent, in fleshy persons : Kali-bi.

Females : See Female Affections.

Increased : Calc; Calc-p; Cam; Cann; CANTH; Carb-v; Con; Flu-ac; Lyc; Lyss; Mos; *Nux-v;* Onos; PHO; PIC-AC; PLAT; *Pul; Sil;* Stap; Stram; *Tub; Zin.*

Emission after : Nat-m; Pho-ac.

Erection, without : Am-c.

Excessive, Maniacal : PHO; *Stram;* Tarn; *Zin.*

Females : See Female Affections.

Old men, in : Flu-ac; Lyc; Sele.

Paralysis, with : Sil.

Physical Weakness, with : Calad; Calc; Con; Grap; *Kali-c; Lyc;* Nat-m; *Pho;* Sele.

Priapism, with : Nat-m; Sil.

Perverted : Agn; Nux-v; Plat; Stap.

Suppressing, ill effects from AGG : Ap; *Cam; Con;* Kali-br; Lyss; Pho; *Pul.*

ENJOYMENT Absent (Males) : Agar; Anac; Calad; Grap; Nat-m; Sep.

Emission, during : Psor.

Females : See Female Affections.

ERETHISM (Children) : Alo.

Climaxis, at : Manc.

Puberty, at : Manc.

EXCITEMENT Easy : Pho; Sumb; Zin.

AGG : *Buf;* LIL-T; Plat; Sars; Senec; Tarn.

Uneasy feeling in body, with : Ant-c.

EXHAUSTION, Excess, After AGG (See Coition Agg) : Calad; Con; Grap; Lil-t; *Lyc;* Nat-p; Nux-v; Onos; Pho; Pho-ac; Sec; Stap; Sul; Symp.

FRIGIDITY (Female) : Ign.

MINDED : Sep; Stap.

NEUROTICS : Sabal.

ORGASMS Easy (Women : Stan.

RESTLESSNESS : Canth; Kali-br; Raph.

THOUGHTS : Grap; Pho; Plat; Stap.

TOUCH, Mere AGG : Con; Grat; Nat-c; Plat.

URGE, Unsatisfied, Futile : Stap.

SHADE In AGG and AMEL : See Twilight Agg and Amel.

SHAKING AGG : See Jarring Agg.

SHALLOW : See Respiration and Ulcers.

SHAMELESS (See Amative) Exposes the person : *Hyo;* Pho; Phyt; Sec; Tarn.

+ **SHAMS** : Op.

SHATTERED, Flying into Pieces, Explosions, as if : Aeth; Ars; *Bell;* Bry; Carb-an; *Cof;* Dig; Glo; *Mur-ac; Nit-ac; Nux-v;* PUL; RHUS-T; Sil; *Stan;* Stap; Sul; Ver-a.

SHAVING AGG : Caps; *Carb-an;* Cic; Ox-ac; Pho; Pho-ac; Plb; PUL; Radm.

AMEL : Bro.

SHIFTING : See Wandering.

SHINGLES : See Eruptions, Zoster.

SHINING, SHINY : See

356

Glistening.

OBJECTS AGG : See Glistening Objects Agg.

SHIVERING : See Shuddering and Chilly.

CONCOMITANT, As a : Saba.

SHOCKS (Through Body) : Amb; Arg-m; *Ars;* Bell; Cic; Cocl; Colch; Cup; Kre; Lyc; Nux-v; Op; Pod;Ran-b; Sil; Stro; Thu; Val; *Ver-a;* Zin; Zin-chr.

ELECTRIC Like :Arg-m; Arg-n; Ars; Buf; Cimi;Mag-m; Nat-p; Radm; Ver-a; Ver-v.

AGG : Pho.

Sleep, during : Ant-t; Arg-n; Ars; Cup; Mag-m; Nat-m; Nat-p; Nux-m; Nux-v; Radm.

Wide awake, when : Mag-m; Nat-p.

INJURY, From : See Nervous and Traumatic.

MENTAL (See also Injuries) : Aco; Ap; *Arn;* Mag-c; Nit-ac; Nux-m; Pho-ac; Pic-ac.

NERVOUS : Aco; Amb; *Arn;* Cam; Carb-v; Cof; Gel; Hyo; Hypr; *Ign;* Iod; Op; Ver-a.

PAIN, From : Arg-n; Cina; Lyc; Plat; Pod; Sul-ac.

PAINFUL : Zin-chr.

SLEEP, On going to : Arg-n; Ars.

SUDDEN : Cic; Ign.

SURGICAL: Aco; Cam; Carb-v; Stro; Ver-a.

TOUCHING Anything : Alu.

TRAUMATIC: See also Injury and Concussion; Aco; ARN; Cam; *Hypr; Lach;* Op; Ver-a.

VIOLENT : Stro.

Pain, as from : Plat.

SHOOTING : See under Pain, Shooting.

SHORT, AS IF, **T**OO : Alu; *Am-m; Caus; Colo;* Dig; Dios; Grap; Guai; Lach; Merc; Mez; Nat-m; Nux-v; *Rhus-t; Sep;* Syph.

SHOULDERS (And Region) : Aco; Bry; Fer; Fer-p; Kali-c; Kalm; Mag-c; Phyt; Pul; Rhus-t; Sang.

RIGHT : Fer; Kali-m; Kalm; Phyt; *Sang;* Stic; Stro.

LEFT : *Fer;* Fer-p; Led; Mag-c; Nux-m; Rum; Sul.

Neck, to : Spig.

Night Agg : Pho.

Right, to : Lyc.

ABDUCTING Arm Agg : Chel.

ALTERNATING : Lyc.

ANKYLOSIS : Cup.

ARM Behind him Agg : *Fer;* Rhus-t; *Sanic.*

Hanging, down Amel : Pho.

CHEST,To : Fer-p.

+ CHILL, Between : Tub.

CHILLINESS : Lept.

COLD : Caus; Kali-bi; Kre; Vio-o.

CONSTRICTION : Cact.

COUGH Agg : Dig; Fer; Lach.

Left Agg : Rum.

Right Agg : Pyro.

CRAMP : Naj.

EMACIATION : Plb.

FINGERS, Along, with : Fago; Fluac.

FLUTTERING, Between : Cup.

HEAVINESS : Anac; Chin; Lach; Pho; Pul; *Rhus-t;* Stap; Sul.

Right, under : Kali-m.

HIGHER, As if, Left : Hell; Merc.

JOINT : Calc; *Fer; Fer-p;* Ign; Kali-c; Nat-m; Pul; Rhus-t; *Sang;* Sep; Stap; Sul.

Cracking, in : Calc; Cic; Croc; Kali-c.

LUMP, Between : Mag-s.

MENSES Agg : Flu-ac; Sang; Ust.

NUMB, Fingertips, to : Ox-ac.

PULSATION : Led.

RAISING ARM Agg : Led; Phyt; Rum; Sang; Sanic.

Amel : Pho-ac.

SENSITIVE : Ap.

SHRUGGING Agg : Calc.

SINGING Agg : Stan.

SPRAINED, As if : Alu; Rhus-t.

STIFF : Calc-s; Rhus-t.

SWELLING : Colo.

TALKING Agg : Pyro.

UNEASY : Ascl.

WIND Blowing on, as if : Lyc.

WRIST, To : Fer-p.

SHRIEKING : See Cries.

HELP, For : Plat.

SHUDDERING (Nervous) : *Aco;* Am-m; ARN; Ars; Bell; Cham;

Cimi; Cina; Cocl; Dios; Gel; Glo; Hell; *Hypr; Ign;* Led; Mez; Mos; Nat-m; *Nux-v;* Phys; Pul; Ran-b; Rhe; Rhus-t; Sep; Sil; Spig; Thu; Zin.

AFFECTED, Part, of : Ars.

AIR, Cold, from : Mos.

COITION, After: Kali-c.

CONTRADICTION, From: Elap.

DEFORMED, Persons, seeing on : Benz-ac.

DISAGREEABLE Things, thinking on : Benz-ac; Pho.

DRAFT Agg : Phys.

DRINKING, When : Caps.

EMOTIONS Agg : Asar.

ERUCTATIONS, With : Dul.

FLOWER, Smell, from: Lac-c.

INTERNAL : Canc-fl.

MENSES. Before : Sep.

PAIN, From : Ars; Bar-c; Caps; Dios; Ign; Mez; Ran-b; Sep.

After : Glo.

PART TOUCHED : Spig.

SLEEP, Falling to, on : Tub.

STOOLS, After : Canth; Rhe.

URINATION, Desire, with : Hypr.

During : Stram.

Urging for, when not attended : Sep.

VOMITING, With : Dul.

YAWNING, When : *Cina;* Old.

SHUT PLACES AGG : See Fear of Narrow or Shut Places.

SHY, TIMID, Mild (See Anthro-

pophobia) : Bar-c; Bor; Calc;
Calc-s; Coca; Cocl; Con;
Crot-h; Gel; Grap; *Kali-c;*
Kali-p; Lyc; Nat-c; Petr; Pho;
Plb; PUL; Sep; Sil; Sul.

SICK FEELING : See Ill Feeling.

SAYS HE is NOT : See Nothing
Ails Him.

SUDDENLY : Con.

SICKLY : See Delicate.

SIDE : See Directions, and
Pain, Goes to side lain on.

STITCHES : Abro; Aco; Bry;
Pul; Ran-b; Sang; Sul.

Right : Chel; Kali-c; Nat-s.

SIGHS, GROANS, Takes deep
breath (See also Respiration
wants deep; Sighing) : Apoc;
Arg-n; Calc-p; *Cimi;* IGN.

INVOLUNTARY : Calc-p; Hell.

LEUCORRHOEA, During : Phys.

MENSES, Before : *Igb;* Lyc.

SWEAT, With : *Bry.*

SILENT : See Taciturn.

SILLY : See Childish.

SINGING, SINGS : Cic; Cocl;
Fer-p; Hyo; Mar-v; Sang *Spo*;
STRAM.

AGG :Arg-m;Aru-t; Carb-v;
Dros;Fer-p; Hep; *Nux-v;* PHO;
Sang; Sele; Stan; Verb.

MENSES, During : Stram.

SLEEP, During : Bell; Croc;
Pho-ac; Sul.

SINGLE PARTS, EFFECTS : Agar;
Alu; Bar-c; Caus; Con; Dul;
Kali-c; Ol-an; Plb; Rhod; Secl
Sul-io; Val.

TURN WHITE And Insensible
: Sul-io.

SINKING DOWN : See Prolapse.

HOLLOW FEELING : See Empty.

SENSATION : Alu; *Bry*; Chin-s;
Cup; Dul; *Glo;* Hell; Hyd-ac;
Kali-c; *Lach;* Laur; Lyc;
Nat-m; *Pho*; Rhus-t; Tab;
Ver-a; Xanth.

THROUGH Floor : Benz; Hyo;
Pho.

UNCONSCIOUS : Glo; Hyd-ac.

SINUS AFFECTIONS, Of : See
Sinus, under Nose.

+ PAINFUL, Inhaled air, to : Syph.

SIT AVERSION To : Iod; Lach.

INCLINATION, To : *Ars;* Caps;
Carb-v; CHIN; *Cocl;* CON;
GRAP; *Guai;* Lil-t; Merc;
Nat-m; NUX-V; PHO; *Pul;*
Scil; Stan.

SITS, BED, In, will not lie
down : Kali-br.

Suddenly, and lies down :
Hyo.

BENT, Forward, straightens
difficulty, with : Lathy.

BREAKS, Pins and sticks : Bell;
Calc.

ELBOWS and Knees, on : Lob.

HANDS, Supporting the body,
with : Berb; Sul.

LEGS Crossed, Uncross can
not : Bell; Ther.

MEDITATING : Calc-s.

Misfortunes, imaginary
over : Calc-s; Lil-t.

QUITE Stiff : Cham; Hyo;
Kali-m; Sep; Stram.

For a long time : Nat-p.

+ SILENTLY : Flu-ac.

+ Speechless, in a corner : Hep.

STILL : Bro; Cocl; Flu-ac; Gel;
Hell; Hep; Plat; *Pul;* Sep;
Ver-a.

As if wrapped in deep and
sad thoughts : Cocl; Plat;
Pul; Ver-a.

Ground, looking at : Stram.

Moody silence, in : Mag-p.

Thinks about little affairs :
Calc.

+ THOUGHT, In as if : Arn.

WEEPING : Amb.

WITH Knees drawn up, resting her head and arms on
knees : ARS.

SITTING AGG : *Agar;* Am-m;
Ap; Ars; Asaf; CAPS; CON; CYC;
DUL; EUPHOR; Fer; Kob; Laur;
LYC; Mag-m; Mur-ac; *Nux-v;*
Pho; PLAT; PUL; *Rhus-t; Rut; Sep;*
Sul; Tarx; *Val;* VERB; Vio-t; ZIN.

AMEL : BRY; Cocl; COLCH;
Cup; Hyo; *Nux-v;* Scil; Sep.

BENT AGG : Ran-b.

AMEL : Lach.

CHAIR, Low Agg : Syph.

CROOKED AMEL : Sul.

DOWN ON First AGG : *Am-m;*
Ant-t; *Spig.*

AMEL : *Caps; Con.*

ELBOWS, Knees, on AMEL:
Kali-c.

ERECT AGG : *Kali-c;* Nat-m; Sul.

AMEL : ANT-T; Ap; Aral; Ars;
Bell; Con; DIG; Gel; *Hyo;*

Kali-bi; Kali-n; Nat-m;
NAT-S; Pho; Pul.

Hand, folded across chest,
with : Ox-ac.

SUPPORTS, Weight, hands on,
with : Sul.

UP IN BED AMEL : *Kali-c;* Samb.

WET Surface, Moist floor etc.
AGG : See Lying on Wet
Surface.

SIZE : See Proportion
Disturbed.

SKIN AFFECTONS In General
: Ap; Amb; ARS; Bell; Bry;
Calc; Caus; Grap; Hep; *Lach;*
Lyc; MERC; Mez; Nit-ac; Petr;
Pho; Pul; Ran-b; Ran-sc;
RHUS-T; Saba; Sars; Sep;
Sil; SUL; Thu; Thyr; Ust;
Vio-o; Vio-t.

ALTERNATING, With : Ant-c;
Ars; Calad; Grap; Hep;
Stap; Sul.

Digestive symptoms, with
: Grap.

Internal symptoms, with
: Ars; Crot-t; Rhus-t.

Joint pains, with : Stap.

BITING : *Euphr; Led; Pul;* Syph.

Scratching, after : Lach;
Old.

BLACK AND BLUE Spots : See
Ecchymoses.

BLEEDS, Scratching, on : Aru-t;
Lyc; Psor.

BLUISH : See Bluish.

Eruptions, after : Abro.

BRANNY (See Desquamation)
: Calc-p; Sanic; Thyr.

BROWNISH : See Brownish.

BUBBLING : Calc.

BURNING, Heat (See Burning) : ACO; Ap; ARS; BELL; Bry; Flu-ac; Kali-bi; *Lach*; Lyc; Pho; *Radm;* Rhus-t; Sil; *Sul; Terb; Ust.*

Coldness, with : Ver-v.

Fever, without : Grap; Lach.

Mustard, plaster, like : Kali-c.

Sparks, as from : Calc-p *Sec.*

Spots : Pho-ac; Sul.

Touch, on : Canth; Fer.

BURNT, Scorched, as if (See Burnt, Scalded): *Ars; Canth;* Ran-b; Ver-a; Ver-v.

CHAFFED, Easily : Old; Rut.

CLAMMY : Aeth; Pho.

COLD (See Coldness) : Cam; Carb-v; Kali-chl; Kali-n; Latro; Med; Mos; Sec; Tab; Ver-*a*.

Agg : Agar; *Hep;* Lac-d; Petr; *Psor; Rhus-t.*

Bathing Agg : *Ant-c;* Thu.

Dry, and: Cam; Nux-m.

Icy : See Coldness, Icy.

CONTRACTED : Rhus-t.

CRACKS : See Cracks.

Deep, Bloody : Nit-ac; Petr.

Itching : Petr.

New Skin cracks and burns : Sars.

Painful : Grap.

Washing, after : Calc; Sep; Sul.

Winter in : Calc; Carb-s;

Petr; Sep; Sul.

Yellow : Merc.

DIRTY Colour: *Ars;* Fer; Fer-pic; Merc; Petr; Pho; *Psor;* Sec; Sul.

DRY (See Dryness) : *Ars; Cam;* Diph; Flu-ac; GRAP; Iod; Kali-c; *Lyc;* Nat-c; *Nat-m;* Nit-ac; *Plb;* Rhus-t; Sang; Sec; Thyr; *Tub;* Vio-o.

Cracking, as if : Murx.

Hot : Ust.

Jaundice, in : Sang.

Sweat : gushing, alternating:Ap.

DUSKY : Ars-io; Calc-p; Merc.

EDGES : Grap; Hep; Nat-p; Nit-ac; Petr; Psor; *Sul.*

Itching : Amb; Caus; Petr.

EXCORIATED, Denuded, Raw : *Arn;* ARU-T; *Aur;* Bar-c; Calc; Calc-s; *Carb-v;* CHAM; *Chin;* GRAP; *Hep;* IGN; LYC; *Merc;* Nit-ac; *Petr; Psor;* PUL; Rhus-t; *Sep;* Sul.

Scratching, after : Grap; Petr.

EXHALATION, Foul (See Sweat Offensive) : Stram.

FILTHY : Psor; Sul.

FLABBY : Abro; Calc; Ver-a.

FOLDS, Flexures : Ars; Calc; Carb-v; GRAP; Hep; Lyc; Merc; *Nat-m;* Ol-an; *Petr;* PSOR; Pul; Sele; Sep; Sil; Sul.

Cracked : Mang.

Pimples, at : Cup.

Rough : Mang.

+ Soreness : Caus.

FORMICATION (See Formication) : Lyc; Pho-ac; Rhod; Rhus-t; Sec; Sul; Tarn.

Between flesh, and : Cadm; Pho; Sec; Zin.

Paralysed parts, in : Cadm; Pho.

FRAGILE : Petr.

FRICTION, Slight Agg : Sul; Vinc.

Clothes, of Agg : Bad; Old.

Constant Agg : Sep.

+ FROZEN, As if : Agar.

HAIRY : See Hair, Body over.

HARD : Ant-t; Calc-f; Cist; Clem; Dul; Grap; Petr; Pho; *Rhus-t;* Sars; *Sep;* Sil.

HEAL Won't, Vulnerable Suppurates, Unhealthy (See Healing difficult) : Ant-c; *Arn; Ars;* Bor; Calc; Calc-s; *Cham;* Con; Grap; *Hep;* Kali-bi; *Lach; Lyc;* Merc; Mez; Petr; *Sil; Sul;* Thu.

Joint,around : Mang.

HIDE Bound, as if : Crot-t.

INACTIVE : *Anac;* CON; *Kali-c;* Kali-p; *Lyc; Pho-ac.*

INDENTED : Ap; Ars; *Bov;* Caps; Pho; Ver-a.

INELASTIC : Bov; Cup; Rhus-t.

INFLAMMED : *Cham; Hep;* Merc; Petr; Pul; Rhus-t; *Sep; Sil;* Sul.

Malignant, oedema, with : Como.

INJURY, Slight Agg : Alu.

IRRITABLE : Radm.

JUMPING, Out, as if : Thu.

LOOSE : Carb-an; Pho.

Torn, bones from, as if : Ol-an.

MENSES Agg : Bor; Calc-p; Carb-v; *Dul; Grap;* Kali-c; Kali-m; Mag-m; *Nat-m;* Sang; Sars; Sep; Stram; Ver-a.

Scanty Agg : Con.

MOIST : Carb-v; *Grap;* Lach; *Lyc; Rhus-t.*

+ MOON, Full and New : *Alu.*

MOTTLED (See Mottled) : Ail; Lach; Pul; Sars; Sul; Syph; Thu.

NODES, on (See Nodes) : Con; Iod; Pho; Sep.

Hard : Kali-io; Nat-s; Sil.

Under : Alu; Kali-ar; Mag-c.

NUMB, Insensible (See Numb-ness) : *Anac;* Arg-n; Con; Nux-v; Old; S*ec.*

Scratching, after : Old.

Spots, in : Buf.

OILY (See Greasy) : Psor; Thu.

OOZING : *Calc; Grap; Lyc; Merc; Petr; Sul.*

PAINFUL : See Sensitive.

Cold, to : Agar; Aur; Plb; Rhus-t

Pressure Amel : Ign.

Scratching, after : Bar-c; Sil; Sul.

PARCHMENT Like : *Ars;* Calc-f; Lyc; Petr; Sil.

Dry : Saba.

PEELING OFF (See Desquamm-ation) : Elap; Thyr; Vip.

As i f : Agar; Bar-c; Lach; Pho; Pho-ac; Phyt;

Rhus-t; *Sul.*

PINCH, Remains raised : Caps.

PRESSURE, Slight Agg : Sul.

PRICKLING, Tingling (See Pain, Prickling): Ham; Kali-c; Lob.

PRURIGO : See Itching.

PUFFED, Bloated : Ant-c; *Ap;* Calc; Caps; Cup; Fer; Syph.

QUIVERING, Twitching : Mang; Pho; Sec; Tab.

ROUGH, Ragged : Ars; Bell; *Calc;* Calen; Flu-ac; *Grap;* Iod; Nit-ac; *Petr;* Phyt; Psor; Saba; *Sep; Sul;* Tub. Knots, small, as from : Hypr.

SCALY, Scurfy (See Desquamation) : *Ars;* Calc; Dul; Kali-m; Kre; Lyc; Manc; Med; Nat-c; Nit-ac; Pho; Rhus-t; Sep; *Sil; Sul;* Thyr.

SCORCHED, As if : See Burnt, under Skin.

SENSITIVE : Ars; Asaf; Bell; Calc; Carb-v; Chin; Coc-c; *Cup; Hep;* Kali-c; *Lach; Merc;* Mang; *Nit-ac; Nux-v;* Nat-m; Old; *Pho-ac;* Plant; Rut; Sil; *Sul;* Tub; Ver-a.

Spots, In : Fer; Hep.

SHINY : Ap; Bell.

SHRIVELLED : See Withered.

SOFT, Boggy : Ars; Caps; Kali-c; Lach; Sil; Thu.

SOGGY : See Withered.

SORE : See Sensitive, and Bed Sores.

Feeling : Cimi; Eup-p; Hep; Merc; Sep; Zin.

SPOTS, Blue, Brown etc. : See under Bluish, Brownish.

Every tint of : Crot-h.

Itching : See Itching.

Pigmented : Iod; Lyc; Sep.

+ Pink : Colch.

White : See Leucoderma.

STICKY : Pho.

STIFF: Kalm; *Rhus-t;* Ver-a.

STINGING (See Pain, Stinging) : Asaf; Ham; Stap; Ther; Thu; Urt.

STRIPES, Streaks, on : Bell; Buf; *Carb-v;* Cep; *Hep;* Merc; Myg; *Pho;* Sabi; Sil.

STROPHULUS (Dentiton during) : Bor; Cham; Merc; Sul.

SWELLED : Syph.

SWELLING, On (See Nodes) : Ant-c; Arg-m; Ars; Bar-c; Grap; Thu.

SWOLLEN, As if : Bell; Pul; Rhus-t.

TANNED : Tub.

TENSE : Cact; Caus; Meny; Nit-ac; *Pho;* Stro.

THICK : Ant-c; Cast-eq; Cist; Dul; *Grap;* Hydroc; Petr; Radm; *Rhus-t; Sep;* Sil; Sul.

Purple : Sep.

Scratching, after : Rhus-t.

UNDER : Aco; Aesc; Agar; Alu; Bell; *Bro;* Cic; Coca; Euphor; Lach; Pho; *Sec;* Thu; *Zin.*

Crawling, like a Bug or Worm : Calc; Cocain; Oenan; Stram; Vario.

Clothes, touch Agg : Oenan.

Heat : Terb.

Nodules, small : Kali-ar.

Thin Cord, as if : Euphor.

+ Worm, moves away, when touched : Coca.

URINARY, Affections, with : Vio-t.

WASHING, Bathing Agg : Ars; Sul.

WIND Agg (See Wind AGG) : Psor.

WINE COLOURED : Sep.

WINTER Agg : Alu.

WITHERED, Shrivelled : Abro; Ars; Bor; *Calc; Chin; Cocl;* Cup; *Iod;* Lyc; Phyt; Rum; *Sec;* Sil; *Ver-a.*

WORMS : Ars; Coca; Merc; Nat-c; Nit-ac; Sele; Sil; Sul.

WRINKLED : *Calc;* Cam; Pho-ac; Sars; SEC; Sep; Ver-a.

YELLOW See Yellowness : *Merc*

SKULL: See under Head, External.

SLEEP AFTERNOON AGG : Bry; Lach; Pul; *Stap;* Sul.

BEFORE AGG : *Ars;* BRY; CALC; *Carb-v; Lyc; Merc; Pho;* Pul; *Rhus-t;* Sep; Sul.

DURING AGG : *Aco;* Arn; *Ars; Bell; Bor; Bry;Cham; Cina;* Con; *Hep; Hyo;* LACH; *Merc;* Op; *Pul; Sil; Stram; Sul;* Zin.

FALLING To, or First AGG : Aral; Ars; Bell; *Bry;* Carb-v; Crot-h; *Grind;* Kali-c; LACH; Op; Pul;Samb; *Sep;* Sul.

AMEL : Merc.

Waking or Both *Agg* : Stan.

HALF Asleep, when AGG : Cam; Nit-ac; Saba; Val.

AMEL : Sele.

AMEL, Loss of AGG : Ars; Calad; Carb-v; Cimi; *Cocl;* Cof; Colch; Cup; Kali-p; Lac-d; Laur; Med; Merc; Myg; Nit-ac; *Nux-v;* Pall; PHO; Pul; Sang; Sele; Sep; Zin.

AFTER Waking From AGG : See Awakening after Agg.

ANXIOUS : Aco; Ars.

BROKEN : See Unrefreshing.

CAN NOT FALL To: Laur; *Pho.*

Unless legs are crossed : Rhod.

CAT NAPS, In : See Awakes, Frequently.

CHATTERING, During : Pul.

COMATOSE, Deep : Aeth; *Ant-t;* Arg-n; Arn; *Bap; Bell;* Chin; Con; *Croc;* Grap; *Hell;* Kre; *Nux-m; Nux-v;* OP; *Pul;* VER-A.

Chill, violent, during : Op.

Menses, during : *Nux-m;* Pho.

Old people, in : Op.

Snoring, with (Children) : Chin.

Spasms, during : Op.

Vomiting, After : Aeth.

Yawning, with : Cimi.

EYES, Half-open : Ip.

Open, with : Cadm.

JERKS, Starts, On falling to : Aco; Ars; *Bell;* Bor; Bry; Calc; Cham; Cina; Ign; Kali-c; Lyc; Nit-ac; Op; *Pul;* Sep; Sil; Stram; Zin.

Air, wanting, as if from : Calc-s.

During : Carb-v; Dig; Hell; Hyo; Kali-c; Op; Rhe.

Fear, with : Sabal.

+ LAUGHS and Weeps : Lyc.

LIGHT, Hears every sound : Aco; Alu; Am-c; Ars; Cof; Ign; Lach; Merc; Op; Pho; Sele; Sul.

LITTLE, Enough : Rhe.

PAINS, During : *Ars;* Aur; Bell; Carb-an; Cham; Grap; Lyc; Merc; *Nit-ac;* Nux-m; Rhus-t; Sul; Sul-ac; Til.

Abdomen, in : Ant-t.

After : Phyt.

RESTLESS, Tossing about : Aco; *Ars; Bar-c;* BELL; Carb-an; *Chin;* Cina; Cocl; Cup; Grap; Lyc; Op; *Pul;* RHUS-T; SIL; *Sul.*

Heat of body, from : Bar-c; Mag-m.

Sexual thoughts, from : Aur; Canth; Kali-br; Raph.

+ Shocks, from : Mag-m.

+ Voluptous dreams, from : Bism.

+ Whining and Crying: Rhe.

ROUSED From AGG : Spo.

SHORT AGG : Aral.

AMEL: Calad; Flu-ac; Kali-bi; Meph; Nux-v; Pho-ac.

Seems too long but Amel : Med.

SIDE, Not lain on, as if : Flu-ac.

+ SOBS, During : Aur; Hyo; Nat-m.

STARTING Up : See Jerks.

STUPID : See Sleep, Comatose.

+ TALKS : Carb-an.

UNREFRESHING, Awakes tired : Bry; Chin; Con; Hep; *Lach; Mag-c;* Mag-m; Nit-ac; Op; Pho; Rhus-t; Sul; Zin.

Though sound : Pic-ac.

WALKING, In : See Somnambulism.

+ YAWNING : Cimi.

SLEEPINESS (By Day): Aeth; Am-c; ANT-C; *Ant-t;* Ap; Ars; *Bap;* Bell; Calc; Carb-v; Caus; *Chel;* Chin; Clem; *Croc; Fer-p; Gel;* Grap; Lach; Lept; Merc-c; Mos; NUX-M; NUX-V; *Op;* Pho; *Pho-ac;* Pic-ac; Pod; *Pul; Sul; Terb;* Thu.

ACCOMPANIED, By : Ant-t; Nux-m; Pul.

AFTERNOON : Chin; Nux-v; Rhus-t; *Sul.*

CAUSED By other complaints: Ant-t; Nux-m; Op; Rhus-t; Ver-a.

COITION, During : Bar-c; *Lyc.*

CONSCIOUSNESS, Losing, as if with : Phys.

COUGHING, With : *Ant-t;* Ip; Kre.

After : Anac; *Ign.*

EATING, On: Agar; Calc; Caps; Chin; *Kali-c;* Nux-v; Pho; Rhus-t; *Sul.*

EXERTION Agg : Ars; Bar-c; *Nux-m;* Sele.

Mental Agg : Ars; Gel; Hyo; Kali-c; Nux-m; Pho-ac;

Saba; Sele.

EVENING : Amb; Am-m; Ars; *Calc*; Calc-s; *Kali-c* NUX-V; Pul.

FEVER, During : Ant-t; Calad; Eup-p; Gel; Lach; Lyc; Mez; *Nat-m*; Pho; Pho-ac; Pod; Samb.

Paroxysms after : Pod.

Septic : Stram.

FORENOON : Ant-c; Saba.

INTOXICATED, As if : Led; *Nux-m*.

LAUGHING, After : Pho.

LYING, Left side, on : Thu.

MENSES, During : Kali-c; Mag-c; *Nux-m*; Pho; Sul.

Absent, with : Senec.

MIGRAINE, Then : Sul.

MORNING : Calc; Calc-p; Con; Grap; Nux-v; Sep; Sul.

+ MOROSE, And : Cyc.

OCCUPATION, Literary Amel : Croc.

OVERPOWERING : Nux-m;Op; Phys.

PAINS, After : Phyt.

During : See under Sleep.

PARTURITION, After : Phel.

PNEUMONIA, In : *Ant-t;* Chel; Op; Pho.

PREGNANCY, During: Helo; Nux-m.

READING, While : Bro; Colch.

SEWING, While : Fer.

SITTING, While : Fer; Nat-p; Nux-v.

Sleepless, lying when : Cham.

STANDING, At Work, while : Phel.

STOOL, After : Aeth; Nux-m; Sul.

STUDENT, In: Fer; *Gel*; Mag-p.

SUDDEN : Rum.

SWEAT, With : Rhus-t.

TALKING, Speaking while : Chel; Mag-c; Plb.

TWILIGHT : *Am-m.*

URINE, Retention, with : Terb.

VOMITING, After : Aeth; Ant-t; *Ip*; Sanic.

WRITING While : Pho-ac.

YET SLEEPLESS, At night : Fer; Mag-c; Mos; Op; Pho-ac; Pul;Rhus-t; Sul.

SLEEPING SICKNESS : Ars; *Atoxy;* Gel; Nux-m; Op.

SLEEPLESSNESS (Insomnia) : Aco; Anac; Arg-n; ARS; *Bell*; Bels; Bry; Cact; *Calc; Cham*; Chin; Cocl; COF; Hep; HYO; *Kali-c; Lach; Merc;* Merc-c; Mos; NUX-V; Op; Ox-ac; *Pho*; Plb; PUL; *Rhus-t;* Senec; *Sep; Sil;* Stan; Stap; SUL; Syph; Thu; Zin-val.

ACHING Body, from : *Stap.*

Bones, from : Daph.

ALTERNATE, Night : Anac; Lach.

ALTHOUGH Sleepy : Ap; *Bell;* Cham; Chel; Hep; Op; Pho; Pul; Sep.

CAUSED By : Ars; Bry; Calc; *Cham*; Chin; Cof; Merc; Pho; Pul; Rhus-t; Sep.

+ Horrible dreams : Adon.

Nervous excitement : Scut.

+ Rambling thoughts : Adon.

CONVERSATION, After : *Amb.*

DRUGS and Liquor habitues : Sec.

DRUNKARDS: Lach; Nux-v; Op.

EXHAUSTION Agg : Avena; Chlo-hyd; Coca; Cocl; *COF.*

EYES Won't stay shut : Pho.

GRIEF, From: Ign; Kali-br; *Nat-m.*

+ HEARING, Acute, from : Op.

HEART Symptoms, from: Cratae; Tab.

HOMESICKNESS, From : *Caps.*

IDEAS, Fixed, from : Calc; Grap; Pul.

LASTING, Several nights : Anac.

LYING, Left side, on : Card-m, Thu.

MENSES, During : Agar; Senec.

MIDNIGHT, Before (Sleeps after) : Amb; *Ars; Bry; Calc;* Calc-p; *Carb-v; Chin;* Cof; Con; *Grap;* Kali-c; Lyc; Mag-m; *Merc;* Nat-c; *Nux-v; Pho;* Pic-ac; PUL; *Rhus-t; Sep;* Sil; Sul.

After (Sleeps before) : Ars; *Caps; Cof;* Hep; *Kali-c;* NUX-V; Pho-ac; SIL.

1 A.M. : Bels; Mag-c; Nux-v; Sep.

NERVOUS Excitement, From : Aco; Calc; Chin; COF; Gel; Hyo; Lach; Lyc; Mar-v; Mos; *Nux-v; Plat;* Stic.

NEURITIS, Multiple, from : Con.

NICOTINISM, Chronic, from : Plant.

OLD AGE : Bar-c.

ONCE Awakening, on : Ars; Lach; *Nat-m; Nux-v;* Sil.

OPERATION, Surgical, after : Stic.

PERSISTENT : Thu.

PRODROME, As a : Chin.

RESTLESSNESS, From : Aco; Ars; Cham; Iod.

RETIRING, After, but Sleepy before : *Amb.*

RUSH Of IDEAS, From : Ars; Calc; Cof; Gel; Hep; Hyo; Ign; Nux-v; Op; Pul.

SEXUAL : Canth; Kali-br; Raph.

TWITCHINGS, From : *Ars;* Bell; Ign; Pul; Sul.

UTERINE, Complaints, from : Senec.

WEANING of Child, from : Bell.

YAWNING, With : Cimi.

SLEEPS, ABDOMEN, On: Bell; Colo; Med; Stram.

ARMS, Abdomen on : Cocl; *Pul.*

Apart : *Cham;* Plat; Psor.

Head Over : Ars; Cimi; Lac-c; Nux-v; *Pul.*

under : Ars; Bell; Plat.

BACK, On : *Bry;* Colch; Merc-c; *Pul; Rhus-t;* Stram.

Knees Drawn up, with : Bry; Hell; Lach; Merc-c; Stram.

and spread apart : Plat.

CURLED Up Like a dog : Ars;

Bap; Bry.

+ DAY All, Cries at night : Lyc.

KNEES, Chest, on : Med.

ODD Position, in : Plb.

ONE LEG Stretched out, and the other drawn up, with: Lac-c; Stan.

SIDE, On : *Bar-c*; Colch; Pho.

Not lain, as if : Flu-ac.

SITS Up and, again : Hyo.

STRANGE, Position, in : See Attitude Bizarre.

SLIDES DOWN IN BED : See Bed.

SLIGHT CAUSES AGG : Amb; Amy-n; Carb-an; Cocl; Kali-p; Mag-c; Nit-ac; Nux-m; Pho.

SLIMY : See Discharges.

SLOUGH : See Phagedena.

SLOVENLY : See Indolent, Gait.

SLOW (Comprehension, Thinking etc.) : Amb; Anac; Ars; BAR-C; Bry; *Carb-v*; Cocl; *Con;* Echi; HELL; Kali-bi; Kali-m; Lycps; Old; Onos; Op; Pho; *Pho-ac;* Plb; Pul; SUL.

Motion : Cocl; Pho.

+ **SLOWED DOWN** EVERYTHING : Aesc.

SLUGGISH : See Indolent.

+ ORGANS And FUNCTIONS : Eup-p.

PROCESSES : Sil.

+ RESPONSES : Hell.

SLY : *Tarn.*

SMALL AS IF (Object, Roomsetc.) : Berb; Carb-v; Cyc; Merc-c; Nat-c; Plat.

SMALLER, SEEMS (Body, Limbs

etc.) : Agar; Cact; Calc; Carb-v; Croc; Glo; Kre; Saba; Tab; Tarn.

CRANIUM : Chel; Glo; Grat.

SMALL POX: Ant-t; Ars; Bap; *Merc; Pul; Rhus-t;* Sul; *Thu; Vario.*

SMARTING : See Pain Biting.

SMEGMA INCREASED : Canth; Caus; Nux-v.

FOUL : Sul.

SMELL (See also Odour)

AFFECTIONS IN GENERAL : Aur; BELL; Calc; *Colch;* Grap; Hep; Lyc; Nat-m; NUX-V; PHO; *Pul; Sep; Sil;* SUL.

ACUTE: Aco; *Ars; Aur; Bell;* Carb-ac; *Chin; Cof;* COLCH; *Grap;* Ign; *Lyc;* NUX-V;Op; PHO; Saba; *Sep;* SUL.

DIMINISHED, Wanting, Weak : Anac; *Bell; Calc;* Calc-s; Cyc; Hep; *Hyo;* Mar-v; *Merc; Nat-m; Plb;* Pho; PUL; Sang; *Sep;* SIL.

Epilepsy, with : Plb.

Taste, and : Anac; Crot-t; Just; Mag-m; *Nat-m; Pul;* Sil.

Coryza, with : Med.

after : Mag-m.

ILLUSORY : Anac; Bell; Calc; Manc; Par; Sul; Val.

Agreeable : *AGN;* Pul.

Burnt feathers : Bap.

Cabbages : Benz-ac.

Catarrh, as of : Grap; Pul; Sul.

+ Cheese, old like : Nux-v.
Dung : Manc.
Dust : Benz-ac.
Earth, as of : Calc; Ver-a.
Foul : *Bell*; Benz-ac;
Kali-bi; Meny; *Par*; Pho;
Pul; Sul.
Gun Powder : Manc.
Onions, roasted, like : Sang.
Sulphur, as of : Nux-v.
PREVERTED : Anac; Mag-m;
Mag-p; Sang.
SMILE, DOES NOT : Alu; Amb.
FOOLISHLY : Bell.
SLEEP, In : Cadm.
SMOKE AGG : Ars; Chin;
Euphr; Kali-bi; Lyc; Pho; Sep;
Spig.
TOBACCO, Inhalation AGG : Bro.
SMOKE AS OF : See Vapour,
Respiration, Smoke.
HOT, Coming through all
orifices, as if : Flu-ac.
SMOKING AGG : See Tobacco.
SMOOTH : Alu; Pho; Terb.
SNAKES, IMAGINES : Lac-c; Tub.
SNAPPISH : Lil-t; *Stap.*
SNEEZING AGG (See Jarring)
: Ars; Bell; Bry; Kali-c; *Lyc*;
Pho; Rhus-t; SUL; Verb.
AMEL : Chlo-hyd; Lach;
Mag-m; Naj; Thu.
SNEEZING (Remedies in
General) : *Ars*; Ars-io; Bry;
CARB-V; CEP; *Cina*; Coc-c;
Eup-p; *Gel*; Ign; Ip; Kali-io;
Kali-p; Merc; *Nat-m*;
NUX-V; *Pul*; RHUS-T; Rum;

Saba; Sang; Scil; Senec;
Seneg; *Sil*; SUL.
ABORTIVE : Ars; Calc-f;
Carb-v; Nux-v; *Saba*; Sil.
Agg Sneezing : Carb-v.
BLOWING, Nose Agg : Carb-v.
COMBING or Brushing the
hair, from : Sil.
CORYZA, Without : Agar; Calc;
Cic; Merc; Nit-ac; Stap.
COUGH, Before : Ip.
Whooping, with : Cina.
With : Agar; Bad; Bell; Just;
Psor; *Scil.*
DIZZY, Until : Seneg.
EAR, Itching in, with : Cyc.
EYES, Closed, with : Gamb.
Opening, on : Am-c; Grap.
HEAD Thrown, backwards
while : Lyss.
LARYNX, Irritation, from :
Carb-v.
MORNING Agg : Am-c; Cam;
Caus; Kali-bi; Nat-m;
Nux-v; Sil.
Waking on : Am-c; Grap.
MUCOUS, Secretions, profuse
with: Solid.
NIGHT, At : Aru-t.
NOSE, Burning in, with:
Senec.
ODOURS, Fron : Pho.
PAINFUL : Dros.
PERSISTENT : Cyc; Saba; Sang.
For Hours, with weakness :
Petr.
PUTTING Hands, water in, on
: Pho.

RAPID And Continued : Ver-v.

SALIVATION, With: Flu-ac.

SLEEP, In: Bar-m; *Nit-ac*; Pul.

SUNSHINE, In : Agar; Aur; Merc; Sang.

TALKING, Prevented : Rhus-t.

THROAT Pain, with: Pho.

TWO A.M. : Kali-p.

UNCOVERING Least, on : Hep; Nux-v; Pyro; *Rhus-t;* Sil.

UNSATISFACTORY *:* Ars-io.

VIOLENT : Agar; Cep; Kali-io; Nat-c; Nux-v; Rum; Saba; Scil; Seneg.

Day time only : Gamb.

WAKES Him, Sleep, from : *Am-m.*

WIND, Cold, every from: Hep.

YAWNING, With: Bry; Cyc; Lob.

SNOW AIR AGG : Agar; Calc; *Con;* Form; Lyc; Mag-m; Pho; Pho-ac; Pul; Rhus-t; *Sep;* Sil; Sul; Urt; Vib.

LIGHT AGG : Aco; Cic; Glo.

SNUFFLING (See Nose obstructed) : Kali-bi; Med; Merc; Osm; *Samb;* Vib.

+ **SOBBING** LIKE A Child : Lob.

SOCIETY, SOCIALFUNCTIONS AGG : Coca; Pall.

AMEL *:* Bov.

GIRLS, Modern : Amb.

ILL AT EASE : Coca.

+ PREFERS : Lil-t.

SOLES : Cup; Pho-ac; Pul; Tarx.

ACHING: Rhus-t; Sul-io;Zin-ar.

Standing, when: Sul-io;

Zin-ar.

Tired, when : Zin-ar.

Walking, while : Rhus-t.

BOILS : Rat.

BURNING : Calc; *Lach;* Lyc; Psor; Sang; Sanic; SUL; Sul-io.

Bed, in: Cham; Sul.

Amel : Nat-c.

Itching : Psor.

Walking Agg : Nat-c.

CALLOSITIES *:* *Ant-c;* Ars; *Bar-c;* Grap; Sep; SIL; Sul.

COLD, Icy : Nit-ac.

Bed, in : Sul.

CRACKS *:* Ars; Merc-c.

CRAMPS *:* *Calc;* Carb-v; Caus; Cup; Nux-v; Sil; Stro; *Sul;* Ver-v.

DESQUAMATION : Manc.

DRY : Bism; Manc.

FORMICATION : Caus.

ITCH :Cimi; Hydroc; Med; Tarn.

KNEES, To : Lith.

NEEDLES, At : Bry; Nat-c.

NUMB *:* *Cocl;* Raph; Sep.

PAINFUL (See Aching) : Caus; *Kali-c;* Kali-p; Led; *Lyc;* Med; Pul; Syph; *Thu.*

Contractive feeling, with : Syph.

Feet, swollen, with : Saba.

Pavement, walking on Agg : Alo.

PRESSURE Amel : Zin-ar.

RUBBING Amel : Chel.

SOFT, Furry : ALU; Ars; Cann;

Cocl; Helo; *Xanth*; Zin.

STICKING : Bor.

SWELLED : Fer; *Lyc*; Pul.

TENDER, Sore : Alu; *Ant-c*; Bar-c; Calc; *Led*; MED; *Nat-c*; Sul-io; Thu; Zin.

Balls of : Med.

THICK Skin : *Ars.*

TINGLING : Sil.

VESICLES: Kali-bi; Manc; Merc; Nat-c; Nat-s.

VIBRATIONS : Old.

WITHERED : Ant-c.

WOODEN Sensation : Ars.

SOMEONE ELSE : See Duality.

SOMNAMBULISM (Walking in Sleep) : Aco; Art-v; Bry; Dict; Kali-br; Kali-p; Nat-m; *Pho*; Op; Sil.

CHILDREN, In: Kali-br.

EMOTIONS, Suppressed, from : Zin.

HONOUR, Wounded, from: Ign.

SOOTY : See Nostrils.

SORE : See Pain, Bruised.

SORROW (See Grief) : Aco; IGN; *Nat-m; Pho-ac; Pul; Stap.*

SOUR, SOURNESS, Acidity : CALC; Chin; *Grap*; Hep; Iris; Kali-c; Kob; Lapp; Lith; *Lyc*; *Mag-c*; Merc; Nat-c; Nat-m; Nat-p; Nat-s; NUX-V; Ox-ac; *Pho*; Pho-ac; Pul; Rhe; Rob; Sep; Sil; SUL; Sul-ac; Tarx.

ALL OVER : Mag-c; Rhe.

BITTER : Iris; Nux-v.

+ **BODY** Of : Sul-ac.

+ Children : Cina.

FOOD, All turns : Lapp.

+ Tastes, good : Radm.

KRAUT Agg : See Food.

+ **SMELLS**, Sensitive, to: Dros.

SPASMS : See Convulsions.

SPARKS, SENSATION : See Electric Sparks.

SPEAKING, TALKING AGG : Aco; Alu; Amb; Am-c; *Anac*; Arg-n; *Am; Ars*; Aru-t; *Calc*; Cann; Chin; COCL; Dros; *Ign*; Iod; Mang; *Nat-c; Nat-m*; Nux-v; PHO; *Pho-ac; Rhus-t*; *Sele; Sep*; Sil; *Spo; Stan*; SUL.

LONG AGG : Nat-m.

SPEECH, AFFECTED (See also Voice) : Arg-n; *Bell; Caus*; Coll; Crot-c; *Gel; Glo; Hyo*; Kali-br; Kali-io; LACH; Lyc; *Merc*; Merc-c; Nat-c; Nat-m; Nux-m; *Nux-v*; Pho; Stan; STRAM.

BABBLING : Hyo; Lyc.

CHOREA, In : Caus.

DEVELOPMENT, Retarded: Pho.

DIFFICULT : Bell; Cocl; Dul; Gel; Kali-br; Lac-c; Lach; Lol-t; Nat-m; Op; Stan; Stram.

Menses, during : Ced.

Though, she tries : Cimi.

FALTERING, Hesitating : *Arg-n*; Nux-m.

FOREIGN Tongue, in : Lach; Nit-ac; *Stram.*

HASTY : Ars; Bell; Cocl; Hep; Hyo; Lach; Lyss; Merc.

+ **INDECENT** : Cam.

INDISTINCT : Cocl; Glo; Lyc.

Excitement, from : Laur.

JERKY : Agar; Caus; Myg.

LISPING *:* Ars; Ver-a.

LOST, Wanting : Bar-c; Bell; Bothr; Caus; Cheno; Cup; Kali-cy; Laur; Lyc; Merc; Naj; Nit-ac; Old; Onos; Plb; Stram.

  Amnesic : Kali-br; Plb.

  Fright, from : Hyo.

+ Inteligence, intact: Kali-cy.

  Stomach pain, from : Laur.

  Typhoid like fevers, in : Ap; Ars; Op; *Stram.*

  Uterine displacement,in : Nit-ac.

NASAL : Bar-m; Bell; *Kali-bi;* Lac-c; Lach; Pho-ac.

  Tonsils, enlarged, with : Stap.

PLAINTIVE *:* Crot-h.

+ RAPID *:* Ars.

SLOW : Thu.

  Hunts, for words : Thu.

+ SPASMODIC : Mag-p.

+ SPOONERISM : Caus;Chin.

STRAMMERING : Agar; *Bell;* Bov; Buf; *Caus;* Cocl; *Hyo;* Kali-br; *Merc;* Nux-v; Spig; *Stram;* Ver-a.

  Children : Bov.

  Coition, after : Ced.

  Every word, loudly : Hyo.

  Last word : Lyc.

  Suddenly : Mag-c.

  Talking, Fast, when : Lac-c.

    strangers to, when : Dig.

  Typhoid, in : Arg-n; Lyc; Ver-a.

+ STUTTERING : Cann.

THICK: Agar; Bap; Caus; Dul; GEL; *Lach;* Nux-v.

  Blundering : Lach.

TRIES, To, But can not : Cimi.

UNDERSTAND, Can not, but can speak : Elap.

UTTERS, Every word, loudly: Hyo.

WHISPERS *:* Ol-an.

WORDS, Can not form rightly : Aesc.

  Convulsive motions of head and arms, every with : Cic.

+ Right, cannot find : Dul.

  Roll out, tumbling over each other : Hep.

+ Says, not intended : Cup.

SPERMATIC CORD : Berb; Ham; *Pul;* Rhod; Spo.

ABDOMEN, To : Rhod.

ACHING *:* Clem; Sars.

BURNING : Berb; Pul; Spo.

COITION, Emission Agg : Mag-m; Nat-p; Sars; Ther.

HEAT, In, seminal discharge with : Sabal.

INDURATED, Hard : Pho-ac; *Syph.*

INFLAMMATION : Pul; Spo.

NODES : Syph.

PAINFUL, Sore : Berb; *Clem;* Ham; Kali-c; Ox-ac; *Phyt.*

RIDING, Carriage Amel: Tarn.

SWELLED : Pul; Spo.

  Inguinal glands, with : Clem.

Sexual excitement, after :
Sars.

TENSION : Clem; Pul; Sul.

THICKENING: *Clem;* Rhus-t; Sul.

THIGHS, To : Rhod.

TUBERCLES : Pul; Sil; Spo.

TWITCHING : Mang.

URINATION Agg : Polyg.

SPHINCTERS: Laur; Sil; Stap.

+ RELAXED : Pod.

SPINA BIFIDA: Bry; *Calc-p;*
Psor; Tub.

SPINAL CORD : Med; Ox-ac;
Pic-ac; Plb; Sec.

CALCAREOUS, Deposits, in : Vario.

SPASMS, From : Pic-ac.

SPINE (See Back) : Par; Ther;
Val; Vario.

ACHING: Agar; Lac-c; Nux-m;
Syph; Tell; Zin.

AIR, Can not bear a draft of :
Sumb.

Warm streaming up, into
head : Ars; Sumb.

ALONG, Legs, down : Kob.

BREATHING Deep Agg : Chel;
Rut.

BURNING :Alu; Ars; Cocl; Glo;
Kali-bi; Lach; *Lyc;* Med;
Pho; Pho-ac; Phys; Pic-ac;
Sec; Tab; Zin.

+ Right, side : Kali-c.

COITION Agg : Nit-ac.

COLDNESS (Interscapular) :
Agar; *Am-m;* Arg-n; Caps;
Helo; Hyo; Lachn; Med;
Petr; Rhus-t; Sec.

Creeping up : Ox-ac.

CONCUSSION : See Injuries.

CONGESTED : Gel.

CRACKING : Agar; Sec.

CURVATURE : Aur; *Calc;*Calc-f;
Calc-s; *Lyc; Merc;* Merc-c;
Pho-ac; PUL; Sil; SUL.

Lies, back, on knees drawn
up, with : Merc-c.

Painful : Aesc; *Lyc; Sil.*

CUTTING, Up : Elap; Nat-s; Polyg.

DOWN : Pic-ac; Tab; Tell.

Epileptic Aura : Lach.

Feet, to : Kob.

EATING Agg : Kali-c.

ERUCTATION Amel : Zin.

FORMICATION : *Aco; Agar;* Ars;
Lach; Nux-v; Pho-ac; Sal-ac.

HOT IRONS : *Alu;* Buf; Cam.

INJURIES, Concussion : Arn;
Bels; *Con;* HYPR; *Nat-s;*
Nit-ac; Sil; Zin.

Lies, Back on, jerking head,
backwards : Hypr.

Lifting, from : *Calc; Rhus-t.*

Old : Ign.

Spasms, from : Zin.

Wounds : Rut; Symph.

JARRING Agg : *Bell;* Grap; Sil;
Ther; Thu.

LOWER Bulged, backwards, as
if : Aur.

NEEDLES, Icy, in : Agar; Cocl.

NUMBNESS, Creeping down :
Phys.

PAIN, In, Relieves the
headache : Kali-p.

Sciatica, during : Petr.

PARALYTIC : AESC.

THIGHS, To : Rhod.

TUBERCLES :Pul; Sil; Spo.

TWITCHING : Mang.

PRESSURE Agg : Bell; Lac-c; Tarn.

Amel : Ver-a.

Pain in remote parts, on : Sil; Tarn.

PULSATING : Arg-n; *Lach.*

SENSITIVE, Sore : AGAR; *Bell; Chin;* CHIN-S; *Cimi;* Grap; *Hypr; Ign;* Kali-p; LACH; Lyss; Med; *Nat-m;* Nat-p; *Nux-v; Pho;* Phys; Rut; Sil; Stram; Tarn; Tell; *Ther; Zin.*

Fever, during : Chin-s; Cocl.

Leaning against chair Agg : *Agar; Ther.*

Pressure, slight Agg : Stram.

Stretching Agg : Med.

SEXUAL Excess Agg : Calc; Croc; *Nux-v; Pho-ac; Sele.*

SHORT, As if : Agar; Sul.

SHUDDERING,Along haematuria with : Nit-ac.

SITTING Agg : Pho-ac; Rut; Zin.

Amel : Mur-ac.

SPOTS, In : Agar.

STANDING Agg : Nit-ac; *Pho-ac;* Zin.

Amel : Mur-ac.

STOOPING Agg : Agar.

SWALLOWING Agg : Caus.

TICKLING : Sumb.

TREMBLING : Lil-t.

TUMOUR, Of : Tarn.

UP and DOWN : Gel; Phyt.

Occiput, to : Petr.

VERTEBRA Absent, as if : Mag-p.

Cracking, in: Ol-an.

Rub against, each other as if : Ant-t.

Single, Heat, sensitive to : Agar.

Tuberculosis of, Pott's disease. (See Caries of Bones) : Aur; Calc-p; Iod; Pho; Pho-ac; Stan; Syph; Tub.

lies, back, on knees drawn up, with : Merc-c.

WALKING Agg : Grap; Mur-ac; Rut; Sul.

Amel : Gel; Hyds; Pho-ac.

WEAK : See Back.

Sitting Agg : Calc; Sul; Zin.

Standing,impossible : Sul-ac.

Support body, can not: Ox-ac.

Typhoid fever, after : *Sele.*

SPITEFUL : See Revengeful.

SPITTING, SPITS : Ant-t; Bar-c; Cam; Lyss; Stram; *Tab;* Zin-chr.

AGG : Led; Nux-v.

BILE, Of : Sang.

COMPLAINTS, Other, with : Tab.

+ CONSTANT Desire: Coc-c.

+ CONSTANTLY : *Lyss.*

FOOD : Fer.

IN FACE OF PEOPLE : *Bell;* Calc; Cup; Pho; Stram; Ver-a.

ON THE FLOOR And Licking it up : Merc.

SPASMODIC : Lyss.

SPLASHING, SWASHING, As of
water : Ars; *Bell;* Carb-ac;
Carb-an; *Chin; Crot-t;* Dig;
Glo; *Hep; Hyo;* Kali-c; Nat-m;
Pho-ac; *Rhus-t; Spig.*

HOT : Chin; Hep; Sumb.

SPLEEN (Left Hypochondria)
: Alu; Am; Ars; Asaf; *Carb-v;*
Cean; CHIN; Con; Flu-ac;
Ign; Iris; Helian; Kali-bi; Naj;
Nat-m;Nat-s; Nit-ac; Ran-b;
Rut; Scil; *Sul;* Ther.

BREATHING, Deep Agg :
Card-m; Kob; Sul.

BULGING : Tub.

BURNING, Heat : *Asaf;* Coc-c.

CHEST, To: Bor.

COUGHING Agg : Bell; Card-m;
Chin-s; Scil; Sul-ac; Sul.

ENLARGED : Ars; Bro; *Cean;
Chin;* Chin-s; *Iod;* Mag-m;
Nat-m; Scil; Sul-ac.

GURGLING : Verb.

HARD, Indurated : Ars; Bro;
Chin; Sul-ac.

HEAVY : Kali-io; Sul.
Walking, when : Mag-m.

INFLAMMATION : *Chin.*

PAINFUL : *Cean; Chin;* Scil.
Chill, during : Chin-s; Pod.
Diarrhoea, with : Cean.
Dyspnoea, with : Cean.
Fever, during : *Carb-v;*
Nat-m; Nux-v.
Menses, profuse, with :
Cean.
suppressed, with : Cean.

SORE, Tender : *Chin; Rhus-t.*

STITCHING : Agar; *Ars;* Card-m;
Cean; Sil; Sul.
+ Eating, while : Am-m.
Headache, with : Urt.
+ Lumbar Region, to :
Kali-bi.
Running Agg : Agar; Tub.
Walking, Fast Agg : Rhod.

SWELLING : *Chin.*
Painful : Rut.

SPLINTER: See Pain, Stiching,
Needle like.
+ PROMOTES Expulsion : Anac.

SPLITTING : See Pain, Bursting.
AS IF : Thyr.

SPOKEN To Or Addressed AGG
: Cham.

SPONDYLITIS CERVICAL : Pho-ac.

SPOONERISM (See Speech)
: Caus; Chin.

SPOTS, (Symptoms, Sensations
Occur in General) : Agar;
Alu; Arg-m; Ars; *Berb;* Buf;
Calc-p; Caus; *Cist;* Colch;
Con; Flu-ac; Glo; Hep; Ign;
KALI-BI; LAC-C; Lil-t;
Nat-m; Nux-m; Ol-an; Ol-j;
Ox-ac; Pho; Rhus-t; Sars;
Sele; *Sep;* Sil; SUL; Thu; Zin.
COLD : Calc-p; Petr; Sep;
Tarn; *Ver-a.*
HECTIC : See Face, Hectic Spots.
MOIST : Petr.
PAINFUL, Sore : Arn; *Glo;*
Kali-bi; Lith; Merc; Pho;
Ran-b; Saba; Sul.

SPRAINS AND STRAINS (See

Lifting **A**GG) : Agn; Arn; Bels; Calc; Calc-f; Carb-an; Con; Grap; Kali-m; Lach; Mill; Onos; Petr; Rut.

CHRONIC: Am-m; Nat-m; Stro.

EASY : Carb-an; Pho; Rhus-t.

LAMENESS, After : Rhe; Rut.

PARTS, Lain on : Mos.

SPRING (Season) **A**GG : Amb; *Bell*; Bry; Calc; Calc-p; Carb-v; Cep; Con; Crot-h; *Gel*; Iris; Kali-bi; LACH; *Rhus-t*; Sars; Ver-a.

SQUATTING AGG : Calc; *Colo*; Grap; Syph.

SQUEEZING : See Pain, Sqeezing.

SQUINT: See under Eyes.

SQUIRMS : Val.

STAGE F**RIGHT** : See Fear of, Appearing in Public.

STAGGERING : See Reeling and Gait Staggering.

STAINS :See under Discharges, Menses, Leucorrhoea, Urine, Stool.

STAMMERING : See under Speech.

STANDING A**GG** : Alo; Berb; Bry; Cocl; Con; Cyc; Ign; Lil-t; *Nat-m*; Nat-s; Plat; Pul; Rhus-t; *Sep*; SUL; Tarx; *Val*.

A**MEL** : *Ars*; BELL; Colch; Led; Pho; Ran-b; Scil; Sul-io.

E**RECT** A**MEL** : Ars; Bell; Ced; *Dios*; Kali-p.

Impossible : Aeth; Cocl; Hydroc; Kali-br.

falls, after : Arg-n.

EYES Closed, with **A**GG :

Arg-n; Calad; Iod; Lathy.

INABILITY To remain : Chin-s.

LEGS Keeps wide apart, when : Pho; Pic-ac; Terb.

TIP TOE, On **A**GG : Cocl.

STAPHYLOMA : Ap; *Euphor*; Pul.

STARE, STARING : See under Eyes.

+ C**ONSTANTLY** : Hyo.

EVERYTHING At, as if : Med.

+ F**RIGHTENED,** As if : Zin.

+ O**NE** P**OINT** : Bov.

+ P**ERSONS** At, who talk to him : Merc-c.

+ S**TUPID** : Hell.

+ T**HOUGHTLESS** : Guai.

VACANTLY : Bov.

STARTLED E**ASILY** : See Frightened easily.

STARTS : See Jerks.

EASILY : Med; Saba; Zin.

INVOLUNTARILY, Violent : Stro.

NOISE, Least, from : Ant-c; Sil.

PAIN Agg : Arg-n; Lyc.

SLEEP, In : See Sleep, Jerks during.

TOUCH, On : Kali-c; Mag-c.

TRIFLES, At : Bor; Ther.

Unexpected, from: Arn.

STARVING : Ign.

HE MUST : Kali-m.

STEALS MONEY : Calc.

NECESSITY, Without : Art-v; Cur; Nux-v; Tarn.

STEAM AGG : Kali-bi.

Aᴍᴇʟ : Ars-s-fl; Lyss.

STEPPING Bᴀᴄᴋᴡᴀʀᴅs : See Gait.

Dᴏᴡɴsᴛᴀɪʀs Aɢɢ : Stram.

High, Steps, from Agg : Phyt.

Hᴀʀᴅ ᴀɢɢ : See Jarring Aɢɢ.

Hɪɢʜ : See Gait.

Pᴇʀsᴏɴs, Are, as if : Alo.

STERILITY : See under Female Affections.

STERNUM Bᴀᴄᴋ To: Kali-bi; Kali-io; Merc-sul.

Aʙᴅᴏᴍᴇɴ, To : Stic.

Cᴀʀɪᴇs : Con.

Cʟᴏsᴇ, Too, back to : Cina.

Cᴏʟᴅ : Cam; *Ran-b.*

Cᴏᴜɢʜɪɴɢ Agg : *Bry; Caus;* Kali-bi.

Exᴏsᴛᴏsᴇs : Merc-c.

Fᴏʀᴍɪᴄᴀᴛɪᴏɴ : Ran-sc.

+ Iᴛᴄʜɪɴɢ, Lungs in, behind : Iod.

Pʀᴇssᴜʀᴇ, Behind : Pho-ac.

Sᴘɪɴᴇ, To : Con; Stic.

+ Sᴛᴏɴᴇ, As if, in middle : Arg-n.

Tʜʀᴏʙʙɪɴɢ : Lach; Sil.

Abdomen, to : Stic.

Tᴡɪsᴛɪɴɢ : Pho-ac.

Uɴᴅᴇʀ: Am-c; Aur; Calc; *Caus;* Cham; Gel; Iod; Pho; Rhus-t; *Rum;* Sang.

Aching : Manc; *Rum.*

Axilla, to : Kali-n.

Burning Sang.

Food has lodged, as if : Led; Lyc.

Heaviness (crushing

weight) : Aur.

ascending Agg : Aur.

Lump : Aur; Bur-p; Chin; Echi; Gel; *Pho;* Pul; Sil.

Rawness : Kali-bi.

Sore : Ran-sc.

Ulcer, as if : Psor.

Wᴀʀᴛs, On : Nit-ac.

STERTOR : Op.

STICKY, Sᴛʀɪɴɢʏ, Pasty : See Discharges.

STIFFENING OUT (Of Body) : Cam; Cham; *Cina;* Cup; *Ign; Ip;* Just; Pho; Stram.

STIFFNESS, Rɪɢɪᴅɪᴛʏ : Aesc; Ap; Bell; Bry; *Caus;* Chel; *Cic;* Cimi; Dros; Dul; *Guai;* Ign; Kalm; Lach; Led; Lyc; *Med;* Nux-v; Old; Onos; Phys; Rat; RHUS-T; Sec; *Sep;* Sil; Stic; *Sul;* Sul-ac; Terb.

Cʀᴀᴍᴘ, From : Sele; Ver-a.

Mᴏᴠᴇ, Can not : Spo.

Pᴀɪɴ Agg : Nit-ac; Onos.

Pᴀɪɴʟᴇss : Old.

STIFLING : See Pain, Strangling.

STINGING : See Pain, Stinging.

Bᴇᴇs, As if : Ap; Gel.

STINGS (Of Bᴇᴇs, Iɴsᴇᴄᴛs) : Ap; Hypr; Latro; Led; Pulex; Urt.

STITCHES : See Pain, Stitching.

Pᴀɪɴғᴜʟ : Stap.

Sɪᴅᴇs, In : See Side.

STOMACH (Affections In General) : Aeth; Arg-n; ARS; Bry; *Calc;* Carb-v; *Chin;* Colo; Ip; Lach; LYC; NUX-V;

PHO; PUL; Sep; Sil; *Sul;* Ver-a.

ACIDITY, Hyper, alternating with Hypo : Chin-ar.

ALTERNATING, Head or Face with : Bism.

Skin, with : Grap.

ANXIETY, Emotions, felt in : *Ars;* Colo; IGN; Kali-c; Mez; Nat-m; *Tarn.*

Head, rising, into: Nat-m.

ATROPHY : Bism; Kre; Ox-ac.

AXILLA, And upper arm, to : Am-m.

BACKWARD : Berb; Bism; Con; Kali-c; Sul.

Bending Amel : Bism.

Reverse, or : Berb.

Shoulders, between : *Bell.*

BEHIND : Arn; Cact; Ham; Kali-c; Stram.

BITTER, Something, as if in : Cup.

BREATHING Deep Agg : Arg-n; Caus; Pul.

Amel : Rum.

BUBBLING : Caus; Lyss.

BURNING : Am-m; ARS; *Canth;* Caps; *Carb-v; Cic;* Colch; Merc-c; Pho; Ran-b; Rob; SEC; Sep; SUL; *Ver-a.*

Breathing, deep Agg : Calad.

+ Painful : Kali-io.

Spot : Gymn.

CANCER : Am-m; Ars; Bism; Cadm; Carb-ac; Carb-an; Con; Hyds; Kre;Lach; *Lyc; Pho.*

CARRYING, Burdens Agg : Cadm.

CHURNING, In : Lyc.

COLDNESS (See Abdomen) : Ars; Cam; Caps; Chin; Cist; Clem; Lyc; Meny; Ol-an.

Cold, Drinks, after : Chin; Elap.

water, as from : Caps; Grat.

Eating, before and after : Cist.

Fruits, after : Elap.

Icy : Aco; *Caps;* Caus; Colch; Pho.

lump : Bov.

oesophagus, to : Meny.

pain, with : Colch.

rubbing and pressure Amel : Carb-an.

sweat, with : Zin-io.

CONTRACTED: Ars; Carb-v; Cup.

CRAMP, Constrictional squeezing : Asaf; Chel; Grap; Kre; Rat; Rob.

Fluid passing through, intestines, as if, with : Mill.

CRAVING At, menses before : Spo.

CUTTING : Dios; Rat.

DEATH Like sensation : Ars; *Cup.*

DIGESTION Disordered : See Indigestion.

DISTENDED (See Abdomen) : Cic; Rat.

DRINKS Agg : Apoc; Rhod.

Cold milk Agg : Kali-io.

DRYNESS, In : Calad.

EATING Amel (See Abdomen)
: *Chel; Grap;* Hep; Petr.

Every bite, hurts : Ars;
Calc-p.

Too much Agg : Ant-c;
Cof; Ip; *Pul.*

EMPTY, Hollow, Sinking,
Weak feeling : Ant-c;
Ant-t; Carb-an; Cocl; DIG;
Hell; Hyds; Ign; Ip; Lac-c;
Lob; Merc; Murx; *Nux-v;*
PHO; *Pod;* Pul; SEP; *Stan;*
Stap; *Sul;* Sul-ac; *Tab;* Tell;
Tril; Ver-a; *Zin.*

At 9-10 A.M. : Hep.

At 11 A.M. : Ign; Petr; Pho;
Sep; *Sul.*

Amel : Dig.

+ Brandy Amel : Old.

+ Deep breath Amel : Ign.

Eating, Not Amel, by :
Carb-an; Cina; Ign; Lach;
Lyc; Mur-ac; Pho; Sep;
Ver-a.

after : Grat; Old; Sars.

Epilepsy, before : *Hyo.*

Extending, heart, to : *Lob.*

Fasting, as from : Sars.

Food, thought of, from : Sep.

loathing of, with : Hyds.

Headache, during : Sep.

Heart weak or dilated,
with : Chlo-hyd.

Hunger, without : Lach.

Milk, sips in, Amel : Diph.

Nausea, during : Pho.

+ No desire to eat : Am-m.

Nursing, after : *Carb-an;*
Old.

Pressure Agg : Merc.

Stools, after : Mur-ac; Sul-ac.

Talking Agg : Rum.

Urination after : Apoc.

Walking, fast Amel : Myr.

ENLARGED : Bar-c; Sil.

EPILEPTIC Aura : Calc; Cic;
Nux-v; Sil; Sul.

Extending head, to : *Calc.*

EXTENDING, To: Bism; Colch;
Dul; Kali-bi; Lapp.

FASTING And Eating, after Agg
: Bar-c.

FEVER Agg : Ip; Ver-v.

FLAMES, As of : Manc.

FLOATING In, Water, as if :
Abro.

FLUTTERING, In : Calad.

FULLNESS : *Carb-v;* Caus; *Chin;*
Kali-c; LYC; Nux-m; Pho;
SUL.

Full Of Dry food, as if :
Cadm.

Water, as if : *Kali-c;* Ol-an.

GNAWING : Aesc; Am-m;
Arg-m; Cina; Colo; Lith;
Sep; Stan.

+ Drinking hot water Amel
: Lyc.

Eating Amel : Anac; Kali-p;
Lach; Lith.

Returns, few hours after :
Lach.

Temple (L) with : Lith.

GRIPING : See Cramps.

GOUT, Alternating, with :
Ant-c; Nux-m.

GURGLING : Cup.

Drinking, when : Cup; Hyd-ac.

after : Pho.

HANGING Down, as if : Bism; Hep; Ign; Ip; Pho; Stap.

Stools, after : Amb.

HARD, Body, rolling about : Lil-t.

Spot, painful, at : Kre.

HEAD,To : Calc.

HEAT, Flushes of : Ars; Bry; Nux-v.

HEAVY Weight, Oppression : Bry; Chin; Kali-c; Lyc; Nux-v; Pic-ac; Pul; Sul.

Back, of : Ham.

Cold drink, from : Rhod.

Eating, after : Hep; Kali-bi.

+ Eructation Amel : Par.

Loose : Grat.

Night, at : Kali-m.

Spot, one, in : Bism.

Stone, as from : Par; Pul.

HORRIBLE Feeling, in A.M. drunkards in : Asar.

ICY : See Coldness, Icy.

water Agg : Caus.

INJURY, After : Nux-v.

INFLAMMATION: See Gastritis.

LIFTING, Heavy Agg : Bor.

LIMBS, To : Kali-c.

LUMP, Ball etc. as if in : Ab-n; Arn; Bell; Bov; Lob; Nux-m; Osm; *Pul;* Sanic.

Hard : Nux-m.

Hot, burning : Bell.

Icy : Bov.

Rising up into throat : Lach; Senec.

Sharp : Hyds.

LYING Amel : Grap.

Side, on Amel : Lyc.

Left Amel : Scil.

Legs drawn up, with Amel : Chel.

MILK Amel : Grap; Merc; Merc-cy; Mez; Rut.

+ Cold Agg : Kali-io.

+ Desire, for : Sabal.

OVER LOADING Agg : *Nux-v;* Stap.

+ As if : Ant-c.

PASSES or Pressed against spine, as if : Arn; Ver-v.

PILES, Operation, after : Croc.

PLUG : Chel.

RAW : Carb-v; *Nux-v.*

REFLEXES, From : Ol-an.

REPLETE, As if : Merc.

ROLLING, Over in : Pho.

SCRAPING, In : Ars; Pul.

SHOULDER, Right, to : Sang.

SOUR, Acidity (See Sour) : *Calc;* Caps; Carb-v; Chin; Kob; *Lyc; Mag-c;* Nat-m; *Nat-p; Nux-v; Pul;* Rob; Sep; Sul; Sul-ac.

Alternating with decreased : Calc-ar.

SPINE, To : Arn; Ver-v.

SPOT, In : Arg-n; Bar-c; Bism; Kali-bi; Lyc.

SQUEEZING, In : Rob.

STITCHING : Ars.

Motion Agg : *Bry;* Pul; Spig.

STONES In, as if : Ant-t; Ars; Bar-c; Bry; Calc; Cocl; Manc; Naj; Nux-m; Nux-v; Osm.

Cold : Sil.

Eating Amel : Ptel.

Eructations Amel : *Bar-c;* Par.

Pressure. as from : Aesc; Bro; Cham; Scil.

Rubbing together : Cocl.

Sharp, as if : Hyds.

STOOLS Agg : Amb; Pul; Sul-ac.

Amel : Chel.

SUMMER Agg : Guai.

SWIMMING, In Water, as if : See Floating.

TALKING, Sensitive, to : Caus; Hell; Kali-c; Rum.

TENSION : Carb-v; Lyc; Nux-v; Rut; Stan.

Milk Amel : *Rut.*

THROBBING, Pulsations : Aco; Ant-t; *Calc;* Chin; Cic; Glo; Kali-c; Nat-m; Ol-an; *Nux-v;* Pho; PUL; *Sep;* Sil.

Back, of: Kali-c.

Eating Agg : Sele.

Eructation Amel : Sep.

TREMBLING, Quivering : Calc; Iod; Nux-v; Pho; Sang.

Extends all over body : Lyc.

TWISTING, Throat, rising to : Sep.

ULCERS : Hyds; Kali-bi; Lyc; Pho; Ran-b; Symp.

+ Cancer : Acet-ac; Carb-v; Crot-h.

UPSIDE, Down : *Aeth.*

UPWARD, From : Kali-m; Pho.

URINATION Agg : Laur.

UTERUS, Reflex from : Bor.

VOMITING Agg : Sep.

Amel : Hyo.

WALKING Agg : Hep.

WARM, Something rises up, causing suffocation : Val.

WATER, As of : Ol-an.

+ WINE Amel : Aco.

WORM, Crawling up throat : Zin.

Morning, in : Cocl.

YAWNING Agg : *ARS;* Phyt.

Amel : Lyc; Nat-m.

STOMATITIS : See Mouth, Aphthae.

STONE CUTTER'S PTHISIS : Calc; Lyc; Sil.

STOOL BEFORE AGG : Alo; Calc; Dul; Merc; *Nux-v;* Sul; *Ver-a.*

DURING AGG: Ars; Cham; *Merc;* Nit-ac; Nux-v; Pul;Sep; Sil; Spig; *Sul;* Ver-a.

+ Remains, as if : Lyc.

AFTER AGG : *Caus;* Merc; *Merc-c;* Nit-ac; Nux-v; *Pho;* Pod; Sele; Sil; Sul.

FROM AGG : Dios; Merc; *Merc-c;* Paeon.

AMEL : Bor; Colo; Gamb; *Nat-s; Nux-v;* Ox-ac; Pall; Pho-ac; Rhus-t.

LOOSE AMEL : Abro; Nat-s; *Zin.*

PRESSING AT AGG : Agar; Bell;

Carb-an; Ign; Nux-v; Pul; Rat; Rhus-t; Sep; Tell.

Leans far back, for   : Med.

STOOLS ACRID : Arn; *Ars;* Carb-v; Chin; Colch; Gamb; Ign; Iris; **MERC**; Nat-m; *Pul;* Rhe; Scop; SUL; Ver-a.

Hair, destroys : Coll.

A**SHY**   : See White.

B**AD ODOUR**, Foul, Putrid : *Ars;* Asaf; Bap; Benz-ac; Bor; Calc-f; *Carb-v;* Chin; Grap; Kali-p; Nux-v; *Pod; Psor;* Pul; Sil; Stram; Sul; Sul-ac; Tub.

Cheese, Rotten : *Bry; Hep;* Sanic.

Eggs, rotten : Ascl; Cham; Psor.

Penetrating : *Pod; Psor;* Stram.

Sour : See Sour.

B**ALLS**, Like : See Sheep Dung.

B**ILIOUS** : Cham; Crot-h; *Iris; Merc;* Nat-s; Pod; *Pul;* Sang; *Ver-a.*

Warm Drinks Agg : Flu-ac.

B**LACK** : *Ars;* Coll; *Lapt;* Merc; Merc-c; Plb; *Op;* Stram; Sul-ac; *Thu;* VER-A.

Foul : Chio; Crot-h; Lept.

Tarry : Chio; Lept; Phys; Ptel.

B**LADDER** Symtoms,with : Merc-c.

B**LOOD** Only (See Haemorrhage) : Aco; Alu; Erig; Ham; Merc-c; Rhus-t; Tril.

B**LOODY** : Alu; Ars; *Canth;* Caps; Chin; Colch; Colo; Elap;

Ham; Ip; Jalap; Merc; MERC-C; NUX-V; PHO; Pul; Rhus-t; Sec; Senec; Terb.

Clots   : Cadm.

bright : Alu.

End, at   : Daph.

Tarry : Ham.

frothy : Elap.

Water : Fer-p; Merc-c; Pho; *Rhus-t.*

B**LUE** : Bap; Colch; Pho.

B**REAKFAST** Agg : Nat-s; Thu.

B**RIGHT** : Sul-io.

B**ROWN** : Arg-n; Ars; *Bry;* Grap; Ip; Kre; Lyc; Merc; Nux-v; *Psor; Rhe;* Scil; Sec; Tub; Ver-a.

Gushes   : Ast-r; Kali-bi.

B**URNING**, Hot : Alo; *Ars;* Ascl; Bell; Bry; Caps; Cham; Gamb; IRIS; Kali-p; *Merc-c;* Pic-ac; Pod; Saba; Scop; Strop; Sul.

C**HANGEABLE** : Cham; Dul; Pul; Sanic; Sul.

C**HILL**, With : Ars; Colo; Lac-c; Merc; *Pul;* Sul; Ver-a.

C**HOPPED**, Hacked : Aco; *Cham;* Nat-p; Sul-ac.

Eggs, like   : Merc; Pul.

C**LAYEY** : Chel; Chio.

C**OLD** : Con; Cub; lyc.

C**OLDS** Agg : Calc; Rum; Tub.

C**OLOURS**, Several : Aesc; Colch; Euon; Kali-p; Menis; Sul; Zin-cy.

C**ONSTIPATED** : See Constipation.

+ CORN MEAL, Like : Aru-t.

CRUMBLING :*Am-m; Mag-m;*
Merc; *Nat-m;* Sanic.

CURDLED, Cheesy : Calend;
Iod; Tab; Val.

Screaming, with : Val.

DARK : Alu; Bap; Chin; Grap;
Kali-n; Scil; Stram.

DIAPER, Running through:
Benz-ac; *Pod.*

DIFFICULT : See under
Constipation, Inactivity,
from.

DIRTY Water, Muddy : Ars;
Bro; Fer-p; Jalap; Lept;
Ox-ac; Pho-ac; Pod.
White : Pho-ac.

DRY : *Bry;* Lac-d; Lyc;
Nat-m; Nit-ac; Nux-v;
Op; Pho; Sil; Zin.

Hard, and : Ascl.

DYSENTERIC : See Dysentery.

FATTY : See Oily.

FILAMENTS, Like hair : Sele.

FLAKY : Ver-a.

FLAT : Merc; *Pul;* Sul; Ver-a.

FLATULENT, Gassy, Noisy,
Spluttering : Agar; Alo;
Apoc; *Arg-n;* Colo; Crot-t;
Fer; Gamb; *Ign; Nat-s;*
Nux-m; Strop; Thu; Thyr;
Tub.

FLATUS Passing, on, Agg : Alo;
Ars-io; Caus; Mur-ac;
Nat-p; Old; Pho-ac; Pod;
Ver-a.

FLOATS : See Scum, Floating.

FLOCCULENT : Kali-m.

FOAMY, Frothy : Arn; *Colo;*

Form; Iod; *Kali-bi; Mag-c;*
Merc; Pod; Rhus-t; Saba;
Scil; *Sul.*

Bloody, black : Elap;

Fluent Coryza, with : Calc;
Canth; Cham; Chin;
Colo; Iod; Lach; Mag-c;
Merc; Op; Rhus-t; Rut;
Sul; Sul-ac.

Gushing : Chin; Crot-t;
Elat.

FOUL : See Bad Odour.

FREQUENT : Aco; Ars; Ascl;
Calc; Caps; *Cham;* Elat;
Kali-io; Merc; MERC-C;
NUX-V; Pho; *Pod;* Ver-a.

Bloody water : *Fer-p.*

But scanty : Ars; Merc;
Nux-v.

Causing unfitness for
work : Ascl.

Normal : Psor.

GELATINOUS : *Alo;* Asar; Colch;
Colo; Hell; Kali-bi; Mag-c;
Rhus-t.

GLISTENING : Alo; Alu; Calc;
Caus; Mez.

Particles : Cina; Mez; Pho.

GRANULAR, Sandy : Ap;
Arg-m; Bell; Cup; Hyds;
Lac-c; Lyc; Mang; Mez;
Pho; Plb; Pod; Sars; Zin.

GRAY : See White.

GREEN (See Green) : Colo;
Crot-t; Gamb; Grat; Merc-c;
Nat-m; Pod; *Rhe;* Sec;
Sul-ac.

Dark : Ars.

Grass : Aco; ANT-T; ARG-N;

Calc-p; Cham; *Ip;* Iris; *Mag-c;* Merc; Merc-d; Thu.

mucus stains skin around anus and scrotum, coppery : Cinb.

Scum : Ascl; Bry; Grat; *Mag-c;* Merc; Sanic.

Tea : Gel.

Turns : Arg-n; Bor; Calc-f; Nat-s; Psor; Rhe; Sanic.

blue : Calc-p; Pho.

yellow : Ip.

Water : Cup; Kali-br.

GURGLES, Pops, out.: Alo; Crot-t; Gamb; Grat; Jatr; Pod; Thu.

GUSHING, Pouring : Alo; Apoc; Ast-r; Bry; Calc-f; *Crot-t;* Cup; Elat; Fer; Gamb; Grat; *Jatr;* Kali-bi; Nat-c; Nat-m; POD; Psor; Sang; *Sec; Ver-a.*

ALL at once in somewhat prolonged effort : *Gamb.*

Torrent, in : Nat-c.

HACKED : See Chopped.

HARD : *Alu;* Alum; BRY; Calc; Card-m; Coll; GRAP; Lach; *Mag-m; Nat-m; Nit-ac;* Nux-v; Op; Pho; *Plb;* Sele; Sep; *Sil;* Stan; Stro; Sul; Ver-a; Verb; Zin.

First, then fluid : *Bov; Calc; Lyc;* Nat-m; Sul-ac.

black, then white and soft : Aesc.

Menses, during : Ap.

Thin first, then : Euphor.

HEAD Washing Agg : Tarn.

HEAVY : Sanic.

HOLDS Back : Nit-ac; Sil; Sul; Thu.

HOT : See Burning.

IMPACTED : Calc; Nat-m; Sanic; Sele; Sep; Sil.

INVOLUNTARY, Hurried : ALO; Ap; ARN; Bar-c; Bell; Gel; *Hyo; Mur-ac;* Nat-m; Nat-p; Old; Op; *Pho; Pho-ac;* Pod; Pyro; Rhus-t; Sec; Stram; *Sul;* Tab; Thu; *Ver-a.*

Although Solid : *Alo;* Ars; Caus; Colo; *Hyo.*

Bloody : Hyo.

Convulsions, during : Cup.

Coughing, when : Pho; Scil; Sul.

Flatus, every time, with: Old; Pho-ac.

Foetus, movement from: Pho-ac.

Fright, from : Op.

Headache, with : Mos.

Laughing on : Sul.

Lying when : Ox-ac.

Moved, when (Children): Pho-ac.

Sleep, during : Arn; Bry; Con; Mos; *Pod; Psor.*

Sneezing, on : See Coughing.

Stooping : Rut.

Urine and : Ail; *Mur-ac.*

Urinating, when : *Alo;* Alu; Ap; Hyo; Mur-ac; Scil.

Vomiting, during : Arg-n

Ars.

Walking, while : Alo.

Yellow, watery : Hyo.

KNOTTY, Lumpy : See Sheep dung, like.

LARGE Caliber : Alum; BRY; Calc; Elat; *Grap; Kali-c;* Kali-s; Lac-d; Lept; *Lyc;* Mag-m; Mez; Nat-s; Nux-v; SANIC; Sep; Sul; *Ver-a.*

Burnt, as if : Bry.

Hard : Bry; Lac-d.

MEALY : Pod; Stro.

MEAT WATER, like : Canth; Pho; Pod; Rhus-t.

MEMBRANOUS : See Shreddy.

MENSES Agg : See Diarrhea.

MILK Agg : Nat-c; Sep.

MILKY : Calc; Chel; Chin; Dig; Merc; Pod; Sanic; Tab.

MISSHAPEN, Angular, Square, etc. : Nat-m; Plb; Sanic; Sele; Sep.

MOLASSES, Like : Ip.

MUCUS : Arg-n; ARS; Asar; Bor; CAPS; CHAM; *Colch;* Coll; Gamb; GRAP; *Hell;* Ip; Kali-m; Kali-s; *Merc; Merc-c; Nux-v; Pho;* PUL; Rhe; Rhus-t; Solid; Spig; SUL; Ver-a;

Balls, of : Ip.

Bloody : Colch; *Merc; Merc-c;* Nat-c; Nux-v; Pod.

Coated : Am-m; Cham; *Grap;* Hyds; Nat-m; Pul.

Copious : Terb.

involuntary : Solid.

Green : Aco; *Arg-n;* Ars; Castr; *Cham;* Dul; *Gamb;* Iris; Laur; Mag-c; MERC; Merc-c; Pul.

Jelly, like : Asar; Colch; Hell; Sep.

Lumps, of : Alo; Cop; Grap; Ip; Mag-c; Pho; Spig.

Offensive : Sep.

Only : Ant-c; Asaf.

Stools, after : Bry; Sep; Thu.

Tenacious : Asar; Canth; Hell.

Transperant : Bor; Colch; Hell.

White : Bor; Kali-chl; Nat-m.

milky : Kali-chl.

Yellow : Asar; kali-s.

MUDDY : See Dirty Water.

MUSHY : Bry; Chin; Nit-ac; Onos; Pho; Pul; Rhus-t; *Sul.*

Yellow : Bry.

MUSTY : Colo.

NARROW, Long : See Slender.

NERVOUS : See under Diarrhea.

NIGHTLY : See under Diarrhea.

NOISY : See Flatulent.

NOON, At : Radm.

ODOURLESS : Ap; Kali-bi; Pho-ac; Ver-a.

OILY, Fatty : Ascl; Caus; Dul; Iod; Iris; *Mag-c;* Nat-s; Pho; Pic-ac; Tarn; Thu.

ORANGE Colour, or pulp : Ap; Nat-c.

PAIN, Long after : See under

Rectum.

PASTY : See Sticky.

PURULENT : Arn; Merc; Pul.

PUTTY Like : Dig; Plat.

RECEDING : See Constipation, Stool recedes.

RED : Chel; Lyc; Merc; RHUS-T; Sul.

REMOVED, Must be : See Constipation.

RETAINED : *Cocl*; Sil; *Stram*.

Pain from : Sil.

RICE WATER : Ars; *Cam*; Cupars; Jatr; Pho-ac; *Ver-a*.

RUMBLING, With : Colo; Strop.

SAGO-LIKE : Colch; Pho.

SAND, In: See Stool, Granular.

SCANTY : Am-m; Merc; Nux-v; Plb; Sil; Sul.

SCRAPING of intestine, like : Canth; Colch; Colo.

SCUM Floating : Ascl; *Bry;* Colch; Grat; *Mag-c*; Saba; Sal-ac; Sanic.

SHEEP DUNG : *Alu; Alum; Chel; Grap;* Hyds; Lyc; Mag-c; MAG-M; *Merc; Nat-m;* Nit-ac; OP; PLB; Pyro; Sanic; Sep; Sil; Stan; Stro; *Sul;* Syph; Thu; Verb.

Chalky : Bell; Calc.

Green : Chin; Stan.

Tallow, like : Mag-c.

SHREDDY : Arg-n; Canth; Carb-ac; Colch; Colo; Merc-c.

SHOOTING : See Gushing.

SLENDER, Narrow : Bor; Caus; Grap; Mur-ac; *Pho;* Sul.

SOFT : See Mushy.

First part, then hard : Nux-v.

SOUR : *Calc;* Colo; Dul; Grap; Hep; Jalap; Mag-c; Merc; Nat-p; Rhe; Sul.

Milk, Like : Tab.

SPRAYING : Thu.

STANDING Amel : Alu; Caus.

STARCH, Like : Arg-n; Bor.

STICKY, Pasty : Bry; Chel; Colo; Crot-t; Kali-bi; Lach; Merc; Merc-c; *Plat*; Pod; Rhe; Rhus-t; Sul.

STRINGY, Tough : Colch; Grap; Lept; *Pho.*

SUDS, Like : Benz-ac; Colch; Elat; Glo; Iod; Sul.

SWEETISH, Odour : Mos.

TARRY : See Black.

TEARING Anus : Mez; Nat-m.

Though, soft : Nit-ac.

+ TOMATO-SAUCE Like : Ap.

UNDIGESTED : *Ars;* Bry; CALC; Calc-p; CHIN; Chio; *Fer; Grap;* Mag-m; *Old; Pho;* Pho-ac; Pod.

Brown : Kre; Psor.

Milk : Mag-c.

One day; before, of : Old.

URINOUS, Pungent odour : Benz-ac.

WATERY, Thin : Ant-c; Apoc; Asaf; Benz-ac; Calc; Calc-p; Chin; Cina; Colch; *Colo;* Dul; Gamb; Hell; *Iris;* Jalap; Kali-p; Kre; Nat-s; Old; Pho; Pic-ac; Pod; Rhus-t; Sec; Sul; Thu;

Tub.
Black : Ars.
Bloody : See under Bloody.
Brown: Ars; Ast-r; *Grap;*
Kali-bi.
Green : Cham; *Grat.*
Hard, although, or : Hyo.
Jaundice, with : Berb.
Lumpy, and : Ant-c; Lyc;
Sanic.
black, with : Thu.
Muddy : Lept.
Rice Water : See Rice Water.
Yellow : Dul; *Gamb*; Grat;
Old; *Pod*; Stro; Thu.
Waxy : Kali-bi; Lept.
Wheyey : Cup; Iod.
White, Gray, Ashy: Ars;
Benz-ac; Calc; Canth;
Chel; Cina; Dig; Kali-c;
Lach; *Merc;* Nat-m; Op;
Pho; Pho-ac; *Pod;* Pul; Stil;
Tarx; Urt.
Chalk, like: Calc; Pod;
Sanic.
curdy: Calend.
Egg white, like boiled : Urt.
Glassy : Ars-io.
Parts, in : Pho.
Putty like : Mag-c.
Yellow : Apoc; Ars; Colo;
Crot-t; Merc; *Pod.*
Bright : Aeth; Alo; Chel;
Colch; Gel; *Kali-p; Nux-m;*
Pho; Pho-ac; Pod; Sul-ac;
Sul-io.
+ Green : Aeth.
Saffron, like : Sul-ac.

Whitish : Pho-ac.
STOOP, Inability, To : Bor.
Coccyx, Fall on, from : Hypr.
Shouldered : Sul; Tub.
STOOPING Agg : Aesc; Agar;
Am-c; Bell; BRY; *Calc;* Caus;
Lyc; *Mang;* Merc; Nux-v; Pul;
Ran-b; Sep; Sil; *Spig; Sul;*
Tell; Ther; *Val.*
Amel : Cina; COLCH; Con;
HYO; Ign; *Iris;* Pul; Ran-b.
Easy, Stretching difficult :
Nat-m.
Prolonged agg : Asar; Bov;
Caus; Hep; Plat.
STORMS Agg (See Change of
TemperatureAgg) : Hyd-ac.
After agg : Calc-p; Rhus-t.
Before agg : *Elap;* Med; Rhod;
Rhus-t; Sul-io.
STOVE HEAT Amel : See
under Heat.
STRABISMUS : See Squint,
under eyes.
STRAINING : See Pain Pressing.
STRAINS : See Sprain.
STRANGE Positions, In Amel
: See Attitude, Bizarre.
Does, Thing: Arg-n; Cact; Sep.
Everything, Seems (See
Bewildered) : Cic; *Med;*
Plat; Val; Tub.
Disagreeable, and : Val.
Terrible, and : Cic; Plat.
Notions, Pregnancy, during
: Lyss.
STRANGER, In Presence of
Agg (See CompanyAgg)

: *Amb; Bar–c;* Carb–v; Caus; *Lyc;* Petr; Pho; SEP; STRAM; Tarn; Thu.

AMEL : Thu.

AMONG, As if : Ast–r.

MENSES, During Agg : Con.

ONE WERE, As if : Val.

STRANGLING SENSATION : Sul; Val.

SLEEP, Falling to, on : Val.

STRANGURY : See Urination, Difficult.

STREAKS : See Pain, Linear, Red and Skin.

STRENGTH SENSATION, Of : See Vigour.

CHANGING Suddenly : Tarn.

+ SINKING, Suddenly : Grap.

STREPTOCOCCUS INFECTION : Ail; Arn; Sul–ac.

STRETCH, IMPULSE To : *Alu; Am–c; Ars;* Bry; Carb–v; CAUS; Cham; Grap; Guai; Lyc; Mar–v; Meph; NUX–V; Pul; Rhus–t; Rut; Scil; Zin.

Abdominal troubles, in : Plb.

Chill, with : Eup–p; Fer–p; Nat–s.

Drowsiness, with : Pod.

Enough, can not : Grap.

Hiccough, with : Amy–n.

Hours, for : Amy–n; Plb.

Urination, before : Pul.

Yawning, with : Amy–n.

STRETCHES, TWISTS, Turns (See Stiffening out) : Alu; *Bell; Calc;* Chel; *Cina;* Colo; Ign; Mar–v; Nux–v; Plb;

Rhus–t; Sul.

CONVULSIONS, Before : Calc.

COUGH After : Merc.

STRETCHING, Extending limbs Agg and Amel : See under Bending.

FORCIBLE AMEL : Sec.

PARTS AGG : Stap.

STRICTURE : Canth; Cic; *Clem;* Con; Flu–ac; Guai; *Merc;* Nit–ac; Nux–v; Petr; Pul; Rhus–t; Sil; Sul–io.

DILATATION, After : Con; Mag–m.

INFLAMMATION, After : Rhus–t.

STRIKES : Arg–m; *Bell; Cham;* Cina; Hyo; Kali–c; Lyss; Plb; Stram; Tarn.

STRINGY: See Discharges, Sticky.

STROPHULUS: See under Skin.

STUBBING TOE Agg : Colch.

STUBBORN, OBSTINATE : Agar; *Alu;* Anac; Ant–c; Ant–t; Arg–n; Aru–t; *Bell;* BRY; *Calc; Cham;* Chin; Cina; *Hell;* Kre; NUX–V; Sanic; Sil; Tarn.

MENSES, Before : Cham.

STUDY (See Mental Exertion) AGG : Ars–io; Mag–p.

STUFFED UP : Anac; Coc–c; Med; Spo.

STUMBLING (See Jarring) AGG : Bry; Caus.

STUMPS PAINFUL : See Pain, Stumps in.

STUNNED, STUPEFACTION : See Dull.

STUNNING: Flu-ac.

STUPID (See Childish) : Merc-c; Rhod.

STYES : See under Eyelids.

SUBARACHNOID : Gel.

SUBINVOLUTION: See under Uterus.

SUBSULTUS TENDINUM : See under Twitchings.

SUCKLING : See under Children.

AGG : See under Mammae.

SUDDEN EFFECTS, Symptoms : Aco; Ap; Ars; *Bell*; Colo; Con; Cup; Hyd-ac; Lyc; Mag-c; Mag-p; *Mez*; Nat-s; Pho; Radm; Tab; Tarn; Tarn-c; Val; Ver-a.

CHANGING About : Amb; Berb; Cimi; Dios; Val.

SUFFOCATION : See respiration, Difficult.

SUICIDAL DISPOSITION, Weary of life : Am-c; ARS; AUR; Aur-m; Chin; Dros; Lach; Meli; Merc; Naj; Nat-m; *Nat-s*; Nit-ac; *Nux-v; Pho*; Psor; Pul; Sul; Thu; Tub.

BLOOD, Seeing on : Alu.

BROODING : Naj.

BY DAGGER : Ars; Bell; Nux-v.

BY DROWNING : Dros; Hyo; Rhus-t; Sec; Sil; Sul.

BY HANGING : Ars; Bell.

BY POISON : Ars; Bell; Pul.

BY SHOOTING : Anac; Ant-c; Nat-s.

BY STARVING : Merc.

CARS, Under : Ars; Kali-br; Lach.

EROTO MANIA, In : Orig.

HEIGHT Leaping, from : Arg-n; Gel; Iod; Lach; Sul.

HOMESICKNESS, from : Caps.

KNIFE, Seeing on: Alu.

LOVE Disappointment, from : Bell; Caus; Stap.

MENSES, During : Merc.

MUSIC, From : Nat-c.

PAIN, From : *Aur*; Nux-v.

WEEPING Amel : Merc; Pho.

SULCI, MEMBRANES of : Kali-bi.

+ **SULKY** (See Morose) : Ant-c.

SUMMER AGG (Hot Weather AGG): Aeth; Ant-c; Bell; Bry; Carb-v; Cup; Dul; *Flu-ac*; Gel; *Glo*; Grat; Iris; *Kali-bi*; Lach; Nat-c; Nat-m; POD; Rhe; Sele; Ver-a.

AMEL: Alu; Aur-m; Calc-p; Fer; Sil.

OVER COAT, Wears in : Hep.

SUNBURN: See under Burns.

SUN HEAT, Exposure to AGG (See HEAT of Fire AGG) : Cact; Cadm; Cocl; Kob; Murx.

AMEL : Anac; Cinb; Con; Crot-h; Iod; Kali-m; Pic-ac; Plat; Rhod; *Stro*; Tarn.

LIGHT AGG : *Ant-c*; Bell; Euphr; *Glo*; Kali-bi; Lith; *Nat-c*; Pru-sp; Sele.

Blinds: Lith.

AMEL : Rhod; Thu.

PAINS : See Directions, Increasing gradually.

RISE, After AGG : Cham; Nux-v.

389

SLEEPING, In AGG : Aco.

SUNSET AGG : Aur; Kre; *Merc;* Phyt; *Syph.*

AMEL: Coca; Lil-t; Med;Sele.

To SUNRISE AGG : Colch; *Syph.*

SUNSTROKE (See also Heat exhaustion) : Aco; Ant-c; Arg-m; *Bell;* Cact; Cam; *Gel; Glo;* Hyo; Lach; Nat-c; Nux-v; Op; Stram; Ther; Ver-v.

EFFECTS, Chronic : Nat-c.

SUPERSTITIOUS : *Con;* Zin.

SUPPORT AMEL : Fer; Kali-c; Lil-t; Nat-c; Nat-m; Pho-ac; Sep.

SUPPRESSIONS (See Discharges Amel) : Mez; Stram; Thu; Ver-a.

SUPPURATION : See Abscess, and Pus.

STUBBORN : Kali-bi; Nit-ac; *Sil.*

SURGINGS : See Waves.

SURPRISE AGG : Gel.

PLEASANT AGG : Cof.

UNPLEASANT : Gel.

SUSPENDED : See Hanging down, as if.

SUSPENSE AGG : Arg-n.

SUSPICIOUS DISTRUSTFUL : Aco; Anac; Ars; Aur; BAR-C; Bry; *Calc;* Cann; CAUS; CIC; Cimi; Crot-h; Dig; *Hyo;* Kali-br; *Lach;* LYC; Merc; Nat-s; Nux-v; PUL; Rhus-t; Sec; Stram; Sul; Thyr.

FOOLISHLY : Ap.

LOOKS ON ALL SIDES : Kali-br.

PEOPLE Are Talking about her : *Bar-c;* Hyo; Ign; Pall; Stap.

WALKING, While: Anac.

SUTURES : See Fontanelles under Children.

PAINFUL : Stap.

SWALLOW CONSTANT DISPOSITION to : Bell; *Caus;* Con; Cub; Grap; Lach; Merc; Merc-c; Saba; Senec; Sep.

CHOKING, From : *Grap;* Lyc; Merc; *Merc-c;* Sep.

With : Bell.

DRINK Must, to : Bar-c; *Bell; Cact;* Calad; Guai; Kali-c; Nat-c; Nat-m.

EATING Amel: Caus; *Merc-c.*

EXCITEMENT Agg : Stap.

FOREIGN Body, as from : Ant-c.

HASTILY, Anger with : Anac.

INVOLUNTARILY : Cina; Mur- ac; *Sep;* Stap.

LUMP, Large, as of a, from: Cep.

SLEEP, In : Calc; Cina.

SOUR, Bitter fluid, Vertigo with : Caul.

SPEAKING, While : *Cic;* Stap; Thu.

WALKING In Wind, while : Con.

SWALLOWING AGG (Also Painful, Difficult) : Am-c; Ap; Bar-c; BELL; Bro; Bry; Canth; Caus; Chin; Cina; Cocl; *Gel;* Grap; Hep; Hyd-ac; *Hyo;* Kali-c; Lac-c; LACH; Laur; Lyss; Meph; Merc; Merc-c; Merc-i-f; *Nit-ac;* Nux-m; Pho; Phyt; Plb; *Rhus-t; Stram;* Sul; Sul-io.

AFTER AGG : Cadm; Vinc.

AMEL : Alu; Amb; Arn; *Caps;*
IGN; Lach; Led; Mang; Mez;
Nux-v; Pul; *Rhus-t;* Saba;
Spo; Zin.

CHOREA, In : Art-v.

CONTINUOUS AMEL : Ign.

EMPTY AGG : *Bar-c;* Bell; Bry;
Cocl; Grap; Hep; *Kali-c;*
LACH; Merc; Merc-c;
Merc-i-r; Nux-v; Pul; Rhus-t;
Saba; Sul; Tell.

AMEL : Alu; Ip.

Eating drinking Amel :
Ol- an; Tell.

EYES Open, while, coma
during : Terb.

FOOD, Goes Wrong way,
while : *Anac;* Caus; Hyo;
Kali-c; Lach; *Meph;* Nat-m;
Op.

Large piece of, as if : Cep;
Phys.

Pushed up, when : Fer-io.

Stops, and while : Con.

+ Turns like cork-screw :
Elap.

Warm Agg : Gel.

Amel : Hyo.

HASTY : Anac.

AGG : Ars; *Nit-ac;* Nux-v ; *Sil.*

HEAD, Bends forwards and
lifts his knees up, while :
Bell.

IMPEDED : Nat-s

LIQUIDS AGG : Arg-n; Ars;
BELL; Bro; *Canth;* Chin;
Crot-t; Ign; LACH; Lyss;
Merc; *Merc-c;* Nux-v; *Pho;*

Stram; Ver-a.

AMEL : Alu; Nit-ac; Nux-v.

Cold Agg : Kali-c.

Hot Agg : Phyt.

Warm AMEL :Alu; Kali-c;
Nux-v.

+ LUMP, Painful, swallow
cannot : Gel.

+ NAUSEA, Prevents : Arn.

NECK, Twists to get it down :
Kali-m.

NOISY : Arn; *Ars;* Caus; Cina;
Cocl; Cup; Gel; Hell;
Hyd-ac; Lach; *Laur; Pho;*
Thu.

PAINFUL : Ant-t; Ars; Bell;
Canth; Lac-c; *Lach;* Mer-c;
Phyt; Sil; Sul; Sul-io.

Nose to ears : Elap.

PAINLESS : Ap; Carb-ac.

PARALYTIC : Caps.

PUNGENT, Acrid things AGG : Lach.

SMALL Morsel, at a time : Alu.

SOLIDS AGG : Alu; Ant-t; Ap;
Bap; Bar-c; Crot-h; Kali-c;
Lac-c; Merc-i-r; Plb; Sil.

AMEL : Bro; Fer; *Hyo; Ign;*
Kali-bi; Lach; Merc-cy;
Rhus-t; Sanic.

Lying down, when Agg :
Cham.

Reach a certain point, and
are violently rejected :
Nat-m.

SOUR AGG : Ap.

SWEETS AGG : Bad; Lach;
Sang; *Spo.*

AMEL : Ars.

STRANGLING : Ant-t; Dig.

WON'T Go Down: Bar-c; Calc; Grap; *Hyo;* Lac-c; Lyc; Naj; Nit-ac; Sep; Stram.

Even a teaspoonful : Lyc; *Nit-ac.*

nausea, as from : Am.

SWASHING : See Splashing.

SWAYING AGG : See Car Sickness, Rocking.

AS IF : See Vertigo, Swinging.

SWEAT, In GENERAL, Easy Tendency, to : *Agar;* Ant-t; *Calc;* Calc-s; Carb-v; *Chin; Fer; Grap;* Hep; Ip; *Jab;* Kali-c; Kali-s; Lach; *Lyc;* Med; Merc; Merc-cy; *Nat-c;* Nat-m; Nit-ac; *Nux-v;* Op; *Pho; Pho-ac;* Psor; Samb; *Sep;* Sil; Stan; *Sul;* Tub; *Ver-a.*

AGG (Sweats without relief) : Ars; BELL; Benz-ac; *Caus;* Cham; Chel; Chin; Dig; Form; Hep; MERC; *Nux-v; Op;* Pho; *Pho-ac; Pyro; Rhus-t; Sep; Stram; Sul;* Tarn-c; Til; Tub; Ver-a.

AFTER AGG *:* Chin; Pho-ac; Sep.

AMEL (See Discharges Amel) : Bap*; Bry;* Canth; Cham; *Cup;* Eup-p; *Gel;* Iod; *Nat-m;* Psor; Rhus-t; Tarn.

Headache, Except : Eup-p.

ABSENT (See Skin Dry) : Bell; Bry; Calc; CHAM; CHIN; Colch; Colo; *Dul;* Lach; Psor; RHUS-T; Scil;*Sil; Sul; Stram.*

ACRID : Cham; Flu-ac; Tarn.

AFFECTED Parts, on : Amb; Ant-t; Cocl; Flu-ac; Kali-c;

Merc; Rhus-t; *Sil;* Tarn-c.

ALTERNATING, Sides on : Agar.

ANGER, From : Sep.

AROMATIC : Benz-ac.

AWAKE, Only, while : SAMB; Sep.

BLOODY *:* Crot-h; Lach; Nux-m.

BURNING : See Hot.

With : Mez; *Nat-c.*

CAN NOT : Apoc.

CHILL, Alternating, with : Ars; Chin; Mez; Nux-v; Sang.

Followed, by : Carb-v; Hep; Nux-v.

with : Tab.

CLAMMY : Ars; Cam; Cham; Cup; Fer; Fer-p; *Lyc; Merc; Pho;* Pho-ac; Tub; Ver-a; Ver-v.

COITION, After : Grap; Nat-c; Sep.

COLD : Am-c; *Ant-t; Ars; Cam;* CARB-V; Castr; *Chin;* Cocl; Cup; Dros; Fer; Hep; Ip; Lyc; *Merc;* Merc-c; *Sec;* Sep; Tab; Ther; Tub; VER-A; Ver-v.

AMEL : Nux-v.

Clammy, Haemorrhage, with : *Chin.*

Convulsions, with : Stram.

Cough, during : Ant-t; Ver-a.

after : Dros.

Easily, excited : Ther.

Exertion, slight, mental or

physical: Hep; Sep.

Loquacity, after : Cup.

Mania, with   : Stram.

Nausea, with: Ant-t; Lob; Ver-a.

Palpitation, with   : Am-c.

Stools, during : Plb.

Sudden, Attacks of : Crot-h; Tab.

+ Thighs, on : Caps.

Urination, after : Bell.

COLDS, From   : Nit-ac.

COLLIQUATIVE : Agar; Ant-t; Ascl; Chin; *Jab.*

COMA, With : Benz-ac.

COMPANY Agg   : Thu.

COUGHING Agg : Ars; Calc-s; *Carb-v;* HEP; Pho; Samb; Sep; *Tub.*

COVERS, Heat Amel (Uncovering Intolerance of) : *Clem;* Grap; Hep; Nat-c; NUX-V; Rhus-t; *Samb; Stro.*

CRITICAL : Pyro.

DEBILITATING : Bry; Calc-p; Cam; Carb-an; Chin; Chin-s; Fer; Iod; Merc; Nit-ac; Pho; Psor; Samb; Sep; Tub.

Delivery, after   : Samb.

Fever, after : Castr.

Foul : Croc.

Spinal injuries, from : Nit-ac.

DIARRHOEA, With : Aco; Ascl; *Ver-a.*

DYSPNOEA, With : Ars; Carb-v.

+ EASY : Ox-ac.

EATING Agg : Benz-ac; Carb-an; Carb-v; Cham;

Nat-m; Nit-ac; Sul-ac.

Amel : Lach.

Food, warm Agg : Pho; Sul-ac.

EGG, Rotten like, smell : Stap.

EMISSION, After : Phys; Rhus-t; Sep.

EVERY Thing, excites : Berb.

EXERTION, Slight, from : Aeth; Caus.

EXHAUSTING : See Debilitating.

EYES, Closing, on: Bry; *Con;* Lach.

FACE, Except : Rhus-t; Sec.

FLATUS, Passing, while : Kali-bi.

FLIES, Attracting : Calad.

FRIGHT, From   : Anac; *Op.*

GUSHING : Amy-n; Ap; *Bell; Colch;* Ip; Jab; Lach; Merc-cy; Nat-c; Pho; Samb; Tab; Thu; *Val.*

Alternating, with dry hot skin : Ap.

Company Agg   : Thu.

+ Influenza, after : Amy-n.

Suddenly : Val.

HEAD Except : Rhus-t; Samb; Thu.

HEART Symptoms, with : Spo.

HOT, Burning : Aco; BELL; CHAM; Con; *Ign; Ip;* Nat-c; Nux-v; OP; Psor; *Saba;* Sang; *Sep; Stan; Stram;* Til; Vio-t.

Unconsciousness, with : Calc; Sep.

ITCHING, Causing : Cham; Op;

Rhus-t.

LYING, Right side, On Agg : Lach.

MENSES Agg : *Grap*; Nux-v; Ver-a.

MICE, Like odour : Sil.

MORE Pain, More : Cham; Til.

MOTION Agg : *Chin*; Hep; Merc; Merc-c; Psor; Sep; Stan; Ver-a.

MUSK, Like Odour : Ap; Mos; Sul.

MUSTY : Cimx; Ol-an; Psor; Pul; Stan; Thu; Thyr.

NECK, About : Lach.

NERVOUS (See Fright from) : Jab; Rhus-t; Sep.

NIGHT, At: Agar; Ars; *Calc*; Carb-an; Carb-v; Caus; Con; *Hep; Kali-c*; Kali-s; Lach; *Merc*; Merc-c; *Petr*; Pul; *Pru-sp; Samb*; Sep; *Sil*; Stro; Sul; Tarx; Thu.

Climacteric : Stro.

Phthisis of : See under Night.

OFFENSIVE, Foetid, Putrid : Arn; *Bap; Bar-c*; Carb-an; Carb-v; Con; Croc; Grap; Hep; Led; Merc; Merc-c; Nit-ac; Nux-v *Petr*; Psor; Pul; Sec; Sep; Sil; *Stap; Sul*; Thu; Vario.

Coughing, after : Hep.

OILY, Greasy: Bry; Chin; Flu-ac; Mag-c; *Merc*; Stram; Thu; Thyr.

ONIONS, Garlic Like : Art-v; Bov; Kali-p; Lach; Lyc; Thu.

Convulsions, after : Art-v.

PAIN Agg : *Cham*; Lach; *Merc*; Nat-c; Pul; *Rhus-t*; Sep; TIL.

After : Chel.

PAINFUL Parts, on : Kali-c.

PALPITATION, With : Calc.

PARTIAL, Single Parts : Ap; Bar-c; CALC; Carb-v; Caus; Guai; Ign; Merc-c; Mez; Nux-v; Pho; *Pul*; Sele; SEP; *Sil; Sul; Thu;* Ver-a.

Front of the body : Arg-m; Cocl; Pho; Sele.

Lower part of the body : Croc.

Parts Lain on: Chin; Nit-ac.

not lain, on : Aco; *BENZ*; Nux-v; Thu.

Upper Part: Asar; Calc; Kali-c; Op; Par; Sil; Spig; Tub.

PROFUSE, Drenching : Bell; Benz-ac; Calc-hyp; *Carb-an*; Caus; CHIN; Coca; Guai; Hep; Jab; *Pho-ac*; Psor; Sele; *Sil*; Sul-ac; Tarn; Thyr; Til; Tub.

Delivery, after : Samb.

Diarrhoea, chronic; in : Tub.

Fainting, with : Hyds.

Mania, with : Stram.

Many Symptoms : Samb.

Nausea, with : Lob.

PROLONGED, Long Lasting : Caus; Fer; Hep; Merc; Samb.

PUNGENT : Flu-ac; Thu.

RED : Lach; Nux-m.

RELIEF, Without : See Sweat Agg.

RHEUMATISM, With : Ascl.

ROOM, In : Ip; Pul.

SADNESS, From : Calc-p.

SALTY Deposit : Nat-m; Sele.

SCANTY : Alu; Grap; Sang.

SENSATION, As if about to sweat but no moisture appears : Ign; Stan.

SHIVERING, With : Nux-v.

Slight, after : Bothr.

SITTING, While : Ars.

SLEEP, During : Bell; Cham; Chel; Chin; Con; Hyo; Mez; Lach; Plat; Pul; Rhus-t; Sele; Sil; Thu; Til.

Deep, in : Pul.

waking, from : Rum.

Eyes closing on, even, when : Carb-an; CON.

Falling, on : Ars; Merc; Mur-ac; Sul; Tarx; Thu.

SPASMS, During : Bell; *Buf.*

SPOTS, In : Merc; Petr; Tell.

STAINING The Linen: Bell; Lach; Mag-c; Thu.

Bloody Red : Lach; Nux-m.

White : Sele.

Yellow: Bell; *Carb-an; Grap;* LACH; MERC; *Sele;* Thu; Tub.

STEAMING : Psor.

STICKY : Kali-bi; Lyc.

STIFFENS, Hair: Sele.

Linen : Merc; Nat-m; Sele.

STOOLS, Before Agg : Merc; Tromb.

During Agg : Merc; Ver-a.

After : Caus; Nat-c; Plb.

STRANGERS, In presence of : *Bar-c;* Sep.

SUDDEN : Carb-v; Crot-h; Ip; *Tab.*

And disappearing suddenly : *Bell;* Colch.

Chill, with : Tab.

SUPPRESSED AGG : Aco; *Bell; Bry;* Calc; CHAM; CHIN; Colch; *Colo; Dul;* LACH; Psor; RHUS-T; Sep; *Sil;* Stram; SUL.

SWEETISH: Calad; Merc; Thu.

UNCOVERING Amel: Cham; Led; Lyc; Sec.

UNILATERAL, One sided : Bar-c; Jab; NUX-V; Petr; Pul; *Sul;* Thu.

Right : Pho; Pul.

Left : *Bar-c;* Chin; *Pul.*

URINATION, After : Merc.

URINOUS : Canth; Colo; Nit-ac.

VINEGAR, Smell, of : Iris.

WAKING, On : Dros; Par; *Samb;* Sep; Sul.

WALKING Amel : Pul; Thu.

WARM Amel : Aco.

WASH Can not : Mag-c; Merc.

WASHING Amel : Thu.

WRITING, While : Hep; Kali-c; Psor; *Sep;* Sul; Tub.

SWEETISH : Thu.

SWEETS, Body were made of : Merc.

SWELLED, As if : See Enlarged, as if.

SWELLING : Aco; *Ap;* Ars; Bar-c; *Bell; Bry;* Calc; Cham; Grap; Hep; *Lach;* Led; Lyc; *Merc;* Nit-ac; Nux-v; Pho; PUL;

RHUS-T; SIL; SUL.

ABSENT In, Affected or Inflammed parts : Ars; Cam; Carb-v; Con; Laur; Op; Pho-ac; Sul.

BAGGY : Ap; Ars; Kali-c.

BODY, Whole of, as if : Buf.

CHRONIC : Cist.

COLD : Asaf; *Cocl*; Con; *Dul*; *Merc*; *Sul*.

CORDLIKE: Dul; Iod; Rhus-t.

DARK RED : Asaf.

GLANDS, Of : See under Glands.

GLANDULAR : Lap-a.

*H*ARD : Ars; Bell; Chin; Con; Hep; Iod; Lach; Merc; Pul; Rhus-t; Sil; Spo; *Tarn-c*.

Here and there : Pho.

MENSES, During : Kali-c; Lac-c.

NODES, Like : Bry; Nit-ac.

PALE : Bar-c; *Bry*; Lach; Lyc; Rhus-t; *Sul*.

RECEDING : Ars; Calc; Hep; Kre; Lach; Lyc; Merc; Sep; Sil.

RED, Shiny : Sabi.

SACCULAR : Ap; Ars; Kali-c; Rhus-t.

VASCULAR : Lyc.

SWIMMING or Falling into water : Ant-c; Bels.

While AGG : Cocl.

SWINGING AGG : See Carsickness, Rocking.

AS IF : See under Verhgo.

SYCOSIS (See Gonorrhoea) : Ap; Arg-m; Ars; Calc; Grap; Kali-io;Kali-s; Kalm; MED; Merc; NAT-S; *Nit-ac*; Pho-ac; Pul; Saba; Sabi; *SARS*; Sele;

Sep; Stap; Sul; THU.

SUPPRESSED : Merc; Nit-ac; Stap; Thu.

SYMMETRICAL : Arn; Kali-io; Lac-d; Syph; Thyr.

SYMPATHETIC : Caus; Ign; Nat-m; Nux-v; *Pho.*

SYMPATHY AGG : Ars; *Bell*; *Calc*; IGN; Kali-s; *Nat-m*; *Plat*; Sabal; Sep; *Sil*.

AMEL : Asaf; Pho; *PUL*.

BARS, Against friend : Arg-m.

RESENTS : Cof; Syph.

SYMPTOMS BEGIN On one side; goto other and there

AGG : See under Pain.

ALTERNATE : See Alternating Effects.

BETTER, Worse and without any Cause : Alu; Psor.

BROODS Over his own: Sabal.

CHANGE Constantly : Berb; Croc; Sang; Tub.

Places, suddenly : Amb; Berb.

DIVERSE, Many : Agar; Kali-io; Merc; Syph; Tub.

EVERY, Is a settled disease : Lac-c.

GROUP, Recur (See Relapses) : Anac; Caus; Cham; Cocl; Cup; Plb; Sil.

Alternating : Cimi.

MAGNIFIES, Her : Asaf; Buf; Cham.

OR SENSATIONS, Appear on side lain on, Not lain on etc. : See under Directions.

THINKING, Of AGG : See

Thinking of it Agg.

SYNALGIAS (Sexual) : Ap; Tarn.

SYNCOPE : See Fainting.

SYNOVITIS : See under Joints.

CREPITATION : Nat-p.

SYPHILIS : Asaf; *Aur; Carb-an; Cinb; Iod;* Kali-bi; *Kali-io;* Kali-s; *Merc;* Merc-c; Merc-i-f; Merc-i-r; *Nit-ac; Phyt;* Sars; Sil; Still; Syph; Thu.

+ FEAR OF : Hyo.

INFANTS Of : Bad.

TABES DORSALIS : See Locomotor Ataxia.

TACHYCARDIA : See Pulse Rapid, Fast.

TACITURN SILENT, Reticent : Ant-c; Ars; Aur; *Bell;* Bry; Carb-an; Caus; Cocl; Glo; Hell; *Ign;* Mag-c; Mez; MUR- AC; Pho; PHO-AC; Flat; Plb; *Pul;* Stan; Thu; *Ver-a;* ZIN.

ALTERNATING With, Quarrelsomeness : Con.

Mania : Ver-a.

TALK CAN NOT (See Voice Lost) : Dig; Pho; Stan; Sul.

Weeping, without : Med.

DESIRE, To : Arg-m; Arg-n; Stic.

HEARING OTHERS AGG : Amb; Am-c; ARS; Cact; Chin; *Hyo;* Mag-m; *Mang;* Mez; *Nat-v; Nux-v;* Rhus-t; *Sep;* Sil; Stram; *Ver-a;* Zin.

MUST : Frax; Stic.

SAME Over and over again : Med.

TALKING AGG : See Speaking AGG.

OTHERS, About her : *Bar-c;* Hyo; Ign; Pall; Stan; Stap.

PAINFUL : Cep.

PLEASURE, Takes in his own : Nat-m; Par; Stram.

UNPLEASANT Things of AGG : Calc; Cic; Mar-v.

TALKS ALWAYS About her pain : *Mag-p.*

+ CHANGES, Subjects rapidly : Agar.

DEAD People, with : *Calc-sil;* hyo.

EXCITEDLY : Mos.

FAST : Bell; Calc-hyp; Thu.

FAULTS, Of others about : Ver-a.

HIMSELF, To : Ant-t; Aur; Chlo-hyd; Hyo; Kali-bi; Mag-p; Mos; Pyro.

Gesticulates, and : Mos.

Loudly : Nux-m.

+ INCOHERENTLY : Agar.

NONSENSE, Then angry, if not understood : Buf.

NOSE Through (Children) with : Bar-m; Lac-c.

PERSONS, Imaginary, with : Chlo-hyd; Hyo.

SENSELESS : Anac.

SLEEP, In : Ars; Bar-c; *Bell;* Carb-an; Cina; *Kali-c;* Lach; Nux-v; Pul; Pyro; Sil; Sul.

Eyes open, with : Diph.

Loudly : Nux-m; Sep; Sil; Sul.

Old Men : Bar-c.

SPIRITS, With : Nit-ac.

THROUGH HIM, Other persons as if : Alu; Cann.

TROUBLES, Of Her : Arg-n; Asaf; Mag-p; Nux-v; Zin.

VERSES, In : Ant-c; Nat-c.

VOICE LOW, Soft, in : Vio-o.

TALL : Calc-p; Mag-p; Pho.

TAPE WORMS : See Worms.

TARRY : See Discharges, Menses, Stools.

TARSI (Edges of Eyelids) : Bor; Merc; PUL; Stap; *Sul;* Val.

BLUE : Bad; Bov; Phyt.

BURNING : Ars; Euphr.

ECZEMA : Bacil; Tub.

INFLAMMED : Clem; Grap; Mag-m; Petr; Pul; Sanic. Sul.

ITCHING: Calc; Pul; Saba; Stap.

PUSTULES : Ant-c.

RED : *Ars; Euphr;* Grap; Merc; Pul; Saba; Sep. SUL.

SCALY : Ars; *Grap;* Mag-m; Med; Merc; *Sep.*

THICK, Swelled : Alu; Calc; EUPHR :Grap; Hep; Merc; Pul; Tell.

TUMOURS : Mar-v; Sep.

ULCERS, On : Clem; Sanic.

TASTE ACUTE : Chin; Cof; Nat-c.

AFTER TASTE, Of food, eaten : Ant-c; Caus; Dios; Nat-m; *Pho; Pho-ac;* Pul; Sil.

ALKALINE : Kalm.

ALTERED, In General : Chin; *Pul;* Rhus-t.

AROMATIC : Glo.

ASTRINGENT : Alu; Arg-n; Ars; Chio; Grap; Hyd-ac; *Merc-c; Pho.*

BAD, Foul, Repulsive, Nauseous : Anac; *Arn;* Calc; Caps; Grap; *Merc.* Nat-s; NUX-V; PUL; Psor; *Rhus-t;* Stap; Sul; Syph; Vario.

Coition, after : Dig.

Eating, after : Lyc.

Amel : Lil-t.

impossible : Myr.

Epilepsy, before : Syph.

Everything, to : Pod.

Fever, during: *Arn;* Ars; Pul.

Sweets, from : Lac-c.

Menses, during : Kali-c.

Morning, in : Ars; Bry; Calc-p; *Nat-s;* NUX-V; PUL.

Waking, on : Val.

Water, to : Aco; Ap; Ars; Aur; Bell; Bur-p; Fer; *Kali-bi; Nat-m; Pul; Sil.*

BANANA, Like : Mag-p.

+ BEER, Like honey : Mur-ac.

BITTER : Aco; Ant-c; *Ars;* BRY; Carb-v; Cham;Chel; *Chin;* Colo; *Lyc; Merc;* Nat-c; Nat-m; *Nat-s;* NUX-V; Pho; Pod; PUL; *Sep;* Solid; *SUL;* Tarn; *Ver-a.*

Bread, to : Pul; Rhus-t; Scil.

Butter, to :Chin; Pul; Rhus-t.

Coffee, to : Sabi.

Continuous : Colo; Solid.

Drinking Agg : Ars; Bry; Chin; *Kre;* Pul.

Amel: *Bry*; Psor.

Eating Agg : Ars; Pul.

Everything, even saliva : Bor; Kre.

except water : *Aco; Stan.*

Food, to : Chin; Iod; Nat-c; *Pul;* Rhe; Stram.

but not drinks: Iod.

swallowing, when : Kre.

Head ache, with : Calc-p.

Menses, at : Calc-p; Caul.

Milk, to : Sabi.

Morning : *Cham; Pul.*

waking, on : Helo; Kali-io; Sul.

Night, at : Solid.

Plums, to : Iod.

Smoking Agg : Cocl; Pul.

Amel : Aran.

Sour : Arg-n; Asar; Cup; Lyc; Merc; *Nux-v*; Pho; Sep; Stan.

milk after : Amb.

Sweet things, sugar: Rhe; Sang.

Thirst, with : Pic-ac.

Tongue, cold with : Kali-m.

Water, to : ARS; Calc-p; Chin; *Chin-ar*; Ver-a.

BLOODY : Am-c; Ars; Bell; Fer; Ham; Ip; Lil-t; Nat-c; Pul.

Coughing Agg : *Bell;* Kali-bi; *Rhus-t.*

Pregnancy, during : Zin.

CHALKY : Nux-m.

CHEESY : Aeth; Lyc; Sep.

COUGHING Agg : Lach; Nux-v; Sang.

DULLED, Flat, Insipid Watery : Anac; *Bry;* Chin; Ign; Merc; *Pul*; Stap.

+ Everything to : Mos.

Food, to : Cup; Stro.

Water, to : Aco.

EARTHY : Fer; Ip; Nux-m; *Pul.*

EGGS, Like Rotten : *Arn;* Bur-p; Grap; *Merc; Mur-ac;* Pho-ac; Psor.

Coughing, when : Sep.

EVERY thing, inclination, to : Bell.

FISHY : Sep.

FLAT : See Dulled.

GREASY, fatty : *Alu;* Asaf; Caus; Iris; Kali-p; Mang; Petr; Pul; Tril; Val.

HERBY : Nux-v; Pho-ac; Rhus-t; Sars.

Food, to : Stram.

ILLUSIONS, Of : Val.

INKY : Calc.

INSIPID : See Dulled.

LOST, Wanting : Anac; *BELL;* Cyc; Hyo; Mag-m; NAT-M; Pho; Pod; *Pul*; Sil.

Cold, during : Nat-m; Pul.

after : Mag-m.

Food, to : Hell; Nat-m; Pul.

Salt, to : *Calc;* Canth.

METALLIC, Coppery : Bism; Cimi; *Cocl;* Cup; Hyd-ac; Iod; Kali-bi; MERC; *Nat-c;* Nux-v; Radm; *Rhus-t; Seneg;* Thyr; Vario; Zin-chr.

Tip, at : Thyr.

MILKY : Aur; Pho.

MUSTY : Led; Lyc; Mar-v; Stap.

Coughing : Led.

OILY : See Greasy.

ONIONS, Like : Aeth.

+ **P**ALATABLE, Extremely : Cann.

PEPPERMINT, Like : Ver-a.

PEPPERY : Echi; Hyds; Lach;
Mez; Radm; Sul; Xanth.

PERFUME, Like : Bell; Cham;
Coc-c; Glo.

Water, to : Med.

PERVERTED : Mag-m; Nat-c.

PUSSY : Hyd-ac.

RANCID: Alu; Carb-v; Cham;
Kali-io; Mur-ac; Syph; Thu;
Val.

Drink and food, after :
Kali-io.

Sweet **A**GG : Lac-c.

SALTY : A*rs*; Chin; Con; Cyc;
Kali-io; Lyc; *Merc*; Merc-c;
Nat-m; Pho; Pul; *Sep.*

Every thing : Sep.

Food only, tastes natural :
Lac-c.

Food, to : Chin; Cyc; Pul.

more : Cop; Cyc; Sul.

not enough : Calc; Cocl.

Sour : Cup; Lach.

Sweet : Croc; Pho.

water, to : Bro.

SAWDUST Like : Cor-r.

SEMEN, Odour like : Ver-v.

SLIMY : Kali-bi; Merc; *Pul*; Val.

SOUR : *Arg-n*; Bell; Bism;
CALC; Chin; Grap; Ign; Kob;

LYC; *Mag-c;* Nat-c; NUX-V;
Ox-ac; Pho; Pul; Rhe;Rob;
Stan; Sul; Tarx; Zin-val.

Drinking, after : Nux-v.

Every thing : Pod.

Food, to: *Am-c*; Calc;
Caps; Lyc; Mur-ac.

Meat, to : Lapp.

Milk, after : Amb; Pho; Sul.

to : Calad.

Putrid, or : Pod.

Salty : Cup; Lach.

Sweets, after : Calc.

STRAW, Like : Cor-r; Stram;
Sul.

SWEET : Bism; Calad; Cup;
Dul; Iris; Lil-t; Merc; Pho;
Plb; *Pul*; Pyro; Saba; Scil;
Sele; Stan; Sul; Thu.

+ Beer : Cor-r.

Bread, to : Cor-r; Merc.

Butter, to : Mur-ac; Ran-b.

Coughing, when : Pho.

Every thing : Mur-ac;
Phel.

Food, to : Scil.

Hunger, with : Nit-ac.

+ Metallic : Coc-c.

Morning, in : Aeth; Ars.

Mouth, back of : Lil-t.

Salivation, with : Dig.

Tobacco smoking, after :
Dig.

Tongue, tip, on : Plat.

Water, to : Form.

URINOUS : Psor; Seneg.

WATERY : See Dulled.

WOODY : Rut.

TEARING : See under Pain.

TEARS : See Lachrymation.

THINGS, Himself, etc. : *Bell;* Cann; Kali-p; Sec; *Stram;* Tarn; Ver-a.

TEETH : ACO; *Ant-c;* Bell; Bry; *Calc;* Calc-p; *Caus;* CHAM; Chin; Cof; Kre; *Lach;* MERC; Mez; Nux-v; Plant; Pod; PUL; *Rhus-t;* SEP; Sil; Spig; STAP; *Sul.*

RIGHT : Bell; Flu-ac; Stap.

LEFT :Caus; Cham; Clem; Euphor; Mez; Sep;Sul; *Thu.*

ALTERNATING, Sides : Amb; Am-m; Caps; Chel; Iod; Kali-n; Lyc; Psor; *Pul;* Stram; Sul; *Zin.*

Between upper and lower : Aco; Laur; Nat-m; Pul; Rat; Rhod.

Breast (L) with : Kali-c.

CHANGING About : Bry; Cyc; Hyo; Hypr; Kali-bi; Kali-c; Mag-c; Mang; Nat-m; Nux-m; Pru-sp; Pul; Rhod; Sil; Thu.

RADIATING : MERC.

ROW In a **W**HOLE : Ars; Aur; Carb-v; Glo; Lach; Mag-c; Mag-p; *Merc;* Nat-m; *Nux-v;* Psor; Sep; Spig; *Stap;* Zin.

UPPER : Am-c; *Aran;* Bell; Carb-v; Chin; Kre.

LOWER : Bell; Canth; *Cham;* Nat-c; Plb; Stap.

CANINE : Calc; Nux-v; Sep; Sul-ac.

INCISORS : *Colch;* Sul.

Behind : *Pho.*

MOLARS: Bry; KRE; Stap;Zin.

ROOTS : Mag-c.

ABSCESSED, Roots : Calc; *Hep;* Kre; Pho; SIL; Stap.

ACIDS Agg : Arg-n; Mur-ac.

Amel : Pul.

AIR, Cold Agg : Calc; Caus; Cham; Merc; Rat; Sul; Tub.

Amel : Clem; Mez; Nat-s; Nux-v; *Pul;* Sele.

BEER Amel : Cam.

BITING Agg : Am-c; Mez; Sep.

Amel : Bell; Caus; Chin; Mur-ac; Ol-an; *Phyt;* Pod; Pru-sp.

Mouth, empty, with : Cocl.

Suddenly, involuntarily : Ap.

BLACK : Chin; Flu-ac; Kre; *Merc;* STAP.

Spots, in : Kre; Scil.

BLUNT : Am-c; Mez; Ran-sc; Rob; Sul-ac.

BRUSHING Agg : Bry; Coc-c; *Lach;* Stap.

BURSTING : Sabi.

CARIES : See Decay.

CHATTER : Lach; Nux-v; Radm.

Coldness, internal with : Radm.

Fear, from : Elap.

Nervous : Kali-p.

Speak, attempting to, on : Cocl.

Trembling, inward with : Ant-t.

CHEEK, Rubbing Amel : *Merc;*

Pho.

CLENCH, Inclination, to : Hyo;
Lyc; Merc-i-f; *Phyt*; Pod.

COATED, As if : Colch; Dios; *Pho.*

COITION Agg : Daph.

Amel : Cam.

COLD : Carb-v; Mez; Nit-ac;
Pho-ac; Rhe; Spig; Sele.

Air, coming from, as if : Rat.

Edge, at : Gamb.

Tips : Ol-an.

COLD Things Agg : Ant-c;
Arg-n; Hep; *Kali-c;* Lach;
Merc-i-f; *Nat-m;* Rhod;
Rhus-t; Sep; Stap; Thu.

Food Agg, not by cold drinks
: Con.

AMEL : Bism; *Bry;* Chim; Clem;
Cof; Fer; Nat-s; *Pul.*

Hot, or Agg : Carb-v; Merc;
Merc-i-f; Lach; Syph.

Rinsing, water, with Amel
: Rum.

COLDS Agg : Mag-c; Sep.

CRAWLING : Bar-c; Cham.

CRUMBLING: Euphor; Med;
Plant; Stap; Thu.

CUPPED, Children, in: Syph.

DECAY, Caries; Hollow : Ant-c;
Bell; Bor; *Calc;* Cham;
Euphor; Flu-ac; *Kre;* Lach;
Merc; Mez; Nat-c; Plb; Sep;
Sil; *Stap;* Syph.

Children, in: Calc-p; *Kre;*
Stap.

Diabetes, in : Sul-ac.

Gums, edge at : Syph; Thu.

Long too, as if : Hep.

Rapid : Flua-ac; *KRE;* Sep.

Roots, at : Flu-ac; Thu.

Sides : Mez; Stap; Thu.

DENTAL Operations after :
Alum; *Arn;* Calen; Ham;
Merc-i-f; *Nux-v;* Stap;
Thu.

+ Extraction, convulsions
after : Buf.

+ Extraction, persistent
bleeding : Pho.

DWARFED : Syph.

EATING Agg : Ant-c; Chim;
Kali-c; Merc; Stap.

Amel: Cham; Ign; Ip;
Plant; *Rhod;* Spig.

Dinner Amel : Rum.

EDGE On: Calc; Chio; Dig;
Grat; Iris; Lyc; Merc-i-f;
Rob; Sul-ac.

ELONGATED, As if : Alu; Ant-t;
Ars; Berb; Caus; Cham;
Colo; Lach; Mag-c; Merc;
Merc-i-f; Mez; Plant; Sil.

Dull, and : Mez.

ENAMEL, Deficient : *Calc-f;*
Flu-ac; Sil.

EXERTION Agg : Chim.

EXTENDING to Ear or Face :
Alu; Ant-c; Cham;
Kali-bi; Lach; Mang; *Merc;*
Mez; Plant; Pul; Rhod.

Finger tips, to: Cof.

FISTULA : Caus; Flu-ac;
Nat-m; Stap.

FOOD, Touch, on Agg : Mag-m.

FRUITS Agg : Nat-c; Nat-s.

GRINDING: Ap; *Ars;* BELL; Cic;
Cina; Crot-h; Cup; Hell;

Hyo; Lyc; *Phyt*; Pod; Sul; Ver-a; Zin.

Convulsions, during : Buf; Cof; Hyo.

Frightful : Plb.

Sleep, in : Ars; Bell; Calc; Cann; CINA; Ign; Tub.

sitting posture, in : Ant-c.

HEAVY : Flu-ac; Ver-a.

HOLLOW : See Decay.

HOT Things Agg : Calc; Dros.

ICE Water Amel : Clem; Cof; Fer.

INTO, Pains go : Chin; Fer; Kali-bi; Merc; Mez; Stap; Thu.

ITCHING : Kali-c.

JAMMED : Lach; Merc-i-f; Tub.

JERKING : Calc; Chaml; Euphr; Ip; *Merc;* Pul; Rhod.

Tobacco chewing,

smoking on : Bry.

LARGE, Too : Berb; Calc; Sil.

LONG Too : See Elongated.

LOOSE : Am-c; Bor; Bry; Calc-f; Carb-an; Carb-v; *Caus*; HYO; MERC; *Merc-c; Nit-ac*; Nux-v; Psor; Rhus-t; Sil; Zin.

LYING Agg : Aran; Benz-ac; Rat; Sep.

Amel : Spig.

painful side on Amel : Hypr.

MENSES Agg: Bar-c; Calc; *Carb-v; Cham;* Cof; Lach; Sep; Stap.

Before Agg : Ant-c.

MUSIC Agg : Pho-ac.

NIGHT Agg : *Cham Grap; Lyc*; Mag-c; MERC; Rat; Sul.

NOISE Agg : Cof; Plant; Ther.

NUMB : Chin; Dul; *Pho;* Plat; Rhus-t.

OILY, As if : Aesc.

OUT Of Place, As if : Syph.

PAIN Ceases suddenly Agg 2 or 3 hours after : Rhod.

PEGGED : Kre.

PICKING Agg : Pul; Sang.

Amel : Bell; Cep; Pho-ac.

PREGNANCY Agg : Chin; Kali-bi; *Kre;* Lyss; Mag-c; Nux-m; *Sep.*

PRESSURE, Cold hand , of Amel : Rhus-t.

Hard Amel : Stap.

PULLED, As if: Calc; Chim; Mez; Nux-m; Pru-sp; Rhus-t.

Cold water Amel : Chim.

QUIVERING : Phys.

RADIATING. Pain : Kali-bi; MERC; Mez; Nux-v; Stap.

Glands, swelled with : Kali-bi.

ROUGH : Phys.

SALIVA Flows, during pain : Cham; Dul; Merc; Nat-m.

SALTY Things Agg : Carb-v.

Amel : *Carb-an*; Mag-c.

SCREWED Toghether, as if : Euphor; Stro.

SENSITIVE, Tender: Gel;Lach; Sul.

SERRATED : Med.

SMOKING Agg : Bry; Clem.

Amel : Bor; Spig.

SMOOTH, As if : Aesc; Colch; Dios; Pho; Sul-io.

SOFT, Feel : Calc-p; Caus; Med; Nit-ac; Sul-io.

SORDES, On : Ail; Ars; Bap; Bry; Chin; Hyo; *Pho; Pho–ac; Rhus-t.*

Black : *Chin;* Con; *Flu–ac.*

Brown : Bap.

Slimy : Rhus-t.

STICKY : Arg-m; Crot-h; Lach; Psor; Sang; Syph.

SUCKING Agg : Bov; Carb-v; Chin; Mang; Nux-m.

Amel : Cep; Clem.

In, Air, Amel : Mez.

SUCKLING When Agg : *Chin.*

SWEETS Agg : Merc-i-f; Mur-ac; Nat-c.

TARTAR : Ars; Ascl; Bacil; Calc-ren; Calend; Carb-s; Chin; Epip; Merc; Plb; Thu.

TEA Agg : Sele.

TEMPLES, To : Merc; Mez.

TENSION, In : Pul.

TOUCH Of Tongue Agg : *Ant-c;* Merc; Mez.

Food Agg : Mag-m.

WARM, As if : Flu-ac.

WISDOM Teeth, Eruption from Agg : Calc; Flu-ac; Mag-c; Sil.

WORM, In: Syph.

+ wriggling, in : Kali-io.

YELLOW : Cep; Iod; Lyc; Med; Merc; Sil; Thu.

TEMPERATURE CHANGE Of AGG : See Change of Temperature AGG.

EXTREMES *OF* AGG : Ant-c; Carb-v; Caus; Ip; Lach; Sul-ac; Syph.

TEMPLES : *Anac; Arg-m;* BELL; CHIN; Cyc; Glo Kali-c; Kre; Lyc; Nux-m; Par; Pho-ac; Plat; *Pul;* Rhus-t; Sabi; Thu;Verb; *Zin.*

BITING, Chewing Agg : Zin.

BLOW, On : Lyc; Plat; Sul-ac.

BOLT, Passed through, as if : Ham.

BURNING : Colo; Lyc; Mez; *Pho.*

COLD : Berb.

COUGHING Agg : Lyc.

Holds, while : Petr.

+ CRUSHED, As if : Pho-ac.

+ CUTTING : Nat-p.

EMPTY Sensation : Cyc.

FINGER Tips, pressing, as if : Epip.

HAMMERING (L) : Ham.

HEAVY : Zin.

+ MENSES Agg : Lyc.

NECK And FACE, to: Tarn.

+ PLUG, Driven in, as if: Sul-ac.

+ SCREWED, Together : Lyc.

SHOCKS, Blows : See Blow.

+ SQUEEZED In Vise, as if : Dios.

STOMACH, Pain, with: Lith.

TEMPLE, To : Chin.

THROBBING : Aur; *Bell;* Glo; Zin-chr.

TWITCH : Chin; Psor; Spig.

VEINS : Ars; Cup; Flu-ac; Glo; am; Pul; Sang; Vip; Zin

Swollen : Ars; Cub; Glo;
Sang.

WET WEATHER Agg : Bor.

TEMPESTUOUS ACTION : *Aco*;
Glo; Tab.

TENACIOUS : See Discharges,
Sticky.

TENDER : See Delicate, Pain
bruised.

TENDO ACHILLES : Anac;
Benz-ac; Kali-bi; *Mur-ac*;
Sep; Val; *Zin*.

CONTRACTED : Cimi.

CRAMP : Caus.

PAINFUL : Benz-ac; Kali-bi.

Stepping, on : Rhod.

Swelled : Kali-bi.

SHORT, As if : Dios.

STIFF : Cimi; Sul.

Walking, when : Ant-t.

WALKING Agg : Am-m; Ant-t;
Cinb; Colch.

TENDONS : See Fibrous Tissue.

CRACKLING, In : Kali-m.

FLEXURE : Rut.

INJURED : Anac.

JERKING, In : Sul-ac.

PAINS, In : Rhus-t; Sabi.

SHEATH, Of : Bry; Iod; Rhus-t.

SWOLLEN, Hard : Calc-f.

TENSE, Short : Am-m; Caus;
Dios; Grap; Guai; Nat-m; Ol-j.

TENESMUS : See Pain,
Pressing down.

TENSION TIGHTNESS :
Am-m; Asaf; Bar-c; Bell; *Bry*;
Cact; Caus; Colo; Con; Kali-m;

Lyc; Mag-p; *Nat-m; Nux-v;*
Par; PHO; Plat; PUL; Ran-b;
RHUS-T; Senec; Sep; Stro;
Sul; Verb; Vio-o; Visc.

ALL OVER Body : Ars; Bar-c;
Cact; Grap; Sul.

TERROR : Aco; Spo; Stram;
Tarn.

SUDDEN : Glo.

TESTES : Arg-m; Arn; *Aur;* ·
Clem; Iod; Merc; Nux-v;
Pul; Rhod; Rhus-t; Sep;
Spo; Stap.

ALTERNATELY : Berb; Rhod.

ATROPHY: Ant-c; Iod; Kali-io;
Sabal.

Sexual excess, after : Stap.

BRUISED : Thu.

BURNING, Heat: Nit-ac; Nux-v;
Pul.

CANCER : Spo.

COITION Agg : Mag-m; Pho-ac.

COLD : *Agn*; Merc.

CRAMP : Psor.

Emission, after : Caps.

CRUSHED : Arg-m; Ox-ac;
Rhod.

DRAWN Up: See Retraction.

ENLARGED, Swelled : Bro;
Clem; Dul; Mez; *Pul;* Rhod;
Spo.

Alternately : Ol-an.

Pain, griping with : Dul.

Sexual passion, unrequited,
from : Iod.

HANGING Low : Calc; Clem;
Pul; Pyro; Sul.

Right : Crot-t.

INDURATED : Aur; Bro; *Clem;*
CON; Iod; Med; *Rhod;* Sil;
Spo; Sul.

Jarring, slight Agg : Bro.

Painless : Bro.

Small : Iod; Pul; Sil; Spo;
Tub.

INFLAMMED (Orchitis): *Aco;*
Arn; Bap; *Clem;* Con; Ham;
PUL; Rhod; Rhus-t; Spo.

Epididymis : Pul; Rhod; Spo.

Mumps, after : Jab; Plb; *Pul.*

Sitting on cold
pavement from : Pul.

NEURALGIA : Berb; Ham; Zin.

Nausea, with : Ham.

Supra-orbital pain, with :
Lycps.

NODULES : Psor; Syph.

PULLED UP : Arg-n; Berb; Cic.

As if : Ol-an.

PRESSING : Caus; Pul; Zin.

PRESSURE Of Clothing Agg :
Arg-n.

RETRACTION : Arg-n; Aur; Berb;
Cic; Clem; Ol-an; Plb;
Rhod; Sabal; Zin.

External ring, to : Cic.

Left: Crot-t.

Painful : Sabal.

SEXUAL Excitement,suppressed,
Agg : Mag-m.

SOFTENING : Caps; Sul-io.

SQUEEZING : Spo.

STITCHING : Caus; Spo.

THROBBING : Ox-ac; Spo.

TUBERCLES : Iod; Pul; Sil; Spo;
Tub.

TUMOUR : See Sarcocele.

Indolent : Tarn.

UNDESCENDED, In Children :
Thyr.

UNDEVELOPED, Punny boys,
in: Aur.

UNREQUITED, Sexual Passion
Agg : Mag-m.

URINATING Agg : Polyg.

Amel : Kob.

WALKING Agg : Zin.

TETANUS : Bell; Cic; Cocl;
Cup; Hyd-ac; Hyo; Ign; Nux-v;
Op; Passif; Petr; Stram; Stry;
Tab; Ver-v.

LASTING For days : Latro.

TOBACCO, Swallowing, from
: Ip.

TETANY : Calc; Cocl; Grap;
Lyc; Merc; Plb; Sec; Sol-n.

COLD Agg : Thyr.

TETTER : See Eruptions.

THICK, THICKNESS : See
Discharges, Thick.

THIGHS : Ars; Chin; Clem;
Guai; *Merc; Nat-m;* Phyt;
Plb; Pyro; Sep.

ANTERIOR : Anac; Bels; Cimi;
Spo; Xanth.

Cramps, Menses, before :
Dict; Xanth.

Weak : Lapp.

INNER : Petr; Rhod; Stan; Sul.

Red and swollen : Stram.

MIDDLE, Knee to : Ind.

OUTER : Caus; Helo; *Pho-ac;*
Phyt.

POSTERIOR (See Sciatica)

Colo; Gnap; Mang; *Rhus-t*;
Sul; Zin.

BANDAGED : Plat.

BLUE : Bism.

BOILS : Hyo; Ign.

BONES Painful: Euphor; Guai;
Rut.

Dislocated, as if while
sitting : Ip.

BROKEN, As if : Rut; Sul; Tub.,

CHANGE Of Weather Agg :
Phyt.

COLD : Berb; Spo.

Colic, with : Calc.

Menses, after: Coll; Colch.

CONTRACTION : Rhus-t.

Walking, while : *Nux-v.*

CRAMPS : Ant-t; Chel; Colo;
Cup; Meny; Naj; Sul.

Sitting Agg : Mag-m; Meny.

CROSSING Agg : Agar.

+ DROPS Of Water, flowing
down : Aco.

EMACIATION : Calc; Nit-ac;
Sele.

EXCORIATION, Easy, walking
on : Aeth.

FORMICATION : Guai; Nat-c;
Pall; *Sec.*

ITCHING : Bar-c; Calc; Sul; Zin.

MENSES Agg : Mag-m; Meny;
Xanth.

PAINFUL : Anac; Plb; Pyro;
Rhus-t.

PAINS, Into: Cham; *Stap;*
Xanth.

+ Ovaries settling in: Sabal.

PULSATION *(R)* : Ver-v.

RACKING, Violent in marrow
: Naj.

SHOCKS : Agar.

SHORT, As if : Guai; Kre.

SITTING Agg : Lyc; Mag-m;
Pyro.

STOOLS Agg : Rhus-t.

SWEAT : Amb; Ars; Thu.

Cold : Caps; Merc; Sep; Spo.

TENSION : Am-m; Caus; Guai;
Mag-m; Pul.

Sitting Amel : Guai.

TINGLING : Merc.

TWITCHING : Kali-c; Kali-m.

URINATION Agg : Berb.

WATER, Warm, running down
: Bor.

WEAK : Cocl; Con; Eup-p; *Gel;*
Lapp; *Mur-ac;* Nat-s; Stan;
Urt.

THIN: See Discharges, Watery.

THINGS LOOK STRANGE : See
Strange, Bewildered.

THINKING AGG : Par.

ABOUT His own wrongs Agg
: Iod.

BAD ACT, Has comitted, as if :
Cyc.

DIFFICULT : *Anac;* Bap; Berb;
Con; *Gel; Lyc;* Nat-c;
NUX-M; NUX-V; Old; *Op;*
Pho; PHO-AC; Pic-ac; Sep;
Zin.

DISEASE, Is incurable : Cact;
Lac-c; Lil-t.

DUTY, Her, not done : Cyc.

EVERY One is looking at her
: Meli.

FLUIDS Of Agg : Lyss.

HIMSELF, Too little : Kob; Lac-c.

HIS Own sufferings, of : Sabal.

OF IT AGG : *Amb;* Arg-n; Aur;
Bar-c; Calc-p; Caus; Colch;
Gel; Helo; Lycps; Med;
Nat-s; *Nit-ac;* Nux-m; *Ox-ac;*
Saba; Spig; Spo; Sumb;
Thyr; Tub.

AMEL : *Cam; Cic;* Hell.

THINNESS, SPARE HABIT
: Amb; Arg-n; Calc-p; Kre;
Mag-p; Nat-m; Nit-ac;
Nux-m; Nux-v; Pho; Psor;
Rat; Sanic; Sars; Sec; Sul.

THIRST : Acet-ac; ACO;
Arg-n; *Arn;* ARS; *Bell;* BRY;
Calc; Calc-s; *Caps;* Caus;
CHAM; CHIN; *Cina;* Croc; *Dig;*
Eup-p; Hell; Iod; *Lyc;* MERC;
NAT-M; Op; *Pho;* RHUS-T; Sec;
Sep; Sil; STRAM; SUL; Tarn;
VER-A.

ALTERNATING, With Aversion to
drink : Berb.

+ BEER, For : Petr.

BUT Drinks, Aversion, to : Ars;
Hell; Nux-v; *Stram.*

+ Causes shuddering: Caps.

Fears to drink : Lach.

CHILL, Before : Ars; Carb-v;
Chin; Eup-p; Pul.

During : Ap; Arn; BRY;
Caps; Cina; Eup-p; IGN;
NAT-M; Nux-v; Pyro; Sep;
Sil; Tub; Ver-a.

After : Ars; Chin; Dros; Pul.

COLD Drinks, for : Aco; ARS;
Bism; Bry; Calc; Chin; Diph;

Dul; Merc-c; PHO; Rhus-t;
Thyr; VER-A.

Coldness of body, with :
Carb-v.

Icy: Mag-p; *Pho;* Rut.

Night, at : Calc.

CONSUMPTION, In : Nit-ac.

HEADACHE, With: Mag-m;
Pulex.

HEAT, During : Aco; Ars; Bell;
Bry; Eup-p; Nat-m; Nux-v;
Tub.

+ KNOWS not for what, all
drinks are offensive : Arn.

LARGE Quantity, for : Ars;
Bry; Lil-t; Nat-m; Pho; Sul;
Ver-a.

Long intervals, at : *Bry.*

+ Often : Coc-c.

LITTLE And OFTEN, For : Aco;
Ant-t; Ap; ARS; Bell; Chin;
Hyo; *Lyc;* Rhus-t.

MORNING : Nit-ac.

MOUTH, Bitter, with : Con;
Pic-ac.

Heat, in : Hypr.

MUCH, Eats little : Dig; Sep;
Sul.

NIGHTLY : Calc; *Cham;* Sil.

PAINS, With : *Cham;* Nat-c.

STOOLS, After : Caps.

SWEAT, With : Ars; Chin;
Nat-m; Stram; Ver-a.

SYMPTOMS,Severe, before :
Lil-t.

UNQUENCHABLE : Jatr; Sec.

VERTIGO, With : Ox-ac.

VIOLENT, Burning : Acet-ac;

*Aco; Ars; Bry; Colo; Cup;
Eup-p; Merc; Merc-c; Nux-v;
Pho; Pyro; Saba; Tam; VER-A.*

THIRSTLESS, Aversion to
Water, Drinks : Aco; Aeth;
Ant-t; AP; Bell; Canth;*Chin;*
Colch; Fer; GEL; *Hell;* Hyo;
Ign; Ip; Meny; NUX-M;
Pho-ac; *Pul; Saba;* Sele;
Sep; STRAM.

For **D**ays : Calad.

Heat, During : *Ap;* Carb-v;
Cham; Cina; *Gel;* Hell; Ign;
Ip; Nux-m; *Pul;* Saba; Sep.

THOUGHT, Buried, In : Carb
an; *Hell; Mez; Nux-m; Sul.*

As to what would become
of him : Nat-m.

Horrid : Psor.

Menses, During : Mur-ac.

Strange, Pregnancy during :
Lyss.

Unpleasant Subject, fixed on
: Cocl.

Vanishing, Of : Manc; Nit-ac;
Ol-an.

THREAD Sensation (See Pain
Fine, and Hair) : Lach; Osm;
Plat; Saba; VAL.

Stretched, Head to arm etc.
: Lach.

THREATENING : Hep; Stram;
Tarn.

THROAT (Including inner
Mouth): *Ap;* Arg-n; Aru-t;
Bar-c; BELL; Caus; Gel;
Hep; Kali-bi; Lac-c; LACH;
Lyc; MERC; *Merc-c;* Merc-cy;
Merc-i-f; Merc-i-r; Nit-ac;

Nux-v; *Pho;* Phyt;Pul;
Rhus-t; Sul.

Right : Agar; Am-c; *Ap; Bell;*
Bry; Carb-ac; *Ign;* Kali-m;
Kre; LYC; *Merc;* Merc-d;
Merc-i-f; Phyt; Sang; Stan;
Sul; Syph; Tarn.

To left : Ap; BELL; Calc;
Caus; LYC; MERC-I-F; Pho;
Saba; Sang; Sul-ac; Syph.

Left : Calc; Caus; Crot-h;
Diph; Fer; Hep; Kali-c;
Lac-c; LACH; Mar-v;
Merc-c; Merc-i-r; Naj; Petr;
Pho-ac; *Rhus-t; Saba; Sep;
Sil;* Til.

In A.M. : Cimi; Rhus-t.

To right: Calc; LACH;
Merc-i-r; RHUS-T; Saba;
Stan.

Air, Feels cold : Ol-an.

Amel : Diph.

Alternating Sides : *Alu;* Arn;
Cocl; Colo; LAC-C; Pod; Pul;
Sul.

Back, Of : Aco; Cocl; Kali-c;
Merc; Nit-ac; Rhus-t.

Angina (Simple Sore Throat)
: Aco; Arg-n; Bap; Bell; Ign;
Lach; Lyc; Merc; Merc-c;
Merc-i-f; Pho; Rhus-t; Sep;
Sil; Sul-ac.

Chilliness, with : Mag-p.

Colds Agg : Sil.

Diphtheria, after : Phyt.

Morning, in : Rhus-t.

Nervous : Mag-p.

Operation, after : Fer-p.

Singers : Fer-p.

Smokers : Caps.

Speakers: Coll; Kali-io.

Winter Agg : Mez.

APPLE CORE, Choke Pear etc. as if : Aral; Merc; Nit-ac; Pall; *Phyt;* Plant; Ver-a.

BITTER : Chin; Con; Kre; *Pho;* Sil; Spo; Ver-a.

Food, swallowing, on : Kre.

BOILING Water rising in, as if : Stram.

BURNING, Heat, in : Aco; ARS; *Aru-t;* Canth; Caps; Caus; Cub; Euphr; Iris; Lac-c; Lach; Lyc; Mez; MERC-C; Nux-v; Oenan; Petr; *Pho;* Phyt; Ran-b; *Sang; Sul; Ver-a.*

Air cold Amel : Sang.

Eating, drinking when : Par.

Pepper, like : Radm.

Swallowing, when : Ars; *Bar-c;* Hep.

  compels : Strop.

Sweets Agg : Sang.

Vapour, hot, as of : Merc.

CHEST, To : Sang.

CHOKING, Constriction, Spasm, Narrow as if : Alu; Arg-m; Bap; BELL; Cact; Canth; *Caus; Cham; Hyo;* IGN; Lac-c; LACH; *Laur; Lyc;* Lycps; Merc-c; Merc-i-r; Mos; NAJ; Nux-v; Pho; *Plb;* Rum; *Spo;* Stram; Strop; *Sul; Sumb;* VER-A.

Ascends speaking when : Manc.

Bending head backwards,

Amel : Hep; Lach.

Breathing, when : Chel.

Contraction of fingers and toes, alternating with : Asaf.

Cough, inclination, with : Cocl.

Eat, when attempting to : Zin-val.

Goitre, from : Grap.

  exophthalmus, with: Meph.

Hawking, when: Amb; *Arg-n;* Nux-v.

Large morsel, as if from : Chel.

Sleep, during : Lach; Spo; Val.

Speaking when : Manc.

Swallowing, when : Grap; Lyc; Mur-ac; Pul; *Stram.*

  compels him to retch, while : *Grap;* Merc-c.

  food : Carb-v; *Pul.*

  hasty, as from : Chel.

  liquid, drops of, when: Merc-c.

  lump, as from, on empty : Grap.

  urging to, with : Caps.

Valve rolling and closing, as from : Fer.

Walking, while : Nat-s.

    Amel : Dros.

Warm Drinks Amel : Calc-f.

Water, from : Bap; Bell; Canth; Hyo; Nat-m; Stram; Sumb.

Word, every uttered with :
Dros.

Writing, while : Bar-c.

CLOSED, As if : Calc-f; Carb-v.

Something by, preventing
speech : Nat-p.

CLOTHES Agg : *Kali-c; Lach.*

CLUTCHES, At : Bell.

COATED Feeling : Carb-v; *Pul.*

COLD Agg : Alu; *Ars;* Hep;
Lac-c; Lob; LYC; Manc;
Merc-i-r; Nux-v; Rhus-t;
Saba; Sil; Syph.

Amel (Heat Agg) : *Ap;*
Arg-n; Calc; Diph; Ign;
Kali-m; *Lach;* Merc-c;
Merc-d; Merc-i-f; Pho;
Phyt; Sang.

Air penetrating, as if :
Ol-an.

wants : Diph.

Drinks, seem warm : Nat-m.

Warm, or Amel : Lac-c.

COLDNESS:Cep;Cist; Kali-chl;
Lyc; Ol-an.

Peppermint, like :Sanic;
Ver-a.

COLDS Agg : Bell; Cist; *Dul;*
Lach; *Merc; Nux-v.*

CONSTRICTION: See Choking.

COPPERY : Kali-bi; *Merc.*

COTTON, As if, in : Pho.

COUGHING Agg : Arg-m;
Aru-t; Caps; Cist; Ol-an.

CRAMPS : Gel; Grap; Sars.

CRAWLING : *Carb-v; Kali-c;*
Kali-m; Lach.

CUTTING : Manc; Merc-c; Nit-ac.

Cold drinks Agg : Manc.

DARK : Aesc; Ail; Arg-n; Bap;
Crot-h; *Lach; Phyt.*

Red : Arg-n; Bap; Cham;
Merc-i-r.

DRINKING Amel : Tell.

Sips, in Amel : Cist.

+ water runs out, seems :
Ver-a.

DRY : Aco; *Aese;* BELL; *Bry;*
Calc; Caus; *Lyc; Merc;*
Mur-ac; Nat-m; Nux-m;
Petr; Pho; Pho-ac; Pul;
Rhus-t; Saba; Sang; *Sep;*
Stic; *Stram; Sil;* Sul-io;
Thyr; *Ver-a;* Ver-v.

But no thirst : See Mouth.

Singer's : Sang.

+ Spot : Cist.

+ Stiff, and : Onos.

Swallows, saliva
constantly : Cub.

Thirst, with : Stram.

EAR, Extending to : Gel; Guai;
Hep; Kali-bi; Kali-m; Lach;
Merc; Merc-c; Merc-d;
Phys; Phyt; Sang; Stap.

Yawning, on : Hep.

EATING Amel : Benz-ac; Tell.

EMPTY : See Hollow.

ENLARGED, As if : Sanic.

ERUCTATION Agg : Phys.

EXERTION Agg : Caus; Lac-c.

FISSURES, Cracks : Aru-t; Bell;
Elap; Kali-bi.

FOOD Lodges In, Swallowing
when : Arg-n; Ars; Bar-c;
Caus; *Chin;* Grap; Ign;

Kali-c; *Lyc; Nat-m;* PUL; Sul.
+ As if : Pall.

Returns Through nose :
Aru-t; *Cocl;* Gel; Hyo;
Lach; *Lyc;* Merc; Op; *Pho;*
Sil; Sul-ac.

FOREIGN Body, as if, in : Ant-c;
Aral.

FULL : Arn.

Speaking Agg : Iod.

GLISTENING, Glazed : Ap;
Kali-bi; LAC-C; Nat-m; Petr;
Pho; Stram.

GRASPS, The : *Aco;* Aru-t; Asaf;
Cep; Dros; Iod; *Naj;* Pho.

GRAY : Phyt.

HAIR In (See Sensation under
Hair and Thread) : Kali-bi;
Saba; Sil; Sul; Val.

Back of : Coc-c.

HANGING, Loose, as if, in : Alu;
Berb; Iod; *Lach;* Merc; *Pho;*
Plat; Saba; Sul; Val.

Hyoid bone, near: Pall.

HAWKS : See Hawking.

HOLLOW, Empty : Calc-p;
Flu-ac; Iris; Lach; Lob; Phyt;
Rum; Sanic; Xanth.

Swallowing, on : Lyc.

HOT SOMETHING Rises, in :
Caps; *Merc;* Fright from,
anxiety with : Hypr.

INFLAMMED: Aco; Alu; Am-m;
Ap; Arg-n; Bap; *Bar-c;* Bell;
Bro; Bry; *Caps;* Cham; Chin;
Cocl; Cof; Dul; Fer-p; HEP;
Ign; *Lach;* Lyc; Mang; *Merc;*
Nit-ac; Pho; Pul; *Rhus-t;*
Petr; Sul; Sul-ac; Ver-a.

Painless : Bap.

IRRITATION Agg : Coc-c.

ITCHING : Ap; Aru-t; Caus;
Con; *Nux-v.*

Coughing, when : Zin-io.

LIFTING Agg : Caus; SIL.

LUMP, Ball, Plug, Globus :
Asaf; Coc-c; Hep; IGN;
Lach; Lob; Naj; Nat-m;
Par; Psor; *Pul;* Saba; Sep;
Ust.

Coughing Agg : Lach.

Amel : Kali-c.

Eructation Amel : Mag-m.

Hard : Nux-m.

Hawks : Merc-i-r.

Hot : Lach; Phyt.

Left side : Lach; Sil.

Rises and is swallowed
again : Alo; Asaf; Bar-c;
Calc; Cam; Chel; Con;
Kali-c; Lac-c; *Lach;*
Lil-t; Plb; Spo; *Rum.*

Rolling, and : Fer.

Sleep, in : Lach; Nux-v.

Soft : Lach.

Something, in : Merc.

Soreness, with : Nat-m.

Speech, preventing : Nat-p.

Sticks, and : Lyc.

Swallowed, as if : Phys.

Swallowing, impeding :
Lob.

empty Agg : Fer; Grap.

LYING Back, on Amel : Lach;
Spo.

MENSES, During Agg : See
under Menses, Throat

Agg.

Morsel, As if, in : Saba.

Mouldy, Taste, in : Mar-v.

+ Mucous, Constant, in : Eucal.

+ Glairy : Pall.

Narrow, As if : See Choking.

Neck and Shoulders, to : Kali-bi.

Nose, Ascending into : *Bro*; Lac-c; Merc; Sep.

Numb : Bap.

Odour, From : Petr.

Open, Wide, as if : Bar-m.

Painful : See Angina, Raw, Sore.

Paralysis : See Swallowing Noisy.

Pepper, As if, in : Radm.

Pressure Towards : Asaf.

Puffy : Arg-n; Lact-ac; Phyt.

Purple : Ap.

Raw, Sore : *Arg-m; Arg-n;* ARU-T; Bap; *Bell;* Calc; Carb-v; Caus; Chin; Ign; Lach; *Lyc;* Merc; Merc-c; *Nit-ac;* NUX-V; *Pho;* Radm.

Clergyman's : Alu; Aru-t.

Onions from : Alu.

Streak : Ol-an.

Rough, Scraping : Anac; Arg-m; *Chin;* Mez; *Nux-v;* Sul; Ver-a.

Sing, attempting, on : Agar.

Talking Agg : Seneg.

Sipping Water Amel : Cist.

Skin, Hanging, as if : Saba.

Slimy : Am-m; Bell; Caps;

Chel; *Lach;* Merc; Petr; PUL.

Smoker's Of : Arg-n; Caps; Nat-m.

Smoking Agg : Caps; Coc-c; Tarx.

Sneezing Agg : Hypr; *Pho;* Poth.

Soppy : Sul-ac.

Sore: See Angina, and Raw.

Spasms : See Choking.

Speaking Agg : Aco; Alu; Bar-c; Bry; Dul; Ign; *Kali-io;* Mang; Merc; Pho; Rhus-t; Sul.

Amel : Kali-bi.

Splinter, Stick, as of a : Alu; *Arg-n; Hep;* Ign; Kali-c; Nat-m; *Nit-ac; Phyt;* Sul; Thyr.

Across : Thyr.

Breathing Agg : Arg-m.

Eructation Agg : Arg-n.

Neck, moving Agg : Arg-n.

Speaking Agg : Mag-c.

Swallowing Agg : Arg-n; Mag-c.

Amel : Hep.

Spongy : Cist.

Spot, Dry, Sore etc. : Ap; Caus; Cimi; *Cist;* Con; Crot-h; *Hep; Hyo;* Lac-c; LACH; Lith; Merc-cy; *Nat-m;* Nit-ac; *Pho;* Phyt; *Sil.*

+ Sticks, Full Of : Alu.

Sticky, Clammy, Pasty : Aesc; Bap; Chel; KALI-BI; *Lach;* Myr; Pho-ac; Pul; Sec; Sul-ac.

Stiff, Rigidity : Chel; Lach;

Merc-i-r; *Rhus-t*

Sᴛᴏᴏᴘɪɴɢ Agg : Caus.

Sᴡᴇᴇᴛ Agg : Bad; Lach; Sang; Spo.

Amel : Ars.

Sᴡᴇʟʟᴇᴅ: Ail; AP; Hep; *Lach*; MERC; Merc-c;Nux-v; Phyt; Spo.

As if : Lach; Pul.

Tᴀsᴛᴇ In : Nux-v; Sil.

Bitter, low down : Kre.

Coughing Agg : See Hawking.

Eating Agg : Hell.

Hawking Agg: Mar-v; Nux-v.

Mouldy : Mar-v.

Tᴇɴsɪᴏɴ: Merc; Merc-i-f; Rhus-t; Senec.

Yawning Agg : Arg-m.

Tʜʀᴇᴀᴅ, Hanging as if : Coc-c; Pulex; Saba; Val.

Salivation, with : Val.

Vomiting, with : Val.

Tɪᴄᴋʟɪɴɢ : Stic. (See Itching Internal)

Coughing Agg : Zin-io.

Lachrymation, with : Cocl.

Lungs, down : Ver-a.

Tᴏɴɢᴜᴇ Protruding Agg: Kali-bi; Saba.

Tᴜʀɴɪɴɢ About, In : Lach.

Uʟᴄᴇʀs : *Ap; Ars;* Bap; Hep; Kali-bi; Kali-io; Lach; Merc; *Merc-c;* Mur-ac; *Nit-ac;* Nux-v; Rhus-t; Sul-ac; THU.

Uᴘᴡᴀʀᴅ Through or from : *Aco;* Ars; BRO; Calc; Carb-v; Fer; Kali-bi; *Kali-c;* Lac-c; *Lyc;* Merc; Nat-m; Nux-v; Pho; *Sep.*

Vᴀᴘᴏᴜʀ, In : Ap; Fer; Ol-an; Sul.

Coughing, when : Ol-an.

Sulphur, as of : Pul.

Vᴇsɪᴄʟᴇs, Full of : Canth.

Vᴏɪᴄᴇ, Overuse Agg : Bar-c.

Wᴀsʜ ʟᴇᴀᴛʜᴇʀ : Phyt.

Wᴇᴀᴋ : Lac-c; Stan.

Wʜɪᴛᴇ Wᴀsʜᴇᴅ : Sul-ac.

Wɪɴᴛᴇʀ Agg : Mez.

Wᴏʀᴍ, Wriggling in : Hypr; Pul.

Yᴀᴡɴɪɴɢ Ag : Arg-m; Arg-n; Nat-c; Zin.

Amel : Manc.

THROAT EXTERNAL : Bell; Lyc.

Rɪɢʜᴛ: Caus; Flu-ac; Lyc; Merc; Nat-c; Nat-m; Nit-ac; Sil.

Lᴇғᴛ : Asaf; Calc; Con; Sul.

Aʟᴛᴇʀɴᴀᴛɪɴɢ Sides : Am-m ; Calc-p.

Cᴀʀᴏᴛɪᴅ Arteries, Throbbing of : Aur; *Bell;* Cact; Chin; Glo; Pru-sp; Spig; Ver-v.

Cʟᴏᴛʜɪɴɢ Agg : See Sensitive.

Cᴏʟᴅ : Spo.

Wind blowing on, as if : Old.

Cᴏɴsᴛʀɪᴄᴛɪᴏɴ: Lach; Stram.

Gʟᴀɴᴅs : Am-m; *Bar-c;* Bell; Bro; Calc; Calc-f; Calc-io; Calc-p; *Cham;* Grap; Hep; *Ign; Iod;* Lach; Lyc; Nat-m; Rhus-t; *Spo;* Stap; Sul; Vip; Zin-io.

Air passing through, breathing on, as if : Spo.

Right: Ars; Kali-c; *Merc;* Nit-ac; Sil; Zin-io.

ITCHING : Alu.

LARYNX, Motion of : Stram.

NUMB : Spo.

RED : Bell; Grap; Sul; Ver-a.

SENSITIVE To Touch, Pressure Clothes: Ant-t; Ap; Bap; Crot-h; Crot-t; Lac-c; LACH; Merc-c; Nux-v.

SWALLOWING Agg : Zin.

SWEAT : Mang; Rhus-t; Stan.

SWELLING : Lyc; Rhus-t; Tarn.
Goitre, like : Vip.
Speaking, loudly, when : Iod.

TENSION : Nux-m.

TUMOURS : Bar-c; Bro.

TWITCH : Agar.

UNCOVERING AGG : Hep; Kali-c; Nux-v; Rhus-t; Scil; Sil; Zin.

THROAT PIT : Ap; Arg-m; *Cham;* Chlor; Hep; Kali-bi; Pho; *Rum;* Sang; *Sep;* Zin-chr.

CONSTRICTION : *Bro.*

CRAWLING, Formication, causing Cough : Sang.

FULLNESS : Lach.

IRRITATION : Ign; Rum; Sang.

LUMP, In : Lob.

PAINFUL : Caus; Lach.
Hawking, when : Caus.

PRESSURE : *Bro;* Calc; *Lach.*

SORE : Ap; Arg-n.
Back, of : Lach.

STITCHING : Spo.

SWOLLEN : Lach.

THROBBING : See Pulsation.

THROMBOSIS : Ap; Arn; Ars; Both; Ham; Lach.

THROWS THINGS AWAY : Agar; Caus; Colo; Dul; Kre; *Stap;* Tarn; Thu; Tub.
BUGS, Handfuls, in : Ars.

THRUSTS, Stings, as of : *Ap;* Arn; Cina; Plat; Rut; Sul-ac; Thu.

THUMBS ACHING : Sang.
Ball, with : Sang.
BENT, Backwards : Cam; Lyc; Merc.
CLENCHED : Cup; Hyo; Merc.
Convulsions, with: Stan.
Palms, into : Hell.
CRAMP, Writing, when : Mur-ac.
Contraction, Index finger with : Cyc.
LAME : Calc-s.
PAINFUL : Anac; Kre; Menc; Ox-ac.
SPRAINED, As if : Grap; Pru-sp.
STIFF : Kre.
Writing, while : Kali-c.
SUCKING : Calc-p; Nat-m; Sil.
SWELLING : Sang.
ULCER, Turning yellow : Kali-io.
UP, Arms to shoulder: Ced; Naj.

THUNDERSTORMS AGG (See Change of Weather AGG) : Nat-c; Nat-p; *Pho;* Psor; Rhod; Syph.
AMEL : Rhus-t.

THYROID : See Goitre.
  DYSFUNCTION : Calc.
  PINCHED, As if : Nat-ar.
TIBIAE : Agar; *Asaf;* Calc;
  Carb-v; Cinb; Lach; Merc;
  Mez; *Pho;* Phyt; Pul; Stil.
  BURNING : Zin.
  CARIES : Sil.
  COLD *;* Mos.
  COPPERY, Spots : Nit-ac.
  EXOSTOSIS : Merc-c; Nit-ac.
  LYING Agg : Pul.
  NODE: Calc-f; Cinb; Sul-io.
  OSTEO SARCOMA, Middle, in :
    Syph.
  PAIN, In: Cast-eq; *Lach;* Pho;
    Phyt; Stil; Sul-io.
    Digging : Mang.
    Spots : Amb.
    Stretching, while : Aur.
    Throat, with : Lach.
  + PERIOSTEUM : Mang.
  SPONGY *;* Guai.
  STICKING : Pul.
  SYPHILITIC: Merc; Phyt; Stil;
    Sul-io.
  ULCER, On : Flu-ac.
TIC : Arg-n; Ars; Hyo; Laur;
  Lyc; Ran-b; Sep; Tarn; Zin.
TICKLING : See Itching Internal.
  AMEL : Sep.
TIGHTNESS : See Tension.
TIME AGG AND AMEL
  MORNING AGG (4 A.M. to 9 A.M.)
    : Agar; AM-M; ANT-T;
    Arg-m; Ars-io; AUR; Bor;
    Bov; *Bry;* CALC; Calc-p;
    Cann; Carb-an; *Carb-v;*

Castr; Cham; CHEL;
Cina; Con; *Croc;* Echi;
Elap; Hep; *Ign;* Kali-bi;
Kali-c; Kali-n; LACH; Naj;
Nat-s; *Nat-c; Nit-ac;*
NUX-V; Onos; Petr; PHO;
Pho-ac; *Pod;* Pul; *Rhod;*
RHUS-T; Rum; Saba;
SCIL; *Sep;* Spig; SUL; Val.
AMEL : Chel; Merc; Zin.

Bed, in Agg : Alo; *Amb;*
  Am-m; Bry; Con; *Kali-c;*
  Lyc; Nux-v; Pho; Sep; *Sul.*

Evening, and Agg : Alu;
  Bov; *Calc;* Caus; Coc-c;
  Grap; Kali-c; Lach; LYC;
  PHO; Psor; *Rhus-t;* Sang;
  SEP; *Stram; Stro; Thu;*
  Ver-a.

One day, Evening, next
  day : Eup-p; Lac-c.

6 A.M. Agg : Alo; *Alu;* Arn;
  Bov; Fer; *Hep;* Lyc; *Nux-v;*
  Sil; Sul; VER-A.

7 A.M. Agg: *Eup-p;* Hep;
  Nat-c; *Nux-v; Pod;* Sep.

8 A.M. Agg : *Eup-p;* Nux-v.

8 A.M. to 12 Noon Agg :
  Cact; *Chin-s; Eup-p; Gel;*
  Nat-c; NAT-M; Nux-v;
  Pho; Saba; Sep; Stan; Sul.

9 A.M. Agg : Bry; *Eup-p;*
  Kali-bi; Kali-c; Lac-c;
  Nat-m; Nat-s; Nux-v;
  Sep; Sul-ac; *Verb.*

To 4 P.M. Agg : Verb.

FO RENOON AGG (9 A.M. to
12 Noon : Arg-m; CANN;
Carb-v; Guai; Hep; Laur;
NAT-C; NAT-M; Nux-m;

Pod; Ran-b; Rhus-t; SABA; SEP; Sil; STAN; SUL; Sul-ac; Val;Vio-t.

AMEL : Alu; Lil-t; *Lyc.*

10 A.M. Agg : *Ars; Bor;* Chin; Chin-s; *Eup-p;* GEL; *Iod;* Med; NAT-M; Petr; *Pho; Rhus-t;* Sep; Sil; *Stan; Sul;* Thu.

10 A.M. to 3 P.M. Agg : Chin-s; Nat-m; Tub.

11 A.M. Agg : Ars; Asaf; Bap; *Cact; Chin-s;* Cocl; *Gel; Hyds;* Hyo; Ip; *Lach;* Mag-p; Nat-c; NAT-M; Nat-p; *Nux-v; Pho; Pul; Rhus-t; Sep; Stan;* SUL; Zin.

12 Noon Agg : Ant-c; *Arg-m;* Chel; Chin; Elap; *Eup-p* Gel; Kali-c; Lach; *Nat-m; Nux-v;* Pho; *Sil;* Spig; Stram; *Sul;* Val; Verb.

To 4 *P.M.* Agg : Alu; Ars; Bell; Lach; Lyc; Pul; Sil; Thu; Zin.

Eating, after Amel : *Chel.*

To Midnight Agg : Lach.

AFTERNOON AGG (12 Noon to 6 P.M.) : Agar; Alo; *Alu;* Amb; Ant-c; AP; Asaf; BELL; Bry; Chel; *Chin; Cimi;* Colo; *Dig;* Hell; *Ign; Kali-n;* LYC; PUL; *Rhus-t; Sep; Sil; Sul;* Thu; ZIN.

AMEL : Cinb; Gel; Nat-s; Phyt; Rhus-t; Sep.

1 P.M. Agg : *Ars;* Cact; Chel; Cina; Grat; Kali-c; *Lach;*

Pho; *Pul.*

2 *P.M.* Agg : Ars; Chel; *Eup-p;* Fer; Gel; *Lach;* Mag-p; Nit-ac; *Pul.*

3 *P.M.* Agg : Ant-t; *Ap; Ars;* Asaf; BELL; Ced; Chel; *Chin-s;* Con; Samb; Sang; *Stap; Thu.*

3 *P.M.* to 5 *P.M.* Agg *:* Sep.

4 *P.M.* Agg : *Aesc; Anac; Ap;* Ars; Cact; Caus; *Ced; Chel;* Chin-s; *Colo Gel;* Hell; Ip; LYC; Mang; Nat-s; Nit-ac; Nux-m; *Nux-v; Pul;* Rhus-t; Sul; Verb.

4 *P.M.* to 8 *P.M.* Agg : *Ap; Caus;* Colo; Hell; Hyo; LYC; Nit-ac; Nux-m; Pho; Plat; *Pul; Rhus-t;* Sul; THU; Tub; Val.

To day light Agg : Syph.

5 *P.M.* Agg : Alu; Bov; Caus; Ced; *Chin;* Colo; Con; *Gel;* Hep; Hypr; *Kali-c; Lyc;* Nat-m; Nux-v; *Pul; Rhus-t;* Sul; *Thu;* Tub; Val.

EVENING AGG (6 P.M. to 9 P.M.: ACO; Alu; Amb; *Am-c; Ant-c; Ant-t;* Arg-n; *Arn;* Ars; BELL; *Bry* Calc; *Caps;* Carb-an; Carb-v; *Caus;* Cep; Cham; *Colch;* CYC; EUPHR; Flu-ac; *Hell; Hyo;* KALI-N; Kali-s; Lach; LYC; *Mag-c;* MENY; *Merc; Mez;* Nat-p; NIT-AC; *Pho;* Pho-ac; PLAT; *Plb;* PUL; *Ran-sc; Rum;* Rut; SEP; Sil; *Stan;* STRO; SUL; Sul-ac;

Syph; Val; *Zin.*

AMEL : Alu; *Aur;* Bor; Med; Sep..

MID-NIGHT, Until Agg : Anac.

6 *P.M.* Agg : Ant-t; *Ced; Hep; Kali-c;* Nat-m; NUX-V; Petr; *Pul; Rhus-t; Sep; Sil;* Sumb.

To 4 A.M. : Guai.

To 6 A.M. : Kre.

7 P.M. Agg : Alu; Bov; *Ced;* Chin-s; Fer; Gamb; Gel; *Hep; Ip; Lyc;* Nat-m; *Nat-s; Nux-v;* Petr; Pul; Pyro; *Rhus-t;* Sep; Sul; Tarn.

8 *P.M.* Agg : Alu; *Bov ;* Caus; Cof; Elap; Hep; Mag-c; Merc; Pho; *Rhus-t;* SUL.

8 P.M. to 12 midnight Agg : Arg-n; *Bov;* BRY; Carb.v; Gel; Lyc; Mur-ac; Pho; Pul; Rum; Stan; Sul.

NIGHT **A**GG (9 P.M. to4A.M.) : ACO; Arg-n; *Arn;* ARS; Ars-io; Bell; Calc; Calc-p; Calc-s; Carb-an; CHAM; CHIN; *Cimi; Cof;* COLCH; Con; Cyc; *Dul;* FER; GRAP; HEP; *Hyo; Iod;* Ip; Jal; Kali-bi; Kali-c; KALI-IO; Lach; Lil-t; MAG-C; *Mag-m; Mang;* Meph; MERC; NIT-AC; *Pho;* PLB; PSOR; Pul; *Rhus-t;* Rum; Sep; SIL; STRO; SUL; SYPH; Tell; ZIN.

9 *P.M.* Agg : Ars; *Bov;* BRY; *Gel;* Merc.

10 *P.M.* Agg : *Ars; Bov;* CHIN-S; *Grap;* Ign; Lach; Petr.

11 P.M. Agg : Aral; Ars; Bell; CACT; Calc; Carb-an; Rum; Sul.

Amel : Bor.

12 **M**IDNIGHT Agg : *Aco;* Arg-n; ARS; Calc; Calad; Canth; *Caus; Chin;* Dig; *Dros; Fer;* Kali-c; Lach; Lyc; Mag-m; Mur-ac; Nat-m; Nux-m; Op; Pho; *Rhus-t; Samb;* Stram; Sul; Ver-a.

After Amel : Anac; Form; LYC; Ran-sc.

To 4 *A.M.* Agg : Am-c; *Ars;* Caus; Ced; Dros; Kali-bi; Lach; *Nat-m;* Nux-v; POD; Rum; *Sul;* Ver-a.

To Noon Agg : Ars.

Amel : Pul.

1 A.M. Agg : ARS; Carb-v; Mag-m; *Pul.*

2 A.M. Agg : ARS; *Benz-ac;* Canth; *Caus;* Como; Dros; Fer; Grap; *Hep;* Iris; Kali-ar; KALI-BI; *Kali-c;* Kali-p; Lach; Lachn; Lyc; Mag-c; Mez; Nat-m; Nat-s; *Nit-ac;* Ptel; *Pul;* Rum; Sars; *Sil;* Spig; Sul.

3 A.M. Agg : Am-c; *Am-m;* Ant-t; *Ars; Bry;* Calc; Canth; *Ced;* Chin; Fer; Iris; KALI-C; Kali-n; *Mag-c;* Nat-m; *Nux-v;* Pod; *Psor; Rhus-t; Sele;* Sep; Sil; *Sul; Thu.*

4 *A.M.* Agg : *Alu;* Am-m; Anac; Ap; *Arn; Bor; Caus;* CED; Chel; Colo;

Con; Fer; *Ign*; Kali-c; *Lyc*; *Mur-ac*; *Nat-c*; Nat-ac; Nit-ac; NUX-V; *Pod*; *Pul*; Radm; Sep; Sil; Stan; *Sul*; Ver-a.

To 4 P.M. Agg : Kali-c.

4 A.M. To 8 A.M. Agg : Alu; Arn; Aur; Bry; Chel; *Eup-p*; Hep; Kali-bi; Lach; *Nat-m*; Nux-v; POD; Rum; *Sul*; Ver-a.

5 A.M. Agg : Alo; Ap; CHIN; Dros; *Kali-c*; Kali-io; *Nat-m*; Nat-p; Pho-ac; Rum; Sep; Sil; *Sul*.

TIME SENSE CHANGED : Alu; Cann; Lach; Merc.

PASSES Too Slowly : Alu; Amb; Arg-m; Arg-n; Cann; Glo; Med; Merc; Nux-m; Nux-v; Pall.

Too Quickly : *Cocl*; Ther.

TIMID : See Shy.

TIMOROUS : Alu.

TINGLING (See Itching Internal) : Aco; Kalm; Sec.

PAIN, After : Sec.

TINNITUS: See Hearing Illusory Noises, And Meniere's Disease.

VERTIGO Then: Chin.

TIRED : See Weakness.

ACTS, As if born : Onos.

+ ALWAYS, Women : Alet.

OF LIFE : See Death; Desires and Suicidal Disposition.

TO AND FRO : See Altern ations.

TOBACCO AGG: Ars; Ars-io; *Cam*; Gel; *Ign*; Nux-v; Pho;

Plant; *Pul*; Radm; Sele; Spig; Spo; Stap; Strop; Ver-a.

AMEL : Aran; *Hep*; Naj; Plat; Sep; Stro; Tarn.

AVERSION, To: *Calc*; IGN; Lob; Nat-m; *Nux-v*.

Addicted, though : Lob.

+ BITTER Taste : Cocl.

CHEWING AGG : *Ars*; Lyc; Plant; Ver-a.

+ DISGUST, For, produces: Plant.

+ SMOKE Agg : Aco; Cic.

SMOKERS AGG : Sec.

SMOKING, When breaking off : Calad.

TOES : Arn; *Caus*; *Grap*; Plant; Pul; Ran-sc; Sabi; *Sul*; Thu.

BALLS, Of : Berb; Led; Petr; Pul; Spig.

Painful : Med.

BEND, Walking, while : Bad; Lyc.

BLUISH : Sec.

BROKEN : Cocl; Lach.

BURNING : Ap; Tarx.

COLD : Abro.

CORNS : See Callosities.

CRACKED : Saba; Sars.

Between : Saba; Sil.

Under : Saba.

CRAMPS: Calc; Caus; Cup-ac; Pho; Ver-a; Zin-chr.

Dysmenorrhoea, alternating with : Dios.

DRAWN, Down : Ars; Colch; Cup; Hyo.

Up : Cam; Cic; Lach.

ECZEMA, Nails loss of, with : Bor.

ENLARGED, As if : Ap; Laur.

GLISTENING: Sabi.

GOUT : See Gout.

GREAT (Toe) : Arn; Asaf; Caus; Kali-c; Nat-s; Plat; Radm; Sabi; Sil; Zin.

Felon : Caus.

Inflammed : Ran-sc.

Needles, at : Ran-sc.

Numb: Ars; Calc; Cham; Nat-s.

Swelled : Led; Sabi.

HIPS, To : Pall.

INFLAMMED : Sil.

INSTEP, To : Anac.

JERKING : Agar; Calc; Merc.

JOINTS : Aur; Caus; Kali-c; Led; Mar-v; Sabi; Sep; Sul; Zin.

NAILS (See Nails) : Grap; Saba.

Under : Ant-c; Flu-ac; Grap; Mar-v.

pricking : Elap.

NUMB : Abro; Grap; Pho; Sec.

Extending to other parts : Thal.

PAINFUL : Phyt; Rhod.

PRICKING : Abro.

RED : Sabi.

SORENESS, Between : Nat-m.

SPASMS : Chel; Cup; Sec; Zin.

Stairs, ascending, on : Hyo.

Walking, on : Hyo.

SPREAD Apart : Glo.

STUBBING Agg : Colch.

SWELLED : Grap.

As if : Zin.

THIGHS, To : Nux-v; Thal.

TIPS, Of : Kali-c; Thu.

Aching : Zin.

Blisters : Nat-c.

Formication : Thu.

Painful : Kali-c; Zin.

Wind Blowing through, as if : Cup.

TREMOR : Arn; Mag-c.

ULCERS On : Sil.

VESICLES : Sec.

WHITE, Becomes, sweat from : Grap.

TONGUE : Bell; Hyo; Merc; Mur-ac; Nux-v; Pho; Plb; Pul.

ACROSS : Acet-ac; Asar; Kali-p; Kob; LACH; Merc.

APHTHAE : Bor; Carb-v; Kali-chl; Merc; Mur-ac; Sul; Thu.

ATROPHY : Mur-ac.

BITES : Buf; Dios; Ign; Thu; Vip.

Sleep, in : Cic; Pho-ac.

Talking, while : Hyo.

Tip, of : Ther.

BLACK : Arn; Ars; Carb-v; Chin; Crot-h; Dig; Gymn; Hyo; Lept; Lyc; Merc; Op; Pho; Radm.

Centre, down : Lept.

Gangrenous : Bism.

+ BLEACHED, As if : Ver-v.

BLEEDING : Aru-t; Bor; Sec.

BLUE : Ant-t; Ars; Dig; Gymn; Mur-ac.

White : Ars; Gymn.

BROAD : Mag-m; Merc; Nat-m; Pul.

As if : Nat-m; Par; Plb; Pul.

BURNING, Burnt etc. : Aco; Adon; Ap; Ars; Bap; Bell; Calc-p; Hyds; Ign; *Iris;* Kali-io; Mag-m; Mur-ac; Nat-s; Plat; Pod; Ptel; *Pul;* Saba; Sang; Sanic; Ver-v.

Stomach, to : Bro; Mez.

CANCER : Kali-cy; Mur-ac.

CATCHES, Teeth, on protruding : Ap; Hyo; LACH.

CENTER, Down (strips) : Ant-t; *Arn;* Ars; *Bap;* Caus; Iris; Lach; Malan; Merc-c; *Pho;* Pyro; *Rhus-t;* VER-V.

Furrow : Nit-ac.

Pea like elevation : Castr.

CLEAN : Cina; Dig; *Hyo;* Ip; Mag-p; Sec.

Edges : Arg-n.

Menses, during : Sep.

Urine, profuse, when : Solid.

COATED : Bell; *Bry;* Chin; Merc; *Nux-v;* Pho; Pul.

Diagonally : Rhus-t.

Edges clean with: Arg-n.

Green, base at : Caps.

salivation, with: Nit-ac.

One side : Daph; Mez; Rhus-t.

White : ANT-C; Ant-t; *Ars; Bell;* Bism; Bry; Calc; *Chin;* Hyds; Hyo; Kali-bi; *Kali-m;* Merc; Nit-ac; Pho; *Pul; Sul;* Tarx.

centre : Petr.

Yellow : Bry; Chel; Chin; Hyds; Kali-p; MAG-M;

Merc; Nux-m; Ol-j; Pul; Rhus-t; Spig.

edges indented, with : Chel; Hyds.

greenish : Chio.

moist, filmy : Merc-i-f; Nat-p.

mustard were spread on, as if : Kali-p; Pod.

patchy : Lil-t.

COLD : Cam; Carb-v; Cist; Iris; Kali-chl; Naj; Ver-a.

CONTRACTED : Carb-v; Merc-c.

Cylindrical : Cina.

CONTROL, Loss of : Aesc.

CRACKS, Fissures : Ail; Ars; *Aru-t;* BELL; Benz-ac; Bor; Flu-ac; *Hyo;* Iod; **KALI-BI**; Kali-io; Lyc; *Nit-ac; Pho;* RHUS-T; Sec; Spig; Sul.

Across : Kob.

Bleeding : Aru-t.

Centre : Nit-ac; Syph.

Directions, in all: Flu-ac; Nit-ac.

Middle of : Mez.

Peeling, off: Ran-sc.

CRAMP : See Spasm.

CRAWLING : Plat; Sec.

CUTTING, Asthma, before: Bor.

DIAGONALLY : Rhus-t.

DIRTY : Cean; Chin; Hyds; Nat-s.

DISTORTED : Con.

DOTTED : Ant-t; Bell; Grap; Stram.

DRAWN, Backward : Tarn.

Up : Chin.

DRY : *Ars;* BELL; Bor; *Bry;*
Calc; Hell; Hyo;Lyc; Nux-m;
Pho; RHUS-T; Sul.

As if : Nat-m; Nux-m.

+ Brown : Ail.

Half : Bell; Sang.

Middle : Ant.t.

ECCHYMOSES : Pho.

EDGES, Of : Ap; Nat-m; Phyt.

Aphthae : Arg-n.

Beads, Foam, on : Am-c;
Ap; Iod; *Nat-m;* Pho.

Dark, streaked : Petr.

Indented : Ant-t; Chel.

Needles, at : Nux-v.

Painful, sore : Ap; Zin.

Red : *Ars;* Bell; Bry; *Chel;*
MERC; Sul.

centre : Rhus-t.

tip, and : Ap; Sul.

Turned up : Sanic.

Ulcer, right : Sil; Thu.

left : Ap.

Vesicles, on : Am-c; *Ap;*
Lach; Nat-m; Pho.

white : Thu.

ERUPTIONS, On : Nat-m; Sars; Zin.

Psoriasis : Cast-eq.

Ringworm : Nat-m; Sanic.

FILMY : Merc-i-f.

FLABBY : Cam; Dig; Hyds; Merc;
Pod; Sanic.

FORMICATION : See Crawling.

+ FUR, Dots, thick white : *Grap.*

+ White : Guai.

FURROW Across : Merc.

Centre : Nit-ac.

FURRY : Merc.

GLISTENING : Ap; Ars; Cist;
Kali-bi; Lach; Pho; Sul-io;
Terb.

GRAY : Chel; Kali-c; Kali-m.

GREENISH At base : Caps.

HAIR, On : All-s; Kai-bi;
Nat-m; Nat-p; *Sil.*

Reading while : All-s.

HANGS, Out of mouth : Ap;
Stram. '

HEAVY : Bell; *Gel;* Glo; Kali-bi;
Lach; Lyc; Mur-ac; Nat-c;
Nat-m; Nux-m; Nux.v.

HYPERTROPHY, Of : Iod.

INDENTED : *Ars;* Bor; *Chel;*
Hyds; Kali-io; Mag-m;
MERC; *Pod;* Pul; *Rhus-t;*
Stram; Syph.

INDURATION : Hyds; Hyo;
Merc-d; Nux-m.

Knotty : Carb-an.

INFLAMMED : Aco; *Ap;* Bell;
Crot-h; Lach; MERC; Merc-c.

JERKING, In : Cham.

LARGE, As if : Par.

LEATHER, Like, hard : Aur.

Burnt : Hyo.

LOLLING : See Oscillating.

LONG, As if : Aeth; Mur-ac.

LUMPS, Hard : Mur-ac.

MAPPED : See Patchy.

MOTION Of, difficult : See
under Protruded.

Lapping : Buf.

NEURALGIA : Ap; Crot-t;
Kali-ar; Mang.

NODES, On : Iod; Mang;

Mur-ac.

NUMB : Aco; Echil; GEL; Hell; Nat-m;; *Nux-m;* Old; Pul.

One side : Nat-m.

vertigo, with : Agar.

OILY, Greasy : Iris; Phys.

OSCILLATING : Hell; Hyo; Lach; Lyc.

Spasms, during : Sil.

PAINFUL : See Sore.

PALATE, Sticks to : Bry; Kali-p; Nux-m; Sanic.

PAPILLAE, Showing (Strawberry) : Arg-n; Ars; Aru-t; *Bell;* Caus; Kali-bi; Terb.

PARALYSIS : Bar-c; CAUS; *Gel;* Hyo; Lach; *Op; Plb;* Sec.

Creeping : Kali-p.

PATCHY, Mapped, Spots : *ARS;* Dul; Hyds; Kali-bi; Lach; Merc; Merc-c; NAT-M; *Nit-ac;* Ran-sc; *Rhus-t;* Sep; Syph; *Tarx;* Tub.

PEA, Like bodies, red centre with : Castr.

POINTED : Chel; Ip; Lach; Petr.

PRICKLING, Under : Lyss.

PROTRUDED: Ap; Bell; Crot-h; Cup; Phyt; Vario;Vip.

Brain affections, in: Ap; Hyd-ac.

+ Cannot be : Merc-c.

Difficulty, with: Ap; Caus; Gel; Hyo; Lach; Myg; Pho.

drawing, in : Hyo.

jerk, with : Kali-br.

sore throat, with : Saba.

+ Pain, then : Kali-bi.

Rapidly, Darting in and out like a snake : *Cup;* Lach; Lyc; Merc; Vip.

Side, right : Crot-h; Op.

Sleep, in : Vario.

To keep it cool : Sanic.

PROTRUDING AGG : Cocl; Cist; *Kali-bi; Phyt;* Syph.

AMEL : Med.

PUCKERED, As if : Ars.

PUFFY : Bor.

RATTLES : Hyo.

RAW : Carb-v; *Nux-v;* Sil.

RED : Ant-t; AP; *Ars;* Bell; Hyo; *Kali-bi;* Lach; Merc; *Pho;* Rhus-t; Sang.

Base at : Bry.

Centre, along : Ver-v.

Cracked, dysentery, in: Kali-bi.

Dots, fine : Stram.

Fiery : Ap; Pyro; Sang.

Stiff, painful, moving when : Merc-i-r.

Streak, centre down : Caus; Ver-v.

middle : Ant-t; Cham; Pho-ac.

+ Stripe down centre, widens at tip : Calad.

ROOT, Of : Bap; Kali-bi; Kali-io; Lach; Nat-s; Phyt.

Burning : Med.

Green : Caps; Chio.

yellow : Nat-s.

Swelling : Caus.

Tension : Kali-io.

Tickling : Stan.

White : Kali-m; Nat-m; Sep.

Yellow : Merc-i-f; *Nat-p;* Nat-s; Phyt.

ROUGH : Aru-t; Pod.

SANDY : Ap; Cist.

+ SCALDED, Feeling : Adon;Aesc; Colo; Hyds; Ol-an; Phys.

SCALLOPED : Mag-m.

SHRUNKEN : Mur-ac.

SIDE, One : Bell; *Calc;* Lob; Mez; Nat-m; RHUS-T; Sang; Sil; Thu.

SKIN,Covered with, as if : Rhus-t.

SLIMY : Eucal; *Pul.*

SMOOTH, Glazed : Ap; Lach; Pyro; Sul-io; Terb; Tub.

SOFT *:* Merc; Rhus-t; Stram.

SORE, Painful : Agar; Calc; Caps; Carb-v; Ign; *Nit-ac;* Pul; Saba; Sep.

Root at, yawning when : Lach.

Spots, on : *Agar;* Ant-c; Sil; Tarx.

SPASMS *:* Arg-n; Cocl; Con; Lyc; Syph.

Causing embarassment of speech : Rut.

+ SPONGY : Benz-ac.

STIFF : Anac; Ap; *Bell;* Hyo; Lac-c; Merc-i-r; Mur-ac; Nat-m; RHUS-T.

STITCHING : Merc.

STRAWBERRY : See Papillae Showing.

STRIPE : See under Red.

SWELLED *:* *Aco;* Anac; *Ap;* Ars; Bell; Canth; Caus; Crot-h; Dul; Hyds; Lyc; *Merc;* Polyg; Zin.

Small, round, middle in : Dros.

TEARING : Merc.

THICK, As if : Bap; *GEL.*

TICKLING : Alu; Stan.

TIP, Of : Kali-c; *Rhus-t;* Sul; Thyr; Zin.

+ Burns like pepper: Coc-c.

Burnt : Calc; Caps; Chin; Colo; Nat-s; Psor; Terb.

+ Clean, white at back : Hypr.

Cracked : Lach.

Needle pricks : Merc.

Pimple, painful : Buf.

+ Pricking : Radm.

Red : Arg-n; *Ars;* Ip; Merc-i-r; *Phyt;* RHUS-T; *Sul.*

painful : Arg-n.

triangle : Arg-n; *Rhus-t;* Sep.

Spot, dark red : Diph.

Sweet : Plat.

Vesicles : Ap; Caus; Kali-c; Lyc; Nat-c.

TREMULOUS : Agar; Ap; Cam; Canth; Gel; Hell; *Lach;* Lyc; *Merc;* Pho; Plb; Sul.

Protruding, when : Bell; Gel; Hell; Hyo; *Lach;* Plb.

TUMOUR, were forming: Kali-m.

TWITCHING : Castr; Glo; Sec; Sul.

ULCERATED: Arg-n; *Bap;*
Carb-v; Kali-io; MERC;
Psor.

Jagged : Cund.

Yellow : Hell.

UNDER : Flu-ac; Grap; *Lyc;*
Nat-c; *Sanic.*

VEINS, Distended : Dig; Thu.

WARM, As if : Cimi.

WARTS, On : Aur.

WEAK : Bar-c; Caus; Con.

WHITE : See Coated.

WOOD, Made of, as if : Ap.

WRINKLED: Calc-p; Merc-i-r;
Pho; Sul-ac.

YELLOW : See Coated.

TONSILS : Bap; *Bar-c;* BELL;
Calc; *Calc-p;* Guai; Hep;
Lac-c; LACH; Lyc; *Merc;*
Merc-d; MERC-I-F; MERC-I-R;
NIT-AC; Pho; *Phyt;* Sil; Sul;
Tub.

CHAMOIS Skin, Wash leather
: Phyt; *Rhus-t.*

CHRONICITY : Bar-c; Bar-m;
Bro; Hep; Kali-io; Lyc; Mez;
Nat-m; Sul-io; Thu.

+ Hardness of hearing with
: Hep.

CRYPTS, Greyish white :
Calc-io; *Ign.*

Mucus plug of, constantly
form : Calc-f.

ENLARGED : BAR-C; *Bar-m;*
CALC-F; CALC-I; CALC-P;
Con; Ign; *Lach;* Lyc; Merc;
Merc-i-f; *Merc-i-r;* Nit-ac;
Stap; Syph; *Tub.*

Coryza, after : Saba.

+ Deafness with, children :
Kali-bi.

Mouth, opening Agg :
Calc-p.

Pus, plugs of, with: Calc-f.

FOUL : Ail; Bap; *Lach;* Lyc;
Merc; Nit-ac.

GLISTEN : Ap; Lac-c.

GRAY : Kali-m; Merc-cy.

INDURATED : Alu; *Bar-c; Bar-m;*
Phyt.

LACUNAE : Ail; Merc-i-f.

MENSES, At Agg : Lac-c.

+ PRICKING, Pin, as of : Sil.

RECURRENT : Guai; Phyt.

RED, Bright : Aco; *Bell;* Phyt.

Dark : Aesc; Bap; Carbac;
Lach.

SUPPURATING (Quinsy) :Bar-m;
Bell; Guai; HEP; Lach; *Lyc;*
Merc; Nat-m; Phyt; Psor;
SIL; *Tarn.*

Chronic : *Bar-c.*

THROBBING, In : Am-m; Phyt.

ULCERS (See Throat) : Ail.

Behind : Ars; Merc.

TOPER (See Alcoholic Drink
AGG) : Caps; Ran-b; Sele;
Stram; Sul-ac.

ABSTAINING, After Agg: Calc-ar.

TORMENTS EVERY BODY, With
Her Complaints: *Zin.*

TORN LOOSE, As if : See under
Bones.

+ OFF, As if : Ap.

OUT, Feeling : Alu; Bry; Calc;
Elap; *Pru-sp;* Rhus-t.

PIECES, To : See Shattered.

TORPID : Asaf; Dros; Kali-s; Led; Nat-m; Nux-m; Op; Sil.

TORTICOLLIS : See Neck, Wry.

TOSSING About : See under Restlessness.

Convulsions, During: Bar-m.

Suddenly : Chin.

TOUCH Agg : See Sensitive, and Touchy.

Amel: *Asaf; Bism; Calc; Cyc;* Grap; *Mur-ac;* Pall; Sang; Stap; Tarx; *Thu.*

Each other (Of arms, fingers etc.) Agg : Lac-c; Psor; Sanic.

Hair, Even of a : Ap.

Pain Amel but appears somewhere else : Asaf; Sang; Stap.

Sense Of, disturbed : Par.

Slight Agg : Aco; Ap; *Bell;* Chin; Ign; LACH; Merc; *Nit-ac; Nux-v.*

Hard pressure Amel : Bell; *Castr; Chin;* Ign; *Lach; Nux-v;* Plb; Psor.

Things Impulse, to : Bell; Lycps; Sul; *Thu.*

Inability to do so : Sul.

TOUCHED When Agg : See under Fear.

TOUCHING Anything Agg : *Cham.*

Amel : Spig.

Cold Things Agg : Hep; Mang; Merc; Nat-m; *Rhus-t; Sil.*

Warm Things Agg : Sul.

TOUCHY (Mentally and Physically) : Aco; Ant-c; Ant-t; Cham; Cimi; CINA; Hep; Pul; Sanic.

TOURIST : Coca; *Plat.*

TOUSY, Dishevelled : Bor; Flu-ac; Med; Sul.

TOXAEMIA : See Blood Sepsis.

Pregnancy, Of: See under Pregnancy.

TRACHEA : See Larynx.

TRAIN SICKNESS: See Car Sickness.

TRANQUIL : See Placid.

TRAUMATISM : See Injuries, Shocks.

TRAVEL *DESIRE,* To : *Calcp;* Iod; Lyss; Tub.

+ Far Away Places : Merc.

+ Ill Effects, of : Ars.

TREMBLING,Tremors : Amb; Agar; Anac; Ant-t; ARG-N; *Ars;* CALC; *Cic; Cimi;* Cocl; *Con;* GEL; Grap; Hyo; IOD; Jab; Kalm; *Lach;* Lil-t; Lycps; Med; MERC; Mos; Naj; NUX-V; Ol-an; *Op;* Phys; *Plat; Pul;* RHUS-T; Saba; Sang; Stan; Stap; *Stram;* Stro; Sul; Sul-ac; Tab; Ther; Tub; Ver-v; *Zin.*

Air, Open Amel : Clem.

All Over : Bro; Visc.

Amorous, Caressing during : Caps.

Anger, From : Nit-ac; Ran-b.

Anxiety, With : Samb.

As If : Seneg.

Burns, After : Calc.

Cold Drinks, Amel : Pho.

Concomitant, As a : Calc-p.

CONVULSIONS, Before : Abs;
Ver-v.

COUGHING Agg : Cup; Just; Pho.

DELIRIUM, With : Aco; Ap; Ars;
Bell; Bry; Calc; Chin; Hyo;
Ign; Nat-m; Op; Phys; Plat;
Pul; Rhus-t; Saba; Samb;
Stram; Sul; Ver-a; Ver-v.

DIRECTION, Downward : Iod;
Merc.

Upward : Sil; Spig.

ELECTRIC Shock, through
body, with : Buf.

EMOTIONS, From : *Cocl*; Mar-v;
Plb; Psor; *Stap*.

EXERTION, Slight, from : Anac.

EXOPHTHALMOS, With : Meph.

FEAR, From : Elap.

HANDS and FEET: Ap;Ox-ac.

HEADACHE, With : Bor.

HERE and THERE : Ver-v.

HUNGRY, When : Alu; Crot-h;
Sul; Zin.

INTENTIONAL : Arg-n; *Cocl;
Kali-br*; Rhus-t; *Sec;* Zin.

INTERNALLY : Calc; Caul; Diph;
Grap; *Hep;* Iod; Mar-v; Med;
Rhus-t; Stan;Stap; SUL-AC.

Excitement Agg : Mar-v.

LOWER Part : Amb.

MEETING Friends, when : Tarn.

MOTION, Slow Agg : Stan.

MUSIC, From : Alo; *Amb*; Thu.

NERVOUS : Cimi; Cof; Gel;
Lil-t; Mag-p; Pho; *Stap;*
Stram.

NOISE, Sudden, from : Alo;
Kali-ar.

NURSING, Infant, after : Old.

PAINS Agg : Cocl; *NAT-C*; Plat;
Pul; Zin.

PARALYZED Part : CAUS; Merc;
Nux-m; Plb.

PERIODICAL : Arg-n.

SENILE : Bar-c; Con.

SHIVERING, With : Cina.

SIDE, Lain on : Cimi; Clem.

SMOKING, From : Hep; Kali-c;
Nat-m; Nit-ac; Sep.

SPASMODIC: Ign; Nux-v; Saba.

STOOL, After : Ars; CON.

SWEAT, With : Jab; Merc.

+ THUNDERSTORM, From : Nat-p.

TOUCH, Unexpected : Cocl;
Kali-ar.

URINATING With : Gel.

VOLUPTUOUS : Calc.

WAKING, On : Merc; Tarn; Ver-a.

WALK, On Attempting to :
Cup-ar.

While : Stan.

WRITING, While : Pho; Sil.

TRENCH MOUTH : Merc-c.

TRICKLING, DROPPING Or
Flowing as of water :
Arg-n; Buf; *Cann*; Caus; Glo;
Grap; Kali-bi; Lap-alb; Nat-m;
Petros; Pho; Rhus-t; Sep;
Stan; Sumb; Tarn; *Thu;*
Ver-a; Vario.

AFFECTED Part, on : Arg-n.

HOT : Hep; Sep; Stan; Sul;
Sumb.

TRICKY : Cup.

TRIFLES (Mental Symptoms)
AGG : *Ars*; CHAM; Cina;

Cof; Dros; Hep; *Ign;* Nit-ac; NUX-V; SIL; Thu.

SEEM IMPORTANT : Ars; Calc; Caus; Con; *Grap;* *Hep;* Ign; Nat-m; *Nux-v;* Sil; Thu.

TRISMUS: See Jaws, Locked.

TUBE METALLIC : Merc-c.

HOT WATER, Running through, as if, Pain during : Terb.

TUBERCULOSIS : See Consumption.

TUMID : See Puffiness.

TUMOURS: See Growths, New.

+ TUNE OUT OF: Nux-v.

TURGIDITY (See also Puffiness) : Am-m; *Ap;* ARS; BELL; *Bry;* Cham; Kali-c; *Lyc; Merc; Nux-v;* Op; Pho; *Rhus-t;* Stram.

TURNING AROUND AGG : Calc; *Ip;* Kali-c; Par.

AFFECTED Part, *AMEL*: Bell.

FROM LEFT to Right Amel : Lach; Pho.

Right to Left Agg : Scop; Sul.

OVER : See under Bed and Rolling.

RAPIDLY, As if : Mos.

RIGHT, To AGG : Carb-v; Spig.

Before he can rise : Kali-c.

Walking, when : Helod.

SIDEWAYS AGG : Bell; Calc; Kali-c; Nat-m.

SOMETHING by limbs AMEL : *SEP.*

TWILIGHT AGG : *Ars;* Berb; CALC; Caus; Nat-s; Pho; Plat; PUL; *Rhus-t.*

AMEL : Bry; Meny; *Pho;* Plat;

Seneg; Tab.

SEES Things, in : Berb.

TWINGES NIPS : See Pain, Twinging.

TWISTING :Ars; Bell; Calc; Cina; *Colo;* Dios; Elap; Ign; *Nux-v;* Pul; Rhus-t; SIL; VER-A.

TWITCHING(See Convulsions) : Agar; Amb; Asaf; Cina; Gel; Hyo; Ign; Iod; Kali-c; Laur; Mez; Mos; Nat-c; Saba; Sec; Stram; Strop; Tarn; Zin.

COLDNESS, With : Amb.

CONVULSIONS, Before : Ast-r.

ONE SIDE, Other side lame : Ap.

PAINFUL : Agar; Meny.

After : Sec.

With : Meny.

PARALYSED Parts, of : Arg-n; Merc; Pho; Sec; Stram.

SLEEP, During : Ars; Bar-c; Op; Sul.

SUBSULTUS TEDINUM : Ars; *Hyo; Iod;* Lyc; Mur-ac; Pho; Pho-ac; *Zin.*

TYMPANUM : See under Ear.

TYPHOID (See Blood Sepsis) : Ars; Bap; Bell; *Bry;* Kali-c; Mur-ac; Op; Pho; Pho-ac; Pyro; *Rhus-t;* Sul; Tarx.

ABORTING : Bap; Pyro.

+ VACCINATION, Ill effects : Bap.

TYPHUS FEVER : Ars.

UGLY (In Behaviour) : Bry; Buf; *Cham;* Cina; *Nux-v.*

ULCERS : *Arg-n;* ARS; Ars-io; *Asaf;* Calc; Calc-s; Carb-v; Caus; *Hep; Kali-bi;* Kali-chl; Kali-s; *Lach; Lyc;* MERC; *Nit-ac;* Pho; Pho-ac; Phyt; PUL; Rhus-t; Sep; SIL; *Sul;* Sul-io; Syph; Vip.

AREOLA, Edges, Margins, with : Ars; Asaf; Hep; Lach; Lyc; Merc; *Pul; Sil.*

Dark : Aesc; *Lach.*

Elevated : Ars; Asaf; *Merc; Sil.*

indurated, and : Ars; Lyc; Sil.

Eruptions, Pimples etc. in : Carb-v; *Hep;* Lach.

Fungoid : Lach.

Hanging, over : Kali-bi.

Hard : Flu-ac; Grap; Pul; Sil.

red : Pul.

Sensitive : Asaf.

Shiny : Pul.

Small ulcers, over : Calc; Hep; Mez; Pho; Rhus-t.

Zigzag, irregular margins, with : *Merc;* Nit-ac; *Pho-ac.*

ATONIC, Indolent, Painless : ARS; Carb-v; Con; Hep; Hyds; *Lach;* LYC; Op; PHO-AC; Sec; *Sil; Sul.*

Tumours, removal after : Hyds.

BED Sores : See under Bed.

BLACK : Anthx; Ars; Bism; Carb-v Kali-ar; Lach; Lyc; Sec.

BLEEDING: Arn; Ars; Bur-p; Carb-v; Hep; *Lach;* Lyc; Merc; Nit-ac; *Pho;* Pho-ac; Sul-ac.

Menses, during : Pho.

BLOODY Water, from : Carb-ac; Kali-ar; Rhus-t.

BLUISH : Ars;Asaf; Crot-h; *Lach;* Mur-ac; Sil; Tarn-c; Thu; Vip.

BOILS, Around : Hep.

BREAK AND HEAL, Recur : Carb-v; Kre; Vip.

BURNING : Anthx; *Ars;* Carb-v; Caus; Kali-ar; Lyc; Merc; Plb; Pul; Rhus-t; *SIL;* Sul.

+ CANCEROUS : Aur.

COITION Agg : Kre.

COLD Feeling, in : Ars; *Bry;* Rhus-t; Sil.

CUTTING : Bell; Kali-ar; Merc.

DEEP, Perforating: Ars; *Calc;* Calc-s; KALI-BI; Kali-c; Lach; Merc; Merc-c; Mez; *Mur-ac; Nit-ac; Pul;* Radm; Ran-b; Rat; Sil; Sul; Tarn.

Hard and : Mez.

DIRTY : Lach; Merc; Nit-ac.

DOTTED: Arg-n; Ars; Kali-bi; Med.

DROPSICAL Persons, in : Ars; Grap; Hell; Lyc; Merc; Rhus-t; Scil; Sul.

DRY, Hard : Mang.

FLOWING : Kali-ar; Kali-s; Nat-s; *Rhus-t;* Zin-s.

Yellow water : Kali-s.

HEAT Agg (Cold Application Amel) : Cham; Flu-ac; *Led;* Lyc; *Pul.*

Amel : Ars; Clem; Con; HEP; *Lach;* Rhus-t; *Sil;*Syph.

HONEYCOMBED : Cinb.

INDOLENT : See Atonic.

INJURY, Slight, after : Mang.

IRREGULAR : Ars; Kali-bi; Merc; Phyt; Sars; Sil.

ITCHING : Kali-ar.

MAGGOTS, With : Saba; Sil.

MUSTARD Poultice, from:Calc-p.

OFFENSIVE, Foul : Carb-v;Hep; Kali-ar; Mur-ac; Sec; Sil.

Asafoetida like : Carb-v.

PAINFUL :Ars; Bell; Carb-v; Grap; Hep; Sabi; Sil.

PAINLESS : See Atonic.

+ PHAGEDINIC : Cist.

PIMPLES, Around : Hep.

PULSATION : Hep.

Walking, when : Mur-ac.

RAPID, Malignant : Arg-n; *Ars;* Carb-an; *Carb-v;* Caus; Chel; Hyds; Lyc; Merc; *Merc-c;* NIT-AC; Petr; Ran-b; Ran-sc; *Sil;* Thu.

Borders, blue with : Mang.

ROUND, Punched: Kali-bi; Merc; Phyt.

SCOOPED,Out : Vario.

SENILE : Tarn-c.

SENSITIVE, Touch causes convulsions : Stap.

SHALLOW, Flat, Superficial : ARS; Hyds; LACH; *Lyc; Merc;* NIT-AC; Thu.

Climaxis, at : Polyg.

SHOES, Pressure, from : Bor; Paeon.

SMALL : See Dotted.

SPONGY : Sil.

SUPPRESSED : Clem; Lach; Sul.

SWELLED : Lyc; *Merc;* Pul; *Rhus-t; Sep; Sil;* Sul.

SYPHILITIC : Ars; Asaf; *Iod;* Kali-io; *Merc;* Merc-c; *Nit-ac;* Phyt; Thu.

TUMOURS, Removal after : Hyds.

VARICOSE : See under Blood Vessels, Distended.

ULNAR NERVE ALONG : Aran; Hypr; Kalm; Pod; Rhus-t; Tub.

UMBILICUS : See Navel.

UNATTRACTIVE, THINGS, Seem : Chin.

UNCERTAIN : Merc.

EXECUTION, Of : Med.

GAIT etc. : Con.

UNCIVIL : See Ugly.

+**UNCLEAN** : See Dirty Habits.

ODOUR, Body, Of : Guai.

UNCONSCIOUS, INSENSIBLE (See Numbness) : Aco; Ars; Bar-c; *Bap;* BELL; *Cam;* Cocl; *Cup;* Hell; Hyd-ac; HYO; Ign; Lach; Mos; Nat-m; Nux-m; OP; PHO-AC; Pul; STRAM.

BECOMING, As if : Cup.

BLOOD, Sight of : Nux-m.

COITION, After : Agar; Dig.

CONVULSIONS, After : *Buf;* Cic;
Oenan; Stan.

Prolonged : Bell.

EMOTIONS, From : Cof; Ign; Lach.

EYES, Closing, on : Ant-t;
Cann.

Open, with : See Coma, Vigil.

FEVER, During : Ap; Arn;
Mur-ac; Nat-m; Op.

FREQUENT Spells : Ars.

MENSES, During : Lach.

Suppressed, from : Nux-m.

ODOURS From : *Nux-v;* Pho.

PAIN, During : Hep; Nux-m;
Val.

PARTURITION, During : Cimi;
Cof; *Nux-v;* Pul; Sec.

PREGNANCY, During : Nux-m;
Nux-v; Sec.

PROLONGED : *Cic; Gel;* Hyd-ac;
Laur.

RUBBING Soles Amel : Chel.

SUDDEN : Canth; Cocl; Kali-c.

SWALLOW, Inability, to: Amy-n.

TALKING, While: Lyc.

TRANCE, As if, in : LACH; Laur.

TRANQUIL : Ign; Pul.

UNCOUTH : Bar-c; Caps.

UNCOVERING AGG : See Heat
Amel and Wind, Draft *Agg.*

AMEL : See Cold Amel.

CHEST AMEL : Sars.

LEAST AGG : Hep; Nux-v;
Rhus-t; *Sil.*

NECK AMEL : Sars.

WANTS, Sleep, in : Plat.

UNDRESSING AGG : See

under Itching, and Wind Agg.

AIR, Open in AGG : Pho.

UNDULATIONS (See Waves)
: Asaf; Grap; Nux-v; Rhod;
Sep; Strop; Zin-io.

UNEASY FEELING : Aeth; Ascl;
Ced; Cup; Dros; Grap; Guai;
Sep; Stan; Val; Ver-v.

KNOWS, Not, What to do, with
himself : Stan.

SEXUAL Desire, with : Ant-c.

UNHAPPY : See Sadness.

UNLUCKY : Ver-a.

UNREAL, EVERYTHING SEEMS :
Alu; Cann; Cocl; *Med.*

+ LIKE *A* DREAM : Anac.

+ **UNPLEASANT THINGS,**
DWELLS on : Benz-ac.

+ **UNRULY** : Am-c.

UNSOCIAL : Anac; *Syph.*

UNSTEADY As If : *Agar;*
Arg-n; Bar-c; Caus; Cic;
Cocl; Kali-br; Lil-t; Nat-c;
Sec; Stan; *Sul.*

LOOK, Eyes roll vacantly :
Lach.

UNSUCCESSFUL, THINKS
HIMSELF : Naj; Sul.

UNTIDY : *Sul.*

UNUSUAL THINGS, From any
AGG : Amb.

UP AND DOWN : See Directions.

UPPER LIMBS : See Arms.

URAEMIA : *Ap;* Ars; Aru-t;
Bap; Bell; Canth; Hell; Hyo;
Op; Pic-ac; Plb; Senec;
Stram; Terb; Urt; Ver-v.

URETERS : Ap; *Bell; Berb;*

Canth; Carb-an *Lyc*; Oci-c;
Par; Polyg; *SARS*; Sep; Terb;
Ver-a.
BURNING : Terb.
CRAMP : Nit-ac; Polyg.
CUTTING: Bell; Berb; Carb-an;
Lyc; Par-b; Polyg; Sars;
Ver-a; Ver-v.
INFLAMMATION : Canth.
SORE : Ap; Berb; Oci-c.
VOMITING, With : OCI-C.

URETHRA : Arg-n; *Cann*;
Canth; Caps; Clem; Lyc; Merc;
Pho; Pul; Sul; Thu.
ABDOMEN, To : Sars.
ABSCESS : Canth; Pul; Rhus-t.
BLEEDS : Merc-c.
+ Bladder pain, with: Ant-t.
 Coition, during : Caus.
 Gonorrhoea, Suppressed
  After : *Pul.*
 Paraplegia, with : Lyc.
 Stools, during : *Lyc*; Pul.
 Urine, first part, with : Con.
 Urination, after : Hep;
  Merc-c; Pul; Sars; Thu.
BURNING : Aco; Ars; Berb; Cam;
Cann; *Canth*; Merc; *Merc-c*;
Nux-v; Pru-sp; Sil; Sul; Thu.
 Coition Agg : Agar; Canth;
  Clem; Sep; *Sul.*
 Emission, during : Ant-c; *Sul.*
 Erection, with :Canth;
  Nit-ac.
 Flatus passing Agg : Lyc;
  Mang.
 Stools, during : Colo.
 Urination, before : Bor;
  Cann; Canth; Caps.

 after Agg : Merc.
 during : Nat-c; Uran-n.
 Amel : Berb; Bry; *Merc*;
  Stap.
 at the end of Agg : Clem;
  Nat-c.
 coition, after : Caus.
CARUNCLE : Arg-n; Ars; *Cann*;
Hep; Nit-ac; Sul; Sul-io.
CLOGGED : Merc; Sep.
COLD Drop of urine,
 passing as if : Agar.
CRAMP : Canth; Chin; Clem.
CRAWLING : Fer-io; Lyc;
Petros; Pho-ac.
CUTTING : Arg-n; Calc-p;
Canth; Con; Thu.
 Glans penis, grasping
  Amel : Canth.
 Seminal discharge, on :
  Con.
 Urination, during : Ant-t;
  Cantth; Con.
 after : Canth; Nat-m.
DISCHARGE Acrid : Arg-n;
Merc-c.
 Bloody : Calc; Canth; Sil.
 Cream, like : Caps.
 Foetid : Benz-ac; Carb-v;
  Hep; Sil.
 Gleety : Agn; Alu; Alum;
  Benz-ac; Kali-chl;
  Kali-io; Nat-m; Petros;
  Sele; Sep; Sul; Thu.
 Milky, white, stools after
  : Iod.
 Mucous : Elap; Sep.
 Night, at : Sep.

Painless : Fer; Nat-s; Thu.

Persists : Alu; Arg-m; Kali-bi; Pho; Sul.

urinating after : Sars.

Thin : Lyc; Nat-m; Nit-ac; Pho; Psor;Sul; *Thu.*

Yellow : Alu; Arg-n; Merc; Pul; Sep; Thu.

stains : Alu; Nat-m; Psor.

DRAGGING : Til.

DRAWING : Flu-ac; Merc.

DROPS, Biting, forcing its way out : Sele.

+ Few pass out as if : Amb.

One remained, urination, after : Kali-bi.

Rolling continuously as if : Lact-v; Sele; Stap.

FLATUS, passing Agg : Mang.

HEAVY : Eup-p; Saba; Til.

HOT Wire, in : Nit-ac.

INDURATED : Arg-n; Clem; Hypr; Merc-i-r.

Whip cord like : Clem.

ITCHING : Merc-c; Nux-v; Rhus-t; Sil; *Sul.*

JERKING : Alu; Cann; Lyc; Petr; Pho; Sars; Thu.

KNOT, Ball, as if, in : Arg-n.

Rolling through : Lach.

NARROW, As if : Arg-n.

NODES, In : Bov.

NUMB : Arg-n; *Caus;* Kali-br; *Mag-m.*

OPEN, As if : Cop.

PULSATION : Merc-c.

RIDING Agg : Stap.

RUNNING OUT, something emission, after : Dig.

STINGING : Sabal.

Flatus passing on : Mang.

STRAW Thrust, as if, back and forth : Dig.

STRICTURE : Canth; Cic; *Clem;* Nat-s; Nit-ac; PETR; Pul; Sul-io.

Dilatation, after : Mag-m.

Drunkards : Op.

Gonorrhoea, after : Sul-io.

Spasmodic : Nux-v.

TINGLING : Clem; Petros.

TRICKLING : Arg-n; Kali-bi; Petros; Stap; Thu.

TUMOUR, Small, in : Lach.

TWITCHING : Cann; Canth; Pho.

ULCERS : Merc-c; Nit-ac.

UNEASY Feeling : Ced.

URINATING Amel : *Merc;* Stap.

WALKING Agg : Stap.

URGING (See Pain, Pressing) : *Canth;* Lil-t; *Merc-c;* Sabi.

URIC ACID DIATHESIS

LITHEMIA (See under Urine, Red Sediment) : Benz-ac; Berb; Bur-p; Coc-c; *Lyc;* Nat-s; Sars; Sep; Thu; Urt.

URINARY ORGANS In GENERAL : Aco; AP; Arn; Ars; Bell; *Berb;* Calc; Cam; Cann; CANTH; *Caus;* Dul; Fer; Hell; Hep; Hyo; Lyc; *Merc; Merc-c;* Nat-m; Nit-ac; *Nux-v;* Op; Par-b; Pho; Scil; Pho-ac; Polyg; PUL; Rhus-t; Sars; Stap; Sul; *Terb;* Til; Thu; Val;

Ver-a.

RHEUMATIC Symptoms, Alternating, with : Benz-ac.

URINATION BEFORE AGG (Crying etc.) : Aco; *Bor;* Canth; *Colo; Lyc;* NUX-V; PUL; Sanic; Sars.

AT START of AGG : *Aco;* Canth; Clem; *Merc.*

DURING AGG : Aesc; Alo; Berb; *Cann; Canth; Hep;* Lil-t; *Lyc;* MERC; Nux-v; *Pho-ac;* PUL; *Sep;* Sul; THU.

AT CLOSE OF AGG : *Canth;* Equis; Merc-c; Mez; Nat-m; Sars.

AFTER AGG : Cann; *Canth; Colo;* Equis; *Hep;* Med; Merc; MERC-C; *Nat-m;* Petros; Stap; THU.

AMEL : Chin-s; *Gel; Ign;* Lith; Lyc; Pho-ac; Sang; Sil; Ver-a.

ABORTION, After Agg : Rhe.

CUTTING : Canth; Sep.

DESIRE, Morbid urging : Ant-t; Ap; Arg-n; Bell; Berb; *Bry;* Cam; Cann; CANTH; *Caus;* Chin; Ip; Kali-c; Lil-t; MERC-C.; Nat-m; NUX-V; *Pho-ac; Pul; Sabi; Sars; Scil;* Sep; *Stap;* SUL; Thu.

+ Absent in Pregnancy : Hyo.

Clots, bloody from vagina Amel : Coc-c.

with : Chim.

Coition, after : Nat-p.

Diarrhoea, during : Ap; Ars; Canth; *Merc-c.*

Fever, during : Ant-t; *Ap;* Bell; Pul.

Fruitless, Ineffectual : Am; *Ars; Canth;* Caps; Caus; Chim; *Dig;* Hell; Hyo; *Merc-c;* Nit-ac; NUX-VOM; Op; Pho; Pho-ac; Pul; *Sars;* Stram.

Heart, affections, with : Dig.

Labour, after : Op; *Stap.*

Lifting weight, on : Bry.

Married women, Newly : *Stap.*

Menses, before : *Kali-io;* Sars.

+ More urine, more urge : Colch.

Night : Dig; Lyc; Sabal; Sil; Sul.

Pain, from : Terb.

Prolapsus of uterus, from : *Lil-t; Sep.*

Rectum, ball, as if in with : Lil-t.

Restricted, causes pain : Petr.

cannot, pain after : Rut.

if, then desire ceases : Sanic.

Stools, before : Rhe.

Thinking of it Agg : Ox-ac; Oxyt.

DIFFICULT, Painful, dysuria, Strangury : Aco; Arg-n; Ars; Bell; *Cann;* CANTH; Caps; *Cham;* Cop; Dig; Dul; Erig; Hyo; *Lil-t;* Lyc; MERC-C; NUX-V; Op; Par-b; Petros; Plb; *Pru-sp; Pul;* Sabal; *Sars; Stap; Sul;*

Terb.

Alcoholic drinks, from : Nux-m.

Attempting to urinate, on : Plb.

Dances around the room, in agony : *Ap*; Cann; *Canth*; Petros.

Delivery, after : Ap; Equi.

Dentition, during : Erig.

Dribbling, with : Bur-p.

Dysentery, in : Arn.

Dysmenorrhoea, with : Nux-m; Senec; Ver-v.

Enuresis, alternating, with : Gel.

Erection, then : Radm.

Feet, wet from : Cep.

Forceps delivery after : Bur-p.

Headache, with (children) : Con; Senec.

Hysterical : Nux-m.

Lying Amel : Kre.

Menses before : Sars.

Neuralgic : Pru-sp.

Pregnancy, during : Equi; Eup-pur; Pho-ac; Plb; Stap.

Presence of others, in : *Amb*; Hep; Mur-ac; Nat-m; Tarn.

Prostate, enlargement, with : Ap; Med; Petros.

Renal colic, with : Coc-c.

Riding on rough ground, from : Eup-pur.

+ Spasmodic : Vib.

Utrine profuse with : Equi

Uterine, complaints, with : Nux-m.

displacement, with : Senec.

Women, plethoric, in : Chim.

+ DOUBLE Up, must, to urinate : Pru-sp.

DRIBBLING : CANTH; Caus; *Clem;* Dig; Kali-m; Lil-t; Merc; *Merc-c;* Nux-v; Pic-ac; Plb; Polyg; *Pul;* Sele; Stap; *Sul;* Tab; Terb.

As if, rest Agg : Sep.

Forceps delivery, after : Bur-p.

Involuntary : Arn; Canth; Caus; Clem; Sele.

angry, when : Pul.

Labour, after : Arn; Tril.

Prostate, enlarged, with : Nux-v.

Retention, with : Caus; Nux-v.

Seat, rising from, when : Spig.

Senile : Bar-c; Cep; Cic; Con; Equi; Nux-v.

Sitting, while : Merc-c; Sars.

Spurts, in, then : Bur-p; Caps.

Stools, after : Nat-c; Sele.

during : Colo.

Urination, after : Cann; Clem; Hep; Sele.

Walking, when: Sele.

Women, in winter, Agg : Rhus-t.

DRINKING, After : Ap; Arg-n; Caps; *Fer-p; Samb*; Sars.

DYSURIA : See Difficult.

FEEBLE, Slow, Weak : *Alu;*
Arg-n; *Arn; Caus;* Clem;
Hell; HEP; *Lyc;* Merc;
Merc-c; Mur-ac; Nat-m; Op;
Rhus-t; *Sars; Sep;* Sul;Thu.

Copious, but : Plb.

Difficulty in breathing and
heart symptoms, with :
Laur

Drops Vertically : Arg-n;
Caus; Gel; *Hep.*

violent pain, in bladder,
with : Calc-p.

FREQUENT: Alu; Ap; *Arg-m;*
Arg-n; *Bar-c;* Calc; Canth;
Caus; Grap; Hyo; Ign;
Kali-io; Kali-n; Kre; *Lyc;*
Mang; MERC; MERC-C;
NUX-V; Psor; Pul; *Rhus-t;*
Scil; Stap; Sul; Thu; Vib.

Constipation, with : Sars.

Day time : Kre; Rhus-t.

night, and : Merc.

Every 10 to 15 minutes :
Bor.

Haemorrhage, with : Vib.

+ Headache, with : Vib.

Hour, every : Calc-ar.

Hysterical : Gel.

Menses, during : Hyo; Vib.

Night more, than day : Ther.

Pain, with : Thu.

Pregnancy, during : Pod.

Prostate, affections, in : Ap;
Fer-pic; Sabal; Stap.

Riding in carriage Amel :
Lyc.

Urine, scanty with : Hell.

HURRIED, Sudden, irresistible
: Arn; Bry; Canth; Clem;
KRE; Nux-v; Petros; Pho;
Pho-ac; *PUL;* Rum; Sanic;
Scil; SEP; SUL; Thu.

Water, Hearing running
or putting hands, in :
Canth; *Lyss;* Sul.

INABILITY To pass, Pain,
during : Con.

INFREQUENT, Seldom : Ap;
Canth; Lac-c; Lob; Nux-v;
Op; Scil.

Daytime : Bor; Lyc; Ther.

twice : Pyro.

but scanty : Pyro.

Once a day but profuse :
Lac-c; Syph.

difficulty, with : Lac-c.

INTERRUPTED, Intermittent :
Agar; Ant-c; Ap; Carb-an;
Caus; *Clem; Con;* Gel;
Hep; Kali-c; Kali-p; Led;
Lyc; Op; Sabal; Sars; Sul;
Thu.

Coition, after : Pho-ac.

Priapism, with : Ant-c.

Spurts in, swelled
prostate with cutting
pain : *Pul.*

Strains a few drops, then
full flow follows: Clem.

Suddenly, pain followed
by : Pulex.

INVOLUNTARY : Ail; Ap; Ars;
Ars-io; Bell; CAUS; Dul;
Fer; Hyo; Lyc; Nat-m;
Nux-m; Pho; Psor; *Pul;*
Rhus-t; Sabal; Sec; Sep;
Stap;Uran-n.

Bed, in : See Bed wetting.

Bladder feels empty, when : Helo.

Coition, fright, from : Lyc.

Constipation, with : Tarn.

Convulsions, during : Buf; Caus; Cup; Hyo; Plb; Zin.

Coughing, on : Ant-c; Ap; CAUS; Kali-c; Kre; Mur-ac; *Nat-m;* Nux-v; PHO; *Pul;* Scil; Sep; Sul; Tarn; Thu; Ver-a; Verb; Vib; Zin.

night, at : Colch.

pregnant, women : Cocl.

Day time only : *Fer;* Flu- ac. and night: Arg-n; Ars; Caus.

Desire, if restricted : Pul; Sul; Thu.

Effort on, no urination flow : Gel.

Exertion Agg : Bry.

Flatus passing, when: Mur-ac; Pul; Sul.

Fright, from : Op; Sep.

Hurry, in, when : Lac-d.

Inattention, from : Sep.

Laughing, when : *Caus;* Nat-m; Nux-v; Pul; *Sep.*

Lying Agg : Bels; *Kre;* Lach; Lyc; Pic-ac; *Pul;* Uva-u.

Menses, during : Hyo.

Noise, sudden : Pul; Sep.

Old people, in : Alo; Carb-ac; Cic; Iod; Sec.

Parturition after : Arn; *Ars.*

Pregnancy during : *Ars;* Nat-m; *Pul;* Sep; Syph.

Prostate enlargement with : Iod.

Putting hands in cold water : Kre.

Riding Agg : Lac-d; Thu.
Amel : Lyc.

Rising seat from Agg: *Mag-c;* Petr; Spig.

Running, while : Arn; Bry; Lac-d.

Sitting Agg : Caus; Nat-m; *Pul;* Rhus-t; Sars.
Amel : Zin.

Sleepy, when : Bell.

Sneezing, when (See coughing) : Alet; *Caus;* Pho-ac; Pul; Zin.

Standing, when : Bell; Fer.

Stools, after : Mur-ac; Zin.

Sudden movement, from : Fer.

Surprise, pleasurable Agg : Pul.

Train catching, whilec : Lac-d.

Uterus, prolapsed, from : Fer-io.

Walking, while : Fer; Lac-d; Mag-c; Nat-m; Pul; Vib; Zin.

amel : Rhus-t.

fast Agg : Alet.

yet attempting to, when standing still, nothing passes : Mag-m.

Jets, In : See Spurts, in.

+ Menses, Before Agg : Kali-io.

+ urging : Sars.

NERVOUS : Cimi; *Ign*; Vib.

NIGHTLY : Calc-f; Hyo; *Lyc*; *Rhus-t*; Spig; Sul; Ther; Uran-n.

ODD Position, in : Zin.

PAINFUL : See Difficult.

PAINS Agg : Calc; *Gel*; Terb; Thu.

PROFUSE, Copious, Polyuria : See Urine Profuse.

Amel : Gel; Ign; Meli; Sang; Solid.

Alternating with scanty urine : See Urine, Profuse.

RETARDED, Must wait for Urine to start : See Feeble.

Bending backwards Amel : Alu.

Doubling up Amel : Canth; Pru-sp.

Dribbling with : Alu.

Hearing, water, running Amel : Lyss.

Lying Amel : Kre.

Odd position, in Amel : Zin.

Presence of others, in Agg : *Amb;* Hep; Mur-ac; *Nat-m*; Tarn.

Pressing hard or Straining at stool Amel : *Alo; Alu;* Caus; Hep; Lil-t; Mag-m; Mur-ac; Op; Tub.

more, less it flows : *Kalia-c.*

prostatic affections in : Ap.

so hard that anus protrudes : MUR-AC.

Sitting Agg : Pul; Sars.

Amel : Caus; Zin.

Spasm of sphincter, from : *Op.*

Standing Amel : Alu; Caus; Con; Hypr; *Sars*; Syph.

day time Agg, but night at, flows freely : Sars.

pavements, cold, on Agg : Carb-v.

with feet wide apart body inclined forward, Amel : Chim.

Stooping Amel: Canth; Par-b; Pru-sp.

SENSATION, Without : Alu; Arg-n; *Caus*; Kali-br; *Mag-m.*

SLOW : See Feeble.

SPURTS, In: Bur-p; Clem; Con; Tub.

STOOLS, With, only : Alo; Ap; Mur-ac.

STOPS and Starts : See Interrupted.

STREAM, Forcible : Cic; Nux-v.

Forked : Arg-n; Merc-c; Pru-sp.

Slender : *Clem; Cop;* Eup-pur; Grap; Nit-ac; Ol-an; Stap.

thread, like : Pru-sp.

Spray, like : Kre.

Twisted : Sul-io.

UNEASY Feeling : Ced; Ver-v.

UNSATISFACTORY, Incomplete : Ars; Caus; Clem; *Hep*; Lach; Mag-m; Sele.

URGING To, stool, with : *Nux-v.*

WEAKNESS, After : See Under Weakness.

WHITE AT CLOSE : Pho-ac; Sars.

URINE ALTERED IN GENERAL :
Pul; Sep; Sul.

ACRID :Arn; Benz-ac; *Hep*;
Laur; Lyc; Med; *Merc*;
Merc-c; *Pul*; Sul; Urt.

ALBUMINOUS :See Albuminuria.

ALKALINE : Bap; Carb-ac.

AMMONIACAL, Strong odour :
Asaf; Benz-ac; *Iod*; Med;
Mos; Nit-ac; Pho; Pic-ac;
Stro.

Menses, during : Nit-ac.

AROMATIC : Eup-pur; Fer-io;
Onos; Terb.

BILE, Containing : Cean; *Chio*.

BITING : Sele.

BLACK : Ap; Ars; Carb-ac;
Colch; Kali-c; *Lach*;
Merc-c; *Terb*.

+ Dung mixed, as if : Ars.
Inky : *Colch*.

BLOODY (See Haematuria and
Haemorrhage) : *Arn*; Ars;
Ip; Merc-c; *Pho*; Sec; Scil;
Senec; *Terb*.

Backache with : Kali-bi.

'Clots : Chim.

Constipation, with : Lyc.

Cramps in bladder, after :
Mez.

Cutting, abdomen in, and
urethra in, with : Ip.

+ First part : Con.

Last part : Ant-t; *Hep*; Mez;

Pul; Sars; *Zin*.

Menses suppressed, with :
Nux-v.

Paraplegia, with : Lyc.

Pathological cause, without
: Bell.

Piles, suppressed, from :
Nux-v.

Sexual excess, after : Pho.

Spine, shivering along
with : Nit-ac.

Urination, after : *Hep*; Thu.

frequent with : Ham.

urging, with : Sabi.

BLUISH : Nit-ac.

BRINY Odour : See Fishy.

BROWN : Arn; Ars; Benz-ac;
Bry; Canth; Chel; Merc-c;
Sep.

BURNING : See Hot.

CAT'S Like, Smell : Vio-t.

CLOUDY : Ap; Berb; Bry; Canth;
Carb-v; Chel; Chin; CINA;
Con; Grap; MERC; Myr;
Pho; Pho-ac; *Saba*; Sep; Sul.

Fever, during : Pho.

Sweat, with : Ip; Merc; Pho.

Turning : Bell; Berb; BRY;
Cham; Chel; Chin;Grap;
Lyc; *Pho-ac*; Terb.

COLD : Agar; *Nit-ac*.

DARK : Aco; Ant-t; Ap; Bell;
Benz-ac; *Bry*; Calc; Chel;
Colch; Lach; *Merc*; Sele;
Sep; Solid; Terb; Ver-a.

Flecks, in : Hell.

DROP, Remains, urination
after : Kali-bi; Mag-m.

FISHY Odour : Ol-an; Sanic;
Uran-n.

FLOCCULENT : Berb; CANTH;

Mez; Sars.

FLOWS, Drops in, then spurts in : Caps.

FROTHY : Aur; Cean; Cep; *Chel; Kali-c; Lach;* Lyc; Scop; Sele; Seneg; *Spo;* Syph; Thu.

FOUL, Offensive: Ap; Arn; Bap; *Benz-ac;* Calc; Carb-v; DUL; Kre; Nit-ac; *Pul;* SEP; Solid; Sul; Tarn; Thu.

Dark red, at night, normal during day : Mos.

Profuse : Rhod.

Putrid : Hyds.

GARLICKY : Cup-ar; Pho.

GASSY : Sars.

GREENISH : Cam; Carb-ac; Cean; Merc-c; Ol-an;Ver-a.

Red sediment, with : Mag-s.

HEAVY : Bur-p; Coc-c.

HORSE'S Like: Benz-ac; Nat-c; Nit-ac.

HOT, Burning : Alo; Ap; *Ars;* BELL; *Benz-ac;* Bor; Cam; *Cann; Canth;* Cub; *Hep;* Lil-t; Med; *Merc; Merc-c;* Nat-c; Nat-s; Nit-ac; Nux-v; Senec; Sep; Sul; Thu; Uva.

Constipation, with : Fer.

Coryza, fluent, with : Ran-sc.

Menorrhagia, with : Fer.

Urination before and after : Seneg.

INDICAN Containing : Nit-ac; Nux-m; Pic-ac.

ITCHING, Causing : Merc; Urt.

LESS, Than, drinks : Kre; Lith; Raph.

MILKY : Ap; Aur; CINA; Hep; Kali-bi; Kali-p; Lapp; Lil-t; Lyc; *Pho-ac;* Vio-o; Visc.

Blood, with : Kali-bi.

Frequent, and : Iod.

Hydrocephalus, in : *Ap.*

Menses, before : Pho-ac.

Stools, after : Iod.

Turns : Cina.

Urination, at close of : Carb-v; Pho-ac; Sars; Sep.

MORE, Than drinks : *Ap;* Bell; Colo; Lac-ac; *Merc;* Nux-v; *Pho-ac.*

MUDDY : Aesc; Kali-c; Nat-m; Rhus-t.

MUSK Like : Oci-c.

ODOURLESS : Ced; Spo.

OILY : Chin-s; Merc-c.

ONIONS, Smell, like : Gamb.

ORANGE Coloured : Lept.

OXALIC Acid Containing (Oxaluria) : Berb; Caus; Kali-s; Nat-p; Nat-s; Nit-ac; *Nit-m-ac;* Ox-ac; Terb.

PALE, Colourless : Cann; *Con;* Gel; Kali-c; Nat-m; PHO-AC; Sep; Stro.

PELLICLE, Cuticle, on : Colo; *Par;* Pho; Psor; Pul; Sep.

Iridescent : Cep; Par; Pho.

Oily : Adon; Crot-t; Iod; Pho;Sumb.

Red : Mez.

PHOSPHATES, Containing : Alfa; Benz-ac; Calc-p;

Lapp; Nit-ac; Pho; *Pho-ac*; Pic-ac; Solid; Stan.

PROFUSE, Copious, Increased (Polyuria) : Acet-ac; Alo; *Arg-m;* Arg-n; Cann; Cep; Cimi; Gel; Kre; Lac-c; Led; *Lyc*; Lycps; Merc; Mos; *Mur-ac;* Nat-c; Nat-s; Ol-an; *Pho; Pho-ac;* Plant; Pul; *Rhus-t; Scil;* Scop; *Spig;* Sul; Thu; Uran-n;Val; *Verb;* Vib.

+ Burning and backache : Ant-c.

Concomitant, as a : Vib.

Coryza, with : Sep.

Dropsy, in : Scil.

+ Frequent, and : Iod.

Haemorrhage, with: Calc; Gel; Ign; Lach; Mos; Sars; Stram; Sul; Vib.

Headache, with : Iris; Lac-d; Mos; Ol-an; Vib.

Heat of body, with : Samb.

Hysterical : Ol-an.

Menses, with : Cham; Hyo; med; *Pho-ac;* Phyt; Vib.

+ Nervousness, with: Fer.

Pain, during : Arg-m; Lac-d.

Scanty and alternately : Bell; *Berb;* Dig; Eup-p; Gel; Nit-ac; Senec.

PURULENT : Arn; Bap; Canth; Clem; Polyg; Sul-io; Uva.

Urination after : Hep.

RASPBERRY, Smell like : Sul-io.

RECEDES : Pru-sp.

RED : Arn; Ars; Benz-ac; Berb; Bry; Canth; Chel;

Lept; Lob; Merc-c; Sep; Stram.

Dark : Phyt.

RESIDUAL : Dig.

RETAINED (In Bladder) : ACO; Am-c; *Ap; Arn; Ars;* Bell; *Cam;* CANTH; Caus; Con; Erig; Gel; Hell; *Hep; Hyo;* LYC; Nux-v; *Op;* Par-b; Pul; Tarn; *Terb.*

As if, urination after : Berb; Hep.

Birth, at : *Aco;* Ap.

Cholera in: Cam; Canth; Carb-v; *Ver-a.*

Cold and wet exposure, from : *Aco; Dul;* Gel; Rhus-t.

Confinement, after : Ars; Bell; *Caus;* Equi; Hyo; Op.

during : Plb.

Dribbling, with : Alu; *Caus;* Gel; *Nux-v.*

Dysentery, in : Arn.

Exertion, after : *Arn; Caps; Rhus-t.*

Fever, during : Fer-p; Op.

Fright, from : Aco; Op.

Hysteria, in : Ign; *Zin.*

Illness Acute, in,(Fever etc.) : Fer-p; Lyc; Op.

Infants : Benz-ac.

nursing angry, nurse, on : Op.

+ Labour, after : Caus.

Locomotor Ataxia, in : Arg-n.

Menses, during : Kali-bi.

Music Amel : Tarn.

441

New born : *Aco;* Ap.

Old men : Solid.

Operations, after : Càus.

Overdistension, with : Hell.

Painful: Canth; Caus; Nux-v.

Painless: Nit-ac.

Paraplegia, with: Apoc.

Pavement, Cold, standing on : Carb-v.

Pregnancy during : Equi.

Presence of others, in: NAT-M.

Prostate enlargement, with : Chin; Dig; Stap.

Sleepiness, with : Terb.

+ Spasm, neck of bladder : Op.

+ Urging, unsuccessful : Sec.

Urging, without : *Ars; Caus;* Pho; Plb.

Water, noise from Amel : Hyo; Lyss; Tarn; Zin.

Whistling Amel: Cyc; Tarn.

SACCHARINE : See Diabetes Mellitus.

SAFFRON, Like : Form; Oci-c.

SALTS, Deficient, in : Led.

SANDY: Am-c; Benz-ac;Coc-c; *Led;* LYC; Pho; *Sars; Sele; Sep;* Sil; Sul-io; Tarn; Zin.

Brown : Sul-io.

Sticky : Pyro; Tub.

Turbid : Chim.

White : Berb; Calc; Grap; Kre; *Pho;* RHUS-T; Sars; Sep.

Yellow : Cimi; Pho; Sep; Zin.

SCANTY : AP; *Ars;* Aru-t; Bry;

CANTH; *Colch;* Con; *Dig;* Dul; *Grap;* HELL; Hyo; Hypr; Kali-n; Led; Lil-t; Lyc; Merc; Merc-c; Nat-s; Nit-ac; *Op;* Pho; Plb; Polyg; Pul; Rhus-t; *Rut;* Sars; Sele; *Sep;* Solid; *Stap;* Sul; Sul-io; Terb; Til; Ver-a.

Agg : Benz-ac; Oci-c; Solid.

Fever, during : Ap; Pul.

Frequent and : Meny; Merc; Ol-an.

Headache, then : Iod; Ol-an.

Menses, before : *Ap;* Sil.

during : Nat-m.

Nervous women : Agar.

Thirst, with : Lith.

SEDIMENT : Amb; Canth; Colo; *Lyc;* Merc; Pho-ac; Pul; Sars; *Sep;* Val; Zin.

Adherent : Ap; Colo; Fer; Pho; Polyg; *Pul;* Pyro; SEP; Tub.

Black : Colch; Lach; Terb.

Bloody : Canth; Chim; Pho-ac; *Pul;* Sep.

Branny : Ant-t; Merc; Pho; Val.

Brick dust : See Red.

Brown: *Amb;* Ap; Arn; Lach.

Cheesy : *Pho;* Pho-ac; Sars; Sec.

Clayey, Earthy : Berb; Zin.

Cloudy : Berb; Pho-ac.

Coffee ground : Ap; Hell; Terb.

Flaky, Flocculent : Berb; Canth; *Mez*; Sars; Zin.

Gelatinous : Berb; Colo.

Gravel : Lyc; Polyg; Sars; Sep.

Limy : Sabal.

Mealy : Ant-t; Ap; Berb; Calc; Chin; Grap; Merc; Nat-m; Pho; Pho-ac; Sul.

Mucous : Benz-ac; *Berb*; Chim; Equi; Merc-c; Nat-m; Par-b; *Pul*; Sars; Sep; Terb.

uterine displacement, with : Senec.

Muddy : Terb.

Red, Brick dust : Arn; Ars; Bry; *Canth*; Chin; Dig; Kali-c; Lob; LYC; Merc-c; *Nat-m*; Par-b; Pho; PUL; Sele; Senec; SEP; Tarn; *Val.*

peppery : Iod.

rosy : Am-ph.

thick : Kali-c.

Shreddy : Seneg.

Sour : Coc-c; Grap; Petr; *Sep*; Solid.

Whooping cough, during : Amb.

Specific Gravity Decreased : Merc-c; Pho; *Plb*.

Increased (See Diabetes Mellitus) : Arn; Chio; Colch.

Stains Diaper, brown : Benz-ac.

Red : Sanic.

Yellow : Phyt.

dark : Chel.

Suppressed : ACO; *Ap*; Arn; *Ars*; Cam; CANTH; Carb-v; Lach; Laur; Lob; LYC; Pul; Sec; Solid; STRAM; Urt; Ver-a.

Cholera, in : *Ars*; Carb-v; Cup.

Concussion of spine, from : Arn; Tarn.

Convulsions, with : *Cup*; Stram.

Dentition, during : Terb.

Fever, during : Arn; Ars; Bell; Cact; Hyo; Op; Stram.

typhoid, after : Zing.

Infants, in : Chim.

Menses, during : Kali-bi.

Spine, Concussion, from : Arn; Tarn.

Unconsciousness, during : Dig; Plb.

Sweetish Odour : Arg-m; Eup-pur; Nux-m; Terb.

Thick : Berb; Coc-c; Merc-c; Nux-v; Raph; Sep; Ver-a.

Valerian Like : Murx.

Violet, Odour like : Cam; Cop; Eucal; Lact-v; Nux-m; Osm; Terb; Thyr.

Viscid : *Colo*; Nat-s; Sep.

Watery : Gel; Ign; Mur-ac; Sep; Scil.

dung mixed, with : Ars.

White : See Milky.

Yellow : Aur; Berb; Card-m; Lach; Sep.

+ Beer like : Chel.

Dark : Sang.

URINOUS ODOUR (of Breath, Secretions etc.) : Benz-ac; Canth; *Colo;* Nat-m; Nit-ac; Ol-an; Sec; Urt.

URTICARIA, HIVES, Wheals : Ant-c; *Ap*; Ars; CALC; Calc-s; *Caus*; Chlo-hyd; Cop; *Dul;* Grap; *Hep*; Lach; Led; Mez; Nat-m; Pho; Polyg; RHUS-T; Sep; Sil; Sul; *Urt.*

ASTHMA, Alternating, with : Calad.

ASCARIDES, With : Urt.

BATHING Agg : Bov.

CHANGE Of Weather Agg : Ap.

CHILL, During : Ap; Ars; *Nat-m; Rhus-t.*

CHRONIC *: Lyc*; Strop.

Children, in : Cop.

Recurring : Hep.

COLD AIR Agg : Nit-ac; *Rhus-t;* Sep.

Amel : Calc; Dul.

Bath Agg : Calc-p.

Drinks Agg : Bell.

COLDS Agg *: Dul.*

DIARRHOEA, With : Bov; Pul.

EVENING Agg : Kre; Nux-v.

EXERCISE, Warmth of, Agg : Con; *Nat-m;* Psor; *Urt.*

Amel : Hep; Sep.

FEVER, During: Ap; Cop; Ign; Rhus-t.

FISH Agg : Ars.

Shell : Terb; Urt.

FLAT, Plaques, in : Form; Lob.

GIANT : Ap; Kali-io.

ITCHING Without : Uva.

LIVER Symptoms, with : Canc-fl; Myr; Ptel.

MEAT Agg : *Ant-c.*

MENSES Agg : Dul; Kali-c.

After Agg : Kre.

Delayed Agg : Pul.

Profuse, with : Bov.

MORNING, Awakening, on : Bov.

NAUSEA, After : Sang.

NIGHT Agg : Chlo-hyd.

NODULAR : Sul-ac.

PALPITATION, With : Bov.

PINWORM, With : Urt.

PURPLE : Chin-s.

RECEDING : Strop.

RESPIRATION, Difficult with : Ap.

RHEUMATISM, Alternating with : Urt.

With : Rhus-t; Urt.

RUBBING Amel : Elat.

SCRATCHING Agg : Dul; Lach; Mez; Rhus-t.

SHUDDERING, With: Ap-g.

SUPPRESSED Agg : Urt.

UNDRESSING Agg : Pul.

WARMTH Amel : Lyc.

WHITE : Nat-m.

Apex *: Ant-c;* Pul.

YEARLY, Same Season : Urt.

UTERUS : Arn; *Bell;* Castr; Caul; Cham; Cimi; Kali-c; Mag-m; Pall; Plat; *Pul;* Sabi; Sec; Sep; Ust; Vib.

ANTEVERSION : See Displacement.

ASCENDING Agg : Plat.

ATONY : Cimi.

BALL : Ust.

Hot, ascends throat, to : Raph.

BEARING Down Pains (See Female Organs): Frax; Pall.

Child nurses, when:Ust.

Colds Agg : Hyo.

Sweat, hot with : Til.

BENDING Double Amel : Cact; Cimi; *Nux-v.*

+ BLOATED, Wind in, as if : Pho-ac.

BURNING : Calc-ar; Lach; Nux-v; Sep; Tarn; Terb.

Limbs. pain alternating with : Rhod.

Parturition, after : Rhod.

BURSTING, Something, in : Elap.

CANCER : Alum; ARS; Ars-io; Aur; Bell; Calc-ar; Carb-an; Chin; Clem; *Con;* Grap; Hyds; Iod; *Kre; Lach;* Lyc; Mag-m; Merc; Murx; Pho; Plat; Sabi; Sars; Sec; *Sep;* Sil; Tarn; *Thu.*

+ CAUSE Of many symptoms : Caul.

CLUTCHED AND RELEASED As if : Sep.

COLD : Petr.

COLDS Agg : Hyo.

CONSCIOUSNESS, Of: Helo; Lyss; Murx.

CRAMP : Cocl; Pul.

CURETTING, After : Bur-p;

Kali-c; Nit-ac.

CUTTING : *Bell;* Cocl; Con; Ip; Pall; *Pul;* Sul.

Stools Amel : Pall.

DISPLACEMENT Of(Anteversion Retroversion) : Ab-c; Bell; Calc; Caul; Eupi; Fer-io; Frax; Grap; Helo; Lach; Lapp; Lil-t; Lyss; Nat-m; Sep.

DISTENDED, As if, filled with wind : Pho-ac.

DROPSY (Hydrometra) : Hell; Lyc.

Limbs in, piercing pain : Hell.

ENLARGED : Aur; Calc-io; *Con;* Helo; Lyc; Mag-m; Plat; Plb; *Sep;* Ust.

FULL, As if : Alo; Bell; Helo.

GNAWING : Thyr.

HEART, Alternating with : Lil-t.

HEAVY : Calc-p; *Chin; Gel;* Helo; Pall; Pul; *Sep.*

Hysteria, after : Elap.

Leucorrhoea, with: Cimi.

HOUR-GLASS Contraction : Bell; Sec.

HYDROMETRA : See Dropsy.

HYPERTROPHY : Cale; Ust.

INDURATION : Aur.

Abortions, repeated after : Aur.

INERT: Alet; Caul; Caus; Cimi; Goss; Helo; Kali-c; Plb; Sabi; Sec; Sep.

INFANTILE : Bar-c; Calc-p; Fer; Helo; Iod; Pho; Senec; Thyr.

INFLAMMED : Ap; Ars; *Bell;*
Canth; Lac-c; Lach; Lyc; Pul;
Rhus-t; Sabi; *Sec; Sep;*
Terb; Vib.

Puerperal : Til.

JERKING : Ast-r.

KNOTTED, As if : Ust.

LYING Agg : Amb.

Back on Amel : Onos.

MOTIONS, In : Tarn.

Foetus, as of a : Nat-c; Tarn.

NUMB : Phys.

NURSING Agg : Arn; *Cham;* Sil.

OPEN, As if : Lach.

OS Rigid : See under Cervix.

PAINFUL : Bell; Colo; Helo; Ign;
Lach; Murx; Nux-v; Pod;
Pul.

PESSARIES, After Agg : Terb.

PROLAPSE (See Prolapse) :
Am-m; Arg-m; Arg-n; Aur;
Cimi; Coll; Fer-io; Frax;
Helo; Lapp; Lil-t; *Pall;*
Plat; Psor; Pul; Rhus-t;
Senec; Sep.

Coition Agg : Nat-c.
Amel : Merc.

Confinement, after : Helo;
Pod; Rhus-t.

Diarrhoea, from : Petr.

Electric shock, down the
thigh : Grap.

Forceps delivery, after : Sec.

Fright, from : Gel; *Op.*

Head holding, and straining
Amel : Pyro.

Hot weather in: Kali-bi.

Lifting Agg : Aur; *Calc;*

Nux-v; Pod; Rhus-t.

Lumbar backache, with :
Nat-m.

Lying Amel : Nat-m; Sep.

back on, Amel: Nat-m;
Onos.

Menses, after : Ip.

during : *Pul; Sep.*

Morning, in : Bell; NAT-M;
Sep.

Standing Agg : Lapp.

Stools Agg : Calc-p; Con;
Pod; Psor; Stan.

straining at Agg : Nux-v;
Pod.

Urination, dribbling with
: Fer-io.

during : Calc-p.

foul, with : Benz-ac.

Walking Agg : Lapp.

Weakness from : Sul-ac.

PULSATION, In : Bell; Cact.

PYOMETRA : Lach; Merc; *Pul;*
Sep.

REACHING High, arms with
Agg : Aur; Grap; Sul.

REFLEX Symptoms, from :
Bell; Cimi; Goss; Helo;
Kali-c; Lil-t; Plat.

SEPTIC : See Puerperal
Sepsis.

SHARP Pain : *Aco;* Con.

SOFT, Softening of : Op.
As if : Ab-c.

SORE : Arn; Aur; Bell; Bry;
Gel; Lach; Lapp; *Murx;*
Til; Ust; Ver-v.

Coition, during : *Pul.*

Riding in carriage Agg : Arg-m.

Squeezed, as if: Bels; Gel; Kali-io.

menses, during : Kali-io.

SPASMS, Menses without : Kali-c.

STITCHING : Aco; Bell; Con; Sep.

SUBINVOLUTION : *Arn;* Cimi; *Frax; Helo;* Kali-br; Pul; SEP; Sul.

Abortion, after : Psor.

SWELLED : Aur; Calc-io; Con; Lap-alb; Lyc; Plat; Sec; Sep.

THIGHS, Anterior, to : Vib.

+ Down : Ust.

THROAT, To : Gel.

TILTED, Left, to : Sep.

Right, to : Murx; Pul.

TUMOURS : See Fibroids.

ULCER : Carb-an; Hyds; Kre; Ust.

Abortions, from : Aur.

UNDEVELOPED: Plb.

UNDRESSING Amel : Onos.

WEAK, As if during Stool and Urination : Calc-p.

UVULA : *Ap;* Kali-bi; Merc; *Merc-c;* Phyt.

BLEEDING : Lac-c.

COUGHING Agg : Ham.

DRIPPING: Aral; Cep; Hyds; Kali-bi; Merc-c; Spig.

ELONGATED, Flaccid : Alu; Bar-m; Caps; Cof; Crot-t; *Hyo;* Kali-io; Lach; Pho; *Sul.*

As if : Coc-c; Croc; Dul.

Hawking constant, from : Coc-c.

Pressing on something hard : Caps.

HANGING To one side : Lach.

Right : Ap; Nat-m.

ITCHING : Saba.

OEDEMA : *Ap;* Kali-bi; Merc-c; Phyt; Rhus-t.

PAINFUL : Ap; Sang.

RELAXED As if : Kali-bi.

Bladder like : Kali-bi.

SENSITIVE : Clem; Sul.

STIFF : Crot-h.

SWELLED : Ap; Caps; Iod; Kali-io; Merc-c; Pho;Sil.

ULCERS : Kali-bi; *Merc-c.*

Eating : Hep.

WHITE, Shrivelled, and : Carb-ac.

VACCINATION, ILL EFFECTS Of

AGG : Ant-t; *Ars;* Hep; Kali-m; MALAND; Mez; Sars; SIL; SUL; THU; Vacci; Vario.

VACILLATING : See Irresolute.

VAGINA : Berb; Calc; Fer; Kali-c; Lyc; Merc; Pul; *Sep;* Sul.

APHTHAE : Caul.

BLOODY Water, from : Nit-ac.

BURNING : Berb; Nit-ac; Pulex; Sul; Tarn.

Coition, after : Lyc; Lyss.

hour, fixed, at : Chel.

CANCER : KRE.

COLD : Grap; Nat-m; Sec.

Icy : Bor-ac.

CONSTRICTION : See Spasms.

CONTRACTION : Kre; Sep.

COTTON *BALL*, as if in : Pulex.

CUTTING : Sil.

Coition, during : Berb.

Urination Agg : Sil.

CYSTS : Lyc; Pul; *Sil.*

Serous : Rhod.

DAMP : See Moist.

DISCHARGE Suppressed Agg : Bur-p.

DRY : Fer-p; Grap; Lyc; Nat-m; Tarn; Zin-chr.

Menses, after : Sep.

Uneasy sensation, with : Zin-chr.

ENLARGED, As if : Sanic.

EXCORIATED : Kali-bi.

FISTULA : Carb-v.

FLATUS, From (Physometra): *Bro*; Lac-c; *Lyc*; Nux-m; Nux-v; Pho-ac; Sang; Tarn.

Abdomen, distended with : Sang.

GANGRENE, Prolapse, after : Sul-ac.

HEAVY, Hysteria, after : Elap.

HOT : Fer-p; Grap; Sec; Tarn.

INDURATION, Painful : Chin.

+ INSENSITIVE, During coition : See Numb.

ITCHING : Calad; Carb-ac; Cof; Hydroc; *Kre*; Med; Nit-ac; Plat; *Sep*; Stap; Sul; Tarn; Thu.

Coition, after : Nit-ac.

Deep in : Con.

Pregnancy, during : Sabi.

Rubbing Agg : Med.

Sexual excitement, with : Canth.

Urinating, when : Kre.

Warm bathing Amel : Med.

JERKING In, upwards, Morning : Sep.

LARGE, As if : Sanic.

MOIST, As if : Ast-r; Eup-pur; Petr.

Ease, feeling of, with : Ast-r.

MUCOUS FLOW, Sexual excitement, from : Senec.

NODULES, In : Agar.

NUMB : Berb; Bro; Pho; Sep.

Coition, during : Fer; Kali-br; Pho.

ORANGE Coloured fluid from : Kali-p.

PAINFUL : See Sensitive.

PRESSING, Upward, sitting on : Fer-io.

PROLAPSE : Bur-p; Fer; Plat; Pod; Psor; *Sep.*

Weakness, from : Sul-ac.

PULSATION : Alu; Merc.

RAW, Sore : Berb; Fer; Kre; Lyss; Sul; Tarn.

Menses, during : Kali-c.

SCRATCHING Agg : Tarn.

Until it bleeds : Sec.

SENSITIVE : Calc; Kre; Lyss; Plat; Stap; Thu.

Coition Agg : Hyds; Sul; Thu.

Urinating Agg   : Coc-c.

SHOOTING Up : Rhus-t; Sabi; Sep.

SITTING Agg : Stap.

SPASMS (Vaginismus) : Bell; *Cact*; Caul; Mag-p; Plat; *Plb;* Sep.

Coition Agg : *Cact*; Gel; Plat.

STITCHES : Kre.

SWOLLEN : Nit-ac.

TEARS : Sec.

ULCERATION : Mez.

URINATING Agg   : Sil.

VEGETATION, Granular : Stap.

VAGINISMUS : See Vagina, Spasms.

VALVE, LEAF, Skin as of a : Alu; Ant-t; *Bar-c*; Fer; Iod; Kali-c; Kali-io; Lach; Mang; *Pho*; Saba; *Spo;* Thu.

VALVULAR DISEASE : See Valves, under Heart.

VANITY : See Pride.

VAPOUR, SMOKE, Fumes as of : Ap; ARS; Bar-c; Bro; *Chin;* Ign; Lyc; *Pul; Ver-a.*

HOT, Through all orifices : Flu-ac.

head, rising to : Buf.

VARICELLA : See Chicken-pox.

VARICOCELE (See Blood vessels Distended) : Coll; Fer-p; Flu-ac; Ham; Pul.

STRAIN, After   : Rut.

VARICOSES : See Blood Vessels distended.

VARIOLA : See Small-pox.

VARNISH, LIKE : Euphr; Grap; Nat-m; Petr; *Rhus-t;* Thu.

VAULTS AGG : See Dampness and Cellars AGG.

VEINS BROKEN : Card-m.

HARD, Knotty : Ham; Nux-v.

HOT Water, as if, in : Syph.

SORE *: Ham;* Pul.

THROMBOSED, Hard : Card-m; Flu-ac.

VARICOSE : Bels.

WHIPCORD, Like : Calc-hyp.

VENOSITY : Carb-v; Pul; Sul.

VERMIN   : Stap.

+ **VERSES** MAKES : Agar.

VERTEBRA ABSENT, As if : Mag-p; Psor.

CRACKING, In : Nat-c; Ol-an; Sul. Cervical : Cocl.

DORSAL, Upper : Kalm. Last : Zin.

GLIDING, Over each other, as if : Ant-t; Sul.

HEAT Agg : Agar.

LOOSE, As if : Calc.

SLIPPING (See Dislocation easy) : Sanic; Sul.

TUMOUR   : Lach; Tarn.

VERTEX : *Cact*; Calc; *Calc-p;* Carb-an; Caus; Cimi; Cup; Glo; Hypr; *Lach;* Lyc; Meny; *Nit-ac;* Pho; Pho-ac; RAN-SC; *Sil;* SUL; VER-A; Ver-v.

ACHING : Ign.

Eyes, between and : Ver-v.

ACROSS (Ear to Ear) : Chel;

449

Kali-m; Naj; Nit-ac; Pall; Phys; Sabal; Sil.

BREATHING Deep Agg : Anac.

BURNING, Heat :Calc; Frax; Glo; *Grap*; Lach; SUL.

Grief, after : Calc; Pho.

Spot : Arn.

BURSTING : Carb-an; Cimi; Sanic; *Sil;* Syph.

Eating Amel : Carb-an.

COLD *: Calc; Calc-p;* Naj; *Sep;* VER-A.

Agg : Naj.

+ Icy : *Calc.*

+ Lump, as if *: Ver-a.*

CONGESTION : Cinb.

COUGHING Agg : Anac.

CRACKING, In : Cof.

CRAWLING *:* Cup.

DRY : Ars; Frax.

FLY OFF, As if : *Bap;* Bur-p; Cann; *Cimi;* Iris *Syph;* Xanth.

Air, cold, letting in : Cimi.

HEAVY : See Pressure.

HOT, As if : Tarx.

ITCHES, Headache during : Ver-a.

JAWS, To : Lach.

LYING Agg: Manc.

MENSES Agg : Fer-p.

NIGHT Agg : Laur.

Amel : Mag-c.

NUMB : Glo; Mez; Plat.

+ **O**PEN And **S**HUT : *Cann.*

PRESSURE, Heavy, Crushing : Alo; Ap; Bell; CACT; Cimi;

Fer-p; Glo; Hypr; *Lach;* Lapp; *Lyc;* MENY; NAT-M; PALL; *Pho-ac;* Plb; Sil; Stan; Sul; Zin; Zin-chr.

Agg : *Chin;* Lach; Phys; Ther.

Amel : Mag-c.

SIDES Down : Fer-p; Hypr.

SLEEP Amel : Calc.

SORE, Painful : Chin; Nit-ac; Sul.

STOOPING Agg : Meny.

SWEAT, Pricking, during each meal : Cep.

TENSION : Lob.

THROBBING :Bry; Caus; Cocl; Lach; Pho; *Sil;* Sul; Syph; Visc.

Sudden : Visc.

VERTIGO :Aco; Agar; Ail; Ap; Arg-m; BELL; BRY; *Calc; Chel;* Chin-s; *Cocl; Con;* Cup; *Cyc;* Dig; Dul; Fer; Gel; Lyc; *Nat-m; Nux-m;* NUX-V; Onos; Op; *Petr;* PHO; PUL; *Rhus-t;* Sang; Sec; Sep; *Sil; Sul;* Tab; Zin-io.

AGG, During : *Aco; Calc;* Cyc; Fer; GEL; NUX-V; *Pho;* Pul; *Stram.*

AIR, Open Agg : Cyc.

ASCENDING An Eminence Agg : Bor; CALC; Sul.

Stairs Agg : *Calc;* Sul.

descending, and : Phys.

AURAL : Aur; Bry; Chin; Nat-sal; Sil.

Noises in ear, with : Iris.

BENDING, Backward Amel :

Ol-an.

BLOOD, Rushing to the head with : Bell; Dig; Glo; Hell; Merc; Ver-v.

BLOWING Nose Agg : Codei; Culex; *Sep.*

BREATHING, Deep Agg : Anac; Cact.

BURDENS Carrying in head Agg : Tarn.

CHILL, with : Cocl.

COITION, After: Bov; Pho-ac; Sep.

COLD Application Amel : Nat-m.
Drinks, from : Colch.

CONSTIPATION Agg : Calc-p.

COLOURED Light Agg : Art-v.

COUGHING Agg : Anac; Ant-t; Cof; Kali-bi; Mos.

CROSSING Bridge Agg : Bar-c; Bro; Lyss.
Running water Agg : Arg-m; Bell; Bro; Fer; Hyo; Lyss; Sul.

DARK, In : Alu; Arg-n; Kali-io; Pic-ac; Stram.

DEAFNESS, With : Merc-c.

DESCENDING Agg : Bor; Con; Fer; Gel; Plat; Sanic; Tarn; Vib.
Spire : Sil.

DRAWN Up and Pitched forward as if : Calc; Euon.

DRINKING Agg : Crot-t.

DRUNK, As if : See Intoxicated.

EATING Amel : Alu; Cocl; Dul; Nux-v; Saba.

EMISSIONS, After : Bov; Caus;

Nat-s; Sars.

EPILEPTIC : Arg-n; Ars; *Hyo;* Sil; Tarn; Visc.
After : Calc.

ERECTION Agg : Tarn.

EXERTION Agg : Cact.
Amel : Pho.
Violent Agg : Mill.

EYELIDS, Twitching with : Chin-s.

EYES, Closing Agg : Ap; Arg-n; Arn; Calad; Chel; Lach; Nat-m; Sil; Stram; *Ther;* Thu.
Amel : Lol-t; Tab; Ver-v.
Focus, out of, when : Alu.
+ Glassy : Pho-ac.
Opening, or : Alu.
+ Opening Amel : Alum.
Wiping Amel : Alu.

FAINT Like : Bry; Cocl; Nux-v; Ther.

FALLS, Backward : Chin; Spig; *Rhus-t.*
Forward : Nat-m; Rhus-t.
Left, to : *Nat-m;* Sil.
Right, to : Calc; Caus; Sil; Zin.
Sideways : Benz-ac; Calc; Cocl; Nux-v.

FASTING Agg : Sul-io.

FEMALE Symptoms, with : Cyc.

FEVERS, With : Carb-v; Cocl; Kali-c; Pul.
+ All stages : Eucal.

FLICKERS, Eyes, before with : Aran.

FLOWERS, Smell, from : Hyo.

FORHEAD, Felt, in : Arn; Croc; Euon; Gel; Pho; Sul.

FRIGHT, After : Op.

FULNESS and Aching in vertex with : *Cimi.*

GAS LIGHT Agg : Caus.

HAIR Binding Agg : Sul-io.

HANDS Raising, head above : Onos.

HEADACHE, With : Ap; Bell; Calc; Con; Croc; Fer; Iod; Lac-c; Lil-t; Nux-v; Onos; Sil; Stro; Sul.

Before : Calc; Plat; Plb; Til.

HEAD, Bent, backwards :Stram.

Big, feels during : Kob.

Holding, still Amel : Con.

Injury, from : Op.

+ Lightness, of : Op.

Pushed, forward, as if : Fer-p.

Resting Amel : Ver-v.

Scratching Agg : Calc.

Sinks, forward : Cup.

Sweat Amel : Nat-s.

Turning, quickly Agg : Adon; Colo.

HEART Symptoms, with : Kali-c; Lach; Pho; Ver-a.

HEELS, Turning on, quickly Amel : Stap.

HEIGHT, Falling from as if : Caus; Gel; Mos.

HIGH Celled room, in : Cup-ar.

INTOXICATED, As if : Gel; NUX-V; Pul.

KNEADING, Motion on Agg : Sanic.

KNEELING Agg : Mag-c; Ther.

LIE DOWN, Must : *Cocl;* Nat-s; *Pho; Pul;* Spig.

LIFTING, Head from pillow : Ant-t.

Weight, on : Pul.

LIGHTNING, From : Crot-h.

LOOKING, + Anything turning : Lyc.

+ Fixedly, at an object : Old.

One object at Agg : Lach.

Running water at Agg : Arg-m; Bro; *Fer;* Ver-*a.*

Sideways Agg : Thu.

Up Agg : Caus; Chin-ar; Grap; Kali-p; Sang; Sil; Thu.

LYING Agg : Ap; Calad; *Con;* Kali-m; Pul; Rhod.

Back, on Agg : Merc.

Left side on Agg : Iod; Lac-d; Onos; Pho; Sil; Zin-io.

Right Side, on Agg : Eup-p; Gel; Mur-ac; Rhus-t.

MENSES, Affections, with : Caus; Cyc.

+ Before and during : Sul-io.

Profuse, with : *Calc;* Ust.

Suppressed, from : Sabi.

MENTAL Exertion Agg : Nat-c.

Amel : Pho.

MOTION (Of Head etc.) Agg : *Bry;* CON; Dig; Kali-br; Lil-t.

+ Least Agg : Thu.

Rapid Agg : Sang.

Shaking Agg : Hep.

NAUSEA AND VOMITING, With : *Chin-s;* Cocl; Fer; Lapp; Lob; Petr; Sele; *Ther.*

NIGHT, At : Tarn.

NOISE Agg : Ther.

+ NOSE Bleed, follows : Carb-an.

OBJECTS, + Far off, seem : Stan.

Whirl around each other, as if : Saba.

OCCIPUT, Felt in : Bry; Carb-v; Con; *Gel;* PETR; *Sil;* Ver-a; Zin.

PAIN Agg : Cimi.

Before : Ran-b.

PALPITATION, With : See Heart, Palpitation.

PARALYSIS, Before : Old.

PERIODICAL: Cocl; *Nat-m; Pho.*

PITCHED, Forward, as if : Euon.

PREGNANCY, During : Alet; Gel; *Nat-m.*

PULSE, Slow, with : Ther.

RAILWAY Travelling Agg : Kali-io.

READING Agg: All-s; Grap; Merc-i-f.

Aloud Agg : Par.

Walking, while Amel : Am-c.

REELING (See Reeling) : Arg-n; Bell; *Gel;* Lol-t; Nux-v; *Pho;* Rhus-t.

Amel : Carb-an.

Coition, after : Bov.

RIDING, Carriage in Agg : Hep.

Amel : Nit-ac.

RINGING In Ears, with : Lith; Pho-ac.

RISING From Bed, Raising up Agg : Adon; BRY; Chel; Cocl; Merc-i-f; Nat-m; Nux-v; Pho; *Phyt;* Ver-v; Vib.

Hand, head above, on : Onos.

ROCKED, As if : See Swinging, as if.

ROCKING Amel : Sec.

+ ROOM and Bed spin around : Cadm.

SCRATCHING Agg : Calc.

SENILE : Amb; Arn; Bar-c; Bels; Bry; Con; Cup; Op; Rhus-t.

SEWING Agg : Grap.

SHAVING Agg : Carb-an.

SITTING Agg : Ap; Meph; *Pho;* PUL; Sul.

Amel : Cyc; Lac-d.

SLEEP, Falling on : Tell.

During, at night : Caus.

SLEEPINESS, With : Aeth; Gel; Laur; *Nit-ac;* Nux-m; *Sil;* Zin.

SMOKING Agg : Gel; Nat-m; Nux-v; Tab.

SNEEZING : Ap; Nux-v; Seneg.

SOUR, Fluid gulping, with : Caul.

SPARKS, Before Eyes : Ign.

+ SPASMS, Before : See Epileptic.

Muscles of, with : Cic.

STANDING Amel : Nux-v; Pho-ac.

STARS White, before eyes,with : Alu; Ant-t.

STOMACH Pain, with : Cic.

STOOLS Agg : Kob.

Amel : Cup; Pho; Zin.

STOOPING Agg : Anac; Caus; Meph; Sul; Ther.

Amel : Carb-an; Petr.

Rising from : Anac; Saba; Sil.

STUPEFACTION, With : Aur; Calc; Zin.

SUMMER Agg : Psor.

SUN FACING Agg : Agar; Glo; Kali-p; Nat-c.

SWEAT Amel : Nat-s.

With : Merc-c; Tab; Ver-a.

SWINGING, SWIMMING As if : Calad; *Merc;* Ox-ac; Petr; *Sul;* Thu.

Left, to : Eup-p.

Lying down, on: Ox-ac.

Swimming vision, with : Strop.

Waking, on : Pho.

SYPHILITIC : *Aur.*

TALKING Agg: Alu; Cham.

TEA Agg : *Nat-m; Sep.*

Amel : Glo.

THROAT, Choking, with : Iber.

TINNITUS, With (See Meniers Disease) : *Chin-s;* Iris.

After : Chin.

TOUCH Agg : Cup.

TREMBLING, With : Crot-h; Gel; Zin.

Internal, with : Cup.

TURNING, As if in Circle : Arn; Bry; *Con;* Cyc; Nux-v; Pho; *Pul;* Rhus-t.

Agg: Con; Hyds; Old.

Amel : Stap.

Heels on Amel : Stap.

Right Agg : Lach.

+ Right side Amel : Alum.

Then headache : Rhus-t.

TURNS, In Circle, as if : Bell; Berb; *Calc;* Caus.

UNCONSCIOUSNESS, Followed by : Sil.

URINATION Urging, when : Hypr.

VERTEX, Felt in : Calc; Chel; Lyss; Med; Scop.

VIOLENT : Meph.

VISION Affections, with: *Cyc;* Fer; GEL; Nux-v; Strop.

VOMITING Amel : Eup-p; Nat-s; Op.

WAKES With, night at : Saba.

WALKING Agg : Anac.

Air open, in Agg : Lach.

Darkness in Agg : Stram.

WALLS, Falling on her, as if : Arg-n; Saba.

WEAKNESS, With : Aeth; Colch; Crot-h; Echi; Sele.

WHIRLING : See Turning in Circle, as if.

WINDOW, Looking out of Agg : Ox-ac.

Standing, near Agg : Nat-m.

WINE Agg : Nat-c.

WRITING, While : Grap;

Kali-bi; Sep.

VESICLES: See Under
Eruptions.

VEXATION : See Anger, **A**GG :
See Mortification Agg.

VIBRATIONS, FLUTTERING
: Am-c;Bell; Bro; Carb-v;
Cimi; *Glo*; Meli; Meph; Old;
Op; *Sang;* Sep; Sul.

   AGG : Colch.

   L**YING** Down, on : Clem.

   S**TEPPING, O**N : Arn.

VICARIOUS : See Discharges,
and Menses.

VIGOUR SENSE, Of : Cof; Nat-p;
Op; Pho; Psor.

   I**NCREASED**, Convulsions,
during : Agar.

VINEGAR APPLICATION Of Amel
: Meli.

VIOLENT : See Pain, Tearing.

   E**FFECTS** *: Aco*; Alu; Anac;
Ars; BELL; Bry;Canth;
Carb-v; CHAM; Cup; Glo;
Hep; *Hyo*; Ign; Iod; *Lach;*
Lyss; Merc; Merc-c; Mez;
NUX-V; Ox-ac; Spig;
STRAM; Sul; *Tarn; Ver-a*.

VISE : See Compression.

VISION, AFFECTIONS Of In G**ENERAL**
: Arg-n; Aur; BELL; *Con; Cyc;*
Gel; Hyo; Jab; *Lyc;* NAT-M;
Nux-v; Op; *Pho;* Pul; Rut; Sep;
Sil; Stram; SUL.

   A**CCOMODATION** Disturbed :
Phys.

   A**CUTE** *: Bell;* Buf; Chin; Hyo;
Nux-v.

   Night at, Hysteria in : Fer.

AMAUROSIS : See Paralysis
of Optic Nerve.

ANIMALS, Bugs Etc. Sees :
Cimi; *Hyo; Stram.*

   Snakes : Arg-n; *Gel.*

ASTHENOPIA :Croc; Fer; *Jab;*
Nat-m; Rut; Seneg.

ASTIGMATISM : Gel; *Lil-t;* Phys;
Tub.

BLACK, Sudden Blind Spells :
BELL; Caps; Cic; *Con;* Cyc;
Glo; Grap; Hyo; Merc;
Nat-m; Old; *Pho;* Pul; Sep;
Sil; S*tram;* Sul.

   Menses, during : Grap; Pul;
Sep.

   Periodical: Iris.

BLINDNESS, Loss of Vision (See
also Paralysis of Optic
Nerve) : Aco; Con; HYO;
Merc; Op; *Pul; Sil;* STRAM;
Syph.

   Alcohol, from : Terb.

   Cause, without : Tab.

   Colour : Bell; Carb-s; Chl-
hyd; Cina; Onos; *Sant.*

   Day : Lyc.

   Epistaxis, with : Ox-ac.

   Eyes, inflammation, from :
Manc.

    over use, from : Crot-h.

   Fainting, suddenly, after :
Plb.

   Grief, from : Crot-h.

   Headache, with : Caus.

    after : Sil.

   Hydrocephalus, in : Apoc.

   Hysterical : Pho; Plat; Sep.

Lightning, from : Pho.

Masturbation, from: Pho-ac.

Menses, before: Dict.

　　　Amel : Sep.

Nausea, with : Sep.

Optic, nerve, atrophy from :
Syph.

Periodical : Merc.

Progressive central scotoma
with: Carb-s; Iodf; Plb;
Tab; Thyr.

Reading, while : Pho.

Retinal haemorrhage, from
: Bothr; Crot-h.

Retro-bulbar, Neuritis from
: Chin-s; Iodf.

Stools Amel: Ap.

Stooping Agg : Fer-p.

Sun, lying in, from : Con.

Tobacco, from: Pho.

Vertigo with : Bell; Gel; *Nux-v.*

White objects, looking
steadily, at : Tab.

BLUE *:* Aur; Cina; Crot-c; Lyc;
Tril; *Zin-chr.*

CIRCLES : See Rings.

COUGHING Agg : Ign; Kali-m.

CROSSED : Con; Kali-bi.

Looking, one eye, with
Amel : Kali-bi.

DARK *:* Psor; Stram; Sul.

DAZZLED, Bright : Bar-c; Con;
Dros; *Kali-c;* Nat-c; *Sil.*

DIM, Blurred : Agar; Aur; Bell;
Calc; CANN; CAUS; Chin;
Con; Cyc; EUPHR; *Gel;*
Hep; Lach; Lyc; Merc;
Nat-m; Nit-ac; *Op; Pho;*

Pho-ac; PUL; Rut; Sep;
SIL; Sul.

Looking sideways Amel :
Chin-s.

Luminosities, after : Ther.

+ Reading, after : Colch.

Twilight Amel : Bry; Lyc.

DIPLOPIA : AUR; Bell; *Cic;*
Cyc; GEL; HYO; Med;
Nat-m; Nit-ac; Pho; Pul;
Stram; Sul; Ver-a; Ver-v.

Bending head backwards
Amel : Seneg.

Blowing nose, on: Caus.

Deafness, alternating
with : Cic.

Diphtheria, after : Lach.

Heart, affections with :
Lach.

Horizontal : Nit-ac; Old.

Looking, right, to Amel :
Caus.

　sideways Agg : Gel.

Lying Amel : Spo.

Masturbation, from : Cina;
Sep.

Measles, after: Caus;
Kali-c.

Nausea, with : Crot-t.

Pregnancy, during : Gel.

Rubbling eye Amel :
Carb-an.

Sexual excess, from : Sep.

Uterine affections, from :
Sep.

Vertical : Atrop; Kali-bi;
Lith; Rhus-t; Seneg;
Stram; Syph.

Vertigo Agg : Bell; Old.

Writing Agg : Grap.

DISTANCES, Misjudging, of :
Cann; Carb-an; Onos;
Stram.

DOWNCAST: Kali-c; Stan; Ver-a.

DROPS, Before : Kali-c.

ERRORS Of : Spig.

Difficult to fit glasses : Spig.

EXERTION, Physical Amel : Aur.

EYES Closing Agg : Bell; Bry;
Calc; Pho; Thu; Ver-v.

Using one Amel : Kali-bi;
Pho; Phys.

FANTASTIC Apparitions : Bell;
Stram; Ver-a.

+ Terrifying, twilight in;
children : Berb.

FAR SIGHT (Hypermetropia) :
Arg-n; *Calc;* Nat-m; SEP;
SIL.

FIELD OF : Flu-ac; Hep; Mang;
Pho; Thu.

One half : Hep.

See objects, besides: Calc;
Cam; Cann; Colo; Grap;
Ign; Lac-c; Nux-m; Nux-v;
Stram; Thu.

FIERY, Bright : *Bell;* Cinb;
Hyo; *Kali-c; Pho; Spig;* Sul.

FINGERS : Psor.

FIXED, Absence of : Spig.

FLICKERING; Flames; Flashes,
Fiery : BELL; Coca; Cyc;
Grap; Hyo; Ign; *Kali-c;*
Lach; Nat-m; *Pho;* Sep;
Spig; Sul.

Borders, black with : Cimi.

Coughing on : Ign.

FLIES : See Muscae Volitantes.

FOGGY : See Misty.

FOUNDRY, Working in Agg :
Merc.

FRINGE, As of : Con.

GLIMMERING, Glittering : Cyc;
Grap; Iod; Lach; Nux-v;
Ol-an; Pho; Strop; Syph;
Ther.

Needles : Cyc.

Stooping, on : Ther.

GREEN: Ars; Cina; Dig; Osm;
Pho; Phyt; Sant;Stram;
Vario.

Rising on : Vario.

Spot, dark, in : Stro.

HAIR As of a : Euphr; Lach;
Plant.

HALO Around the Light : Bell;
Chim; Lach; Osm; PHO; Pul;
Sul.

HEADACHE, Before Agg : Gel;
Glo; Grap; Iris; KALI-BI;
Lach; *Nat-m; Pho;* Pod;
PSOR; *Sep;* Sil; *Sul;* Ther;
Tub.

During Agg : Bell; Iris;
Pho-ac; Pod; *Pul;* Zin.

After Agg : Caus; Con;
Lach; Pho; Sil; *Sul.*

HEMIOPIA :Ars; Aur; Chio;
Cyc; Lach; Lith; *Lyc;*
Mur-ac; NAT-M; Tub.

Right half, lost : Calc; Cocl;
Lith; Lyc.

Left half lost : Calc; Cic;
Nat-c.

Headache, then : Nat-m.

Horizontal : *Ars*; Aur; Tub.

Lower, lost : Aur; Sul.

Menses, during : Lith.

Pregnancy, during : Ran-b.

Upper, lost : Ars; Aur; Cam; Dig.

Vertical : Caus; *Lith* Lyc; Mur-ac; Nat-m.

ILLUSIONS Of, in General : Bry; *Hyo*; Op; Sec; Sep; Spig; *Stram*; Thu; Val; Ver-a.

Operations, after : Stro.

Same person, front and behind : Euphor.

IMAGINARY, On closing eyes : See Eyes closing Agg.

LETTERS Appear Dancing : Bell; Lyss.

Disappear when reading : Cic; Cocl.

Double, writing when : Grap.

Red : Pho.

Run together : Bur-p; Cann; Fer; Grap; *Nat-m;* Rut; *Sil;* Stap; Stram.

+ Smaller, appear : Glo.

LIGHT Agg : Hyo.

Amel : Gel; Stram.

Artifical Agg : Aur; Lyc; Nat-m.

LIGHTNING : Kali-c; Nat-c; Pho; Spig.

LOOKING One eye with Amel : See Eyes using one.

LUMINOUS, Dark, in : Val.

Operations, after : Zin.

MENSES, Before Agg : Dict.

During Agg : Cyc; Grap; Pul; Sep.

MIRAGE : Lyc.

MISTY: Ars; *Calc; Caus; Croc;* Cyc; Gel; Meny; Merc; PHO; Pul; Sul; Zin.

Luminous Yellow, Quivering : Kali-c.

Seminal emissions, after : Sars.

MUSCAE VOLITANTES : Agar; Chin; Cocl; Merc; Nat-m; Pho; Phys; Sep; *Sil; Stram;* Sul.

Brown : Agar.

Right : Chin-s; Cimi; Sele; *Sil.*

Left : Agar; Calc; *Caus;* Merc; *Sul.*

White : Jab; Ust.

NEAR SIGHT (Myopia) : Con; Lil-t; Nit-ac; *Pho*; Pho-ac; Phys; *Pul.*

Head turns sideways to see clearly : Lil-t.

+ NEBULOUS : Mill.

OBJECTS Appear Black : Caps; Stram.

Blood, covered, with : Stro.

Blue : Tril.

Borders, coloured, with : Hyo.

Bright : Hyo; Nat-c; Val.

dark room, in : Val.

Crooked, distorted : Bell; Buf; Nux-m; Stram.

Distant : Anac; Carb-an; Gel; Ox-ac; Stan; Stram; Sul.

yawning, when : Cep.

Fade away, then reappear : Gel.

Glisten : Ol-an.

Half in light, half in dark : Glo.

High, lean forward and about to fall : Arn.

Inverted   : Bell; Kali-c.

Large : Berb; Caus; Euphor; Hep; *Hyo;* Laur; Nat-m; *Nux-m;* Onos; Ox-ac; Pho.

linear : Ox-ac.

Move in circle, on closing eyes : Hep.

to and fro   : Cic.

to right : Nat-sal.

Moving, Dancing : *Arg-n; Bell;* Cic; Cocl; Con; Glo; Psor.

colours, changing : Stro.

Nearer : Bov.

distant seem, yawning on : Cep.

each other, to : Nux-m.

eyes, to : Val.

Persons are, as if : Bell; Calc; Nat-p; Stram.

Round, pass before eyes while lying : Caus.

Run together : Berb; Sil.

Shade, as if, in : Seneg.

Small : Med; Merc-c; Plat; Stram.

+ Tremble, then get dark : Psor.

Turning in circle, as if : Chel; Cyc; Nat-m.

Vibrating : Carb-v.

dark, become, then : Psor.

Whirl, each other, around : Saba.

White   : Chlo-hyd; Grat.

PALE *: Sil.*

PARALYSIS OF OPTIC NERVE : *Bell;* Bov; *Caus;* Con; GEL; Hyo; Kali-io; Nat-m; PHO; *Pul; Sec; Sil; Stram; Sul.*

PERCEPTIVE Power, lost : Kali-p.

PHOTOPSIES *:* See Illusions.

PRESBYOPIA : See Vision, Far.

PURPLE *: Ver-v.*

RAIN Through, Looking, as if : Nat-m.

RAINBOW : Bell; Bry; Con; Pho-ac.

RED : BELL; Con; Hep; Hyo; *Pho;* Rut; Sul; *Ver-v.*

Night, at : Ced.

Spot : Ver-v.

RINGS: Calc; Calc-p; Carb-v; Elap; Kali-c; Psor.

Turning : Kali-c.

SCINTILLATIONS : See Sparks.

SHADE Amel   : Con; Pho.

SHADOWS : Rut; Seneg.

One side of object   : Calc.

SITTING Erect Agg: Kalm.

SNOW, Exposure to, Agg: *Aco;* Cic.

SPARKS *: Bell; Chin;* Kali-m; Lyc; Sec;Sep.

Blowing nose, on : Nat-s.

Dark, in : Bar-c; Bell; Pho.

Eyes closing, on : Hyds.

Headache, during : Chel; *Mag-p.*

White : Alu.

Winking, on : Caus.

Spots, Spotted : Am-m; Cyc; *Kali-c;* PHO; Sil; Sul.

Fiery and : Elap.

Green, dark in : Stro.

Sewing, after : Am-c.

White : Jab.

Stooping Agg : Fer-p; Elap; Ther.

Striped : *Con;* Sep; Sul; Thu.

Green : Thu.

Triplopia : *Bell;* Con; Sec.

Veil, As of a (See Misty) : Pho; Sep.

Violet : Cina.

Wavering : Morp; Nat-m; Ver-v; Zin-chr.

Weak : ANAC; BELL; *Chin;* Con; Nat-m;Op; Pho; Rut; Seneg.

Coition, after : Kali-c.

Headache, with : Zin.

Masturbation, from : Cina.

White : Chlo-hyd; Grat.

Yellow : Alu; Calend; Canth; Cina; Dig; Sep.

Attacks of blindness, after : Bell.

Day during : Ced.

Zigzag : Con; Grap; Lach; Lyc; *Nat-m;* Pho; Sep; Sul-io.

VITREOUS Opacity, Diffusion : Gel; Ham; Hep; Kali-io;

Merc-c; Merc-i-r; Seneg; Sul; Thu.

Turbid : Choles; *Kali-io;* Pho; Pru-sp; *Seneg;* Sul.

VIVACITY : See Cheerful.

VOCAL CORDS : See under Larynx.

VOICE (See also Speech) : Aco; *Bell;* Bro; Canth; *Carb-v; Caus;* DROS; Hep; *Iod;* Mang; *Merc;* PHO; Pul; *Spo;* Stan; *Stram;* Ver-a.

Altered : Ox-ac.

Barking : *Bell; Canth;* Lyc; Spo; Stram.

Breaks, Cracks, Fails, Changes Key : Ant-c; Aru-t; Bell; Con; Grap; Sep; Spo; Stram.

Suddenly, higher tones, in : Stram.

Changeable : Arg-m; Ars; *Aru-t;* Fer; Mang; Seneg.

Colds Agg: Carb-v; Caus; Mang; Merc; Pho Sele.

Control, Lacks, using Amel : Grap.

Creaky : Aco; *Stram.*

Croaking : Aco; Stram.

Crowing : Spo; Stram.

Deep : Carb-v; Dros; Stan.

Distant, Seems : Sabal.

Echoes, Ear, in : Caus; Pho.

Exertion Agg : Arn.

Hissing : Nux-v; Pho.

Hoarse, Croupy : Aco; Arg-m; Arg-n; Ars-io; Aru-t; BELL; *Bro;* Bry; *Calc;* Caps; CARB-V; CAUS; *Cep;* Cham; DROS; *Hep;* IOD; *Kali-bi;*

Kali-m; *Lach;* MANG; *Merc;*
Nat-m; PHO; Sele; SPO;
Stan; Stram; *Sul;* Tell; Verb.
Breathing cold air Agg :
Con.

Children, in : Cham.

Choking : Iod.

Chronic : Mang; Sil.

Colds, from : Arn; Ip; Sele.

Cold water bath, from :
Ant-c.

Coughing and expectoration Amel : Mang; Stan.

Diptheria, after : Phyt.

Evening : *Carb-v;* Caus;
Pho; Rum.

Exertion Agg : Arn.

Heart complaints, with:
Hyd-ac; Nux-m; Ox-ac.

Heated, if Agg : Bro.

+ Larynx, burning in:Am-m.

Laughing, when : Calc-f.

Leucorrhoea, with : Nat-s.

Menses Agg: Gel; Grap;
Lac-c; Spo; Syph.

Morning : Calc; Calc-p;
CAUS; *Mang;* Pho; *Sul.*
evening, and: Caus.

Painful : Iod.

Painless : Calc; Ip.

Periodical, painless: Par.

Reading or reciting aloud
Agg : Calc-f; Seneg.

Sexual loss Agg : Seneg.

Singers : Caps; Hep.

Smoking Amel : Mang.

Sneezing Amel : Kre.

Speakers : Caps; Caus.

Stooping Agg : Caus.

Talking Agg : Coca.
Amel : Caus; Grap; Tub.
painful : Merc-cy.

Walking against the wind
Agg : Euphr; *Nux-m.*

Wet getting, from: Arn;
Merc-i-r.

HOLLOW : Bell; *Dros; Spo;*
Stan; *Ver-a.*

HUMAN AGG : Mur-ac.

HUSKY : *Dros;* Grap; Merc;
Pho.

INDISTINCT : *Bro;* CAUS; Lyc.

LOST, Aphonia : Alum; *Am-Caus; Ant-c;* Arg-m; Arg-n;
Ars-i; Bro; CARB-V; *Caus;*
Colch; Hep; Kali-bi; Kali-p;
Mang; Ox-ac; *Pho;* Phyt;
Stram; Ver-a.

Chronic : Phyt.

Colds Agg : Alu.

Cough, with : Mang.

Epilepsy, before : Calc-ar.

Exertion Agg : *Carb-v.*

Menses, before : Syph.
during : Gel.

Over-heating, from : Ant-c.

Paralytic : Bar-c; Caus;
Kali-p; Ox-ac.

Singers : Arg-m; ARG-N;
CAUS; Mang; Sele.
periodically : Cup.

Sudden : Alu; Bell; *Caus.*

Tongue affections without
: Bothr.

LOUD : Hyo; Nux-m.

LOW : Canth; Hep; Ox-ac; Ver-a.

MALE Agg : Bar-c; *Nit-ac.*

NASAL : Bell; *Kali-bi;* Lyc; Pho-ac; STAP.

OVER USE, Talking, Singing Agg : Ant-c; Arg-m; *Arg-n; Aru-t;* Caps; Caus; *Fer-p; Grap;* Merc; RHUS-T; *Sele;* Seneg; Stan.

ROUGH : Bell; Carb-v; Hyo; Kali-bi; *Pho;* Pul.

+ Over use from : Ant-c.

SCREECHING : Samb.

SHRILL : Aco; Samb; Spo; Stram.

SLOW : Ars; Pho; Thu.

SPEAKING, Mouth full through, as if : Nux-v.

STAMMERING : See Speech.

TONELESS, Loss of Timber : *Dros;* Stram.

TREMULOUS : Merc.

TRUMPET, Like : Verb.

UNSTEADY : Seneg.

USING Amel : Ant-c; Caus; Grap.

WEAK : Alu; Ant-t; Canth; Carb-an; Cocl; Hep; Spo; *Stan; Ver-a.*

Menses, during Plb.

VOICES HEARS : See Imaginations, Voices of.

VOMITING (Remedies in General) : Aco; Aeth; Ant-c; *Ant-t;* Ap; APOC; Arn; ARS; *Bry;* Cadm; Carb-an; *Cham; Cina;* Colch; *Cup; Fer;* IP; Iris; Kre; *Lob;* NUX-V; *Op;* Pho; Plb; *Pul; Sil;* Strop;

Sul; Tab; VER-A; *Ver-v.*

AGG : Aeth; *Ars;* CUP; Dros; *Ip;* Old; *Pul;* Sil; *Sul.*

AMEL : Ant-t; Coc-c; Dig; Eup-p; Kali-bi; Nux-v; *Sang;* Sanic; Sec; Tab; Xanth.

ACRID, Scalding : Chio; *Iris;* Kali-c; Kali-m; *Kre;* Lyc; Med; Rob; *Sang;* Sul.

ALBUMINOUS, Glairy : Jat; Kali-bi.

ANXIOUS : Ars; Tab.

AT ONCE : Apoc; Ars; Cadm; Zin.

BED, After going, to : *Tarn.*

BILIOUS (See Yellowness) : Bism; Flu-ac; Ip; IRIS; Lept; Nat-s; Op; *Sang;* Ver-a.

Amel: Card-m; Eup-p; Sang.

Cramps, with : Cham.

Eating, after : Bism.

Errors, diet of, from : Flu-ac.

Stooping, on : Ip.

BITTER : Bry; Chio; Eup-p; *Iris;* Kali-bi; *Nux-v;* Pho; Pic-ac; Sang.

Drinks, after : Eup-p.

Greenish, cold drinks, after : Rhod.

Water: Lac-d; Mag-c.

BLACK : ARS; *Cadm;* Kre; Mez; NUX-V; Pho; Ver-a.

BLOOD : Arn; Cact; Cadm; *Carb-v; Chin; Crot-h;* Fer;

Ham; Ip; Pho; Sabi; Sec.

At the close of : Ver-a.

Infants : Lyc.

Menses, instead of, in girls : Ham.

Splenic affections, from : Card-m.

Toper's in : Alum.

BLUISH : Kali-c.

BRAIN Affections, in : Bell; Glo; Kali-io; Plb.

BROWN : Ars; Bism; Bry; Carb-v; Mez; Nat-s; Plb; Rhus-t.

BURNING, Hot (See Acrid) : Mez; Pod.

CANCER, From : Carb-ac; Kre.

CHILL, During : Eup-p.

After : Eup-p; Lyc; Nat-m.

COFFEE GROUND : Cadm; Con; Echi; Mez; Pho; Pyro.

COITION, After : Mos; Saba; Sil.

COLIC, With : Hyo.

CONSUMPTION, In : Kali-br; Kre.

CONTINUOUS : Ars; Hell; Ip; Merc; Plb; Pyro; Syph.

CONVULSIONS, Alternating with: Cic.

Before : Hyd-ac.

With : Ant-c; Hyo.

CONVULSIVE : *Bism;* Cup.

COUGHING, After : Sul-ac.

With : See under Cough.

CURDS : Aeth; Calc; Nat-p; Sanic; Sil; Val.

Sour: Calc; Nat-p.

CYCLIC, Infants, in : Cup-ar;

Iris; Kre; Merc-d.

DEATH, Desires, during: Phyt.

DELAYED, After a while : Bism; PHO.

DIFFICULT : *Ant-t;* Ars.

DRINKING Agg : *Ant-c; Ars;* Bry; Kali-bi; Pho; Sil; Tab; Ver-a.

Cold Amel: Cup; Pho; Pul.

Every : Apoc.

Immediately after, even smallest quantity : *Ars; Bism; Bry; Cadm;* Cina; Pho; Pyro; Ver-a; Ver-v; Zin.

Warm after : Bry.

Water, from : Sars.

When it becomes warm, after a while : Kali-bi; PHO; *Pyro.*

EASY : Apoc; *Ars;* Bap; *Cham;* Fer; Ip;Jatr; Phyt; Sec.

EATING, After : Kali-br.

Amel : Ant-t; Nux-v; Pul.

EMOTIONS, From : Kali-br.

ERUCTATION, With : Mur-ac.

Recur, as if would, with : Goss.

Sour, with : Nit-ac.

EXHAUSTING : Aeth; Ant-t; Cadm; Pod; Ver-a;Ver-v.

FAECAL : Op; Plb; Pyro; Raph; Rhus-t; Tab.

FEARFUL : Ant-c.

FEVER, During : Ant-t; Bap; Eup-p; Nat-m.

FLUIDS, Only : Ars; Bism.

FOOD, Every kind of : Acet-ac.

Odour, from : Stan.

FORCIBLE : Aco; Ant-t; Apoc; Con; Nux-v; Petr;Ver-a; Ver-v.

Eating shortly, after : Sanic.

Sudden : Ant-t; Kali-bi; Kali-chl; Pic-ac.

    fever, with : Bap.

FREQUENT: *Ars; Chin;* Con.

FROTHY : Aeth; ARG-N; Ars; *Kre;* Led; Mag-c; Nat-c; Pho; Sil; *Ver-a.*

Hot : Pod.

GREASY, Oily : Iod; Mez; Nux-v.

GREEN : *Ars;* Bell; Cham; *Chel;* Cimi; Eup-p; *Ip;* Merc-d; NAT-S; Stram; *Ver-a.*

Bitter, cold drinks,after : Rhod.

Black : Hell; Mar-v.

Olive : Carb-ac.

HAWKING Mucus, in the morning : Bry; Calc-p; Euphr; Nux-v.

HEADACHE, With: Bry; Caus; *Chel;* Cocl; *Ip; Iris;* Meli; NUX-V; PUL; *Sang;* Sep; Ver-a.

HICCOUGH, After : Jatr.

HOT WATER Amel : Ars; Chel; Sul-ac.

HUNGER, With : Ver-a.

HYSTERICAL : Kali-br.

INCESSANT,Food, connection without : Lac-d.

INGESTA, Food of : *Ars; Bry;* Chin; *Cina;* Eup-p; FER; *Ign;* Kre; Lyc; NUX-V; Pho; PUL; Sang; *Sil; Sul;* Ver-a.

Colic, abdominal, followed by : Manc.

Long after meals : Aeth; Ars-io; *Fer;* Kre; Plat; Pul; Sabi; Sang.

whooping cough, in : Meph.

Milk, except : Hyds.

Night. at : Kali-c.

Smallest quantity : Ver-v.

Water, then : Pul.

bitter : Lac-d.

except : Hyds.

LIFTING Agg : Sil.

LIQUIDS, Only : See Fluids.

LYING, Back, on Agg : Rhus-t.

Left side on Agg : Sul-ac.

Right side on Agg : Crot-h.

Amel : Ant-t.

MENSES, After: Crot-h.

During : Am-m; Apoc; Kali-c; Lach; Pul.

MIDNIGHT, After: Fer.

MILK : Aeth; Calc; Mag-c; Pod; Sanic; Sil; Val; Vario.

Mother's : Sil.

anger, after : Val.

Peristently : Calc-p; Pho-ac.

Undigested : Mag-c.

MILKY : *Sep.*

MONTH, Every : Crot-h.

MORE Than he drinks : Kali-bi.

MORNING : Caps; Cup; Grap; Hep.

Early : Stan.

Sickness, during menses

: Grap.

MOTION, Least Agg : Tab.

MOUTH, Rinsing on : Sep.

MUCOUS : Arg-n; *Dros; Ip;*
Kali-bi; Nux-v; Pho; PUL;
Sul-ac; Ver-a.

Amel : Nat-m.

Bloody : Merc-c.

Green : Kali-chl; Plb.

Sour : Kali-c.

Watery, mass of : Guai.

NAUSEA, Without : Ant-c;
Apoc; Arn; Ars; Chel; Fer;
Kali-bi; Lyc; Phyt; *Ver-v;*
Zin.

NEURALGIA, With : Aran.

NIGHT, At : Kali-c.

OBSTINATE, For days : Oenan.

OFFENSIVE : Ars; Nux-v; *Sep.*
Fluid : Abro.

OPERATIONS On Abdomen,
after : *Bism;* Cep; *Nux-v;*
Pho; Stap.

PAINFUL : Ars; *Ver-a.*

PERIODICAL : Cup; Iris; Plb.

PERITONITIS, In : Op.

PESSARY In vagina, from :
Nux-m.

PREGNANCY Agg : Alet; Anac;
Asar; Chel; Cocl; *Cyc;* Fer;
Goss; Ign; *Ip;* Jab; *Kre;*
Lac-d; LOB; MED; Nat-s;
Nux-m; *Nux-v;* Psor; *Sep;*
Sul; Symph; Tab; Thyr.
Obstinate: Alet; Jab; Psor.

PRESSURE On Spine and Neck,
from : Cimi.

PROJECTILE : See Forcible.

PURGING, With : Aeth; Ant-t;
Ap; Arg-n; ARS; Asar; Bor;
Cam; Cham; Colch; Cup;
Ip; *Iris;* Merc; Pho; *Pod;*
Sec; Seneg; Sul; Sul-ac;
VER-A; Ver-v.

Bilious : Eup-p.

Blood : Erig.

black : Ars.

Fright, from : Op.

Menses, during : Am-m.

Urination, and : Crot-h.

RELIEF, Without : Ant-c.

RENAL Origin, from : Senec.

RESPIRATORY Symptoms, with
: Lob.

RICE, After : Tell.

Water : Cup; Kali-bi; Ver-a.

SALTY : Benz-ac; Iod; Nat-s.

SCRATCHING, When : Ip.

SEPTIC : Bap; Crot-h; Lach;
Vip.

SHIVERING, With : Dul.

SLEEP, Then : *Aeth;* Ant-t;
Cup; Nat-m; Sanic.

SOLIDS Only : Arn; Bry; Cup;
Fer; Sep; Ver-a.

SOUR : Calc; Caus; Chio; Iris;
Lac-d; Lyc; Mag-c; Med;
Nat-p; Nux-v; Pho; Psor;Pul;
Rhe; Rob; Sul; Sul-ac; Tab;
Ver-a.

Chill, Fever, during : Lyc.

Water : Con.

STAINS, Black : Arg-n.

STOMACH, From, full, after
interval of days : *Bism;*
Grat.

STOOLS After : Aeth.

During : Arg-m; Ox-ac.

Straining from : Ther.

STOOPING Agg : Cic; *Ip.*

STRINGY : Croc; Cor-r; Cup; Kali-bi.

SUDDEN, Projectile : Ant-t; Kali-bi; Kali-chl; Pic-ac.

SUGAR Amel : Op.

SWALLOW, Attempting, on : Merc-c.

Empty Agg : Grap.

SWEAT, Cold with: Ars; Cup-ar; Tab; *Ver-a.*

SWEETISH : Iris; *Kre*; Plb; *Tub.*

SYNCOPE, With : Cocl.

TALKING, Loudly, when: Cocl.

TEETH, Sets on edge : Chio; Rob.

THIRST, With : Ars; Canth.

TUMOURS, Cerebral, from : Coc-c; Cocl.

UNCONSCIOUSNESS, During : Ars; Benz-n.

+ UNCOVERING Abdomen, Amel : Tab.

URAEMIC : Apoc; Ars; Samb; Scop; Senec.

URINE, Of : Op.

URTICARIA, Suppressed from : Urt.

UTERINE : Caul; Kre; Lil-t; Senec.

+ VERTIGO During: Nux-v; Tab; Ver-a.

VIOLENT : Ant-t; Ars; Canth; Colch; Crot-t; Cup; Kali-bi; *Nux-v*; Pho; Phyt; Stan;

Tab; *Ver-a.*

Death, desires : Phyt.

+ Nausea, without : Ver-v.

Sitting up, on : Sil.

WATER, Sight of (Must close eyes while bathing) : Lyss; Pho.

Cold Amel : *Cup;* Pho; Pul. Except : Hyds.

WATERY : Ars; *Bry*; Caus; Dros; *Iris*; Rob; Tab; VER-A.

Greenish : Old.

Sweetish : Iris.

Then food : Iod; Nux-v.

WINE Amel : Kalm.

WORMS : Cina; Saba; Sang.

YELLOW : Pho; Ver-a.

Bright : Kali-bi.

VORACITY : See Appetite, Increased, Ravenous.

VULNERABLE : See Skin, Heal Won't.

VULVA (Labia) : Sep; Thu.

ABSCESS : Hep; Lach; Merc; *Pul; Sep.*

APTHOUS : Helo.

CHEESY Deposits, on : Helo.

DRY : Tarn.

Menses, after : Sep.

+ ECZEMA, Around : Grap.

ERUPTIONS : Sep.

Herpetic : Nat-s.

HOLDS : Lil-t; Sanic.

HOT : Carb-v; Tarn.

ITCHING : Amb; *Calad;* Carb-v; Coll; Helo; Senec;

Sil; Stap; Sul; Tarn.

Burning : Calad; Kali-io; Senec; Sul; Urt.

Leucorrhoea, with : Fago; Hyds.

Pinworms, from : Calad.

Sexual excitement, with : Kali-bi.

Urinating, when : Amb; Kre.

OOZING, Constant, from : Aur.

OPEN : Bov; Sabal; Sec; Sep.

PAINFUL, Menses, during: Rhus-t.

RAW : Tarn.

SENSITIVE, Sore : Carb-v; Coc-c; Plat; Stap; Sul; Tarn.

SITTING Agg : Berb; Kre; Stap; Sul.

SWELLED : Carb-v; Hep; Pul; Senec; Sep.

As if : Colch; Coll.

+ Intense itching : Rhus-t.

Pregnancy, during : Pod.

WET, As if : Eup-pur; Petr.

WAKING : See Awakes.

AGG : See Awakening After Agg.

WALKING AGG And *Amel* : See Motion.

BACKWARD AGG *:* Mang.

BARE Feet, With Amel: Psor.

BENT AMEL .: Am-m; Con; Pho; Sul.

BONES Of Legs, on, as if : Cham.

BRIDGE On Narrow or over Water AGG : Ang; *Bar-c*;

Fer; Sul.

CANAL, By·the side of AGG : Ang.

CIRCLE, In : Thu.

COTTON ON, As if : Onos.

CROOKED AMEL : Am-m.

DARK, In AGG : Zin.

EYES, Closed with Agg : Alu; Arg-n; Calad; Iodf; Zin.

Amel : Con.

FEET, Swing, half circle, in : Cic.

Swollen, as if, with : Buf.

FLOOR,On : Ars; Cham.

Hand, Wrings, and : Buf.

FOOT, Left, Can not put on ground, when : Mag-c.

GOES To one side : Amy-n.

GROUND, Level on Agg : Ran-b; Ver-a.

Rough, on Agg : Clem; Hyo; Lil-t.

HARD PAVEMENT, On AGG : Ant-c; CON; *Hep.*

IMPULSE To : Aco; Arg-n; *Ars; Bur-p;* Fer; Flu-ac; Kali-io; Lil-t; Lyc; Mag-c; Merc; Naj; Pho; Sep; Tarn; Thu; Val.

INABILITY, Fall after : Arg-m.

Pregnancy, during : Bels.

INVOLUNTARILY, Quick steps with : Coca.

KNEES, Drawn up, involuntary when : Ign.

On : Med.

legs cut off, feels : Bar-c.

LATE Learning : See Children,

Walk late.

MUST (See Motion Amel) : Ars; Aur; Calc; Dig; Dios; Iod; Murx; Op; Paeon; Rut; Stro; Tarn.

Night, at : Merc.

NEEDLES, On,as if : Eupi; Rhus-t.

PEAS, Hard on, as if : Nux-m.

PITCHES, Forward, as if, on : Terb.

SIDE **W**AY **A**GG :Caus; Kali-c.

To one : Amy-n; Ver-v.

SPONGE On, as if : Helod.

+ **S**UDDEN Loss of Strength : Con.

TOES, On : Crot-h; Lathy.

TURNS, Right to, while : Helod.

VELVET, On, as if : Sec.

WOOL On As if : Xanth.

+ **WANDER** **H**OME **T**O **H**OME, Desire : Elat.

WANDERING : See Pain wandering.

WARMTH, Warm Applications (See Also Heat) **A**GG : AP; BELL; Calc; *Carb-v;* Crot-h; Cup; Flu-ac; IOD; Kali-io; Kali-s; LACH; Led; Lil-t; Lyc; *Merc; Nat-m; Pul;* Sabi; Sanic; *Sec;* Spig; *Sul.*

COVERS Etc. (See also Heat) AMEL : *Hep;* Ign; *Mag-c;* NUX-V; Pul; Rhus-t; *Samb;* Scil; *Sil; Stro.*

WARTS (See Fungus Growth)

BLEEDING : Caus.

FLAT : Berb; Caus; *Dul;* Merc-i-f; Rut.

GRANULAR : Arg-n.

HORNY : Ant-c; Sil.

ITCHING : Kali-c.

LARGE, Soft : Mag-s; Dul.

PEDUNCULATED : *Thu.*

RED : *Calc;* Nat-s; *Thu.*

Body all over : Nat-s.

SHOOTING : Bov.

SUPPRESSED : Meny; Nit-ac; Stap; Thu.

ULCERATING : Caus; Hell.

WASH, **I**MPULSE TO : Psor; Syph.

WASHING : See Bathing.

CLOTHES **A**GG : Pho; Ther.

FLOOR **A**GG : Caus; Merc-i-r.

HEAD **A**GG: Canth; Tarn; Zin-chr.

WATER AGG : See Dampness **A**GG.

BLOODY, Meat washing: See Discharges, Meat water.

CAN NOT Bear touch of it : Am-c.

CHOKES Him: Stram.

COLD, Too : Phys; Ther.

DROPPING or Flowing on part : See Trickling.

FALLING or Swimming, in Agg : Ant-c; Bels.

FORCING, Its way, during pain as if : Coc-c.

+ **F**OUL Agg : Crot-h.

HORROR OF, Cold : Phys.

HOT, Flowing on part : See under Trickling.

LOOKING, Running water **A**GG : See Looking Moving

Objects AGG.

SIGHT, Of, AGG : Bell; Bro;
Canth; Lyss; Stram; Sul.

Pregnancy, during : Pho.

SMELLS, Like old musty rain
water : Sanic.

TASTE Bad, Putrid etc. : See
under Taste.

Sweet : Form.

THINKING, Of It Agg : Ham.

WATERBRASH (See also
Raising Mucus) : *Ars;*
Bar-c; BRY; CALC; *Carb-v;*
Lyc; *Mez;* Nat-m; NUX-V; *Par;*
Petr; PHO; Pul; Rob; *Saba;*
Sang; Sep; *Sil;* Stap; Sul;
Sul-ac.

ALTERNATE Day Agg : Lyc.

BITTER, Nausea, with :
Am-m.

Sour, Stomach pain, with
: Kre.

BURNING : Sumb.

CHILLINESS, With : Sil.

COLD : Caus; Ver-a.

CONVULSIONS, Before : Hyd-ac.

COUGH, After : Ab-n.

HEADACHE, With : Mag-m.

HEAT OF Body, with : Cic.

LYING Down, on : Psor.

MENSES, Before: Nux-m; Pul.

MILK, From : Cup.

NIGHT : Carb-v; Kali-c.

PREGNANCY, During : Nat-m;
Nux-m; Tab.

SALTY : Carb-an; Caus.

SENSATION, Of : Kali-io.

SUDDEN : Bar-c.

+ SWEETISH : Ant-c.

TOBACCO Amel : Ol-an.

TONGUE, Brown, with : Sil.

WATERY : See Discharges,
Watery, Thin.

WAVERING : See Irresolution.

WAVES,Ebullitions, Fluctua-
tions Orgasms : Am-m;
Amy-n; Aur; Bell; Calc; Fer;
Gel; Glo; Kre; LACH; Lil-t;
Lyc; MELI; *Nux-v;* Pho; *Sang;*
SEP; Spo; Stro; Strop; Sul;
Sul-ac.

HEAT, Of : See Heat, Flushes of.

Pain, during : Cam.

WEAKNESS, ENERVATION,

Prostration : Aco; Alu; Am-c;
Anac; *Ant-t;* Ap; Arg-m;
Arn; ARS; *Bap; Bar-c;* Bro;
Bry; *Calc; Calc-p;* CARB-V;
Caus; Chel; *Chin;* Cocl;
Colch; Cup; Dig; *Fer;* GEL;
Grap; Hep; Hyo; Ign; *Iod;* Ip;
Kali-c; Kali-p; Kalm; Lach;
Laur; *Lyc;* Med; Merc; *Merc-c;*
Merc-cy; Mur-ac; Nat-c;
Nat-m; Nat-p; Nat-s; *Nit-ac;*
Nux-v; PHO; *Pho-ac;* Pic-ac;
Psor; Pyro; *Rhus-t;* Scil; Sec;
Sele; Sep; Sil; Solid; *Spo;*
Stan; Stap; Sul; Sul; Sul-ac;
Sul-io; *Tab;* Tarn; Thyr; *Tub;*
VER-A.

ACUTE DISEASES, In : Aeth; Ail;
Ant-t; Ap; Ars; Gel;
Merc-cy; Mur-ac; Strop;
Tarn-c; Ver-a.

After : *Chin;* Meph; Psor;
Sele; Ver-a.

AIR Open Agg : Plat; Spig.

Walking in Agg : Alu; Cocl; Rhus-t.

Amel : Flu-ac; Kali-io; Sul.

APPETITE, Increase with: Sec.

CAUSELESS : Psor.

CHEST, Starts in, as if : Seneg.

COITION After (Males) AGG : *Calc;* Kali-p; *Sele;* Sil.

Shuddering, with : Kali-c.

Females : Berb; Sep.

COUGH, After : Cor-r; Ver-a.

DIE, As if, he would : *Ars;* Old; Vinc.

EARLY, Rapid and : *Merc-cy.*

EATING, After : Zin.

EMISSION Agg : Dios; Kali-p; Kob; Lyc; Med; Nux-v; Pho; Pho-ac; Sil; Stap.

+ EPILEPSY, After, One arm one leg : Cadm; Pho.

EVEN CAN NOT Take food : Bar-c; Stan.

EXCESS, After Any : Plb.

EXERTION Agg : Pho.

+ GOING Downstairs, than up : Stan.

HEAD Resting, closing eyes Amel : Anac.

HEAT, Flushes of, after: Dig; Sep.

INDOLENCE and Luxury from (Women) : Helo.

INFLUENZA, After : Abro; Con; Kali-p; Nat-sal.

INJURY, After : Acet-ac; Sul-ac.

INTERNALLY : See Empty Feeling.

MENSES During : Carb-an; Cocl; Iod; Pic-ac; Sep.

Amel : *Sep.*

After Agg : Alu; Am-c; Cimi; *Ip.*

Scanty, with : Ip.

MENTAL and Physical work from (Women) : Helo.

MORNING : Ars; Carb-v; *Lach; Lyc;* Pho-ac; *Sep;* Stap.

11 A.M. : Pho; Sep; SUL; Zin.

NAUSEA, With : Ant-t.

NURSING Sick persons, after : Cimi; *Cocl;* Nit-ac.

Women, in : Carb-an; *Chin; Pho-ac.*

OPERATIONS, After : Acet-ac; Hypr; Stro.

Haemorrhage, severe, from : Stro.

OUT OF PROPORTION, to disease : Ars; Sul-ac.

PAINS From : Arg-m; *Ars;* Cham; Kali-p; Kalm; Pic-ac; Rhus-t; Ver-a.

PALPITATION, After : Kali-c.

PARALYTIC : Ars; *Chin;* Cocl; *Fer;* Gel; Hell; Kali-c; Kali-p; Kalm; Mur-ac; Pho; Pho-ac; *Sul;* Ver-a.

Pleurisy with : Saba.

Sense of : Stro.

Stiffness, with : Lith.

PERIODICAL : *Arg-n.*

RAPID : *Ars; Bap;* Lyc; Sep; Tub; *Ver-a.*

RESTLESS, And : Ars; Rhus-t; Zin.

RIDING, From : Card-m.

SADNESS, From: Calc-p; Ign; Pho-ac.

SCIENTIFIC, Labour Agg : Grap.

SEA Bathing Agg : Mag-m.

SENSITIVE, And : Terb.

SICKNESS, After : See Acute Diseases, After.

SINGLE Parts in (See Single Parts, effects) : Val.

SINKING, Readily : *Merc.*

SPEAK, Can not, from: Cocl.

STOOLS, After : *Ars;* Bism; Cocl; *Con;* Kali-p; *Merc;* Nat-s; Nit-ac; Pic-ac; Pho; Pod; Sec; Tub; Ver-a.

Mucous, after : Bor.

SUCKLING, After: Carb-v.

SUDDEN (See Collapse): Ars; Con; Crot-h; *Laur;* Pho; Ran-b; Sep.

Vision, illusions of with : Sep.

SYMPTOMS, Few, with : Syph.

TAKES, The Voice away : Canth.

TALKING Agg : Alu; Stan; Sul.

TREMULOUS : Arg-n; Chin; Con; Hep; Nat-m, Old; Ol-an; Petr; Stan.

Smoking, after : Hep.

TRIFLE Causes, from : Am-c; Ars.

UNPLEASANT, Impressions, from : Pho.

UPPER Part of, Trembling of lower, with : Amb.

URINATION After : *Ars;* Caus;

Cimi; Fer; *Gel;* Nux-v; *Pho.*

WAKING, On : Nux-v; Sep; Syph.

WALKING Amel : *Rhus-t;* Rut; *Sul.*

Air open in, after : Spo.

WORKED, Hard, as from : Ap.

WEALTHY, THINKS He is : Cann; Pho; *Plat; Pyro; Sul;* Ver-a.

WEANING, ILL EFFECTS of : Bry; Cyc; Pul.

ERUPTIONS, After : Dul.

WEARINESS (See Weakness) : Cann; Croc; Pul.

EXERTION, Slight, from : Bar-c.

PAINFUL : Rut.

SLEEPINESS, With: Ant-c.

Eating, when : Kali-c.

WEATHER CHANGE OF AGG : See Change of Temperature AGG.

HOT Agg and Amel : See Summer Agg and Amel.

HUMID : See Humid.

ROUGH, Windy AGG. : Rhod.

WET AGG : See Dampness *Agg.*

AMEL : See Air, Cold, Dry AGG.

WEDGE : See Plug.

WEEPING AGG : *Arn; Bell;* Croc; Cup; *Hep;* Mar-v; Stan; Ver-a.

AMEL : Anac; Cimi; Cyc; Dig; *Grap; Lach;* Lyc; Med; Nit-ac; Plat; PUL; Tab.

WEEPS : *Aeth;* Ap; Aur; *Bell;* CACT; Calc; Caus; *Cham;*

Cic; *Cof; Grap;* Ign; Kali-br;
Lac-c; Lil-t; *Lyc;* Mag-m; Med;
Nat-m; NUX-M; Pall; Pho; *Plat;*
PUL; Rhus-t; *Sep;* Spo; *Sul;*
Sul-ac; VER-A.

ALONE, When : Con; Nat-m.

ALOUD : Cup; Lyc.

ANGER, After : Nux-v; Plat.

    With : Ant-t; Ars; Sul; Zin.

BITTERLY : Nat-m.

CAUSE, Without : Ap; Cact;
Grap; Nat-m; Pul; Rhus-t;
Sul; Syph; Vio-o.

    Day and night : Ap.

CHILL, During : Bell; Calc;
Cham; Lyc; Pul; Vio-o.

CHOREA, In : Caus.

CONVULSIVE : Mag-p.

    Asthma with : Bov.

COUGHING, Before : See Cries,
Cough Agg.

    With : Spo.

DAY, During: Stram.

DISCONTENT, Self, with : Nit-ac.

DISEASE, Progressive, with :
Aeth; Calad.

DREAMS, In : Calc-f; Plant;
Spo; Stram; Tarn.

EATING While : Carb-an.

EMOTIONS, From : Ast-r; Kre:
Naj.

+ FREQUENTLY : Ust.

HEAT, During : Aco; Bell; Pul;
Spo.

HOPELESS, From : Arg-n.

IMMODERATELY : Fer.

INVOLUNTARILY : Croc; Ign;
Mang; Nat-m; Plat; Pul;
Rhus-t; Sep.

+ INWARDLY : Ign.

LAMENTING, And : Cof.

LAUGHS, And, by turns : Ign;
Sumb.

LONELY, Feeling, from: Lith.

LOOKED At, when : Nat-m.

MENSES, Before : Pho.

    During : Ars.

MUSIC, From : Amb; Grap;
Kre; Nat-c; Thu.

NURSING, While : Lac-c; Pul.

PAINS, with : Cof; Plat.

    After : Glo.

PALPITATION, with : Pho.

PARALYSIS, In : Caus.

PIANO, Hearing on :Cep;
Nat-s.

PREGNANCY, During : Mag-c.

QUESTIONED, When : Cimi.

READING, When : *Crot-h;*
Lach.

SEXUAL Excitement, with :
Ast-r; Stram.

SILENTLY : Cyc.

SITS, And, for Days : Amb.

SLEEP, In: Carb-an; Cham;
Lyc; Nat-m; Nux-v;Stan.

    Loudly : Kali-io.

    Waking, without : Hyo.

SPASMS, After : Alu; Caus.

SPELLS, Of : Sep.

SPOKEN To, when : Cimi;
Med; Nat-m; Plat; Stap.

STOOLS Agg : Aeth; Bor; Cham.

SWEAT, With : Bell; Cup; Lyc; Op; Spo.

TELLING Of her sickness, when : Kali-c; Med; *Pul; Sep.*

Over again, and : Med.

THANKED When : LYC.

TRIFLES, At (In Children) : *Caus;* Nat-m.

UNDRESSES, And : Thyr.

WEIGHT, As Of A HEAVY : Aco; Ars; Bar-c; Bell; BRY; *Cact;* Dios; Elap; Lach; Nux-m; NUX-V; Petr; PHO; Pho-ac; *Pul;* Sep; Zin.

COLD : Agar.

HANGING To part, as if : Cur; Nit-ac; Rhod; Rut.

TIED UP, To part, as if : Ver-a.

WELL, SAYS HE IS, When very sick: Ap; *Arn;* Ars; Cann; Cof; Iod; Op.

FEEL, Does not, but knows not why : Bro.

+ FEELS, In serious cases : Am.

UNUSUALLY, Then AGG : Bry; Nux-v; Pho; *Psor;* Sep.

+ **WENS** : Bar-c.

WET AGG : See Dampness Agg.

WETTING HANDS AND FEET AGG : See Cold of Single Parts And Wet Feet AGG.

WHEALS : See Urticaria.

WHEEZING : See Respiration Whistling.

WHINING, WHIMPERING :

Ant-t; Ap; Aur; Carb-an; *Cham;* Cic; *Cina;* Merc; Pod; Pul; Senec.

AILMENTS, Little, with : Tub.

ATTACKS Of Sickness, before : Ant-t.

+ **MOOD** : Bar-c.

SLEEP, In : Pod; Rhe.

WHIRLING : See Vertigo.

WHISPERS: Calc; Cup; Fer; Ign; Merc; Ol-an.

EAR In, as if : Anac.

HERSELF, To : Pyro.

SLEEP, In: Pyro.

WHISTLES : Croc; Lach; Plat; Stram.

FEVER, During : Caps.

INVOLUNTARY : Carb-an; Lyc.

LOW, Soft, Voice : Vio-o.

WHITE, WHITENESS (Of Skin Discharges etc.) : Ant-t; Ars; CALC; Carb-v; Chel; *Chin;* Cina; Dig; *Fer; Grap; Kali-m;* LAC-C; MERC; *Nat-m; Pho;* Pho-ac; *Pul;* Sep; Sul; *Ver-a.*

CHALKY : Ant-c; Mez.

MILKY : *Kali-m.*

SPOTS : Alu; *Ars;* Grap; Merc; Nat-c; Sep; SIL; SUL.

SWELLING : See Joints Swelling, pale.

TURNING : Sul-io.

And insensible : Sul-io.

Blue : Calc.

Red : Hell.

WHITLOW : See Fingers, Felon.

WHIZZING : See Humming.

WHOOPING COUGH : See Cough, Whopping.

WIFE IS FAITHLESS : Hyo; Stram.

R**UN** A**WAY**, From him, will : Stap.

WILD FEELING : Ambl *Cimi;* Lil-t; Med.

+ **WILD L**OOK : Val.

WILFUL : See Stubborn.

WILY : See Tricky.

WIND, AIR, **D**RAFT AGG : *Aco;* Ars; *Bell;* Calc; Calc-p; Caps; Cham; *Chin;* Colch; Colo; *Hep;* Kali-c;Lach; Lyc; Mag-c; Mag-p; Med; Nux-m; *Nux-v;* Pho; Pho-ac; Pul; Rhe; *Rhod;* Rhus-t; Samb; Scil; Sele; SIL; Stro; SUL; Verb.

A**MEL** : Fer; Iod; Sec; Tub.

B**LOWING** On part, as of a : See Air Blowing on part, as of a.

N**ORTH** A**GG** : Ars; Asar; Carb-v; Caus; Hep; Nux-v; Sep; Spo; Zin.

S**LIGHT** A**GG** : Caps.

W**ARM** A**GG**˙ : Sele.

   A**MEL** : Thu.

WINE A**GG** *:* See under Food, Wine Agg.

WINKING : See under Eyes.

WINTER AGG (See Cold A**GG**) : *Ars; Aur;* Dul; Flu-ac; Hep; Kali-c; Kalm; Nux-v; Petr; Psor; Rhus-t.

A**MEL** : Sul-io.

WIPING A**GG** : Alo; *Grap;* Lach; Mur-ac.

A**MEL** (Eyes) : Alu; *Calc;* Cina; Croc; Cyc; Euphr; *Nat-c.*

WITHERED, SHRIVELLED : Ars; *Calc; Chin; Cocl;* Cup; *Iod;* Lyc; *Sec; Ver-a.*

WITTY : See Jests, Jokes, Joking.

WOMEN: See Females Affections of, and Old Maids.

A**VERSION** To : Dios; Lach; Pul.

C**HILDLESS** : Arg-n; Cocl.

N**EUROTIC**, High strung : Scut.

+ U**NMARRIED** : Cocl; Sil.

W**IDOWS** : Stap.

WOODEN FEELING : Kali-n; Petr; Rhus-t; Thu.

WOOLENS AGG : Merc; Pho; *Psor;* Pul; Rhus-t; Sul.

WORD HUNTING : Arg-n; Arn; Lach; Pho-ac; *Plb;* Pho.

S**WALLOWS** : *Cic;* Stap; Thu.

WORK DISLIKES, Dread of : See Aversion to Work and Indolent.

WORMS : *Aco;* Art-v; *Calc;* Chin; *Cina;* Cup-ac; Ign; Merc; Nat-p; *Saba; Sil; Spig;* Stan; *Sul;* Vio-o.

F**EVER**, From : Cina.

H**OOK** : Card-m; Chenop; Thymol.

P**IN**, Thread : Calc; Chin; Fer; Ign; *Mar-v;* Naph; Rat; Saba; Sul; Urt.

T**APE** *:* Calc; Grap; Plat; Pul;

Saba; Sil; Sul.

+ **WORN OUT** : Amb.

WORRY : See Care, Grief.

CAUSELESS : Petr.

+ **WORTHLESS** FEELS : Anac.

WOUNDS : See Injuries.

ATROPHY, Of : Form.

BLEED, Edges closed from : *Mill.*

Suppurate and : Pho.

BLUE : Lyss.

BREAK and Heal again (See Ulcers) : Carb-v; Pho.

HEALING Rapid, for : Manc.

POISONED : Cist.

WRAPPED Body etc. as if : Bar-c; Cact;Grap; Med; Nux-v; Sul.

WRAPPING : See Covers.

WRAPS UP, in Summer : Hep; *Psor.*

WRETCHED : Tab.

WRIGGLES : Val.

WRINGING : See Twisting.

WRINKLED : *Calc*; Cam; Pho-ac; Sars; *Sec;* Sep; Vera.

WRISTS : Bov; Calc; Caus; Kali-c; Rhus-t; Rut; Sabi; Sep; Sul.

RIGHT : Ox-ac; Vio-o.

ACHING, Loss of power, with : Fer-p.

BURNING : Nat-c.

COLD : Calc-f; Gel.

Puerperal Sepsis, in : Pul.

CONTRACTED, As if : Bels.

CRACKING : Arn; Con.

GANGLION : Benz-ac;Calc-f.

GRASPING Agg : Fer-p.

KNITTING Agg : Kali-c.

MENSES Agg : Nat-p.

NUMB : Zin.

PARALYSIS : Plb.

PINS And Needles : Colch.

SORE, Bruised : Rhod.

STRAINED, As if : Ox-ac.

TURNING Agg : Merc-i-f.

WEAK : Val.

WRITING Agg : Lyc; *Mag-p.*

WRITING AGG : See Fingers, Writing, and working with.

CRAMPS, While : See Cramps under Fingers.

MISTAKES, In : See Mistakes.

WRONG, CAN NOT TELL, what is : Thu.

DOING, Something: Hell.

EVERTHING, Seems : Naj.

HAD DONE Something : Cina; Ign; *Nux-m;* Rut.

POSITION : See under Position.

WRY NECK : See Neck, Wry.

X-RAY Burns : Calc-f; Pho; Radm.

YAWNING : Ant-t; Ars; CAUS; Chel; Cina; *Croc*; Grap; Hep; IGN; Kali-p; *Kre*; Lyc; Mag-p; Mang; NUX-V; *Op*; Pho; Plat; Pul; *Rhus-t;* Sul; Zin-val.

AGG : Alo; Am-m; Caus; *Cina*; IGN; Kali-c; *Kre*;

NUX-V; *Rhus-t; Sars.*

AMEL: Berb; Chin-s; Croc; Guai; Stap.

ACCOMPANIMENT, As an : Agar; Ant-t; Castr; Cina; Kali-c; Kre; Sars.

Abdominal, symptoms, with : Castr.

CHILL, Before : Eup-p.

With : *Eup-p; Nat-m;* Thu.

COLDNESS, With : Nat-c.

COMA, In : Amy-n.

+ CONTINUOUS: Castr; Lathy.

COUGHING, While : Bell.

After : Anac; *Ant-t;* Ip; Kre; Op.

EATING Agg : Nat-s; Scil; Sul.

ERUCTATIONS, With : Tell.

EVENING : Arn.

FEVER, During : Chin-s; *Rhus-t.*

FREQUENT : Chel; Grap; Sul.

Listening to others, when : Caus; Lyss.

GIRDLE, Sensation, with :Stan.

HEADACHE, And : Form; Stap.

HICCOUGH, With : Amy-n; Cocl.

HYSTERICAL : Kali-p; Tarn.

INCOMPLETE, Fruitless : Lach; Lyc.

INTERRUPTED : Lyc.

JAW, Lower trembling, with : Old.

LAUGHTER, Involuntary, followed by : Agar.

MENSES, Before : Pul.

During : Am-c; Carb-an.

+ MUST, Feels : Guai.

NEAR Onjects, seem distant when : Cep.

PAINS, Before : Agar.

With : Aran; Pho.

PAYING, Attention to others when : Caus; Lyss.

+ PROFOUND, Repeated : Amy-n.

RESPIRATORY, Affections, in : Bro.

SHUDDERING, With: Cina; Hyd-ac; Meny; Old.

SLEEP, Deep, in : All-s; Castr; Cep.

SLEEPINESS, Without : Plat; Rhust.

SLEEPY, And : Kali-n; Kre.

Cough, after : Anac.

+ SPASMODIC : Cocl; Plat.

SPASMS, Before : Agar; Merc; Tarn.

STRETCHING, And : Amy-n; Calc-p; Caus; Cham; Elat; Nux-v; Rhus-t; Stap.

Amel : Carb-v; Guai.

Indoor: Rut.

Wretched feeling, with : Form.

TEARS, With : Mag-p; Stap.

VIOLENT : Hep; Ign; Mag-p; Plat; Rhus-t; Sil; Stap.

Repeated, coma in : Amy-n; Kali-c.

WALKING, Air open, in : Euphor.

YEARLY AGG : See under Periodicity.

YELLOW FEVER : See under Fever.

YELLOWNESS (Of Skin, discharges, etc.) : Aco; *Ars; Ars-io;* Bry; Calc; Carb-an; Cham; CHEL; *Chin;* Con; Crot-h; Eup-p; Fer; Hep; *Hyds;* Iris; Kali-bi; Kali-c; Kali-s; *Lach;* LYC; MERC; Merc-i-f; Nat-s; Nit-ac; Nux-v; *Pho; Plb;* Pod; PUL; SEP; *Sul.*

GOLDEN, Bright or Orange : Aeth; Alo; Alu; Card-m; CHEL; Cina; Colch; Kali-c; *Kali-p; Merc;* NUX-M; Pho; Sang; SUL-AC.

GREEN : Ars-io; Mang; *Merc; Pul.*

Turning : Con.

SPOTS : Arn; Con; Fer; Petr; Pho; Sep; Sul.

Summer, in : Chin-ar; *Chio.*

Vexation, from : *Cham;* Kali-c; *Nat-s.*

STICKY: Hyds; Kali-bi; Sumb.

ZEALOUS : Nux-v.

ZIGZAG : Calc; Rhod; Sars; Sul-io.

ZOSTER : See under Eruptions.

ZYGOMAE : See Malar Bones.

■■

Distributed by:
Aggarwal Book Centre
A-147, Shankar Garden, Vikas Puri,
New Delhi-18 (India)Ph.: 091-11-25612013
E-mail aggarwal@vsnl.com
Website : www.homoeopathic.com